PHYSIOLOGY
& ANATOMY

A HOMEOSTATIC APPROACH

PHYSIOLOGY & ANATOMY
A HOMEOSTATIC APPROACH

John Clancy BSc(Hons), PGCE

Head of Biological Sciences Related to Health
School of Nursing and Midwifery
University of East Anglia, UK

Andrew J. McVicar BSc(Hons), PhD

Senior Lecturer
Anglia Polytechnic-University
Colchester, UK

Edward Arnold
A member of the Hodder Headline Group
LONDON   SYDNEY   AUCKLAND

First published in Great Britain 1995 by
Edward Arnold, a division of Hodder Headline PLC,
338 Euston Road, London NW1 3BH

British Library Cataloguing in Publication Data
A catalogue record for this book is available from the British Library

Library of Congress Cataloging-in-Publication Data
A catalog record for this book is available from the Library of Congress

ISBN 0 340 63190 2

1 2 3 4 5   95 96 97 98 99

Typeset in 10/12 pt Palatino by
Scribe Design, Gillingham, Kent, UK
Printed and bound in Great Britain by
Bath Colourbooks, Glasgow, UK

Contents

Preface **vii**

Acknowledgements **ix**

 1   Introduction to human physiology and homeostasis   **1**
 2   Levels of organization I: The cell – 'the basic unit of life'   **9**
 3   Levels of organization II: 'The chemical basis of life'   **43**
 4   Levels of organization III: Tissues   **63**
 5   Intracellular and extracellular fluids   **86**
 6   Nutrition   **101**
 7   The digestive system   **121**
 8   The cardiovascular system I: Blood   **165**
 9   The cardiovascular system II: Heart and circulation   **201**
10   The lymphatic and immunity systems   **256**
11   The respiratory system   **293**
12   The kidneys: Excretion and body fluid homeostasis   **321**
13   Coordination I: The nervous system   **348**
14   Coordination II: The senses   **399**
15   Coordination III: Hormones   **428**
16   The skeletomuscular systems: Control of posture and movement   **454**

17   The skin: Regulation of body temperature   505
18   Reproduction   524
19   Human development and ageing: Conception to death   561
20   Inheritance   594
21   Pain   613
22   Stress   637
23   Circadian rhythms   659
Appendix A   687
Appendix B   690
Appendix C   694
Appendix D   699
Index   701

Preface

The education of health care professionals increasingly places an emphasis on producing students and staff knowledgeable of the holistic, or physiological, psychological and sociological, requirements of health (i.e. homeostasis), and with an understanding of how their disturbance promotes illness (i.e. homeostatic imbalances). From an academic viewpoint, nursing and other health-related courses frequently lead to a diploma or degree in their specialisms.

Recent developments in the health care professions prompted the writing of this book, *Physiology and Anatomy: A Homeostatic Approach*, which is intended to be of use to diploma students but which also contains sufficient detail to make it suitable for students following degree programmes. This book largely takes a mechanistic approach and aims to provide a greater understanding of the ways in which physiological systems are regulated and how the integration of systemic function is required to maintain body homeostasis. The concept of homeostasis, the most important principle underpinning physiological processes, is applied in a clear, accessible style throughout the book to aid learning, provide an insight into the ways in which disturbances of homeostatic mechanisms promote illness, and to help students appreciate the physiological basis of clinical practice.

Physiology is a 'hard' science, based on facts as well as theories. As with any science there is a body of knowledge that has to be understood, yet the homeostatic processes involved in maintaining physiological function are often logical, particularly if applied to the needs of the basic functioning unit, the cell. In *Physiology and Anatomy: a Homeostatic Approach* the principles behind the functions of a particular system are explained and related to cell requirements. Although each chapter of the book can be individually read, frequent cross-referencing with other chapters is used to highlight where the processes described integrate with those of other systems. However the student is encouraged to first read Chapters 1 and 2, since the principles discussed and, in particular, the inclusion of a simple but unique feature, the homeostatic graph, are the foundations for what follows in the other chapters.

To facilitate learning, most chapters are of the following format.

1. Introduction: relation of the system to cell homeostasis
The involvement of the system under discussion in maintaining cell function is explained, with the aim of reinforcing the association between system physiology and the metabolic requirements of cells.

2. Overview of system physiology

Many existing texts confuse the understanding of physiological mechanisms by using excessive anatomical details. This text is not intended to be an anatomy book but provides sufficient anatomical detail to support the description of functions in the accompanying text. This section also includes an introduction to physiological function by discussing the basic principles involved.

3. Details of system physiology

This section develops the subject of systemic physiology by building upon the information provided in the previous sections. The material follows a strong functional approach and, where appropriate, homeostatic adaptations which enhance function are emphasised.

4. Role of the system in homeostasis

The holistic interaction between system functions is emphasised in this section by considering how the system discussed influences other systems, and vice versa.

5. Examples of homeostatic control system failure and principles of correction

It is not intended that this section provides a comprehensive coverage of disorders of the system. More common disorders are considered, however, in the context of a disturbance in homeostatic control. The basis of clinical intervention in the restoration of normal function, and hence health, is also mentioned.

6. Summary

A summary of the main points covered by the chapter is provided.

7. Review questions

A number of review questions are provided to facilitate learning.

Although the text generally follows a system-based approach, further chapters on topics particularly suited to nursing and other health professions have been included which distinguishes this book from other existing texts. There is a chapter on human development from *Conception to Death*, which includes a discussion of the theories of biological ageing. A chapter on *Inheritance* describes the basic principles of genetics, relates these to the pattern of inheritance of disorder, and goes on to describe some of the recent developments in this field. The chapters on *Pain, Stress,* and *Circadian Rhythms* consider the basis of their subjective, and hence holistic, nature by discussing sociological and psychological interactions with the relevant physiological processes.

First and foremost, *Physiology and Anatomy: a Homeostatic Approach* is intended to be a teaching text. Many students find physiology a difficult discipline, and this is not helped by textbooks that are either too superficial for their clinical needs or too deep. This book takes a different approach to the subject and aims to facilitate the learning of students who have only a basic knowledge of human biology, and to enable them to achieve a depth of knowledge sufficient for them to understand the basis of therapies used in their own specialism. The development of subject matter from basic principles will also make the book of use to those students following Further and Higher Education courses on human physiology.

Finally, we hope you enjoy and benefit from reading this book. We would value comments, both positive and negative, to contribute to the next exciting edition!

Acknowledgements

This book would not have been completed without the help, advice and support of many others. In particular our thanks go to:

Rachel and Penny, whose support and lack of complaint helped to make the work almost bearable.

Our parents, families and friends for their support in the early days of our careers and continued enthusiasm for what we have tried to achieve.

Clare and Lisa, who have continued to grow up in spite of everything!

Our colleagues Sheila Stark and Martin Sellens for their encouragement and helpful comments regarding the script. Thanks for being positive! Adrian Brett and Ted Smith for advice on artwork, presentation and collation; Anglia Polytechnic University and the University of East Anglia for help with resources.

Each other for the initial inspiration in putting pen to paper.

Last, but by no means least, we would also like to thank Richard Holloway at Edward Arnold for his long-standing belief in the project and for his staying power, and Dilys Alam for putting up with our moans and groans!

John Clancy
Andrew McVicar
1995

The authors and publishers wish to express their particular thanks to Professor Dugald Gardner for supplying the photographic material for Figures 4.10, 4.11, 4.13 and 16.16a.

These were originally published in Gardner, D. and Dodds, T.C. (1976) *Human Histology: An Introduction to the Study of Histopathology*, Edinburgh, Churchill Livingstone, and reproduced with kind permission of the publisher.

Introduction to human physiology and homeostasis

Introduction: basic needs of living organisms

Introduction to homeostasis

Summary

Review questions

Introduction: basic needs of living organisms

DEFINITION OF HUMAN PHYSIOLOGY AND HOMEOSTASIS

Human physiology is the branch of biology which is concerned with the mechanisms of human body function. 'Homeostasis' refers to the automatic, self-regulating physiological processes necessary to maintain the normal, or standard state of the body's internal environment. Collectively, physiological function and the maintenance of homeostasis enable the body to attain the basic needs necessary for 'health' and a 'normal' life.

CHARACTERISTICS OF LIFE

All living organisms whether they be unicellular (e.g. amoeba) or multicellular (e.g. humans), have identifiable characteristics of life. These are as follows:

1 Feeding or nutrition. This encompasses the intake of energy and raw materials to maintain life processes such as growth, repair and maintenance.

2 Movement. This is a characteristic of organisms in that they, or some part of them, are capable of changing their position or orientation in their environment.

3 Respiration. This refers to the processes concerned with the production of the energy necessary to maintain life processes and movement. In humans and higher animals it includes breathing (external respiration) and the cellular breakdown of food (internal or cellular respiration).

4 Excretion. This is the elimination of waste products of chemical reactions, and of excesses of certain dietary substances (for example water).

5 Sensitivity and responsiveness. These are the processes concerned with monitoring,

detecting and responding to changes in the internal and external environments.

6 Growth. This generally implies an increase in size and complexity.

7 Reproduction or multiplication. This is necessary for the continuation of the species.

A living organism therefore is a self-reproducing system capable of growing and of maintaining its integrity by the expenditure of energy. The human body is comprised of trillions of microscopic cells (Chapter 2) and each cell can be regarded as a 'basic unit of life', since it is the smallest component capable of performing most, if not all, of the characteristics of life. For example cells can generate energy, grow, excrete, and reproduce. Our genes are the controllers of cellular functions and these act indirectly via their role in enzyme production or synthesis (Chapters 2 and 3).

Humans are, however, complex organisms having cellular, tissue, organ and organ system levels of organization (see Chapter 2, and Figure 2.1). Each level is instrumental in sustaining the functions of life for the human body. Table 1.1 illustrates each organ system's involvement in the regulation of the basic functions of the individual. A more detailed analysis of the role of individual organ systems is discussed in later chapters.

The characteristics of life are interdependent. For example, all organisms must take in the raw materials of food and oxygen in order to provide energy, via the process of cellular respiration. This energy is needed to support metabolic reactions, such as those involved in growth and in the muscle contraction necessary for movement. Consequently, these raw materials can be viewed as being the 'chemicals of life' (Chapter 3). As a result of metabolic reactions waste products are generated and these must be excreted to prevent cellular disturbances. Furthermore, bodily processes respond to changes in the environment and, therefore, one must be able to detect altering environmental stimuli and be responsive to the changes.

The interdependence of the characteristics of life means that a failure of one function leads to a deterioration of others. This is reflected in the diverse symptoms of ill-health. For example, poor nutrition results in the retardation of growth and development, lethargy, poor tissue maintenance, a reduced capacity to avoid infection, and a general failure to thrive.

Introduction to homeostasis

Homeostasis is one of the most, if not the most, important concept in physiological studies. It represents the processes necessary for the maintenance of conditions under which cells, and hence the body, can function optimally. For example, even small changes in body temperature can disrupt biochemical activities within a cell and may even kill it. Because of the interdependency of functioning at all levels of organization of the body, such a disruption could be disastrous for the health of the human if enough cells were affected.

The concept of homeostasis was first discussed in the middle of the nineteenth century by the French physiologist, Claude Bernard, though the term was not coined for another 70 years. He stated:

'la fixité du milieu intérieur est la condition de la vie libre' (the consistency of the internal environment is the condition for free life).

Thus Bernard argued that in order to perform successfully the basic functions of life there

Table 1.1 Organ system involvement in maintaining the basic needs of the body

Basic needs		Systems involved
Intake of raw material	Food	– digestive
	Oxygen	– respiratory
Internal transportation		Circulatory and lymphatic
Excretion		Urinary, respiratory and the skin
Sensitivity and irritability	External environment	– special senses, nervous, skeletomuscular
	Internal environment	– nervous and endocrine
Defence	External environment	– skin and special senses
	Internal environment	– immune, digestive and endocrine
Movement within the external environment		Skeletal, muscular, nervous, and special senses
Reproduction		Reproductive and endocrine

The table demonstrates that all the bodily systems are involved in maintaining the constant environment needed by the cells of the body, so they can perform the characteristics of life.

must be a balance within the body, and in particular of the environment inside cells called the intracellular fluid. This environment is largely kept constant by the regulation of the composition and volume of fluids that surround cells, which collectively are called the extracellular fluids. The main components of these fluids are discussed in detail in Chapter 5 and are as follows:

1 Tissue, interstitial, or intercellular fluid. This is the fluid in which body cells are bathed. It acts as an intermediary between the cells and blood.

2 Blood, or more precisely the cell-free component of blood called the plasma. This fluid circulates through the heart and blood vessels, supplying nutritive materials to cells and removing waste products from them.

The composition of these fluids is kept constant by the intake of raw materials, together with the appropriate rates of excretion of 'waste' products of metabolism or of excesses.

The modern view is that homeostasis is dependent upon an integration of physiological functions. For example, Guyton (1987) stated that

'essentially all the organs of the body perform functions that help to maintain these constant conditions.'

Organ systems therefore are homeostatic control mechanisms which regulate the intracellular environment throughout the body (Figure 1.1). This book concentrates on the homeostatic principles of human physiology, emphasizing the role of each system in the maintenance of an optimal intracellular environment, that is in cellular homeostasis. It also discusses the influence of homeostatic control failure in producing some of the commoner homeostatic imbalances (illnesses). In addition, the principles of clinical intervention are mentioned in relation to the re-establishment of homeostasis and 'health' for the individual.

Homeostasis is usually considered to pertain to physiological or biochemical processes and, for the bulk of this text, we will also apply

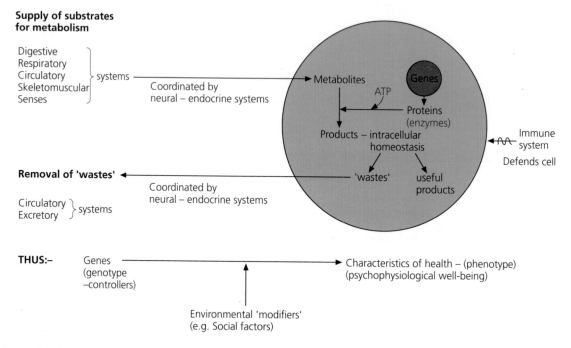

Figure 1.1 Organ systems in the homeostatic control of cellular equilibria.

these principles. It is our intention, however, where appropriate, particularly in relation to stress, pain, and circadian rhythms, to discuss homeostasis as a psychophysiological equilibrium within the body, thus not separating the mind (psychological) from bodily (physiological) functions. Psychophysiological homeostatic processes are measurable and are determined by a person's genes or genotype, which is modified by environmental or social factors. The person and his environment are therefore inseparable and so it is necessary that the sociopsychophysiological implications of a person's health and ill-health should be recognized.

PRINCIPLES OF HOMEOSTASIS

The homeostatic range

The actual term 'homeostasis' was introduced by Cannon in 1932, who defined it as:

'a condition which may vary, but remains relatively constant'.

Physiological parameters are not kept absolutely constant; values fluctuate or 'hunt' about the mean as illustrated in Figure 1.2. This graph, or variants of it, is used throughout this book as a model to explain:

1 homeostatic principles;

2 homeostatic control system functioning;

3 how failure of control results in illness;

4 the principles of clinical interventions used to re-establish homeostasis.

The fluctuations in parameter value above and below the mean represent a homeostatic range within which the value is optimal; the minimum and maximum values of the range exhibit slight individual variations which change with age (Chapter 19). The fluctuations occur as a normal phenomenon as a result of slight disturbances in equilibrium. If, however, the fluctuations are sufficient to cause a devia-

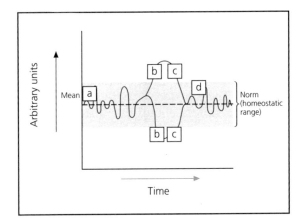

Figure 1.2 Principles of homeostatic control.
a, homeostatic dynamism – constantly fluctuating about the mean.
b, homeostatic imbalance.
c, homeostatic control mechanisms restore balance.
d, homeostasis re-established.

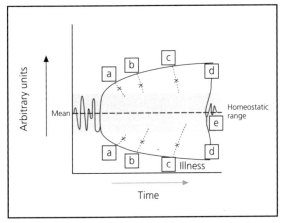

Figure 1.3 Clinical intervention following homeostatic control system failure.
a, failure of short-term homeostatic control system in re-establishing homeostasis.
b, failure of intermediate homeostatic control system in re-establishing homeostasis.
c, failure of long-term homeostatic control system in re-establishing homeostasis.
d, medical and nursing intervention re-establish patient homeostasis.
e, patient's re-established homeostasis.

tion outside the homeostatic range then parameter values begin to be suboptimal, resulting in a homeostatic 'imbalance' or 'disturbance'. Control processes will then act to restore the equilibrium. The greater the effect that fluctuations in parameter value have on physiological function, the narrower the homeostatic range will normally be.

Occasionally, only one homeostatic control mechanism is necessary to redress the balance. For example, when blood glucose concentration exceeds its homeostatic range then this results in the release of the hormone insulin, which promotes glucose utilization. More frequently, however, a number of control mechanisms are involved. For example, the maintenance of body temperature in a cold environment involves heat conservation measures, changes in heat generation by metabolism and behavioural responses (Chapter 17).

These corrective responses are time-dependent; whereas some respond quickly to the imbalance, their failure to re-establish homeostasis prompts other control mechanisms to correct the disturbance. The body therefore has short-term, intermediate, and long-term homeostatic control mechanisms.

Failure of normal control mechanisms results in people exhibiting the signs and symptoms of an illness which will be related to the homeostatic imbalances induced. Medicine employs various treatment/care methods in order to restore homeostasis (Figure 1.3). Some illnesses, such as terminal cancers, are not responsive to treatment and the homeostatic imbalances result in long-term malfunction and eventually death.

Homeostatic negative and positive feedback systems

Most homeostatic control mechanisms operate on the principle of negative feedback. That is, when a homeostatic imbalance occurs, then inbuilt and self-adjusting mechanisms come into effect which reverse the disturbance. The regulation of blood sugar demonstrates the principle of negative feedback control (Figure 1.4); an increase in blood glucose concentration above its homeostatic range sets into motion

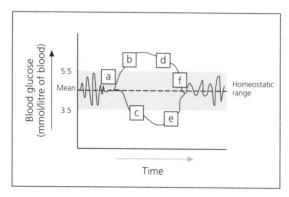

Figure 1.4 Homeostatic scheme for the control of glucose.
a, normal blood glucose level.
b, too much blood glucose (*hyperglycaemia*).
c, too little blood glucose (*hypoglycaemia*).
d, homeostatic control mechanism (insulin) which reverses the hyperglycaemia via negative feedback.
e, homeostatic control mechanisms (glucagon, catecholamines, glucocorticoids, thyroxine, growth hormone, somatomedin and sex steroids) which reverses the hypoglycaemia via negative feedback.
f, blood glucose homeostasis re-established.

processes which reduce it. Conversely, a blood glucose concentration below its homeostatic range promotes processes which will increase it. In both situations, the result is that the level of blood sugar is kept relatively constant over periods of time.

The initial change in a physiological parameter is detected by sensory receptors, sometimes referred to as monitors or error detectors. The function of these receptors is to relay information about the disturbance to homeostatic control centres (analysers or interpreters). These centres interpret the change as being above or below the homeostatic range and determine the magnitude of the change. As a result they stimulate appropriate responses via effectors which bring about the correction of the imbalance by negative feedback, in order to restore homeostasis. Once the parameter has been normalized the response will cease. Thus, a failure of receptor response, control centre activity or effector organs, will prolong the imbalance and may cause illness (Figure 1.5). For example, the failure of the action of insulin, or its deficiency, results in the metabolic disorder diabetes mellitus (Chapter 15).

There are times, however, when actually promoting a change, rather than negating it, is of benefit. For example, a surge in the release

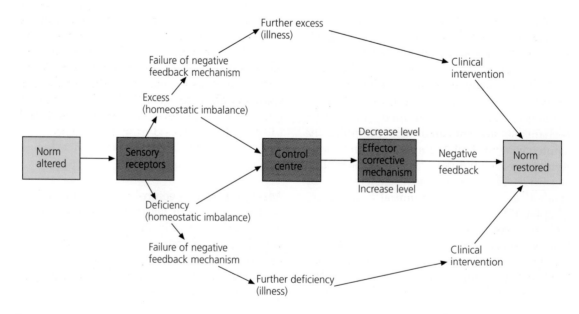

Figure 1.5 Homeostatic negative feedback.

of luteinizing hormone is essential to trigger the release of the egg cell (ovum) from the ovary. For much of the menstrual cycle, however, the high blood concentration of the female hormone oestrogen is responsible for inhibiting (via negative feedback) the release of luteinizing hormone (Chapter 18). At mid-cycle, the inhibitory action becomes a stimulatory one and the presence of the high concentration of oestrogen causes the luteinizing hormone to 'surge'. This effect of oestrogen is called a positive feedback response; however, the effect is short-lived and soon reverts to the negative feedback response. Another example of positive feedback is observed during the clotting process which prevents blood loss from a damaged blood vessel. Thus, the severity of the damage to a blood vessel affects the amount of calcium delivered to this area, and the interaction of platelets with the damaged surface. Calcium is vital for blood clotting, and platelet interaction promotes the intrinsic clotting 'cascade' of reactions (Chapter 8). Hence, the more a blood vessel is damaged, the more calcium is delivered and the greater the clot formation will be.

Since positive feedbacks induce change, the effects tend to be transient; most physiological systems utilize negative feedback mechanisms as a means of maintaining stability. An inability to promote change when necessary can, however, cause a change in health. For example, a failure to ovulate will result in infertility.

Physiological change can also be promoted by another process, that is by altering the mean point about which a parameter is regulated.

Variation of the mean or set-point

The mean value for a parameter is sometimes called the 'set-point'. This term reflects the importance of homeostatic control centres in the determination of the optimal value at which parameters are 'set'. Clearly a modulation of the set-point will either cause responses which promote a change in that parameter, or allow changes to occur uninhibited.

For example, the change in set-point for body temperature that is observed in fever is thought to help prevent proliferation of an invading micro-organism. In this instance a new set-point is recognized by the controlling areas of the hypothalamus at the base of the brain. Accordingly, the 'normal' body temperature is perceived as being below the new set-point and responses occur which cause an elevation in body temperature. Similarly, an increased blood pressure facilitates the supply of blood and hence oxygen to exercising muscles. This involves an inhibition of the 'normal' homeostatic control of blood pressure during exercise.

The capacity to modify set-points, therefore, is essential in certain circumstances and is of benefit, although the high temperature of a fever may not make us appreciate it at the time! Set-point variation and positive feedback responses provide a flexibility to homeostatic processes. As with positive feedback responses, many of the changes promoted by set-point alteration relate to a specific situation and are short-lived. Some resettings are permanent, however, and so promote long-term change. These responses, for example, are vital to human development during the life-span and allow for growth, functional maturation during fetal development and childhood, for pubertal changes during adolescence.

References

Cannon, W.B. (1932) *The wisdom of the body*. New York: Norton.

Guyton, A.C. (1987) *Human physiology and mechanisms of disease*. 4th edition. London/Philadelphia: W.B. Saunders.

Summary

1 Physiology is the study of body functions necessary for expression of the essential characteristics of life.

2 Maintenance of bodily functions regulates appropriate cellular activities, which are determined by enzymes, the products of gene expression.

3 The composition of the intracellular environment will influence the efficiency at which cells operate and, accordingly, it is regulated so as to be optimal. 'Homeostasis' refers to those processes which maintain the equilibrium, or balance, within the body compartments.

4 Homeostatic control relies mainly upon negative feedback mechanisms which act to reverse changes and regulate parameters close to the optimal mean value or set-point.

5 Prevention of parameter variation can be detrimental under some circumstances. The promotion of change via positive feedback mechanisms or through a resetting of homeostatic set-points is then of benefit.

6 Failure of negative feedback processes, of appropriate positive feedback responses, of set-point resetting, or a reduction in their efficacy, leads to illness.

7 Clinical intervention is largely concerned with supplementing normal physiological processes in order to re-establish the homeostatic status of the individual.

Review Questions

1 List the basic needs of the body.

2 Suggest why cells are referred to as the 'basic units of life'.

3 Define homeostasis.

4 Describe how homeostatic negative feedback principles aid intracellular homeostasis.

5 Describe how organ systems, or homeostatic control systems, influence intracellular homeostasis.

6 Positive feedback is usually regarded as a homeostatic failure. Discuss this statement.

7 Give two examples of a positive feedback mechanism in the body which does not result in illness.

8 With the aid of a diagram explain the homeostatic regulation of blood sugar.

9 All illnesses are ultimately a result of cellular imbalances. Discuss this statement.

10 Differentiate between short-term, intermediate-term and long-term homeostatic controls.

Levels of organization I: The cell – 'the basic unit of life'

Introduction: role of the cell in homeostasis

Overview of cellular anatomy

Details of the structure and function of the cell membrane

Cytoplasmic structures and organelles and their roles in homeostasis

Genes and protein synthesis

Examples of homeostatic failure and principles of correction

Summary

Review questions

Introduction: role of the cell in homeostasis

Human physiology is concerned with the 'correct' interdependent functioning of the organ systems and throughout this book each system is considered as a 'homeostatic control system'. Each system has a role to play in maintaining the equilibrium within cells, and hence of tissues, organs and organ systems themselves, because of the interdependency of these different levels of organizations (Figure 2.1). For example, the respiratory system is particularly concerned with maintaining the homeostatic equilibrium of oxygen and carbon dioxide in the blood brought about, primarily, via breathing movements and gaseous exchange between the alveoli and pulmonary capillaries. Thus, aerobic respiration (that is, in the presence of oxygen) by cells throughout the body occurs within its homeostatic range and ensures that sufficient energy is provided to drive metabolic reactions within their normal physiological parameters. The respiratory system is also important in maintaining the pH of body fluids (Chapter 5).

Organ systems cannot operate in isolation; each works interdependently with others to ensure that the intracellular levels of metabolites are maintained and so enable cells to perform the basic characteristics of life. The cell, therefore, is the 'basic unit of life', that is the smallest unit capable of an independent existence given the appropriate environment.

Knowledge of the structure, function and needs of human cells is centred on understanding how tissue and organ dysfunction

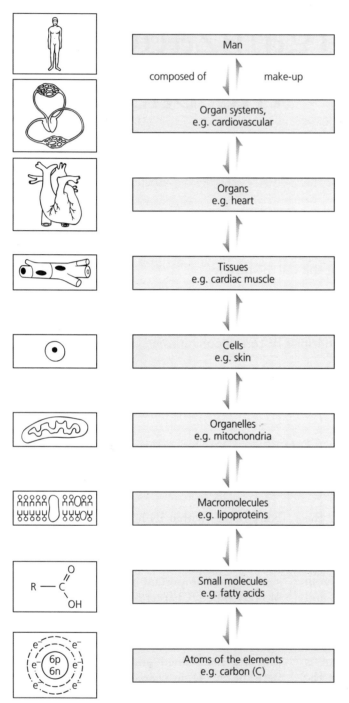

Figure 2.1 The hierarchy of organizational levels of the human organism indicates that specific interactions at each simpler level produce the more complex level above it. C, carbon; e–, electron; H, hydrogen; n, neutron; O, oxygen; p, proton; R, residual group.

results in ill-health, and so provides the rationale for clinical intervention. For example, obstructive respiratory disease induces hypoxia (insufficient oxygen) and may result in cell death. The body attempts to correct imbalances through natural homeostatic regulatory devices, in this instance via an increase in the respiratory rate and depth of breathing. Failure to re-establish gaseous homeostasis necessitates clinical intervention, in order to restore the 'health' of the individual.

The study of cells is called cytology (cyt = cell; logos = study). It investigates how cells are organized, i.e. the structure of cellular components, their role in intracellular homeostasis, how they are controlled and cellular reproduction.

It is argued human life begins as a single cell: the zygote which results from a fusion of the 'ovum' and spermatozoon (Chapter 18). The zygote undergoes multiplication giving rise ultimately to trillions of cells which have undergone specialization and differentiation into the tissues, organs and organ systems of the body. The cells are the basic building-blocks, since the body is composed of them and their substances. Just as the body has organs to perform specialized homeostatic functions, cells have component parts called organelles ('little organs') that have specific homeostatic roles within the cell. Their structures are dependent upon the components from which they are made, mainly macro-molecules, such as proteins, lipids, lipoproteins, and the structures of these in turn are dependent upon their constituent parts, that is amino acids, fatty acids, lipids and proteins respectively (Figure 2.1). These substances are thus referred to as being the 'chemical basis of life' (Chapter 3) and ultimately come from the diet, hence the old adage:

'We are what we eat.'

This, of course, is not strictly correct, since we would be extremely overweight and the food also has to be converted to a form which cells can utilize. Also, we need to remove some of the intake, such as the unstorable, non-transferable materials and waste products of metabolism, in order to maintain cellular, and hence body homeostasis.

Overview of cellular anatomy and physiology

CELL SIZE, SHAPE, AND STRUCTURE

Most cells are microscopic, with the average size ranging from 10 to 30 µm (micrometres; 10–30 thousandths of a millimetre) in diameter. The largest cell in the body is the ovum, which is approximately 500 µm in diameter and is just visible to the naked eye. The erythrocyte (erythro = red, cyte = cell) of blood is the smallest cell, being about 7.5 µm in diameter. The longest cell, up to about 1 m in length, is the neuron (neur = nerve), but even these are microscopically thin (Figure 2.2).

Cellular anatomy or structure varies because cells perform different functions in order to maintain body homeostasis (Figure 2.3). A 'typical' or 'generalized' cell is shown in Figure 2.4, but this is a composite of many types of cells and will share features with most cells within the body without being identical to any of them. Cells have five principal parts:

1 Plasma membrane. This is the outer perimeter of the cell and separates the internal parts of the cell from the tissue fluid bathing it.

2 Cytoplasm. This is the ground material between the nuclear and the plasma membranes.

3 Nucleus. This contains the ground material, or nucleoplasm, in which are suspended the chromosomes that are the 'vehicles of heredity'. These control cell division and

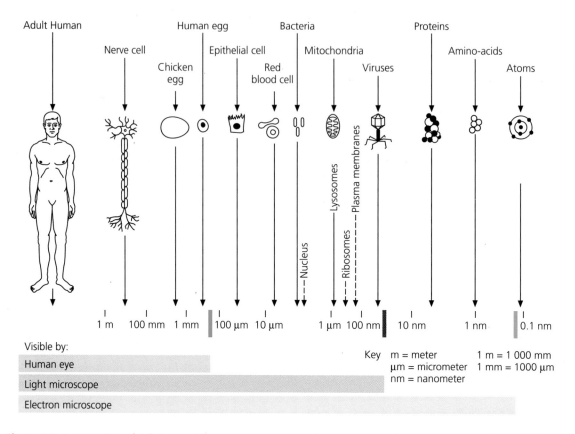

Figure 2.2 A comparison of cell sizes and their components. m, metre; μm, micrometre; nm, nanometre; 1 m = 1000 mm; 1 mm = 1000 μm; 1 μm = 1000 nm.

metabolism and are, therefore, responsible for regulating intracellular homeostasis.

4 Organelles. These small structural components have highly specialized intracellular roles.

5 Inclusions. These include the secretory and storage products of cells.

The homeostatic functions of these cellular components are summarized in Table 2.1, but are considered in detail in the next section.

Details of the structure and function of the cell membrane

The plasma membrane (or cytoplasmic membrane or plasmalemma) provides a selective barrier between intracellular and extracellular compartments. Both compart-ments are aqueous and so the membrane cannot be composed of water-soluble molecules, since it would be permeable to all water-soluble substances and hence prevent

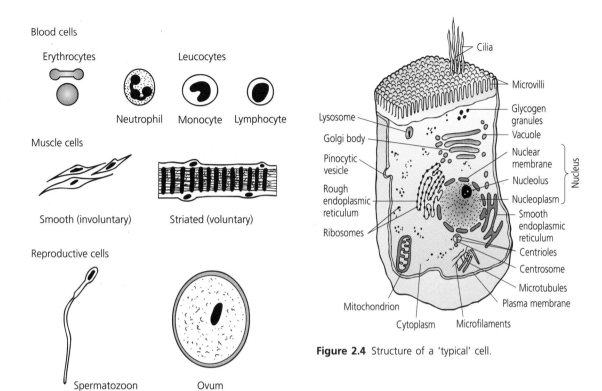

Figure 2.3 Types of cells. The variety of cellular structure reflects their different functions (principle of complementary structure and function).

Figure 2.4 Structure of a 'typical' cell.

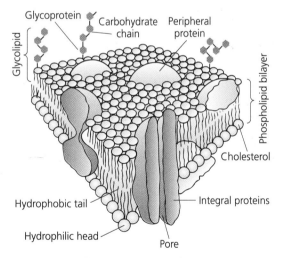

Figure 2.5 The fluid mosaic model of membrane structure.

the regulation of their intracellular concentrations.

The plasma membrane is referred to as a 'unit' membrane, since all membrane-bound organelles have the same structure, and is composed of lipoprotein complexes, that is the main components are lipids and proteins. The main lipids are phospholipids and cholesterol. Phospholipids are polarized molecules, having hydrophilic (hydro = water, philic = liking) and hydrophobic (-phobic = fear or dislike) ends. Each molecule is positioned at right angles to the cell membrane's surface; the hydrophilic heads are exposed to the tissue fluid and the hydrophobic tails are found inside the membrane and thus water or water-soluble substances cannot enter this region (Figure 2.5).

The proteins embedded in the cell membrane are like icebergs floating in a sea of lipid. Integral proteins completely, whereas

Table 2.1 Role of cellular components in homeostasis

Component	Appearance	Description	Homeostatic roles
Plasma membrane		Outer boundary of the cell. Composed mainly of lipids/proteins as lipoprotein complexes. Also, contains carbohydrates as glycoproteins and steroids	Regulates entry/exit of substances. Limits cell size. Important in cell recognition
Cytoplasm		Semi-fluid enclosed within the plasma membrane. Consists of cytosol (fluid) and intracellular substances	Dissolves reactants necessary for enzymatic metabolic reactions. Houses inclusions (contain storage/secretory products)
Endoplasmic reticulum (ER)		A network of membranes throughout the cytoplasm	Rough ER–protein synthesis. Smooth ER–lipid, carbohydrate, and steroid synthesis. ER–segregation of the cytoplasm into different areas of biochemical activity
Golgi-body (apparatus)		Flattened stack of disc-like membranes	Conjugation of cell macromolecules; e.g. lipoproteins, for organelle synthesis and packaging of materials for export
Lysosome		Membranous sacs of digestive (catalytic) enzyme	Intracellular digestion, autolysis, and destruction of worn-out parts of the cell
Mitochondrion		Large, double-membraned organelle, enclosing important respiratory enzymes	Production of a large proportion of the cell's energy (ATP) requirements. Site for aerobic respiration
Cytoskeleton		Microtubules Microfilaments (proteinaceous structures)	Mechanical support for cellular components (e.g. cilia, centrosomes) maintaining their shape. Aids movement of: (i) cellular components for example form spindle for movement of chromosomes during cell division; (ii) substances across the cell's surface (i.e. cilia)
Centrosome (centrioles)		Centralised structure contains centrioles (= bundles of microtubules)	Cell division (see above)
Nucleus		Enclosed by a nuclear membrane. Contains chromosomes	Maintains intracellular homeostasis via expression and non-expression of genes by enzyme production and inhibition respectively. Contains store of hereditary information

peripheral proteins partially, span the membrane. Membrane proteins have the following specialized functions:

1 enzymatic control of metabolic reactions (Chapters 2 and 3);

2 hormonal receptor sites (Chapter 15);

3 antigenic 'markers', important in cell recognition and immunity (Chapter 10);

4 structural support;

5 selective transport properties of membranes.

Some integral proteins form 'pores' or channels extending through the membrane which allow the passage of water and specific electrolytes into and out of the cell without having to cross through the lipid layer (Figure 2.5). Other proteins form 'carriers' by which substances can be transported through the membrane.

The cell membrane also contains carbohydrate molecules that have been conjugated with proteins or lipids, called glycoproteins and glycolipids respectively. They are important in cell recognition, and some are hormonal receptor sites. Their presence is of fundamental importance in sustaining cellular homeostasis.

The plasma membrane is constantly changing its shape as proteins and carbohydrates are mobile within and on the membrane lipids, and because portions of the membrane are continually being removed, recycled, and replaced. Membranes also change their shape and surface area during the processes of exocytosis and endocytosis (see below). The term 'fluid-mosaic model' is often employed to describe the dynamism of the cell membrane structure (Figure 2.5).

Normal cell functions necessitate the movement of substances across the membrane to meet the demands of metabolism, or to secrete metabolic wastes, products or substances in excess. Various factors determine how rapidly such substances are transported, and their mode of transport.

FACTORS WHICH INFLUENCE THE TRANSPORT OF SUBSTANCES ACROSS THE CELL MEMBRANE

The passage of substances across the plasma membrane may be free, restricted or refused. The membrane is, therefore, described as being selectively permeable and the distribution of molecules and ions on either side of the membrane is thus very different. The membrane responds to varying environmental conditions, or intracellular homeostatic requirements, and substances may enter and leave the cell by diffusion through it, or by crossing it via pores or by carrier mechanisms. Factors affecting the passage of molecules across the membrane are as follows:

1 Molecular size. The ability of a substance to enter or leave the cell decreases with its increasing molecular size.

2 Molecular solubility. Oil, or oil-soluble solutes, pass through the membrane more quickly than water-soluble substances because of the arrangement of the membrane phospholipids. The oils probably dissolve through the lipid layer of the membrane.

3 Molecular charge. Uncharged particles enter more readily than charged ones. Anions (negatively charged particles) enter more readily than cations (positively charged particles), since the outer surface of the membrane carries a positive charge and like charges repel each other, whereas opposite charges attract.

4 Temperature. An increase in temperature increases the random movement of molecules and hence promotes the passage of substances across membranes.

The properties of the cell membrane make the distribution of molecules and ions on either side of the membrane very different. The passage of substances across the membrane is a dynamic process, however, and the direction in which they can move across the membrane depends upon their mode of transport. Substances move passively by diffusion, or actively via active transport, pinocytosis or phagocytosis. All of these mechanisms have a role in ensuring that biochemical homeostasis is maintained in body fluids. The active and passive mechanisms involved in transporting substances across membranes are summarized in Table 2.2.

HOMEOSTATIC MECHANISMS BY WHICH SUBSTANCES ARE TRANSPORTED ACROSS THE CELL MEMBRANE

Passive processes

Diffusion

Diffusion is the passage of molecules, or ions, from regions of high (strong) concentration to regions of low (weak) concentration, resulting eventually in a uniform (equal) distribution. For a common domestic example of diffusion, let us consider the making of a diluted orange drink (Figure 2.6). If we put water into the tumbler first, subsequently adding the concentrated orange juice, the orange molecules diffuse outwards from their point of entry. Initially the colour is lighter further away from the juice's entry point, but later the orange solution has a uniform colour, since the orange molecules have moved down their concentration gradient until an even distribution is achieved. In considering the diffusion of molecules across a membrane, the process can be subdivided into that of simple diffusion, and that of facilitated diffusion.

SIMPLE DIFFUSION

Small, uncharged, lipid-soluble substances readily pass across the cell membrane. Diffusion of these molecules is bidirectional and occurs between the intracellular and extracellular compartments. The net passage of molecules depends upon the direction of their

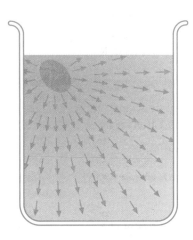

Figure 2.6 Principles of diffusion. Molecules of orange juice (solute = 'orange' molecules) in a beaker of water (solvent) move down their concentration gradient from a region of high concentration to a region of low concentration.

concentration gradient. For example, the movement of oxygen from blood to tissue fluids to intracellular fluid is necessary to maintain levels of cellular energy via aerobic respiration (Chapter 3). Conversely, the movement of carbon dioxide produced by cellular respiration is in the reverse direction and is essential in order to prevent changes in intracellular acidity which could be disastrous for the pH-dependent enzymatic reactions, and hence for intracellular homeostasis.

Other diffusible substances include:

1 Lipid-soluble materials, such as steroid hormones.

2 Small charged particles that are not lipid-soluble, for example, sodium (Na^+), potassium (K^+) and chloride (Cl^-) but which can diffuse through the membrane via channels provided by integral proteins within it.

3 Molecules such as urea, ethanol and water which have a weak charge polarity. Urea

Table 2.2 Processes involved in movement of substances in and out of cells

Process	Description	Factors affecting the rate	Examples in body
Passive process	Substances move down their concentration gradients. No cell energy (ATO) required		
Simple diffusion	Net movement of molecules and ions from regions of a high concentration to regions of a low concentration, until they are evenly distributed (Figure 2.6)	1 Size of molecule 2 Lipid solubility of molecule 3 Charge of molecule 4 Size of gradient 5 Surface area available	Movement of oxygen from lung to blood, from blood to tissue fluid, from tissue fluid to cells. Vice versa for carbon dioxide
Facilitated diffusion	Plasma membrane integral protein carriers allow passage through protein channels (Figure 2.7)	In addition to the above, availability of carrier	Movement of glucose and amino acids into all cells
Osmosis	Water or solvent molecules move from regions of a high concentration of water or solvent molecules through a selectively permeable membrane (Figure 2.8)	1 Concentration gradients (i.e. osmotic pressure gradients) 2 Hydrostatic pressure (can act against osmosis)	Water moves into red blood cells from a hypotonic (weak; high water content) tissue fluid
Filtration	Hydrostatic pressure forces water and small molecules through selectively permeable membranes from areas of high pressure to areas of low pressure (see Chapter 9)	Amount of pressure, size of pores	Capillary exchange when blood pressure if greater than in tissue fluid. Ultrafiltration in the kidney nephron
Active processes	Cell energy (ATP) expenditure allows movement of substances against their concentration gradients		
Active transport	Plasma membrane protein carriers transport ions, molecules from regions of a low concentration to regions of a high concentration (Figure 2.9)	Availability of carrier molecules, transported substance, and ATP	Sodium, potassium, magnesium, calcium in all cases
Exocytosis	Cytoplasmic vesicles fuse with the plasma membrane and expel particles from the cell (Figure 2.11)	Availability of ATP	Neurotransmitter release and secretion of mucus
Endocytosis	Membrane bound vesicles enclose large molecules and take them into the cytoplasm and release them		
1 Phagocytosis	'Cell eating'. Ingestion of solid particles. Phagosomes formed (Figure 2.10a).	Availability of ATP	Phagocytes (white blood cells) ingest foreign bodies (e.g. bacteria)
2 Pinocytosis	Cell drinking. Ingestion of fluid droplets and their dissolved substances. Pinosomes release contents into cytoplasm (Figure 2.10b)	Availability of ATP	Kidney cells take in nephron fluid containing amino acids
3 Receptor-mediated endocytosis	Specific plasma membrane receptors bind with molecules forming ligands and take them into the cell's cytoplasm via endosomes (Figure 2.10c)	Availability of ATP	Intestinal epithelial cells take up large molecules

and ethanol are fat-soluble, and so diffuse through the lipid part of the membrane, whereas water moves across membranes via a special form of diffusion called osmosis.

Rate of diffusion Diffusion across the cell membrane is quicker when the following conditions occur:

1 A greater surface area is available. In certain areas of the body the surface area of tissues is increased by the presence of finger-like processes called villi and microvilli (Chapters 7 and 12). This could be regarded as an evolutionary adaptation for the greater rate of absorption required by large multi-cellular organisms in order to maintain homeostasis. The cell surface of individual cells may also be increased by the presence of protrusions called cilia.

2 A greater permeability of the membrane to molecules. For example, the unstimulated membrane of nerve cells is approximately 20 times more permeable to potassium (K^+) ions when compared with sodium (Na^+) ions. Consequently, potassium diffuses out of the cell more rapidly than sodium diffuses in (their concentration gradients are in opposite directions) and this contributes to the electrical polarization of the cell membrane (see Chapter 13).

3 Increased concentration gradients.

FACILITATED DIFFUSION

Facilitated diffusion is a quicker mechanism than simple diffusion. The facilitated process involves carrier molecules, usually integral proteins, in the membrane which can transport relatively large molecules, such as glucose and amino acids. Glucose is lipid-insoluble, but when combined with a carrier molecule it becomes lipid-soluble. The carrier transports glucose across the membrane, releasing it into the cytoplasm (Figure 2.7).

Rate of facilitated diffusion In addition to those factors which increase the rate of simple diffusion, another important factor in controlling

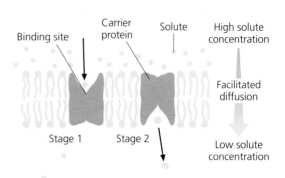

Figure 2.7 A model of facilitated diffusion. A solute molecule (e.g. glucose) is transported across the cell membrane by a carrier protein. Stage 1: carrier molecule binds with the solute, which then changes its shape (stage 2), so that a channel is opened and the solute can pass into the cell's cytoplasm. The process does not utilize metabolic energy; solute molecules pass down a concentration gradient.

the rate of facilitated diffusion is the amount and availability of carrier molecules.

Some carrier-mediated mechanisms are influenced by hormonal actions. For example, insulin is an agent which lowers blood glucose and it is therefore secreted when the blood glucose concentration is above its homeostatic range. Insulin enhances the carrier mechanism and so facilitates the diffusion of glucose into its target tissues, thereby increasing its utiliza-tion. The homeostatic regulation of blood glucose concentration is described in detail in Chapter 15.

Osmosis

Osmosis is the passage of fluid or solvent molecules (in most cases water), from a dilute solution to one of a higher concentration through a selectively permeable membrane. Osmosis is thus a special case of diffusion.

Membranes provide little resistance to the movement of water. Providing that the solute or substance in solution cannot pass through the plasma membrane, then the net effect of osmosis is that more of the water will move to areas of lower solvent concentrations (i.e. higher solute concentration) than in the

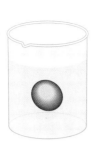

(a)

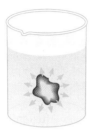

(b)

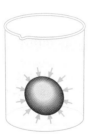

(c)

Figure 2.8 Osmosis and red blood cells. (a) Isotonic solution. The concentration of solute/solvent molecules are the same in the solution surrounding the cell as in the cell. Thus, the net movement of water is zero. (b) Hypertonic solution. The concentration of solute molecules is greater (hence concentration of water molecules is lower) in the solution compared with inside the cell. Thus, the net movement of water is out of the cell (dehydration). The cell shrinks (crenation) and may die, if the solution is extremely hypertonic. (c) Hypotonic solution. The concentration of solute molecules is lower (hence the concentration of water molecules is greater) in solution compared with the inside of the cell. Thus, the net movement of water is into the cell, causing the cell to swell. The cell may burst (lysis) if the solution is extremely hypotonic.

Although the plasma membrane maintains different fluid compositions inside the cell relative to outside it, there is usually no osmotic pressure difference because osmosis will be determined by the osmotic potential of the total solute composition of the fluids. Changes in the total concentration on one side of the membrane can occur, however, if that of individual solutes alter and this will subject the membrane to osmotic effects. It is important, therefore, that cells have relatively constant internal and external osmotic pressures to maintain intracellular and extracellular water balance.

This principle can be demonstrated by suspending erythrocytes in a solution, such as 0.85% sodium chloride, which is isotonic (iso = equal; -tonic = strength) to the intracellular fluid. In such an environment there will be random movement of water into and out of cells, but with the absence of an osmotic gradient the volume moved in either direction will be equal and consequently there will be no net movement (Figure 2.8a).

When extracellular environments are hypertonic (hyper = strong), however, water moves out of the cell by osmosis and causes a decrease in cell volume, with the membrane becoming wrinkled or crenated. This process occurs in the homeostatic imbalance of dehydration (Figure 2.8b). Alternatively, when

opposite direction (Figure 2.8a–c). This occurs until the pressure of the increasing volume of the solution counterbalances the movement. The osmotic pressure of a solution is the force required to stop the net flow of water across the selectively permeable membrane when a membrane separates solutions of different concentrations.

extracellular environments are hypotonic (hypo = weak), water moves into the cell by osmosis and causes an increase in cell volume. If the extracellular environments are sufficiently hypotonic (i.e. diluted) water continues to enter until the intracellular pressure exerted on the cell membrane causes the cell to lyse or burst. The lysis of erythrocytes is termed haemolysis (Figure 2.8c).

Cells, therefore, must maintain their isotonic interdependence, otherwise changes in fluid balance, and the resultant effects on solute concentrations, will disturb intracellular homeostasis. Fluids administered intravenously for clinical reasons are normally isotonic to blood to prevent intracellular fluid imbalance. A common fluid used in clinical practice is 'normal' saline (approximately 0.85% or 0.85 g NaCl per 100 ml of water).

Filtration

The filtration process forces small molecules through pores within the membranes of capillary blood vessels with the aid of water (hydrostatic) pressure. Movement is from regions of high hydrostatic pressure to regions of low pressure. Molecules too large to pass through the filter pores remain within the vessel. Details of the capillary exchange mechanism and of the ultrafiltration process in the kidneys are described in Chapters 9 and 12.

Active processes

Active processes require energy expenditure. This energy is released from the conversion of molecules of adenosine triphosphate (ATP) to adenosine diphosphate (ADP) and phosphate (Pi), i.e.

$$ATP \rightarrow ADP + Pi + energy$$

The energy liberated from ATP breakdown (catabolism) is used to move substances across the membrane. The basic difference between active and passive processes is that in the latter molecules move down their concentration gradient, whereas in the former process molecules can

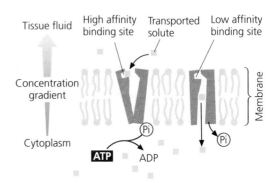

Figure 2.9 Active transport. Phosphorylation of carrier molecules increases their affinity for the specific solute to be transported. Removal of the phosphate from the carrier decreases its affinity for the solute and it is passed into the cytoplasm. Note the use of energy (and phosphate) from ATP which permits transport of solute *against* the diffusion gradient.

move from low to high concentration (i.e. against their concentration gradients or 'uphill'). Active processes include active transport, pinocytosis, phagocytosis and exocytosis.

Active transport

Active transport involves transporting substances across the plasma membrane usually by carrier-mediated integral proteins using the energy released from ATP catabolism as its driving force (Figure 2.9). Active transport carriers are often referred to as 'pumps'. The most cited example is the 'sodium/potassium/ATPase pump'. This active pump compensates for the diffusional exchange of sodium and potassium ions and so maintains their extracellular and intracellular concentrations. Other pumps include that for calcium ions in muscle cells (Chapter 16).

Endocytosis and exocytosis

These active processes transport macromolecules, such as proteins and lipids, and small amounts of fluid into or out of certain cells. Endocytosis involves enclosing the material to be ingested inside a portion of the plasma membrane, and then bringing the substance into the cell (endo- = inside; cyt = cell). The reverse of this process, exocytosis (exo- = outside), is an important mechanism by which cells secrete substances, such as digestive, glandular and endocrine secretions. Exocytosis is important for all cells, in that it is necessary for the elimination of 'waste' products of metabolism and for the removal of excessive substances that cannot be stored, destroyed or transferred into other materials that the cell can utilize.

Endocytosis and exocytosis are therefore instrumental in maintaining intracellular and extracellular homeostatic ranges of metabolites.

There are three types of endocytosis: phagocytosis, pinocytosis, and receptor-mediated endocytosis.

PHAGOCYTOSIS

Phagocytosis literally means 'cell-eating' and begins when the cell membrane encircles the particle to be ingested. For example, a bacterial cell or 'debris' is surrounded by cytoplasmic distensions called pseudopodia. The membrane then folds inwards to form a vesicle called a phagosome which leaves the plasma membrane and enters the cytoplasm. The phagosomal contents then undergo enzymatic digestion by lysozymes (Figure 2.10a). Phagocytic cells are specialized white blood cells, or leucocytes (leuco- = white), which have a role to ingest foreign particles such as bacteria (Chapter 10).

PINOCYTOSIS

Pinocytosis literally means 'cell-drinking'. In this process tiny droplets of fluid and their dissolved components stick to the plasma membrane, which then invaginates forming a

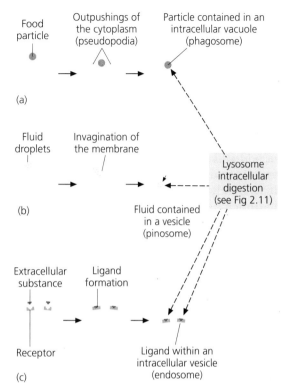

Figure 2.10 (a) Phagocytosis. (b) Pinocytosis. (c) Receptor-mediated endocytosis.

vesicle called a pinosome. This structure separates from the membrane, enters the cytoplasm and the pinosomal contents then undergo lysozymal digestion (Figure 2.10b).

RECEPTOR-MEDIATED ENDOCYTOSIS

This mechanism involves plasma membrane receptors that recognize and bind to specific extracellular macromolecules to form ligands. This area of the plasma membrane then invaginates to form a cytoplasmic vesicle called an endosome. The receptors separate from the ligand structures within the cytoplasm, and are returned to the cell membrane. The ingested molecules are broken down by lysozymes (Figure 2.10c).

Cytoplasmic structures and organelles and their roles in homeostasis

Organelles have specific roles to play in cell function whether it be in the production of energy, in synthetic processes, or in cell division. For convenience they are considered individually in this section but it should be remembered that they function inter-dependently, just as organ systems are inter-dependent in the functioning of the whole body.

ENDOPLASMIC RETICULUM

This is an extensive organelle but its structure and extent varies from cell to cell depending upon the activity of the cell. The endoplasmic reticulum (ER) is a parallel membrane system which forms a network of cavities called cister-nae.

Functions associated with cellular homeosta-sis are as follows:

1　The ER provides passageways through which materials are transported around the cell (Figure 2.11). The organelle makes definite connections with the nuclear and plasma membranes and, thus, may be a link between these two structures, and between adjacent cells.

2　The ER segregates the cytoplasm into areas of different biochemical activity.

3　The ER increases the surface area available for a variety of enzymatic reactions.

4　The cisternae of the ER act as temporary storage sites for specific synthesized chemi-cals, such as glycogen, lipids, and proteins.

There are two types of ER, classified accord-ing to whether or not the membrane is associ-ated with ribosomes (small organelles concerned with protein synthesis). Both types

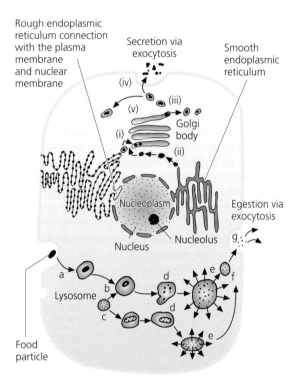

Figure 2.11 The homeostatic roles of the Golgi body and the lysosome. Lysosomal roles:
a, phagosome produced from phagocytosis;
b, lysosome moves toward phagosome;
c, lysosome moves toward 'worn out' organelle e.g. mitochondrion;
d, intracellular digestion of particle and organelle;
e, useful products of this hydrolytic breakdown are absorbed into the cytoplasm;
f, vacuole contains useless (residual) products of this hydrolytic breakdown;
g, exocytosis (egestion) of the residual products.
Golgi roles: (i), protein from rough endoplasmic reticulum; (ii), lipid from smooth endoplasmic reticulum; (iii), conjugated lipoprotein complex in vacuole from Golgi body; (iv), conjugated lipoprotein complex secreted from cell; (v), conjugated lipoprotein complex utilized in cellular metabolism (e.g. production of organelle membrane).

are often continuous with one another and are interchangeable depending upon the metabolic requirements of the cell.

Rough (granular) endoplasmic reticulum

This ER is studded with ribosomes on its outer or cytoplasmic surface. Rough ER is found in all cells since enzymes are proteins which catalyse metabolic reactions and so ensure that the reaction rates are compatible with life processes. It is found in greatest amounts in those cells that are actively engaged in protein synthesis, as in certain hormone-producing cells. The rough ER is therefore an important organelle which contributes to intracellular homeostasis.

Smooth (agranular) endoplasmic reticulum

This membrane is smooth in appearance due to the absence of ribosomes. The smooth ER is concerned with the synthesis of non-protein substances. These substances vary from cell to cell: for example, the smooth ER of secretory cells in the adrenal glands and testes may produce steroid hormones, in sebaceous glands sebum (a lipid) is produced, whilst in liver cells cholesterol may be synthesized. The smooth ER of muscle cells is involved in calcium storage; this ion is important in muscle contraction. In addition, the smooth ER is important in catabolizing potentially harmful substances such as drugs and carcinogens (materials which can produce cancers).

GOLGI COMPLEX

The Golgi complex (body or apparatus) is found in all cells except erythrocytes. It is physically and functionally connected to the endoplasmic reticulum and consists of 4–8 flattened membranous sacs, similar to the smooth ER except that the sacs resemble a stack of dinner plates. The sacs are called cisternae. The apparatus is usually located near to the nucleus, facing the plasma membrane from which the contents of the cisternae may be discharged.

Homeostatic roles of the Golgi complex

The principal homeostatic roles of the complex are to process, sort, and deliver molecules, mainly proteins but also lipids and carbohydrates, to various parts of the cell. In addition, it is responsible for the packaging of secretory products prior to exocytosis. Thus secretory cells, such as neurotransmitter-secreting neurons (Chapter 13), pancreatic enzyme-producing cells (Chapter 7) and pancreatic endocrine cells (Chapter 15) have an abundance of Golgi complexes.

Some vesicles 'pinched off' from the rough and smooth ER fuse together and become Golgi cisternae membranes. Within these proteins, lipids and carbohydrates are modified individually, or are conjugated together to form a variety of compounds, such as lipoproteins, glycoproteins, and glycolipids. Vesicles containing the modified molecules may move to, and fuse with, the plasma membrane, secreting their contents into the surrounding tissue fluid via the process of exocytosis. These secretions may have an extracellular role, for example the action of digestive enzymes (Figure 2.11).

Some Golgi vesicles remain inside the cytoplasm to perform intracellular roles, such as the production of the membranes of organelles and their enzymes, etc. (Figure 2.11).

LYSOSOMES

These organelles originate from the Golgi body. Lysosomes have a thicker 'unit' membrane than the rest of the organelles because they contain approximately 40 different catalytic hydrolases ('digestive' enzymes) which are capable of breaking down nucleic acids (nucleases), lipids (lipases), proteins (proteases), and carbohydrates (carbohydrases). Collectively they are called lysozymes. These enzymes, like most proteins, are synthesized in the rough ER and are transported to the Golgi body for processing into lysosomal vesicles, which become cytoplasmic bound after leaving the Golgi body (Figure 2.11). Sometimes the organelle is referred to as the 'digestive' or 'dissolving body' of the cell. Lysosomes are found in most cells, especially those tissues that experience rapid changes, such as liver cells (Chapter 7), spleen cells, leucocytes (Chapter 10), and osteocytes (Chapter 16).

Homeostatic roles of lysosomes

Intracellular digestion

Any substance that has been ingested by phagocytosis or pinocytosis is taken into the cytoplasm in a membrane-lined vesicle (a phagosome or pinosome). The vesicle coalesces with lysosomes and lysozymes are released into the sac and catabolize the substance mainly into materials that the cell can utilize. These useful products are absorbed into the cytoplasm and may be added to the pool of these specific materials in the cell, if required to maintain their homeostatic ranges, stored in more complex forms, or may be transferred into other chemicals which can be used.

The residue materials that cannot be digested, or utilized, are secreted from the cell in order to prevent a homeostatic imbalance (Figure 2.11).

Destruction of worn-out parts of the cell

Defective or damaged organelles are treated in the same manner as above (Figure 2.11).

Autolysis

Cell death is inevitable and some cells, such as those of the skin, have a very quick turnover rate. Cell death is associated with the release of lysozymes into the cytoplasm and this 'self-destruction' mechanism (called autolysis) accounts for the rapid deterioration of many cells following death. It also ensures that some material (such as lipoproteins, enzymes, etc.) from the dead cells can be re-utilized into the general metabolism. Autolysis therefore has a role in maintaining homeostatic levels of molecules in the body. Lysosomes are often called the 'suicide bags' of the cell because of this autolytic function.

MITOCHONDRIA

The size, shape, and number of mitochondria vary from cell to cell depending upon their metabolic function. Different cell types, however, show the same basic mitochondrial structure of a double-membraned organelle (Figure 2.12a). The smooth outer membrane encloses the mitochondrial contents, and the inner membrane is arranged in a series of shelf-like projections, almost at right-angles to the longitudinal axis of this comparatively large organelle. The function of these folds (called cristae) is to increase the surface area for the enzymatic reactions involved in cellular respiration (Figure. 2.12b).

Homeostatic role of mitochondria

Mitochondria are concerned with aerobic respiration, that is the energy-producing process involving the catabolism of fuel (food) molecules. Some of the energy produced is stored in the form of chemical-bond energy in molecules of ATP. This bond energy is released as required by ATP catabolism (Figure 2.12c). Because of their function mitochondria are often referred to as the 'powerhouses' of the cell; mitochondrial processes provide about 95% of the cell's energy, the remaining 5% coming from cytoplasmic reactions (Chapter 3). Energy from respiration is also liberated as heat and is an important contributor to the homeostatic regulation of body temperature (Chapter 17).

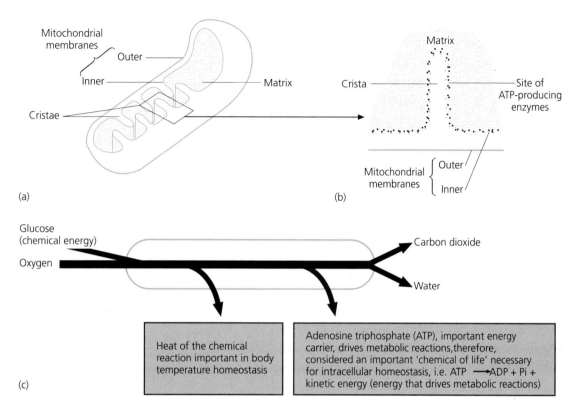

Figure 2.12 (a) Mitochondrion. (b) Magnified view of a crista. (c) Internal (aerobic) respiration.

The number of mitochondria present in a cell varies between cell types and depends upon their energy needs. Inactive cells can have as few as 100 mitochondria, whereas active cells, such as liver, muscle and kidney tubule cells, can contain thousands of mitochondria. The organelles may be scattered throughout the cytoplasm or located at a specialized site in some cells. For example, thousands of mitochondria are contained in the mid-piece of a sperm cell and this region acts as the energy generator for the propulsion of the sperm tail (Chapter 18). Many mitochondria are found close to neuronal presynaptic membranes (Chapter 13). They are numerous in close proximity to plasma membranes involved in active transport, for example in the intestines and kidney.

Mitochondria contain small amounts of deoxyribonucleic acid (DNA) and ribosomes, and as a result they can replicate independently and produce their own enzymes. It is thought that the replication process occurs as an homeostatic response to an increased cellular need for ATP in times of high metabolic demand. Mitochondrial enzymes are involved in the respiration process, and changes in their production or activity have been implicated in the effects of ageing (Chapter 19).

CYTOSKELETON

Within the cytoplasm of most cells there are various sized filaments which form a flexible framework known as the cytoskeleton. There are four types of filaments: microfilaments (the thinnest), intermediate filaments, muscle thick filaments, and microtubules (the thickest) (see Figure 2.4).

Homeostatic roles of the cytoskeleton

Microfilaments are composed of a contractile protein called actin. This substance provides mechanical support for various cell structures and is thought to be responsible for many cell movements.

Intermediate filaments consist of proteins which vary depending upon the cell type; for example, keratin is found in epithelial cells and neurofilaments are present in nerve cells. These filaments help maintain the shape of the cell and the spatial organization of organelles.

Muscle thick fibres are found only in muscle cells and they consist of the contractile protein myosin. Non-filamentous myosin is found in most cells, however, where its function is to produce local forces and movement.

Microtubules are located in most cells and are composed of the protein tubulin. These filaments help to support the shape of the cell and are thought to be an important part of the cell's transporting system, particularly in nerve cells. They are also components of cilia and flagella, and so are involved in cell movements, and of the centriole, which is involved in chromosomal movement during cellular division.

Overall, cytoskeletal structures have important roles in cellular movement and they act as binding sites for specific enzymes.

CENTROSOME AND CENTRIOLES

As its name suggests, the centrosome is an organelle which is located close to the centre of the cell. It is a specialized region of the cytoplasm near to the nucleus, within which are found two small proteinaceous structures called the centrioles, positioned at right angles to one another. Each centriole is composed of a bundle of microtubules (see Figure 2.4 and Table 2.1) and each bundle consists of a cluster of microtubules, arranged in a circular pattern, with a central pair isolated from the rest.

Homeostatic role of the centrioles

During cell division the centrioles move to the opposite poles of the cell and produce a system of microtubules, called the spindle, which radiates to the equator of the cell. Chromosomes become attached to the spindle's equator before migrating to the poles of the cell, seemingly connected to the microtubules (Chapter 20). Failure to form a spindle prevents normal cell replication.

CILIA AND FLAGELLA

These are fundamentally similar structures, differing only in size and their mode of action. The more numerous cilia are generally shorter, often cover the whole surface of the cell, and usually they are used for moving fluids along ducts. The larger flagella are often found singly, or in small groups, and are usually used to move the whole cell, for example, spermatozoon (Figure 2.13 c(i)).

Both organelles, together with microvilli, are extensions of the plasma membrane. They contain microtubules along their length, and in cross-section they show the 9 + 2 pattern (Figure 2.13b). That is, there are nine groups of two tubules arranged in a circle, plus an isolated pair in the centre of the circle. At the base of these organelles is the basal body which controls the activity of the organelle and is probably important in their formation. Below the basal body there is a structure similar to that of the centriole, and it is thought that the centriole produces the flagella of some cells. In other cells the basal body is important in producing the spindle fibres. The longitudinal

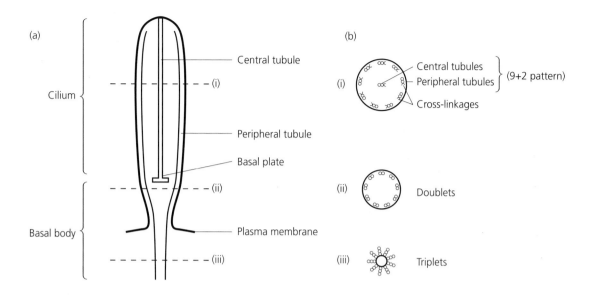

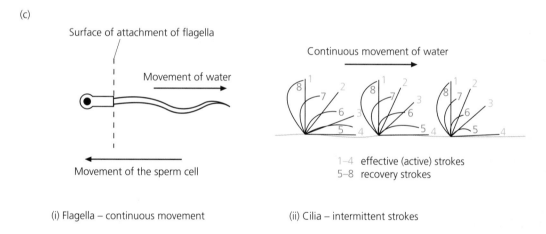

(i) Flagella – continuous movement

(ii) Cilia – intermittent strokes

Figure 2.13 (a) Structure of a cilium. (b) Transverse sections. (c) Mode of action of cilia and flagella.

contractile protein filaments which make up these organelles have ATPase activity, that is ATP is catabolized to provide the energy for the different modes of beating of cilia and flagella.

The beating of cilia is intermittent, and not continuous. It has two phases or strokes, called the active (effective) stroke, which produces movement, and the recovery stroke (Figure 2.13c(ii)).

Ciliary movement is parallel to their surface of attachment. Cilia have a greater density than flagella and this translates the intermittent motion of a single cilium into continuous motion, by determining that each cilium begins its cycle of motion slightly before the cilium next to it. Thus, a wave of effective strokes passes across the surface of the cell (like wind over a field of wheat). This movement is referred to as a metachromal rhythm.

Flagella can contain several waves of contraction at any one time. They therefore produce continuous effective movement. The movement is at right angles to the surface of attachment. Flagella are also capable of the two phase movement of cilia.

CYTOPLASMIC INCLUSIONS

In addition to organelles, the cytoplasm also contains inclusions. These are a diverse group of chemical substances which are usually food, or stored products of metabolism. Thus, inclusions are not permanent cytoplasmic components as they are continually being destroyed and replaced.

Examples of inclusions and their homeostatic roles are:

1 Melanin is a pigment present in skin epidermis. Increasing deposits of melanin causes a tanning of the skin, and occurs as an adaptive protection mechanism against the sun's ultraviolet (UV) radiation. The pigment is also found in the hair and the eyes.

2 Haemoglobin is a pigment present in erythrocytes. The principal homeostatic roles of haemoglobin are to transport respiratory gases in the blood (Chapter 11) and to help regulate blood pH (Chapter 5).

3 Glycogen is a storage carbohydrate in liver and skeletal muscle cells. It is produced whenever the homeostatic range of blood glucose is superseded.

4 Lipids are stored in adipocytes (adipose = fat), whenever the homeostatic ranges of fatty acids and glycerol in blood have been superseded.

5 Mucus is produced in secretory (goblet) cells that line organs. Its functions are to lubricate the epithelial lining of these organs and to contribute to the external defences of the body. For example, the mucus epithelia of the respiratory and female reproductive tracts give protection against pathogenic microbes present in the atmosphere.

NUCLEUS

The nucleus is the homeostatic control centre for cellular operations. It has two principal roles:

1 To maintain intracellular homeostasis by directing cellular metabolic reactions. It does this by expressing the genetic information of DNA in order for the cell to synthesize specific enzymes. Enzymes ensure that the rates of metabolic reactions are compatible with life.

2 To store heredity information (genes), and to transfer this information from one generation of cells to the next, and from one generation of organism to the next.

Most cells possess one nucleus and so are said to be uninucleated, although skeletal muscle cells are multinucleated. Mature erythrocytes lack a nucleus and, therefore, cannot duplicate or produce enzymes. The shape and location of nuclei can vary, but they are mainly spherical, and usually positioned near the centre of the cell. The nucleus is enclosed by a porous double nuclear membrane or envelope. Hence, the fluid of the nucleus, called nucleoplasm, is in communication with the cytoplasm. The nuclear membrane is continuous with the ER, which is also attached to the plasma membrane; as a result the nucleus may also be in communication with the tissue fluid (Figure 2.11).

Prominent structures enclosed within the nucleus are:

1 Nucleoplasm, a gel-like ground substance that occupies most of the nucleus.

2 Nucleolus. There may be one or two nucleoli present. These membrane-bound organelles consist of protein and nucleic acids. Nucleoli are thought to be involved in the initial metabolic reactions involved in the production of ribosomes. Final stages of ribosomal synthesis occur in the cytoplasm.

3 Genetic material. This is in the form of DNA. In a non-dividing cell the DNA

appears as chromatin, a thread-like mass of material. Just prior to cell division the chromatin becomes the rod-like chromosomes.

Chromosomes store the heredity information in segments of DNA called genes. Humans have 46 chromosomes in their body or somatic cells. Sex cells or gametes contain only 23 chromosomes to ensure that, at fertilization, the zygote formed has the full complement of 46. Chromosomes contain the necessary information to maintain homeostasis of all cells, and hence the functional equilibrium of tissues, organs, and organ systems. Interference of this information by genetic mutation may give rise to homeostatic imbalances, resulting in the malformation of organ systems.

Genes and protein synthesis

Genes are segments of DNA that contain the instructions for the manufacture of proteins from amino acids by ribosomes. There is a great variety of proteins and it is this diversity which determines the physical and chemical characteristics of cells and, therefore, the human. Genes control intracellular homeostasis by regulating the production of the enzymes necessary for metabolic processes; since enzymes are the mediators of metabolism they are often referred to as 'key' chemicals of life. Human cells contain between 50 000 and 100 000 genes and these are responsible for the correct numbering, sequencing, and arrangement of amino acids in the required protein.

Most cellular DNA is found in the nucleus, but a small amount is located in the mitochondria. The nuclear DNA is a macromolecule and therefore is too large to pass through the nuclear pores. The gene therefore has to be transcribed, or copied, into messenger RNA (abbreviated as mRNA). The segment of copied DNA is called the cistron and includes non-essential information which is then removed from the mRNA copy. The mRNA can move freely between the nucleus and the cytoplasm.

Protein synthesis requires the involvement of other forms of RNA, called transfer RNA (tRNA), and ribosomal RNA (rRNA); these molecules are responsible for the translation of the original DNA message carried by the mRNA (see below). Protein synthesis occurs at the ribosomes, which are mostly attached to endoplasmic reticulum, although small clusters called polyribosomes are free in the cytoplasm.

In summary:

$$DNA \xrightarrow{\text{transcription}} mRNA \xrightarrow{\text{translation}} protein$$

For an example of genetic involvement in protein synthesis, consider eye colour. This is due to the presence of proteinaceous pigment molecules in the iris of the eye (Chapter 14). The pigment is the product of a long metabolic pathway, which has many intermediate steps. Each step is enzymatically controlled and so the production of this pigment does not involve activation of just one gene for the eye colour, but requires activation of all the genes necessary for the production of the metabolic enzymes required to produce it.

STRUCTURE OF DNA

DNA consists of two polynucleotide chains (each consisting of many nucleotides) coiled around one another in the form of a double helix (Figure 2.14a). Each nucleotide consists of the following (Figure 2.14b):

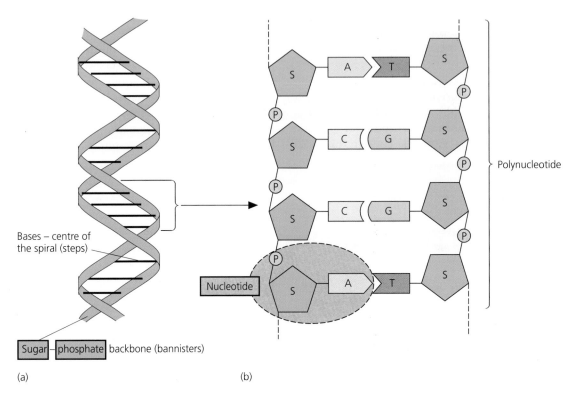

Bases – centre of
the spiral (steps)

Nucleotide

Polynucleotide

Sugar – phosphate backbone (bannisters)

(a)　　　　　　　　　　　　　　　(b)

Figure 2.14 (a) The double helical structure of DNA. (b) Magnified view of DNA components: S, sugar (pentose); P, phosphate; bases – pyrimidines cytosine (C) and thymine (T), purines adenine (A) and guanine (G).

1 One of the four organic bases: adenine, abbreviated as A; guanine, G; cytosine, C; or thymine, T.

2 Sugar: deoxyribose (hence the name deoxyribonucleic acid).

3 Phosphate.

The two strands of DNA are arranged so that one is complementary to the other through specific base pairing: A of one strand specifically pairs with T in the other strand, likewise, C always pairs with G (Figure 2.15a).

A sequence of three of these base pairs provides the code for an amino acid. In fact, since mRNA is a copy of only one of the strands of DNA, only the three bases on this strand forms the code. This group of three bases is referred to as a 'triplet' or codon, and the sequencing of triplets along a portion of DNA which codes for a particular protein is

termed a gene (Figure 2.16a). Smaller genes actually code for polypeptides, which are the subunits of proteins. A typical gene, however, contains a sequence of approximately 20 000 base pairs, although there is considerable variability between genes.

Proteins are made up of their constituent parts or amino acids. There are 20 different amino acids available and, since the four bases can be arranged in 64 different triplet combinations ($4 \times 4 \times 4 = 64$), some triplets must code for the same amino acid (Table 2.3). For example, the triplets CCA, CCG, and CCC all code for the amino acid, glycine. Actually, it is known that only 61 of the 64 possible triplets code for the 20 amino acids, and so the code is said to be degenerate.

The genetic 'blueprint' or code in this triplet form is used by all organisms and always relates to the same amino acids. It is the

Purines   Pyrimidines

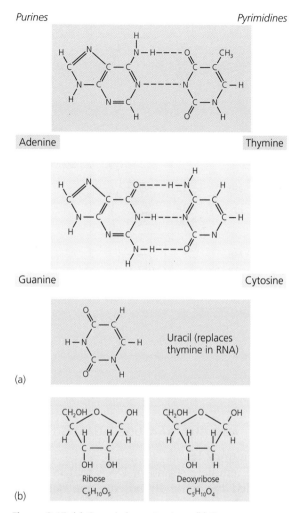

Figure 2.15 (a) Organic base structure. (b) Sugars associated with the nucleic acids.

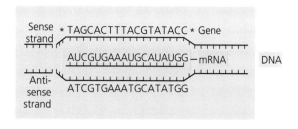

(a)

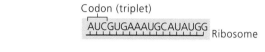

(b)

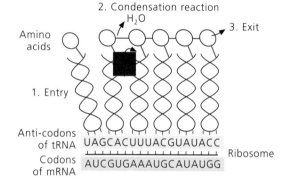

(c)

Figure 2.16 Protein synthesis. (a) Transcription. Messenger RNA synthesis alongside DNA strand in the nucleus. Note the gene is comprised of the triplets from *—* on the sense strand. (b) Messenger RNA passes out of the nucleus to become attached to ribosomes. (c) Translation. Transfer RNA (tRNA) brings the amino acids to the ribosome. E, energy from catabolism of ATP → ADP + Pi + energy. Note that tRNA anticodons are the original triplets on the sense strand of DNA which code for the specific amino acids.

metabolism of these amino acids, however, which varies between different organisms, giving rise to their diversity. This commonality supports the view that all organisms evolved from a common ancestry.

STRUCTURE OF RNA

RNA consists of a single polynucleotide strand. Each nucleotide within this strand is composed of the following:

1 One of the four organic bases: adenine, A; guanine, G; cytosine, C; or uracil, U (replaces the thymine of DNA, but has a similar structure).

2 Sugar: ribose (hence the name ribonucleic acid, see Figure 2.15b).

3 Phosphate.

Table 2.3 The mRNA codons for amino acids

UUU	phe	UCU		UAU	tyr	UGU	cys
UUC		UCC	ser	UAC		UGC	
UUA	leu	UCA		UAA	'stop'	UGA	'stop'
UUG		UCG		UAG		UGG	trp
CUU		CCU		CAU	his	CGU	
CUC	leu	CCC	pro	CAC		CGC	arg
CUA		CCA		CAA	gln	CGA	
CUG		CCG		CAG		CGG	
AUU		ACU		AAU	asn	AGU	ser
AUC	ile	ACC	thr	AAC		AGC	
AUA		ACA		AAA	lys	AGA	arg
AUG	met	ACG		AAG		AGG	
GUU		GCU		GAU	asp	GGU	
GUC	val	GCC	ala	GAC		GGC	gly
GUA		GCA		GAA	glu	GGA	
GUG		GCG		GAG		GGG	

ala, alanine; arg, arginine; asn, asparagine; asp, aspartic acid; cys, cysteine; gln, glutamine; glu, glutamic acid; gly, glycine; his, histidine; ile, isoleucine; leu, leucine; lys, lysine; met, methionine; phe, phenylalanine; pro, proline; ser, serine; thr, threonine; trp, tryptophan; tyr, tyrosine; va, valine.

TRANSCRIPTION OF THE GENE CODE

Transcription is the first stage in protein synthesis and occurs in the nucleus. The process involves copying the sequence of bases encoded in the DNA molecule into the sequenced nucleotides of mRNA using the enzyme RNA-polymerase. The single strand of nucleotides in RNA differs from DNA in that it contains the organic base uracil, rather than thymine found in DNA, but the two molecules are very similar. Consequently, during transcription, the adenine of DNA is complementary for uracil.

For example, a DNA template with the base sequence of

TAG, CAC, TTT, ACG, TAT, ACC

would be transcribed into the complementary strand of RNA as

AUC, GUG, AAA, UGC, AUA, UGG

(see Figure 2.16a).

The template strand of DNA that is copied is called the sense strand, the one not being transcribed is the anti-sense stand, since it complements the sense strand.

TRANSLATION

Once mRNA has been transcribed from DNA, the DNA reassumes its double helical structure. The mRNA leaves the nucleus to become attached to the ribosome (Figure 2.16b, c) and its genetic message is translated. Translation occurs in a number of steps:

1   The process begins when the 'front' end of mRNA has attached itself to a ribosome and begins to move across it (Figure 2.16c). In doing so, the ribosome decodes the message

by reading the triplets (codons). The first codon acts as a 'start' code; subsequent ones code for specific amino acids.

2 Transfer RNA molecules in the cytoplasm are basically anticodons that are a complementary match for the codons on mRNA. Each tRNA molecule combines with a specific amino acid in the cytoplasm and adds it to the growing chain on the ribosome, according to the sequencing required by the arrangement of codons on the mRNA. For example, the mRNA codons for the amino acid glycine are GGU, GGC, GGA and GGG, and thus, the respective anticodons are CCA, CCG, CCU and CCC (Table 2.3). A tRNA molecule which carries glycine from the cytoplasm for incorporation into the growing protein will have one of these anticodons, and will bond only to glycine and no other amino acid. The reader should note that tRNA anticodons are analogous to the original DNA triplets (except that tRNA has uracil in place of thymine). The term 'initiation' refers to the process of positioning the first amino acid at the appropriate mRNA codon site on the ribosome.

3 Following initiation, elongation of the amino acid chain begins with the mRNA moving across the ribosome, one codon at a time. The codon is read by the ribosome, and the corresponding tRNA anticodon brings the specific amino acid and joins it to the previous one. A peptide bond is formed between adjacent amino acids, using energy liberated from ATP catabolism. Further amino acids are added until a terminal 'stop' codon stops the process (Figure 2.16c).

DNA AND CELL DIVISION

All cells originate from the division of the zygote. Cell division, an important characteristic of life, is necessary to maintain cellular homeostasis. It ensures that:

1 Dying cells are replaced, therefore maintaining sufficient cell numbers to ensure adequate tissue functioning. Ageing is a process associated with a decrease in cell numbers, resulting in atrophy of organ systems.

2 Growth of organisms takes place in specific stages of human development, for example, neonate to infant.

3 The development of the organism via cell specialization occurs.

4 The genetic material (the 'blueprint' for homeostatic function) is transmitted from one cell to another, and from one generation to the next.

5 The optimal cell size is not exceeded, since this would lead to intracellular homeostatic imbalances.

Optimal cell size is dependent upon an ideal surface area to volume ratio being achieved. The surface area is the cell's available plasma membrane; this regulates the entry and exit of substances and, therefore, accommodates intracellular requirements. As cells grow, surface area increases at a slower rate when compared with the change in cell volume, since surface area increases to the square of the cell radius whereas the volume increases to the cube of the radius. If the plasma membrane cannot support the increase in volume, intracellular imbalances will occur. Cells, therefore, probably have in-built mechanisms (perhaps a gene or genes), which register the point at which cellular function is impaired and cause cell division to preserve homeostatic function. The dividing 'parent' cells produce 'daughter' cells.

There are two types of cell division, called mitosis and meiosis.

Mitosis

Mitosis ensures that the daughter cells have the same number of chromosomes and identical DNA as the parent cell. For this to occur, the

DNA of the parent cell must first be duplicated so that one copy can be passed on into each daughter cell. Mitosis is sometimes referred to as duplication division.

During the 'resting stage' of a cell's cycle (i.e. a period between cell divisions), the nuclear DNA is in the form of chromatin threads. As the time for mitosis approaches, the strands of the DNA molecule unwind and duplicates are formed by the addition of new nucleotides. In this way the chromatin is duplicated to form identical chromatids; at this point the chromatids remain joined by the centromere. The chromatids coil and fold and eventually the DNA becomes visible in the cell as the chromosomes (see Chapter 20). The nuclear membrane disappears, each centromere divides, and the chromatids of each chromosome separate and move to the opposite poles of the cell. The separated chromatids become the 'new' chromosomes in the daughter cells. Mitosis occurs in all cells except those which give rise to the sex cells. It is, however, limited in skeletal muscle cells and neurons after their specialization because of their complexity.

Although DNA duplication should conserve the genetic make-up of a cell, errors can occur during mitosis with the consequence that daughter cells may exhibit chromosomal abnormalities such as additional chromosomes or chromosomal fragments. Depending upon the extent of the abnormality, these errors during cell division in the adult may not have a great effect on tissue function because this reflects the net effect of thousands of cells. An accumulation of errors with age may, however, contribute to declining function with age or even to the incidence of certain diseases such as cancers. In the embryo and fetus, when tissues are differentiating and growing, errors in cell division can have a pronounced influence on tissue development and function.

Meiosis

Meiosis is referred to as 'reduction' division, since it ensures that the daughter cells have only half of the chromosome complement. That is, the cells will have only 23 chromosomes (called the haploid number) in contrast to the 46 chromosomes (called the diploid number) of the parent cell. Reduction division occurs in the gonads during the production of the sex cells or gametes and is described in more detail in Chapter 20.

Meiosis is necessary so that the 'normal' chromosomal number is restored in the zygote after fertilization. In theory, therefore, all zygotes should have the diploid number of chromosomes in order to perform their homeostatic roles of establishing 'healthy' development. In practice, sometimes this process fails because of gene mutations or chromosomal defects and these are also considered in Chapter 20.

ROLE OF THE NUCLEUS IN CELL HOMEOSTASIS

Many cellular homeostatic reactions are dependent upon specialized organelles and distinct cytoplasmic regions. All metabolic activities directly involve enzymes and thus are indirectly controlled by the nuclear DNA, since genes are responsible for enzyme synthesis.

The availability of enzymes therefore controls biochemical/physiological activities (hence homeostasis). The chemical nature of these reactions means, however, that regulating the availability of raw materials (reactants or substrates) and/or products provides another means of controlling metabolic activities. For example, if we restrict the oxygen supply to cells, ATP levels decrease even though there may be adequate levels of glucose for cell respiration to occur. A decrease in ATP will affect cellular metabolism generally, since it is involved in many chemical reactions. If the levels of oxygen are restored, then (providing glucose levels are adequate) ATP levels will be restored and normal cellular homeostatic activity will be resumed.

HOW ARE GENES CONTROLLED?

Whilst enzymes provide the link between genes and metabolic activity, the question arises as to how it is that gene activity is expressed at the appropriate time. Various models of control have been put forward. These are mainly based on work with bacteria and they suggest how DNA controls enzyme synthesis in response to the presence of substrates (reactants), end products and/or external regulatory mechanisms. Only one model will be discussed, since it is outside the scope of this text to explore the variety of models that exists.

Jacob–Monod operon theory

One way to maintain the steady state (i.e. intracellular homeostasis) is to modulate enzyme production dynamically. For example, when the concentration of the end product of a reaction is above its homeostatic range, enzymes involved in its production could be inhibited and so prevent further increase. The converse is true for an excess of reactants (Figure 2.17); that is, enzymes are produced to remove the excess. The operon theory attempts to explain the regulation of enzyme synthesis.

Jacob and Monod, the proposers of the operon theory in 1961, worked with the bacterium, *Escherichia coli* (*E. coli*). They reported that they could produce several

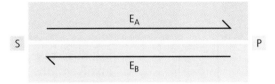

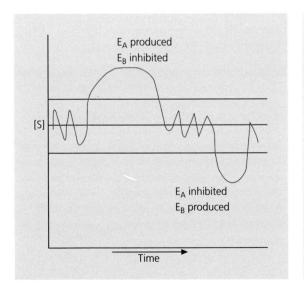

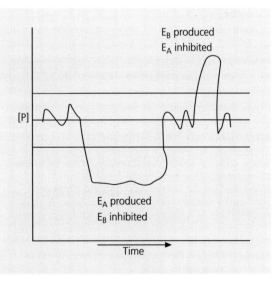

Figure 2.17 Intracellular metabolic homeostasis via enzyme production and inhibition. The reaction goes to the right when there is excess substrate (S) and a deficiency of the product (P). This is controlled by producing and/or activating enzyme A and by stopping producing and/or deactivating enzyme B. The reaction goes to the left when there is an excess of P and a deficiency of S. This is controlled by producing and/or activating E_B and by stopping producing and/or deactivating E_A. The reaction stops when the homeostatic ranges of both S and P are achieved.

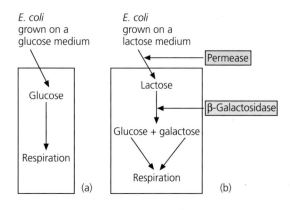

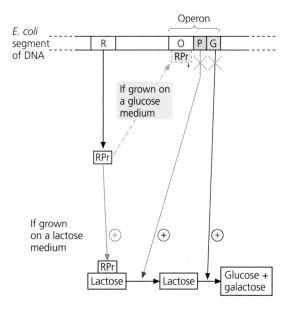

(c)

Figure 2.18 The Jacob–Monod operon theory. (a) *E. coli* grown on a glucose medium. (b) *E. coli* grown on a lactose medium. (c) Enzyme induction and inhibition. R, repressor (or regulator gene); O, operator gene; P, permease and G, β-galactosidase genes (structural genes); RPr, repressor (or regulator) protein; +, enzyme induction; X, enzyme inhibition. Summary: enzyme induction – when grown on a lactose medium; enzyme inhibition – when grown on a glucose medium.

enzymes on demand if the cultured medium of *E. coli* was changed from glucose to lactose, a disaccharide, or double sugar, made of glucose and galactose. When grown on a glucose

medium, *E. coli* was able to use glucose directly in cellular respiration (Figure 2.18a). When grown on a lactose medium, however, the following enzymes were produced:

1 Permease. This enzyme was produced in order to make the membrane more permeable (hence the enzyme's name) to lactose, which is a larger molecule than glucose.

2 Beta-galactosidase. This enzyme was produced in order to convert lactose into its constituents, glucose and galactose (Figure 2.18b)

Jacob and Monod explained enzyme production, or induction, via the operon theory. They argued that there was a linear segment of DNA called the operon which controlled enzyme (protein) synthesis. In this case the operon was composed of three genes:

1 Structural gene. This gene contains the code necessary for the production of the enzyme. In this case two structural genes are involved: the permease gene and the β-galactosidase gene.

2 Operator (or promoter) gene. This gene controls the transcription of the DNA segment of the structural gene.

3 Regulator (or repressor) gene. This gene codes for the production of a regulatory or repressor protein (enzyme) which represses other genes within the operon (Figure 2.18c).

The genes, and their transcribed proteins, therefore interact to provide control over the operon. The overall effects of this interaction are to 'switch on', or express, the structural gene when needed, and to 'switch off', or repress the structural gene when enzyme production is not needed.

When an enzyme is required, for example when there is an excess of the substrate (reactant), the structural gene is expressed in order to reduce the substrate level to within its homeostatic range (Figure 2.17). Enzyme synthesis may be repressed, for instance, when there is an excess of the product, or when there is a low level of the substrate specific for that particular enzyme (Figure 2.17). Using the above example, when *E. coli* is grown on a glucose medium, there is no suitable substrate (i.e. lactose) and so there is no need to express the permease or β-galactosidase structural genes. Consequently, the repressor protein blocks the operator and so represses transcription of the structural gene. This repression prevents the wasteful production of enzymes, a factor which in itself is important in controlling intracellular homeostatic levels of enzymes.

Conversely, when *E. coli* is grown on a lactose medium, permease is produced to allow more lactose into the cell (a build-up of the substrate thus occurs). It then becomes necessary to express the β-galactosidase gene, in order to convert lactose enzymatically into its constituent monosaccharides (Figure 2.18 b, c).

The operon's link with intracellular homeostasis

Enzyme induction and inhibition are directly responsible for maintaining intracellular homeostasis. According to the operon theory, enzyme production involves the activation of the operator gene necessary for that enzyme synthesis. As outlined earlier, enzyme synthesis may be promoted by the following situations:

1 The enzyme availability is below its homeostatic range (see Figure 1.2).

2. The substrate (metabolite) is beyond its homeostatic range. The excess material, therefore, must be removed, using further enzymes in order to remove the homeostatic imbalance. For example, excesses may be removed in various ways:
   (a) storing the substance in a related form. For example, excess intracellular glucose is stored as glycogen.
   (b) transference of metabolites into another form. For example, amino acids may be transferred (transaminated) into certain other amino acids, if their levels have fallen below their homeostatic ranges. The excess amino acids which are not transaminated may be deaminated into energy producing chemicals, keto acids, which are fed into the cellular respiratory pathway, and converted into ammonia, and then urea, which is a metabolic 'waste' product that is excreted (Chapters 7 and 12).
   (c) the excess material which cannot be stored, transferred or destroyed, must be secreted from the cell to prevent intracellular homeostatic imbalances. Some metabolites may require membrane carrier molecules to transport them, and the production of carriers is enzymatically controlled by expressing the relevant enzyme gene(s) to ensure removal of the excess material.

3 'Old' or defective organelles must be broken down and new organelles must replace the loss, to ensure intracellular homeostasis. The metabolic reactions involved require enzymatic synthesis and action.

4 Ultimately, a patient's illness (homeostatic imbalance) requires clinical intervention in order to redress his/her homeostasis. Interventions operate either directly by switching genes on or off, or indirectly by modulating gene expression.

Gene expression and development

The expression or repression of genes can also explain cell specialization and differentiation that occurs during development. In other words how is it that genes which determine a cell will function as, for example, a skin cell are activated whilst those specific to other cell types are repressed? This differentiation occurs during the transition of the morula into the blastocyst and thence into the embryo (see Chapter 19), i.e.

Morula → blastocyst → embryo

All cells appear identical at the morula stage of development and the removal of a cell has no consequences for subsequent development. The blastocyst, however, shows evidence of the first stage of differentiation, since cells specialize into trophoblastic (membrane), or inner mass (embryo) cells. The inner cell mass then differentiates into the three germ layers: the ectoderm, mesoderm, and endoderm.

This differentiation is the second stage of specialization. The germ layers then differentiate into the cells which constitute the specialized tissues and organs of the embryo. The cells of the body therefore undergo many structural and functional developments, and these are enzymatically controlled, and hence genetically controlled. Enzyme production is responsible for changing the expression of genes at the specific transitional periods associated with human development – not just embryonic development but also in the development of the neonate, of the infant and child, of the adolescent, and of the adult.

Each developmental stage has specific psychophysiological characteristics. Such characteristics involve the functioning, or non-functioning, of enzyme systems via gene expression and repression respectively. An individual's genes, or genotype, therefore determines the biophysical and biochemical characteristics, or phenotypes.

Examples of homeostatic failure and principles of correction

Clearly, all disorders involve a disturbance of cell function somewhere within the body. Many examples are provided throughout this book and this section concentrates only on disorders of cell division.

TUMOURS AND CANCER

A tumour is a swelling produced by an abnormally accelerated period of growth and reproduction of cells (called neoplasms). Tumours are classified as benign or malignant.

Benign tumours (non-cancerous)

Benign tumour cells are localized and encapsulated in connective tissue. These cells develop singly, and seldom in small groups, and usually pose no threat to life. They are deemed safe, as long as these tumours do not produce symptoms through pressure on vital tissues or become unsightly. Only a small percentage give rise to 'secondary' growths, or metastases. Thus, these are commonly referred to as 'innocent' tumours and consequently may not be removed. If the size or position, however, impairs tissue or organ function then surgical removal is required. This procedure is straightforward since benign tumours are encapsulated. Post-surgically there is no danger of secondaries and little chance of recurrence.

Malignant tumours (cancerous)

Malignant cells leave the original tumour site and infiltrate other tissues and organs. This spread, or metastasis, is dangerous and diffi-

Table 2.4 Summary of the 'cancer inducers'

Hereditary predisposition
Inherited characteristics make the individual more susceptible. Approximately 19 forms of inherited cancers have been identified to date

Radiation exposure
The governmental health safety standards protect against harmful levels of carcinogenic substances. The problem is that not all the environmental 'pollutants' have been tested for their potential carcinogenicity

Sex
Certain cancers are frequently associated with one particular sex. For example, breast cancer is more frequent in females

Carcinogen-mutagen factors
Many carcinogens are mutagens, since they cause chromosomal changes, for example, insecticides

Chronic tissue damage
Injuries, instead of repairing or regenerating the cells affected, can produce cancer cells. For example, skin cancers due to overexposure to UV radiation (sunlight)

Age
Gene activity changes throughout life, and thus one's susceptibility to certain cancers changes. For example, colonic cancers are more common in the over 40s

Viruses
There are increasing numbers of viruses being linked to certain cancers, for example, the papilloma virus which is responsible for cervical cancer

cult to control, since at their new sites metastatic cells mitotically divide and produce secondary tumours which will affect the functional capacity of the affected tissues or organs.

Cancer refers to a variety of illnesses, many of which are characterized by the appearance of tumours. Cancers are classified according to the type of tissue involved:

1 Carcinoma – malignancy of epithelial cells;

2 Leukaemia – malignancy of certain blood cells;

3 Sarcoma – malignancy of other body cells.

The functions of cancer cells differ from normal cells. They are either abnormally large or small and many have chromosomal abnormalities. Cell division is accelerated and changes in function are largely irreversible. As the number of cancer cells increase, organ function therefore becomes abnormal and homeostatic imbalances associated with that system and interdependent ones become apparent. Also, cancer cells compete with normal cells for nutrients.

Aetiology of cancer

Cancer research has yet to demonstrate why cancer cells behave in the way they do. Nevertheless much is known about the predisposing factors (Table 2.4). In addition, many environmental carcinogens have been identified and include plant poisons, microbial and animal toxins, tar (benzpyrene) in cigarette smoke, food additives, and deficiencies of vital nutrients such as vitamin A.

Specificity is also observed since most carcinogens affect only those cells capable of responding to them, and very few carcinogens, such as radiation, affect cells generally throughout the body.

In general, cells normally capable of rapid division record a high incidence of cancer, since they are more likely to respond to chemical or radiation carcinogens. Consequently, the incidence of epithelial tissue and stem cell cancers is very high, whilst the rates of muscle and nervous tissue cancers are comparatively low.

All cancers show a basic alteration in cellular programming via some change in gene activity. Genetic structural alterations are usually at the molecular level (Chapter 3), but occasionally chromosomal abnormalities are observed. Cancer is not hereditary in the true sense and any hereditary influence is apparently due to some genetically determined variation in the resistance to environmental carcinogens. One could apply the principles of the operon theory to the development of certain cancers. For example, there is a relationship between an overexposure to UV radiation and the occurrence of skin cancers. Perhaps the radiation prevents the repression of the cancer-causing structural genes, consequently causing their expression. Some cancers appear to result from activation of cancer genes, called oncogenes (the study of cancers is called oncology).

Cancer – principles of correction

Because of the incurable nature of some cancers, prevention is paramount and this obviously involves avoiding exposure to known carcinogens. Should a tumour grow, however, then the odds of survival are, in general, markedly increased if the cancer is detected early, especially before it undergoes metastasis. Treatment of malignant tumours must be accomplished by one of the following:

1 Killing of cancer cells. The treatment for early accessible tumours is surgical removal, accompanied by dissection of the related lymph glands, which may contain some migrating cancer cells. Deep x-ray radiation, heating or freezing cells are particularly effective treatments before metastasis.

2 Preventing replication of cancer cells. Drug administration (chemotherapy) kills cancerous tissue by preventing mitotic divisions.

The most effective therapies often involve a combination of these procedures, for example, radiation plus chemotherapy, or surgery followed by radiation and chemotherapy.

At present tumour cells cannot be poisoned without harming healthy cells. Immunotherapy involves administering substances that enable the immune system to recognize and attack just the cancerous cells, and recent advances in producing 'designer' drugs also raise the possibility of specific treatments in the future.

AGEING

Ageing is a natural and progressive process and is considered in detail in Chapter 19. The reader is encouraged to view this process as a homeostatic imbalance, whereby there is a decline in the number of body cells, a decline in cellular function and subsequently decreased functioning of organ systems.

References

Jacob, F. and Monod, J. (1961) Genetic regulatory mechanisms in the synthesis of proteins. *Journal of Molecular Biology* **3**, 318–56.

Summary

1 A cell is the 'basic unit of life', the smallest component capable of performing the basic characteristics of life.

2 Enzymes and ATP are the 'key chemicals of life'. Enzymes regulate the rate of metabolic reactions, so that they are compatible with life. ATP provides the energy to 'drive' metabolism.

3 Cells vary in size, shape, and function. The shape of a cell is closely related to its function, a phenomenon referred to as the 'principle of complementary structure–function relationship'.

4 Intracellular homeostasis is vital to the 'health' of the individual owing to the interdependency of the body's component parts.

5 Each organ system is an indirect homeostatic regulator of cellular metabolism.

6 The cell's passive and active transporting mechanisms are themselves homeostatic control processes since they help determine the concentration of intracellular metabolites, so that the characteristics of life can be performed.

7 Cellular components, organelles, have precise homeostatic functions which are essential in maintaining intracellular homeostasis.

8 The control of organelle function is dependent upon the production of enzymes, the synthesis of which is genetically controlled and environmentally modified; perhaps according to the principles underpinning the operon theory.

9 Homeostatic failures may result from:
   (a) inborn or inherited errors of metabolism (Chapter 20);
   (b) inappropriate numbers of chromosomes (Chapter 20);
   (c) the effects of environmental agents, for example, overexposure of UV radiation can produce skin cancer;
   (d) the ageing process (Chapter 19).

10 Clinical intervention therefore is often based upon correcting the genetic failure directly, for example by chemotherapy or genetic engineering, and/or indirectly, for example by adapting one's life-style to avoid harmful environmental agents.

Review Questions

1 Draw diagrams which reflect the light and electron microscopic views of a typical cell.

2 Give a reason why the following statements are used in Physiology:
   (a) cell – 'the basic unit of life';
   (b) Enzymes and ATP – 'the key chemicals of life';
   (c) mitochondria – 'the power-house of the cell';
   (d) Golgi body – 'the packaging factory of the cell';
   (e) lysosomes – 'the suicide bags of the cell';
   (f) genes – 'the vehicles of heredity'.

3 How are cilia, flagella and centrioles related to one another?

4 Give examples of where you would find ciliated cells. Name the male's flagellated cell.

5 With the aid of a diagram explain how proteins are synthesized, using the following terms: DNA; mRNA; tRNA; codons; sense strand; anti-sense strand; cistrons; anticodons; transcription; translation; amino acids; proteins; nucleus; ribosomes; polyribosomes; endoplasmic reticulum; cytoplasm; peptide bonds; energy; ATP.

6 Describe what is meant by the term 'selective permeability'.

7 List the passive and active homeostatic transport mechanisms of the cell.

8 Explain why osmosis is referred to as a special case of diffusion.

9 Using the principles applied to the operon theory, describe how:
   (a) the levels of intracellular metabolites are controlled;
   (b) cell specialization occurs;
   (c) overexposure to UV light may cause skin cancers;
   (d) drugs may be used to correct homeostatic imbalances.

10 Explain why cancer is considered to be a homeostatic imbalance.

Levels of organization II: 'The chemical basis of life'

3

Introduction: relation of chemicals to cellular homeostasis

Overview of chemical reactions within the cell

The chemicals of life

Energy production by cellular respiration

Examples of homeostatic control failures and principles of correction

Summary

Review questions

Introduction: relations of chemicals to cellular homeostasis

All living and non-living things consist of matter either in gaseous, liquid or solid form. All matter, whether it be animal, vegetable or mineral, is made up of a limited number of chemical elements combined together in ways which ultimately produce the huge diversity of substances that make up the natural world.

Whereas the cell can be considered to be the basic biological unit of life (Chapter 2), it is clear that all cellular structures are made of chemicals, in particular proteins, carbohydrates, and lipids, and that the metabolic processes which take place within cells are reactions between chemicals which result either in the breakdown, or catabolism, of relatively complex chemicals into smaller units, or the build-up or anabolism of new chemicals. Since physiological function of the human body must ensure that conditions within cells are conducive for normal metabolic function, a knowledge of basic chemistry is fundamental to the understanding of physiological processes, and hence of the consequences of homeostatic disturbances (i.e. illness).

Overview of chemical reactions within the cell

INTRODUCTION TO BASIC CHEMISTRY

Elements

Chemical elements are the basic building units of matter. They are substances which cannot be broken down into simpler substances by ordinary chemical reactions. Ninety-two different elements occur naturally but some 15 others too unstable to occur naturally are known to science. The elements are designated abbreviations, or symbols, mostly based on the first one or two letters of the name of the element. This may refer to the Latin name, however, which can add to the confusion. Examples of symbols of elements abundant in the body are C (carbon), O (oxygen), H (hydrogen), Na (natrium = sodium), K (kalium = potassium), Ca (calcium), P (phosphorus) and Fe (ferrium = iron).

Approximately 95% of the weight of the human body consists of carbon, hydrogen, oxygen, and nitrogen, in the form of carbohydrates, proteins, and fats. Another 4% (mainly bone) is made up of phosphorus and calcium. The other 1% consists of about 18 other elements, particularly potassium and sodium but also some which, though essential for life, are found in such small quantities that they are called trace elements (e.g. aluminium and zinc).

The diversity of cell structure and function is made possible because many chemical elements may be combined with others to form a myriad of different substances, the properties of which result in the enormous range of chemical reactions that occur from moment to moment within a cell. To understand how elements interact though, the structure of elements must first be considered.

Atoms

Each element consists of units called atoms. The atoms of one element will be different from those of other elements. Needless to say atoms are minute – the smallest are less than 0.000 000 01 cm in diameter, and even the largest are only about 0.000 000 05 cm in diameter! Some natural substances, such as diamond (a form of carbon) and gold, may be almost entirely comprised of one kind of element. Usually, though, two or more elements are combined together in various proportions.

It can be seen from Figure 3.1 that atoms consist of two parts – the nucleus and its surrounding particles called electrons. Although physicists have identified numerous different nuclear particles, the nuclei of atoms are mainly made up of two kinds called neutrons and protons which are comparatively heavy in relation to electrons. Protons and electrons are electrically charged: by notation protons carry a positive charge, electrons a negative one. Neutrons are uncharged and do not appear to play a role in the chemical bonding between elements.

Electrons spin around the nucleus, and atoms of an element will have the same number of protons and electrons and so the atoms will be electrically neutral (since the numbers of positive particles equal the number of negative ones). Atoms of different elements contain different numbers of protons in their nuclei. For example, hydrogen atoms are the smallest atoms and have only 1 proton, whereas the biggest naturally occurring atoms, those of uranium, have 92. The number of protons in an atom's nucleus is called its atomic number and this is depicted in the 'Periodic Table' of elements as the number above the symbol for each element (see Figure 3.2).

Although atoms of an element have the same number of protons, it is possible for the nuclei to have different numbers of neutrons. This does not influence the chemical activity of the atom but alters its weight or atomic mass since this is equal to the sum of the protons and

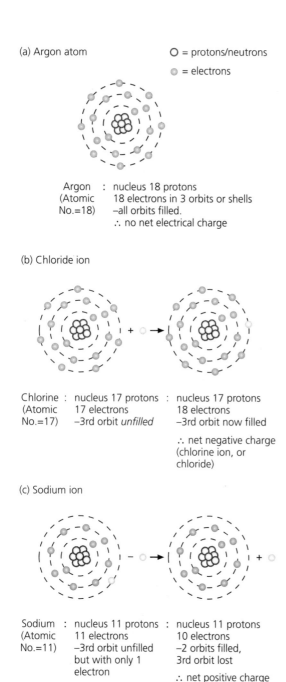

(a) Argon atom

O = protons/neutrons

◉ = electrons

Argon   : nucleus 18 protons
(Atomic   18 electrons in 3 orbits or shells
No.=18)   –all orbits filled.
             ∴ no net electrical charge

(b) Chloride ion

Chlorine : nucleus 17 protons : nucleus 17 protons
(Atomic   17 electrons   18 electrons
No.=17)   –3rd orbit *unfilled*   –3rd orbit now filled

                                    ∴ net negative charge
                                    (chlorine ion, or
                                    chloride)

(c) Sodium ion

Sodium   : nucleus 11 protons : nucleus 11 protons
(Atomic   11 electrons   10 electrons
No.=11)   –3rd orbit unfilled   –2 orbits filled,
             but with only 1   3rd orbit lost
             electron
                                      ∴ net positive charge
                                      (sodium ion)

Figure 3.1 Schematic representation of atoms and ions.

neutrons. The atomic mass is shown in the Periodic Table as the number below the symbol for each element. Forms of atoms of a single element with different numbers of neutrons are called isotopes.

Radioisotopes

Although the number of neutrons in an atom may vary, the nuclei may remain stable. Some isotopic nuclei are so unstable, however, that the nucleus fragments and excess neutrons are emitted as 'radiation'. Such isotopes are called radioisotopes. For example, carbon atoms (atomic number = 6) usually have 6 protons and 6 neutrons (i.e. the atomic mass is 6+6 = 12). Another form of carbon, which must still have only 6 protons in its nucleus actually to be carbon, has 8 neutrons in its nucleus (i.e. the atomic mass is now 6+8=14). This form of carbon is sometimes called carbon-14 to distinguish it from carbon-12. Both forms are chemically identical but the atomic nuclei of carbon-14 are less stable and emit the excess neutrons and so change to the more stable carbon-12.

The emitted neutrons can be detected by appropriate instruments and radioisotopes of various kinds are useful in monitoring the function of tissues. For example, iodine is a constituent of thyroid hormones and radioisotopic iodine is frequently used to assess the functioning of the thyroid gland. In addition, the impact of radiated particles with other atomic nuclei can alter the identity of these nuclei by displacing some of their nuclear particles. This is the basis of atomic weapons, but a more humane application is in the treatment of cancer by radiotherapy, the principle of which is to change the structure of the genetic material of tumour cells and so kill them.

Electrolytes (ions)

Although atoms are electrically neutral some may, under certain circumstances, lose or gain electrons and so disturb the balance between

								1 **H** Hydrogen 1									2 **He** Helium 4
I	II											III	IV	V	VI	VII	
3 **Li** Lithium 7	4 **Be** Beryllium 9											5 **B** Boron 11	6 **C** Carbon 12	7 **N** Nitrogen 14	8 **O** Oxygen 16	9 **F** Flourine 19	10 **Ne** Neon 20
11 **Na** Sodium 23	12 **Mg** Magnesium 24											13 **Al** Aluminium 27	14 **Si** Silicon 28	15 **P** Phosphorus 31	16 **S** Sulphur 32	17 **Cl** Chlorine 35.5	18 **Ar** Argon 40
19 **K** Potassium 39	20 **Ca** Calcium 40	21 **Sc** Scandium 45	22 **Ti** Titenium 48	23 **V** Vanadium 51	24 **Cr** Chromium 52	25 **Mn** Manganese 55	26 **Fe** Iron 56	27 **Co** Cobalt 59	28 **Ni** Nickel 59	29 **Cu** Copper 63.5	30 **Zn** Zinc 65	31 **Ga** Gallium 70	32 **Ge** Germanium 72.5	33 **As** Arsenic 75	34 **Se** Selenium 79	35 **Br** Bromine 80	36 **Kr** Krypton 84
37 **Rb** Rubidium 86	38 **Sr** Strontium 88	39 **Y** Yttrium 89	40 **Zr** Zirconium 91	41 **Nb** Niobium 93	42 **Mo** Molybdenum 96	43 **Tc** Techetium (99)*	44 **Ru** Ruthenium 101	45 **Rh** Rhodium 103	46 **Pd** Palladium 106	47 **Ag** Silver 108	48 **Cd** Cadmium 112	49 **In** Indium 115	50 **Sn** Tin 119	51 **Sb** Antimony 122	52 **Te** Tellurium 128	53 **I** Iodine 127	54 **Xe** Xenon 131
55 **Cs** Caesium 133	56 **Ba** Barium 137	57 **La** Lanthanum 139	72 **Hf** Hafnium 178.5	73 **Ta** Tantalum 184	74 **W** Tungsten 184	75 **Re** Rhenium 186	76 **Os** Osmium 190	77 **Ir** Iridium 192	78 **Pt** Platinum 195	79 **Au** Gold 197	80 **Hg** Mercury 201	81 **Tl** Thallium 204	82 **Pb** Lead 207	83 **Bi** Bismuth 209	84 **Po** Polonium (210)	85 **At** Astatin (210)	86 **Rn** Radon (222)
87 **Fr** Fraicium (223)	88 **Ra** Radium (226)	89 **Ac** Actinium (226)															

58 **Ce** Cerium 140	59 **Pr** Praseodymium 141	60 **Nd** Neodymium 144	61 **Pm** Promethium (145)*	62 **Sm** Samarium 150	63 **Eu** Europium 152	64 **Gd** Gadolinium 157	65 **Tb** Terbium 159	66 **Dy** Dysprosium 162.5	67 **Ho** Holmium 165	68 **Er** Erbium 167	69 **Tm** Thullium 169	70 **Yb** Yttterbium 173	71 **Lu** Lutetium 175
90 **Th** Thorium 232	91 **Pa** Protactin 231	92 **U** Uranium 238	93 **Np** Neptunium (237)*	94 **Pu** Plutonium (242)*	95 **Am** Americium (243)*	96 **Cm** Curium (247)*	97 **Bk** Berkalium (249)*	98 **Cf** Californium (251)*	99 **Es** Einsteinium (254)*	100 **Fe** Fermium (253)*	101 **Md** Mendelivium (256)*	102 **No** Nobelium (254)*	103 **Lw** Lawrencium (257)*

*The relative atomic mass of an element whose isotopic composition is variable is shown in parenthesis. Elements marked with * are those which do not occur naturally on earth.*

59 — Atomic number
Pr (Praseodymium) — Symbol
141 — Relative atomic mass

Figure 3.2 The Periodic Table of the elements. Those highlighted comprise 99% of the body.

positively charged protons and negatively charged electrons. The loss of electrons gives an atom a net positive charge, whilst a gain of electrons gives it a net negative charge.

Electrons spin around the nucleus of an atom in orbits, which for convenience can be visualized as a series of concentric circles around the nucleus (see Figure 3.1). Each orbit has a maximum number of electrons that it can contain: the first orbit at most holds only 2, the second orbit 8, and the third 8 (in smaller atoms) or up to 18 (in large atoms) electrons.

The orbits can be considered to be energy levels or 'shells', the stability of which is determined by how many electrons are present. For example, chlorine (symbol Cl) atoms have the atomic number 17 and so normally have 17 protons and 17 electrons. This means that the third electron orbit will contain only 7 electrons (2+8+7; see Figure 3.1b). For maximum stability the outer orbit might be removed by loss of all 7 electrons, but it is easier for it to fill the orbit instead by accepting another electron. This will produce an atom which will now have 17 protons and 18 electrons and so it will have a net negative charge. Note though that this is still chlorine (or chloride as this form is usually called) as atoms must gain or lose protons to become another element.

In contrast, sodium (atomic number 11) normally would have 11 electrons, with just 1 in its outer orbit (2+8+1; see Figure 3.1c). To achieve maximum stability the atom would need either to acquire another 7 electrons to fill the outer orbit, or to lose the 1 it already has and so lose that orbit completely. Losing the single electron represents the easiest means and this leaves the atom with 11 protons and 10 electrons and hence a net positive charge.

Atoms of an element that have lost or gained additional electrons are no longer electrically neutral and are called ions. The presence of an electrical charge means that a solution of ions will carry an electric current and another term for them is electrolytes. Negatively and positively charged ions are collectively called anions and cations because, when an electric current is passed through a solution of them, they move to the electrodes called the anode and cathode respectively.

Atoms of some elements, such as helium (symbol He), neon (Ne), and argon (Ar), have just the right number of electrons to fill their orbits and do not therefore need to lose or gain electrons for stability. These are called 'inert' elements and do not usually take part in chemical reactions.

Atoms with incompletely filled electron orbits tend to lose or gain electrons by combining with other atoms in chemical reactions to form molecules and compounds.

Molecules and compounds

Molecules are formed when two or more atoms of the same element, or of different ones, combine in a chemical reaction. When two or more different elements are combined the molecule is sometimes called a compound.

For example, oxygen (atomic number 8) has 8 electrons and so has only 6 in its outer orbit (2+6; see Figure 3.3). For maximum stability an oxygen atom therefore needs to gain 2 electrons. This it can do by sharing electrons with another atom such as an oxygen atom. Alternatively, the oxygen atom might 'gain' the 2 electrons by sharing electrons with 2 hydrogen atoms (Figure 3.3). Hydrogen (atomic number 1) has only 1 electron in its outer orbit – remember that this is the first orbit and can maximally hold 2 electrons. By sharing electrons with oxygen the

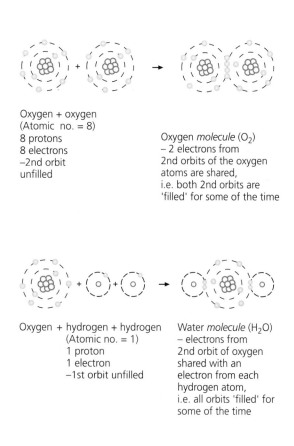

Oxygen + oxygen
(Atomic no. = 8)
8 protons
8 electrons
–2nd orbit
unfilled

Oxygen *molecule* (O_2)
– 2 electrons from
2nd orbits of the oxygen
atoms are shared,
i.e. both 2nd orbits are
'filled' for some of the time

Oxygen + hydrogen + hydrogen
(Atomic no. = 1)
1 proton
1 electron
–1st orbit unfilled

Water *molecule* (H_2O)
– electrons from
2nd orbit of oxygen
shared with an
electron from each
hydrogen atom,
i.e. all orbits 'filled' for
some of the time

Figure 3.3 Covalent bonding to form molecules or compounds.

hydrogen atoms will also 'gain' the extra electron they need for stability.

In these examples the molecule consisting of 2 oxygen atoms is given the symbol O_2 – the subscript number denotes the presence of 2 atoms – and is the form in which oxygen is found in the atmosphere. The molecule or compound consisting of an oxygen atom and 2 hydrogen atoms is given the symbol H_2O. In both examples, none of the atoms actually gained or lost an electron – their electrons are shared. This kind of chemical bond is called a covalent bond. Other kinds of bonds exist (e.g. ionic, hydrogen bonds) depending upon the interaction between constituent atoms but a description of all bond types is beyond the scope of this book.

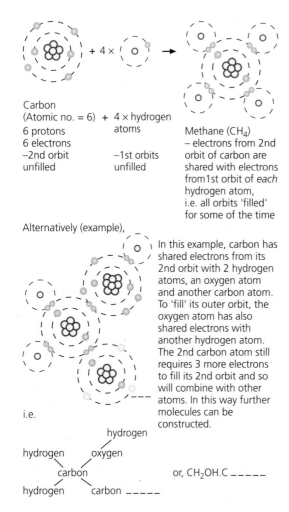

Carbon
(Atomic no. = 6) + 4 × hydrogen
6 protons   atoms
6 electrons
−2nd orbit   −1st orbits
unfilled   unfilled

Methane (CH$_4$)
– electrons from 2nd
orbit of carbon are
shared with electrons
from1st orbit of *each*
hydrogen atom,
i.e. all orbits 'filled'
for some of the time

Alternatively (example),

In this example, carbon has
shared electrons from its
2nd orbit with 2 hydrogen
atoms, an oxygen atom and
another carbon atom.
To 'fill' its outer orbit, the
oxygen atom has also
shared electrons with
another hydrogen atom.
The 2nd carbon atom still
requires 3 more electrons
to fill its 2nd orbit and so
will combine with other
atoms. In this way further
molecules can be
constructed.

i.e.

```
              hydrogen
                  |
hydrogen   oxygen
       \    /
       carbon                or, CH$_2$OH.C _ _ _ _ _
       /    \
hydrogen   carbon _ _ _ _ _
```

Figure 3.4 The versatility of carbon: the building of simple and complex organic molecules.

Although molecules and compounds may simply involve 2 or 3 atoms, others may be more complex. For example a carbon atom (atomic number 6) has 4 electrons in its outer orbit (2+4; see Figure 3.4). To 'gain' the 4 electrons it requires to fill the outer orbit it might share electrons with, for example, 4 hydrogen atoms (to form CH$_4$ = methane) or 2 oxygen atoms (CO$_2$ = carbon dioxide). Alternatively, more complex molecules are possible. For example a carbon atom may share 2 electrons with 2 hydrogen atoms, 1 with an oxygen atom (which might share another

electron with perhaps another hydrogen atom) and 1 with another carbon atom (see Figure 3.4). This latter carbon atom may, of course, combine with yet more atoms to gain the additional 3 electrons it needs for stability, and so the process continues. Potentially such compounds may be very large, involving hundreds of atoms. These compounds are said to be macromolecules (large molecules) and there are many examples of these in cells.

The capacity of carbon atoms to combine with so many other atoms make it a particularly versatile element. In addition, the bonds produced by sharing electrons are relatively easy to form, requiring little energy input, but they are very stable. It is perhaps not surprising, therefore, that carbon-based compounds (= organic compounds) form the chemical basis of living organisms.

CHEMICAL REACTIONS (METABOLISM)

Anabolism and catabolism

What is generally referred to as cell function is, in fact, a complex array of chemical reactions occurring within the cytoplasm of the cell, or within cellular organelles and membranes (see Chapter 2). Since the reactions, and their interactions, in a cell determines that cell's particular role in the body, it follows that there will be many different reactions occurring in the various kinds of cells. Homeostasis can be looked upon as a mechanism which sustains normal cellular function, by maintaining the optimal conditions for the mass of chemical reactions to occur.

Chemical processes within cells fall under the heading of metabolism. They may be divided into those in which new molecules are synthesized by the joining together of atoms and molecules and those in which molecules are broken down into smaller constituent units. 'Anabolism' is a general term for synthetic processes and 'catabolism' is a term applied to the breaking up processes.

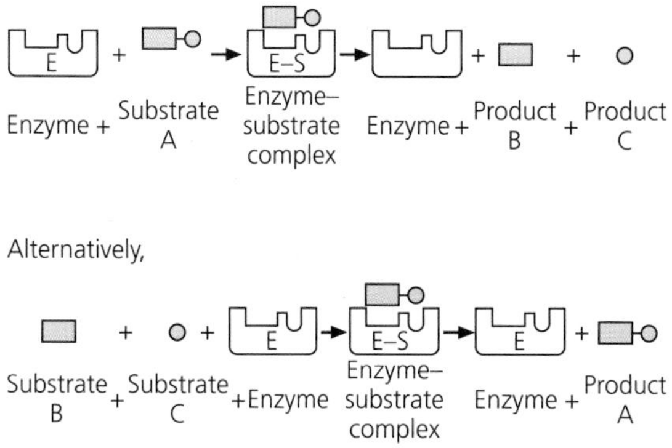

Figure 3.5 Enzyme–substrate interactions.

Anabolic processes involve the formation of chemical bonds between atoms or molecules. They require, therefore, the constituent atoms or molecules (i.e. the substrates) to be present in adequate amounts, together with the provision of energy sufficient for the bonds to be made (Figure 3.5). The energy required comes from that released when chemical bonds are broken, i.e. by catabolism. These energy-releasing processes are collectively called respiration. The release of atoms and molecules by catabolism may also provide some substrates for anabolic reactions.

Clearly, a cell will normally only synthesize those substances required for the structural, or functional, purposes of that cell. Such anabolic processes can only occur, however, if normal catabolic processes are maintained.

Although a degree of recycling of substrates occurs within cells, chemical homeostasis will also depend upon adequate nutritional intake (see Chapter 4), adequate digestive function (see Chapter 7), adequate delivery of materials to cells (see Chapter 9), adequate provision of oxygen (see Chapter 11), adequate cell membrane function and adequate removal of the waste products of metabolism (see Chapter 2). Within cells, the appropriate catabolic and anabolic reactions must proceed in an appropriate way, and at a rate conducive to the demands placed on the cell. The specificity of chemical reactions, and the rate at which they occur, are determined by enzymes.

Enzymes

Enzymes are catalysts: they accelerate a specific chemical reaction but are not changed by the reaction themselves. By promoting a particular reaction, the rate at which products are produced is increased and this effect of enzymes is vital if biochemical processes are to be compatible with life. Cells produce a huge variety of enzymes, some of which are named according to the substrate on which they act. For example, a protease is an enzyme which catabolizes proteins. In fact 'protease' is a term which covers a group of enzymes, each of which acts on a specific bond within a protein molecule. The name of an enzyme can be more specific, e.g. sucrase is an enzyme which breaks down the sugar sucrose into its constituent simple sugar units. Sometimes an enzyme is named after its chemical action, e.g. a dehydrogenase enzyme is one which dehydrogenates (removes a hydrogen atom from) a molecule. Note that enzyme names usually end in the suffix -ase.

Enzymes are polypeptides or proteins. Sometimes an enzyme contains a non-protein cofactor without which it will not function. Some cofactors are ions such as calcium and magnesium whilst others are complex molecules called coenzymes. Some vitamins, such as those of the B-group, are important coenzymes.

Enzymes are produced by anabolic reactions which are controlled by substrate (amino acid) availability, energy availability, and by the genetic information of the cell (Chapter 2). Being an anabolic process, enzyme synthesis is also dependent upon the presence of other enzymes and this is a classic example of the interrelationships which operate in living organisms and contribute to homeostasis.

Role of enzymes in intracellular homeostasis

Interactions between substrate and enzyme availability in regulating a reaction are illustrated diagrammatically in Figure 3.5. In this example an enzyme E combines with a compound A to form an enzyme–substrate complex. According to the 'lock and key' theory the specificity of the enzyme for substance A is made possible by the three-dimensional structure of these molecules – only A will fit into the active sites on the enzyme. By its actions the enzyme promotes the separation of the compound into two of its constituent compounds, say B and C. The reaction may be written as:

$$\begin{array}{c} \text{enzyme} \\ \downarrow \\ A \to B + C \end{array}$$

Because of its specificity in terms of binding to other molecules, the enzyme may also recombine with B and C and promote the reformation of A, as is shown in Figure 3.5. The question then arises as to what factors will determine the direction of the equation and therefore which substance is produced by the enzyme: A or (B+C). Generally it is determined by substrate competition for the binding sites on the enzymes, or by availability of the enzymes.

Competitive binding

If it is assumed that an enzyme can combine equally well with either A or (B+C), it follows that the most frequent combination will be determined by the relative abundance of A, B or C. Thus, if B or C are not utilized by the cell they will become more abundant and the reaction will then favour the reformation of A which in turn will become more abundant and so favour the breakdown to B and C (Figure 3.5). It is unlikely, however, that B or C will not be utilized by, or be removed from, the cell; otherwise, why produce them in the first place! In addition, if that utilization is increased, then the rate of production of B and C will increase

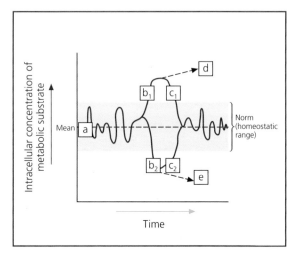

Figure 3.6 Homeostatic maintenance of substrate levels in cells.
a, range of substrate concentration necessary for normal cell function.
b₁, decreased utilization of substrate *or* increased cellular uptake or increased production by metabolism.
b₂, increased utilization of substrate promoted by increased availability of necessary enzyme *or* decreased production by metabolism.
c₁, restoration of normal range by increased substrate utilization either by increased enzyme activity or by a direct effect of substrate availability.
c₂, restoration of normal range by decreased substrate utilization.
d, poor substrate utilization, perhaps due to lack of appropriate enzyme(s) (e.g. inborn error).
e, lack of substrate due to *either* poor cellular uptake *or* lack of its production, perhaps due to enzyme deficiency (i.e. inborn error).

accordingly as there will be fewer molecules of B and C around to compete with A for binding sites on the enzyme, i.e. cellular homeostasis will be maintained. To sustain this reaction, adequate amounts of A must be provided and this in turn may well require yet another enzymatically controlled reaction. Thus enzyme availability is a major determinant in the regulation of intracellular, chemical homeostasis.

Enzyme availability

The conversion of A to B and C, and vice versa, requires the presence of adequate enzyme to catalyse the reaction. Should, for example, a cell require more B and C because of demands placed upon it, this could result from the increased synthesis of an enzyme which will in turn promote the production of the substrate A or, if more than adequate A is already present, might also result from increased production of the enzyme that catalyses A to B and C. The availability of active enzymes will depend upon (1) synthesis of more enzyme, or (2) the release of inactivated enzymes from chemical complexes, or (3) the removal of inhibitory substances. Note that all three of these processes will be dependent upon the presence of further enzymes, i.e. a cell is ultimately dependent upon the synthesis of enzymes appropriate to the functions of that cell.

The process of enzyme or protein synthesis is described in Chapter 2. It depends upon the availability of the amino acids that form the constituent molecules of proteins, and upon translation of the appropriate genetic coding found in the cell's DNA (i.e. the genes). The latter in turn requires the necessary genetic codes to be transcribed, a process which, according to the operon theory (see Chapter 2), is controlled by regulatory genes. The control of gene expression is still poorly understood but it is clear that the 'switching-on' of appropriate genes, and the structural integrity of those genes, plays an essential role in the maintenance of intracellular homeostasis.

The interplay between substrate availability and utilization in maintaining cellular homeostasis is shown diagrammatically in Figure 3.6.

The chemicals of life

The chemistry of cell function is a vast and complex subject area and has its own scientific discipline – biochemistry. Some knowledge of the major chemicals found inside and outside cells, and some of the major chemical processes which constitute metabolism is, however, important for an understanding of physiology. Some of the substances found within cells were described in Chapter 2. This section aims to look at these, and others, in more detail.

Carbohydrates

Carbohydrates are a large group of organic compounds that contain carbon (hence carbo-), hydrogen (hence -hydr-) and oxygen (indicated by -ate) and include substances such as sugars and starch. Carbohydrates have various functions in cells. In particular they form the main substrates for cellular respiration and, therefore, are the primary energy source in cells. Some carbohydrates may also be incorporated into, or combined with, other macromolecules such as DNA, or proteins. Others have roles in membrane functions or are structural components of those membranes. Other carbohydrates, for example glycogen, act as food reserves. The versatility of carbohydrates also means that some may be converted into other essential substances, such as amino acids and fatty acids, and so supplement other sources of these substances.

Carbohydrates can be divided into three main groups: monosaccharides, disaccharides, and polysaccharides. The suffix -ose in the name of a substance denotes that it is a carbohydrate,

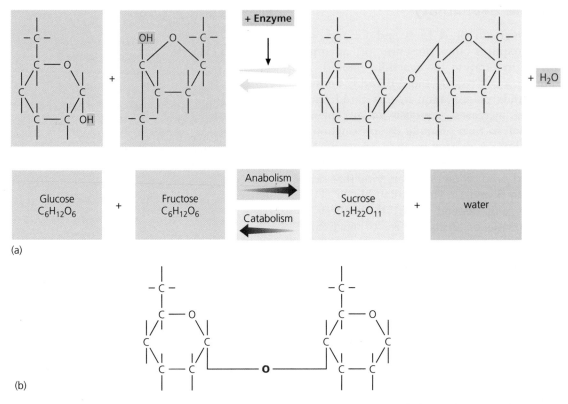

Figure 3.7 Carbohydrates: monosaccharides and disaccharides. (a) Chemical structures of *glucose, fructose,* and *sucrose.* Note that the atoms of glucose and fructose are generally arranged in ring structures. Though both sugars have the same empirical formula ($C_6H_{12}O_6$), their ring structures are different. Sucrose is a *disaccharide* as it contains 2 (monosaccharide) sugar units. For clarity, most H atoms and OH groups found attached to the carbon atoms are not shown. The interacting OH groups of glucose and fructose are indicated. (b) Chemical structure of *maltose.* Note that this consists of 2 glucose molecules joined together (it is a disaccharide) and has the same empirical formula as sucrose ($C_{12}H_{22}O_{11}$), although the structure is different. Numerous glucose molecules joined together like this, including side chains of molecules, form the storage polysaccharide (i.e. many sugar units) glycogen.

although not all carbohydrate names end in this (even starch was once known as amylose).

Monosaccharides

Monosaccharides (mono- = single), or simple sugars, contain from 3 to 7 carbon atoms in their molecules and are highly soluble in water. Trioses (the smallest sugar molecule) have 3 carbon atoms in the molecule, tetroses have 4, pentoses 5, hexoses 6 and heptoses 7. Pentoses and hexoses are of particular physiological importance. For example, the pentose

ribose is a constituent of nucleic acids, and the hexose glucose is the most important source of energy in the cell.

Disaccharides

Disaccharides (di- = 2) consist of two monosaccharides joined together. Sucrose (cane sugar) is a common example of a disaccharide, and is formed by combination of the monosaccharides glucose and fructose. As shown in Figure 3.7 the combination of two monosaccharides also produces a molecule of water; this is called a

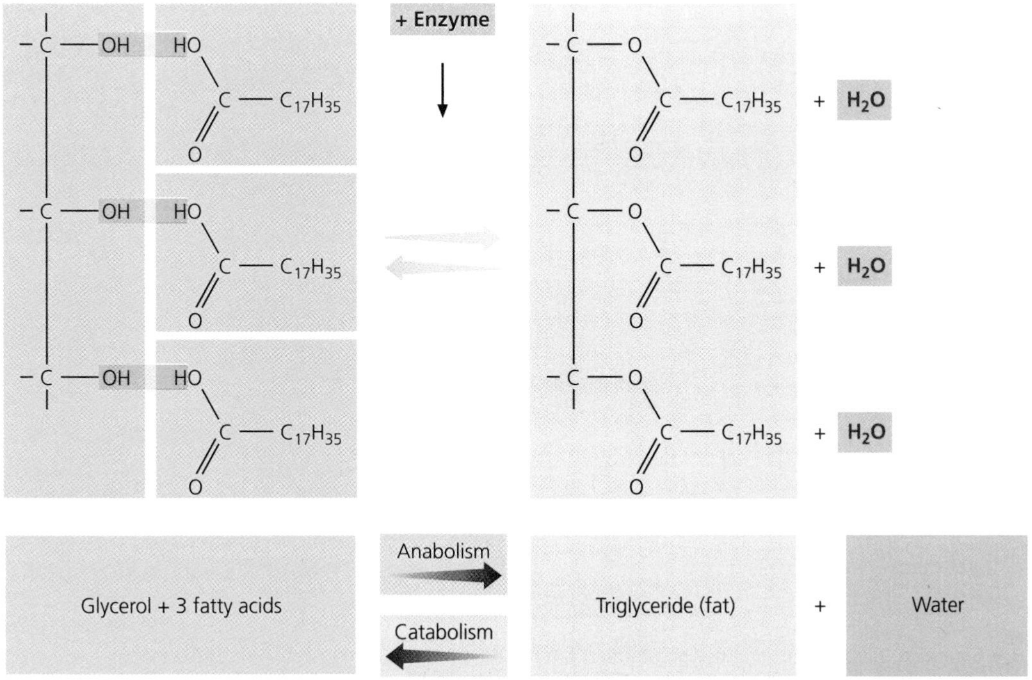

Figure 3.8 Fats: chemical structures of glycerol and fatty acids. Note that a *triglyceride* (fat) molecule is formed from 1 molecule of *glycerol* and 3 *fatty acid* molecules. The interacting OH groups are indicated. Like carbohydrates, fats contain atoms of carbon, hydrogen, and oxygen, but the chemical structures are very different to those of carbohydrates (see Figure 3.7). For clarity, hydrogen atoms attached to carbon atoms in glycerol have been omitted.

condensation reaction. Similarly, the breakdown of a disaccharide into its two constituent monosaccharides requires water for the reaction to proceed; it is a hydrolytic reaction (note: hydro- = water; lysis = breakdown).

Polysaccharides

Polysaccharides (poly- = many) consist of several monosaccharides joined together, and may be broken down to the constituent monosaccharides. Polysaccharides are usually poorly soluble in water, and are important components of cell membranes. Glycogen is a polysaccharide made from numerous glucose units and forms a convenient means of storing glucose in cells, especially in the liver and in skeletal muscle. Starch is the equivalent storage polysaccharide in plants.

Lipids

Like carbohydrates, lipids are composed of the elements carbon, hydrogen, and oxygen. Because of their molecular structure, however, most are insoluble in water. This has physiological implications, for example in the digestion of dietary lipids by the gut and in the carriage of lipids by the circulatory system. Lipids are a diverse group of chemicals, the best known being the fats.

A molecule of dietary fat, or triglyceride (tri =3), consists of a molecule of glycerol combined

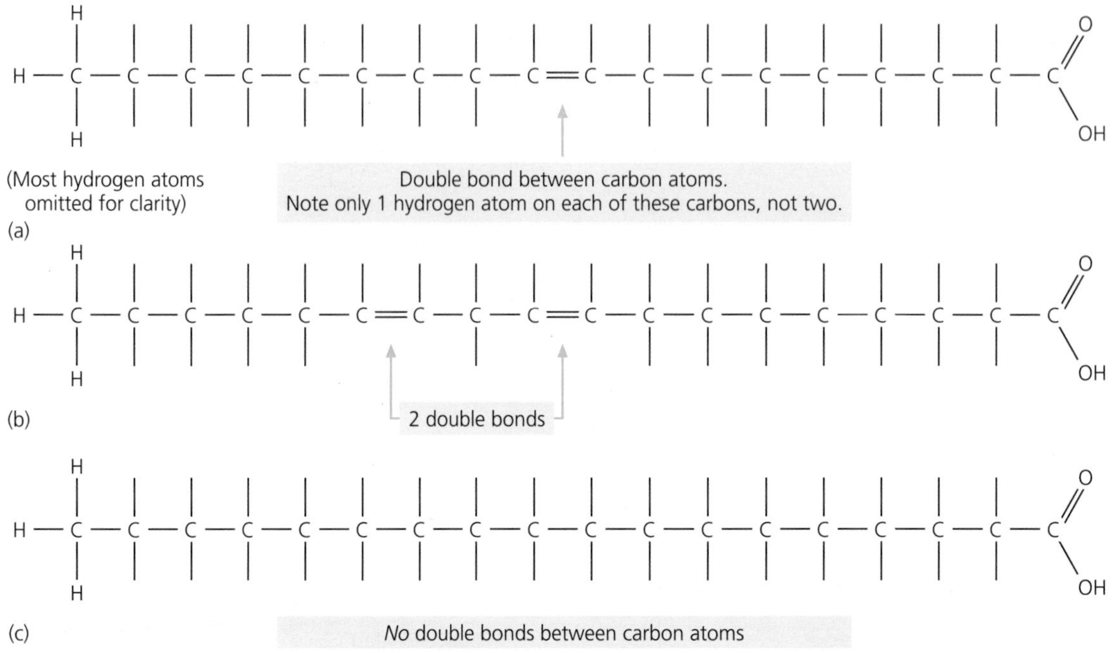

(Most hydrogen atoms omitted for clarity)

Double bond between carbon atoms. Note only 1 hydrogen atom on each of these carbons, not two.

(a)

(b)

2 double bonds

(c)

No double bonds between carbon atoms

Figure 3.9 Saturated, unsaturated, and polyunsaturated fatty acids. (a) Unsaturated, e.g. oleic acid. (b) Polyunsaturated, e.g. linoleic acid. (c) Saturated, e.g. palmitic acid.

with three molecules of fatty acids (Figure 3.8). As with polysaccharides, the fat molecule can be broken down into its component parts.

Fats are important energy stores in the body and contain more than twice the chemical energy of a comparable amount of carbohydrate. Thus, fats contain 9.2 kcal (38.6 kJ) of energy per gram weight, whereas carbohydrates contain 4.2 kcal (17.6 kJ) per gram. This is actually very useful because most of our energy reserves are stored as fat and the consequences regarding body weight and shape would be much more pronounced if that storage was as carbohydrate. Cell utilization of the energy produced by fat catabolism is highly inefficient, however, and fats normally only provide a supplementary source of energy, carbohydrates being the main source.

Saturated and unsaturated fats

Fats are frequently referred to as being saturated, unsaturated or polyunsaturated.

Unsaturated organic molecules are those which contain carbon atoms that are combined with fewer than the maximum of four other atoms (see earlier in this chapter) – in other words a carbon atom must share two of its electrons with only one other atom, and this is called a double bond (Figure 3.9a, b). Potentially this chemical bond may be opened to incorporate another atom into the molecule.

Saturated fats, which include most animal fats, and coconut oil, are those in which none of the constituent fatty acids contain double bonds between carbon and other atoms (Figure 3.9c). In unsaturated fats, such as olive oil, the presence of double bonds means that these may be 'opened' so that some carbon atoms can each combine with another hydrogen atom. In polyunsaturated fats (e.g. sunflower oil, corn oil) two or more further hydrogen atoms could be joined to some carbon atoms. Evidence suggests that polyunsaturated fats reduce the amount of cholesterol (another type

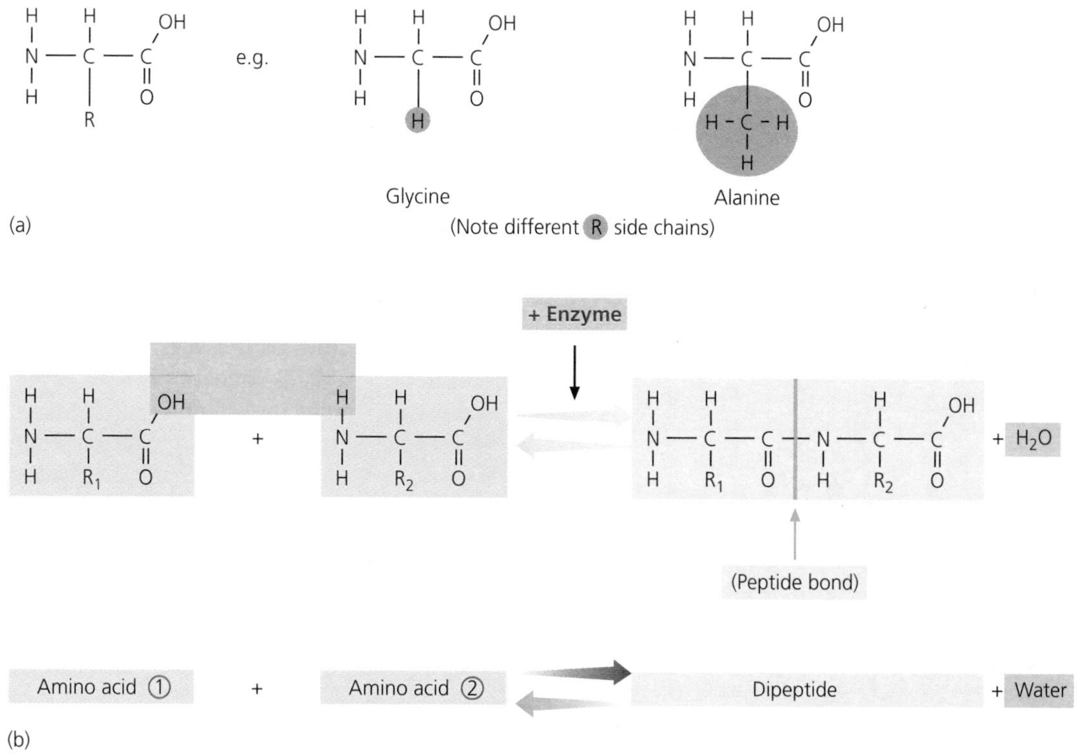

(a)

Glycine

Alanine

(Note different ⓡ side chains)

+ Enzyme

(Peptide bond)

Amino acid ① + Amino acid ② ⇌ Dipeptide + Water

(b)

Figure 3.10 Amino acids and peptides. (a) General amino acid structure: C, carbon; O, oxygen; N, nitrogen; H, hydrogen; R, a side chain of atom(s). (b) Dipeptide synthesis. Note that the side chains R_1 and R_2 do not interact in the formation of the dipeptide. Should more amino acids be joined to the dipeptide to form a polypeptide, interactions *between* the R side chains will cause the polypeptide to bend and fold, i.e. the R side chains largely determine the final 3–dimensional shape of the polypeptide molecule.

of lipid) in blood and so help prevent disease of the heart and circulation.

Proteins

Peptides and proteins have major influences on cell function either as structural molecules, enzymes or hormones. Like carbohydrates and lipids, they are largely comprised of carbon, hydrogen and oxygen, but they also contain nitrogen atoms. Atoms of sulphur and phosphorus are also frequently present.

The basic building units of proteins are called amino acids. These are complex molecules which have the same general chemical formula shown in Figure 3.10a. There are 20 naturally occurring amino acids, and peptides and proteins are comprised of some or all of these, arranged in differing sequences. If the 'chain' is just two amino acids in length the molecule is called a dipeptide (di- = two; Figure 3.10b), if three a tripeptide (tri- =3). Polypeptides may consist of several or perhaps several hundred amino acids, and linkage of two or more polypeptide chains produces a protein. Bearing in mind that polypeptides and proteins may be up to several hundred amino acids in length, the number of possible combinations and permutations of amino acids is colossal. Furthermore, although cells initially synthesize proteins as chains of amino acids

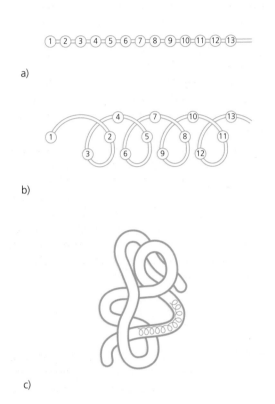

a)

b)

c)

Figure 3.11 Primary, secondary, and tertiary structure of proteins. (a) Primary structure: amino acid chain, determined by the genetic code of the cell. (b) Secondary structure: coiling of amino acid chain. (c) Tertiary structure: further coiling and bending of amino acid chain. Note: (b) and (c) are determined by interactions between side chains of various amino acids.

(this is called the 'primary' structure), the structure may coil (= secondary structure) and bend (= tertiary structure) as chemical bonds are made between component amino acids, so that the final three-dimensional shape of the molecule is also dependent upon the amino acid sequences (Figure 3.11). There is, therefore, tremendous scope for variety in protein molecular size and shape, and this is particularly important considering the need for enzymes to catalyse specific chemical reactions.

The role of enzymes in homeostasis was outlined earlier in this chapter. Their importance cannot be overemphasized since they control the rate of most, if not all, catabolic and anabolic reactions within cells. Protein synthesis is the basis of the expression of inherited characters (Chapter 20), as the kinds of protein manufactured by a cell are ultimately determined by information encoded on the DNA (i.e. by genes).

Nucleic acids

Sometimes called 'key chemicals of life', nucleic acids (DNA and RNA) are macromolecules comprised of a 'backbone' of pentose sugar and phosphate molecules, and sequences of molecules called purines and pyrimidines. Nucleic acids contain the genetic information of the cell and therefore determine which proteins are synthesized by our cells. For further details the reader is referred to Chapter 2.

Adenosine triphosphate (ATP)

The breakage of chemical bonds by catabolic reactions releases energy which cells will utilize to form new chemical bonds in anabolic reactions. Two aspects to the utilization of energy are that released energy may be dissipated as heat, and that energy release may occur in one part of a cell but be required in another part. ATP is a compound which harnesses some of the energy as it is released (a large proportion of it is lost as heat) and acts as an intermediary, carrying the harnessed energy to other parts of the cell. The levels of ATP within a cell must therefore be maintained for normal cellular function, and even increased if the metabolic demands of a cell increase (e.g. in a skeletal muscle cell during exercise).

ATP is produced by combining adenosine diphosphate (ADP) with another phosphate molecule using energy produced by respiration. Thus,

$$ADP + Pi + energy \rightleftharpoons ATP$$

The reaction is reversible which means that, having harnessed the energy, ATP can be broken down again to ADP and phosphate as and when required, so that the energy is released and can be utilized by other reactions. The ADP and phosphate are available for re-use. The initial production of energy by respiration requires the necessary substrates to be available and these are mainly derived from the carbohydrate glucose.

Water

Some 60–70% of our body weight is due to water. All chemical reactions require a medium in which to take place and water is close to being a 'universal' solvent. Indeed, it is because climatic conditions on earth ensure that water exists mainly as a liquid, as opposed to gaseous or solid form, that life can exist on this planet. Changes in water content of the body alter the volume and composition of body fluids and it is not surprising that it is closely maintained (Chapter 12)

Water has the molecular formula H_2O: two hydrogen atoms are bonded to an oxygen atom. Although the sharing of electrons by the hydrogen and oxygen atoms is numerically ideal to achieve stability (see earlier in this chapter), the physical size of the oxygen atomic nucleus relative to that of hydrogen ensures that the shared electrons spend more time around the oxygen nucleus than around the hydrogen nuclei. This results in the water molecule being polarized: the oxygen pole of the molecule carries a weak negative charge, and the hydrogen pole carries a weak positive charge. Thus:

oxygen nucleus = 8 protons
hydrogen nucleus = 1 proton

i.e. electrons will spend more time around the oxygen nucleus than around the hydrogen nuclei.

The polarization of water molecules is sufficient to give water its properties as a solvent.

Mineral salts

Mineral salts such as sodium chloride (= table salt) and sodium bicarbonate (= baking powder) have the property that they dissociate into their constituent ions when dissolved in water. It is in this ionic form that salts are chemically active. Body fluids contain a variety of ions and changes in this ionic environment can have adverse effects on cell function. The concentrations of most ions in body fluids are homeostatically regulated (see Chapters 5 and 12).

Minerals are also important structural constituents. For example, sulphur is an essential constituent of the amino acid cysteine, iron is a constituent of the blood pigment haemoglobin and calcium and phosphorus are constituents of bone. In addition some minerals, for example magnesium, calcium, and iron, are cofactors of enzymes and have a direct input into cellular reactions.

Vitamins

Vitamins are chemicals that are required in small quantities to sustain growth and metabolism (see Chapter 6). Most are coenzymes and their presence is essential for certain reactions to occur. Most cannot be synthesized by cells although some, such as vitamin A, may.

Vitamins are either fat-soluble or water-soluble. The B vitamins and vitamin C are water-soluble and excess quantities consumed are easily excreted in urine. On the other hand fat-soluble vitamins (vitamins A, D, E and K) are stored in (liver) cells and so reserves can be built up.

Intracellular messengers

Many homeostatic responses require the changing of cell function as a result of stimulation by nerve inputs or by interactions with hormones (Chapters 13 and 15). These target cells are equipped with chemical structures, or receptors, which recognize the hormone or chemical released by the nerve ending. In order for cell function to respond to these interactions the 'message' must be conducted through the cell to the appropriate organelles. This is provided by chemicals called, appropriately, intracellular messengers. A number of such 'messengers' have been identified including cyclic adenosine monophosphate (cAMP) and are discussed in more detail in Chapter 15.

Energy production by cellular respiration

The energy required to bond molecules together in anabolic processes is provided by cleaving other chemicals and so releasing the energy from their bonds. The release of energy is called cellular respiration and enzymes play a central role in this process.

Glucose is the main substrate for cellular respiration. Although its metabolism also requires an input of energy, each molecule of glucose generates a net 38 molecules of ATP. Production of 30 of these molecules involves the use of oxygen (aerobic metabolism). This is provided by gas exchange in the lungs, but also requires a normal haemoglobin concentration in the blood for its transportation, and adequate perfusion of tissues with blood for its delivery. Inadequate provision of oxygen (called hypoxia), for whatever reason, makes anaerobic metabolism predominate. Glucose is provided by the digestion of more complex carbohydrates, by its release from stores (i.e. from glycogen by glycogenolysis) or by the synthesis of glucose in the liver from fats and proteins (i.e. by gluconeogenesis). Hormones such as insulin and glucagon are particularly important in these processes. Each system involved in the provision of substrate for metabolism is individually homeostatically regulated, yet an integration of them all contributes to intracellular homeostasis.

Aerobic metabolism of glucose

This part of the text should be read in conjunction with Figure 3.12.

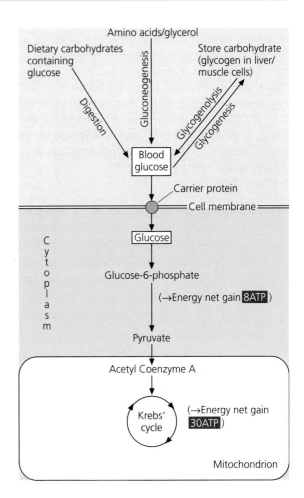

Figure 3.12 Glucose metabolism (cellular respiration). Note that glucose molecules undergo numerous enzymatically catalysed conversions, especially within the Krebs cycle of reactions. Each molecule of glucose generates a net 38 molecules of ATP. See text for description. Overall equation: $C_6H_{12}O_6 + 6O_2 + 38ADP + 38P \rightarrow 6CO_2 + 6H_2O + 38ATP$.

Glucose enters cells via carrier proteins which 'flip' the sugar across the cell membrane. The glucose is immediately converted into glucose-6-phosphate by binding a phosphate molecule to the sixth carbon atom of the glucose molecule. This effectively prevents the glucose from being transported back out again. The molecule is then converted by a series of enzymatically driven reactions to a substance called pyruvic acid, generating eight molecules of ATP in the process. This stage does not require oxygen and so is anaerobic. The pyruvic acid then enters the cell's mitochondria where it is converted into acetyl-coenzyme A, which enters a complex series of enzymatically controlled reactions called the Krebs' cycle (or the tricarboxylic acid – TCA – cycle). This cycle of reactions is important because, although the release of energy from molecules could in theory occur almost instantaneously, the harnessing of the energy as ATP is made much more efficient by releasing the energy in a slower, more controlled fashion. Even so, only some 20–25% of the energy released is utilized. The remainder is lost as heat, the excess of which must be dissipated from cells, and the body, because an elevated body temperature affects the rate of chemical reactions, and so disturbs homeostasis. The Krebs' cycle forms the aerobic part of the respiratory pathway.

One feature of the aerobic metabolism of glucose is that electrons are released which are then transferred from one to another along a series of chemicals found in the membranes of mitochondria, each transfer liberating more energy. These chemicals are called cytochromes (otherwise referred to as the electron transport chain). One of the most important of these is nicotinamide adenine dinucleotide (NAD) which is a derivative of the B-vitamin niacin provided by our diets. Cyanide poisoning results from an inhibition of the cytochrome system.

Aerobic metabolism of glucose produces 'waste' products in CO_2 and H_2O that are excreted via the lungs/kidneys. Homeostatic regulation of the functioning of these organs

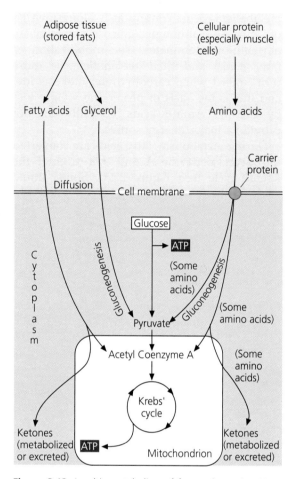

Figure 3.13 Aerobic metabolism of fats and proteins. Note that certain amino acids, and glycerol, by being enzymatically converted to pyruvate, may be used to generate new glucose molecules (gluconeogenesis). The metabolism of fatty acids, and certain amino acids, generates ketones as byproducts, unlike the CO_2 and water produced by carbohydrate metabolism.

ensures that this excretion prevents a build-up of these wastes (see Chapters 11 and 12).

Aerobic metabolism of fatty acids and amino acids

In addition to producing energy from glucose, cells also have the enzymes necessary for the metabolism of fatty acids (from fat) and amino acids (from protein). Indeed, fatty acid metabolism occurs continuously alongside that of glucose, although glucose metabolism normally predominates. The mobilization of fatty acids, and their metabolism, is more pronounced when carbohydrate intake is low and this is the basis of promoting weight loss by dieting. Amino acids normally do not provide a major energy source.

During metabolism, fatty acids are converted into acetylcoenzyme A and thence enter the Krebs' cycle (see Figure 3.13). Some amino acids on the other hand can be converted into either glucose, pyruvic acid or acetylcoenzyme A. In this way they too can enter Krebs' cycle, but can also be used to generate glucose for use elsewhere in the body. One important aspect of the metabolism of fatty acids and certain (especially 'essential') amino acids is that end products called ketones are produced. These cannot be metabolized by the liver but, provided that production is not excessive, the usage of ketones as a source of energy by tissues such as cardiac muscle, and ketone excretion in the urine, prevents their build-up in body fluids.

Anaerobic metabolism of glucose

Although most energy produced by cells involves the use of oxygen, some enzymati-cally mediated reactions are favoured when the oxygen supply is inadequate. These processes constitute anaerobic metabolism.

Anaerobic metabolism is less efficient than aerobic metabolism in that it generates only 8, compared with 30, ATP molecules per molecule of glucose. In addition, the end products are less easily excreted than are those of aerobic metabolism. Thus, metabolic enzymes in the absence of adequate oxygen produce substances such as lactic acid from the glucose. This is highly toxic to cells (as are all acids) and has to be detoxified in the liver by a process which requires oxygen.

Although respiration is predominantly aerobic, all cells exhibit some anaerobic metabolism even though they are not deficient in oxygen. During sharp bursts of exercise, however, the oxygen supply to muscles may not be adequate to maintain aerobic metabolism and so anaerobic metabolism becomes more prevalent. Similarly, exercise which is prolonged and severe will also increase the anaerobic generation of energy by muscle cells. The consequential build-up of lactic acid must be metabolized after exercise has finished, otherwise the resultant accumu-lation of acid will begin to influence enzyme function, and hence homeostasis. The metabo-lism of lactic acid after exercise means that oxygen consumption will have to be greater than is usual at rest – this extra is called the 'oxygen debt'.

Examples of homeostatic control failures and principles of correction

Life requires the maintenance of cellular metabolic activity, and the homeostatic control of systemic functions is central to that mainte-nance (see Chapter 1). For a system to function normally, however, the various cell types of which the system is comprised must also function normally. Thus, there is an inter-dependency between cells by which the function of one cell is determined by the functions of cells elsewhere.

The disruption of chemical composition and utilization by our cells forms the basis of all physiological disorders, and examples of cellular homeostatic failure are extensive. This section describes only some disorders of metabolism and readers are referred to other chapters for further examples of biochemical disturbances.

Reduced glucose availability

Deficiency of glucose, either because of malnutrition or of poor utilization of available glucose, as in diabetes mellitus, necessitates energy production from other sources. Thus, carbohydrate stores in liver and muscle, and fat stores in adipose tissue, will be mobilized. As these are depleted then proteins (especially from muscle) will also be catalysed. The end products of fat and protein metabolism (ketones and keto acids) are toxic in excess, however. In addition, diabetic hyperglycaemia (hyper = greater than normal; glyc- = glucose; -aemia = blood) also influences cell function, particularly of smooth muscle cells of small blood vessels, and of brain cells. Long-term control is aimed at facilitating glucose utilization by cells.

Endocrine disturbances

Metabolism is under hormonal influence. In particular, insulin and glucagon are instrumental in regulating the glucose content of blood and its utilization by cells. In times of stress the actions of adrenaline and cortisol provide additional support, and so increase the metabolic rate. The rate at which glucose is utilized is also influenced by thyroxine and growth hormone.

Metabolic disturbances will result from hypo- (lower than normal) or hyperactivity (greater than normal) of the glands which secrete these hormones. If there is a hormone deficiency then interventions to restore metabolic homeostasis are aimed at correcting the underlying homeostatic disturbance either by the provision of hormone, by agonistic drugs, or by drugs which promote hormone release from the gland. If the hormone is in excess, intervention involves either surgical ablation of or part of the gland or provision of drugs which antagonize or block the actions of the hormone.

Hypoxia

Inadequate oxygen provision, whatever the cause, means that cells must resort to anaerobic respiration. Lactic acid production will then increase and this is toxic. Control is directed at treating the cause of the hypoxia, or alleviating it. Methods will of course depend upon whether the hypoxia is of lung or cardiovascular origin.

Body temperature

Temperature has a pronounced influence on the rate of chemical reactions, either directly or by altering enzyme structure and function (Chapter 17). Hypo- and hyperthermia are therefore life-threatening conditions.

Genetic disturbances

Gene mutations provide novel enzymes or make cells deficient in appropriate enzymes, and the range of genetic disturbances is extensive. A good example is when the enzyme phenylalanine hydroxylase is absent, causing a build-up of the amino acid phenylalanine in cells and thence in blood. Excess phenylalanine is toxic to developing brain cells and the condition, called phenylketonuria (PKU), is therefore damaging to the developing brain of young children. Control of PKU is aimed at compensating for the metabolic accumulation of phenylalanine by reducing its intake in the diet. Screening of babies at risk has greatly reduced the incidence of PKU.

Summary

1 Cells can be envisaged as being complex chemistry sets, with a vast array of interacting chemical reactions, which are directed by genes but which are also influenced by chemical availability and the environment in which the reactions are occurring.

2 Cellular chemicals range from 'simple' ions, in which atoms have gained or lost electrons, to large complex macromolecules involving hundreds of atoms.

3 Much of cellular chemistry concerns 'organic' (carbon-containing) chemicals, the main constituents of which are carbon, hydrogen, oxygen, and, also in proteins, nitrogen.

4 The synthesis of molecules (a process called anabolism) requires energy which is provided by the release of chemical energy during the break-up of others (a process called catabolism) to their constituent molecules or atoms. Together, anabolic and catabolic reactions comprise what is generally called 'metabolism'.

5 Fats, proteins and carbohydrates form the three major classes of organic chemicals synthesized by cells. All have structural and functional roles, and all may be utilized to provide energy via respiration, although carbohydrates are normally the main source.

6 Respiration is most efficient if it is aerobic (i.e. utilizes oxygen) but many cells (not brain cells) are capable of functioning using anaerobic respiration for a limited time. Accumulation of metabolic products of anaerobic metabolism, such as lactic acid, will eventually suppress metabolism.

7 Physiological systems are largely directed at maintaining cell metabolism throughout the body but the complex interactions of systemic functions means that disturbance of the biochemistry of cells in one tissue will disturb the functions of cells elsewhere. Systemic homeostasis will therefore be disrupted which will in turn exacerbate disturbances of chemical homeostasis in cells throughout the body.

Review Questions

1 Name the basic molecular units of proteins, lipids, and polysaccharides.

2 Compare and contrast the structure of carbohydrates, lipids, and proteins.

3 How is the structure of a protein related to its function?

4 Distinguish between catabolism and anabolism.

5 Explain the role of condensation in the anabolism of a lipid, and of hydrolysis in the catabolism of a complex carbohydrate.

6 Name the 'key chemicals of life' which are:

   (a) responsible for controlling the rate of metabolic reactions;
   (b) 'driving' metabolic reactions.

7 What is meant by the term 'denaturization'?

8 Some vitamins are coenzymes. What does this mean?

9 What is the difference between saturated and unsaturated fats?

10 The cell is the 'basic unit of life' which is in turn dependent upon its molecular components. Discuss the roles of these components in maintaining intracellular homeostasis.

Levels of organization III: Tissues

4

Introduction: the need for tissue specialization

Details of the anatomy of tissues

Homeostasis at tissue level: wound healing

Examples of homeostatic disturbance

Summary

Review questions

Introduction: the need for tissue specialization

The structure of the body can be described on five levels: the chemical level (described in Chapter 3), the cellular level (Chapter 2), the tissue level, and the organ and organ system levels (Chapters 7–18). This chapter is concerned with the tissue level of organization.

A tissue is defined as a collection of similar cells and their component parts which perform specialized homeostatic functions. There are many different types of tissues and so it follows that there must be different cell types which comprise these tissues, bearing in mind the definition.

Each cell type differentiates during embryonic development from the three embryonic germ layers (endoderm, mesoderm and ectoderm – Chapter 19). The process of specialization is controlled by the expression and non-expression of developmental genes (Chapter 2). That is, a muscle cell is formed by the expression of genes concerned with the structural and functional development of this cell type, and by the non-expression of other developmental type genes, for example, blood cell genes.

Functional specialization is necessary as each cell type has an important homeostatic role to play in the person; there is a 'division of labour', so that the individual can carry out the characteristics of life described in Chapter 1. For example, muscle tissue specialization is necessary so that the individual can carry out movement (Chapter 16). Other cell-tissue specializations are necessary to support the body (skeletal tissues), whereas others are important as secretory cells which release enzymes or hormones (glandular tissues), and some are involved in the defence of the body (vascular tissues). Once they have specialized some cells lose their ability to perform other functions. For example, the mature red blood cell is concerned with the transport and exchange of respiratory gases, but as a result of this specialization it loses its capacity to divide. Nerve and muscle cells generally also lose this replication function once they become specialized, with the consequence that if such tissues are damaged they are capable of only limited regeneration.

The study of tissues is called histology (histio = tissues; logos = study) and is concerned with the broader patterns of cellular organization, investigating how tissues are structured, and how this structure is important in determining the tissue's homeostatic functions in the organization of the whole person. Tissues produce a good example of the interplay between form and function.

Details of the anatomy of tissues

Clearly the entire body is formed of one tissue or another but structurally and functionally there are only four main types. These are:

1 Epithelial tissues,

2 Connective tissues,

3 Nervous tissues,

4 Muscular tissues.

The body also contains a number of membranes but these are formed from epithelial cells supported by connective tissue.

This chapter is particularly concerned with the details of epithelial and connective tissues, a comparative description of muscle tissue types, and a description of the types of membrane found in the body. Nervous tissue, skeletal muscle tissue, and specialized connective tissues, such as bone and the vascular tissues, are described in more detail in later chapters and are only briefly mentioned here.

EPITHELIAL TISSUES

There are three types of epithelia:

1 Simple epithelia. These are just one cell thick.

2 Compound epithelia. These are more than one cell thick.

3 Glandular epithelia. These produce the secretions of the body.

All are derived from the embryonic germ layers and, since they have different structures, they have different functions.

Homeostatic functions of epithelia

1 Protection. The simple (to a limited extent) and compound epithelia protect the underlying tissues from pathogenic invasion, desiccation, and harmful environmental factors, such as ultraviolet radiation.

2 Transport. The simple epithelia have important roles in controlling the transport of substances across membranous surfaces.

3 Lining. Simple, compound and glandular epithelia line internal cavities and tubes of the body, such as the respiratory and digestive tracts.

4 Secretory. Glandular epithelia are responsible for producing a variety of substances (sebum, sweat, tears, etc.) that have particular homeostatic functions. For example, the production and secretion of sweat are important thermoregulatory mechanisms (Chapter 17).

Epithelial tissues consist of flat sheets of cells. All epithelia have a basement membrane, that is, a thin layer of 'cementing' material on the underside of the tissue which holds the cells together.

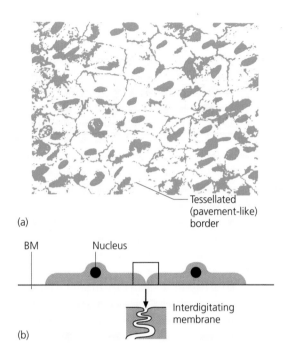

(a)

Tessellated (pavement-like) border

(a)

BM   Nucleus

Interdigitating membrane

(b)

Figure 4.1 Squamous (pavement) epithelium: (a) a surface view; (b) a side view – BM, basement membrane

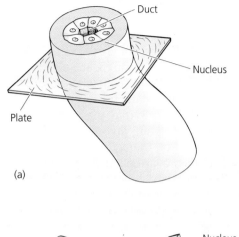

Duct

Nucleus

Plate

(a)

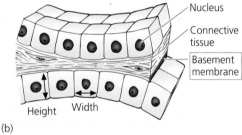

Nucleus

Connective tissue

Basement membrane

Height   Width

(b)

Figure 4.2 Cuboidal epithelium: (a) a surface view; (b) a side view.

Simple epithelia (or covering and lining epithelia)

Simple epithelial cells are arranged as a single or unicellular layer, and these tissues are located in areas where they can carry out their homeostatic functions of absorption or filtration (for example, respiratory surfaces of the lung).

Pavement (squamous) epithelia

Figure 4.1a is a surface view which illustrates how these cells are connected together via interdigitating junctions, giving a tessellated (pavement-like) border appearance. The side view (Figure 4.1b) demonstrates that this tissue is made up of very thin, flat cells. Squamous epithelia are not found in areas where there is wear and tear, but will be located in areas which are adapted for the homeostatic functions of rapid diffusion, osmosis, and

filtration. Examples of location are the alveoli of the lungs, the double membranous Bowman's capsule of the kidney nephrons, the internal lining of the blood vessels and the inner surface of the heart, the lining of lymphatic capillaries, and the serous membranes of the body (see later).

These epithelia generally have fluid on one side and blood vessels on the other, so transport can occur between the two. They allow a frictionless flow of fluids across their surfaces.

Cuboidal epithelia

Figure 4.2a illustrates that this tissue has a hexagonal or pentagonal prism shape when viewed from above. The side view, illustrated in Figure 4.2b, demonstrates the cubic shape of the cells. These cells are slightly thicker than the 'pavement' tissues, but are still thin enough for substances to pass through, and this type of tissue is typically concerned with absorption and secretory homeostatic functions. Examples of location are the thyroid gland and sweat glands, the germinating layer of the skin, the anterior surface of the lens of the eye, the surface of the ovaries, and the proximal tubules of the kidneys where it bears microvilli which increase the surface area for absorption of water. The nuclei of both squamous and cuboidal epithelia are centralized and are either round or oval in shape.

Columnar epithelia

The surface view of this epithelium is similar to the cuboidal type, but the side view (Figure 4.3a) shows that these cells are in fact taller or thicker than the cuboidal cells. Their nuclei are oval and are situated near the base of the cell. Examples of location are the lining of the digestive tract from the small intestine to the anus, and the lining of the gall bladder.

The homeostatic functions of columnar epithelia are varied. They provide a smooth area over which food can pass without friction, protect underlying tissues, and aid food absorption (the cells in the ileum possess microvilli which increases their surface area). Additional functions are to act as a lubricant: some intestinal cells are modified columnar cells called goblet or mucus secreting cells and their secretions lubricate or moisturize food to aid both its passage and the physical and chemical digestive processes. Some columnar and cuboidal cells have cilia on their free surfaces (Figure 4.3b) and these facilitate the movement of materials along the duct.

Examples of ciliated epithelia are the lining of the airways where ciliated cells move dust particles and microbes from the trachea and areas beyond to the oesophagus so that they can be swallowed, and the lining of the Fallopian tubes where the cells waft the

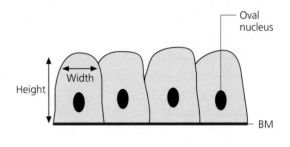

(a)

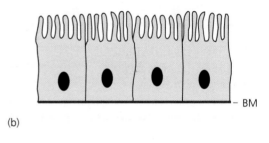

(b)

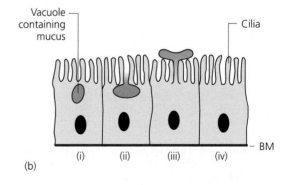

(b)

Figure 4.3 Columnar epithelium: (a) a side view – BM, basement membrane; (b) bearing microvilli; (c) containing goblet cells bearing cilia:
(i) goblet cell producing vacuole of mucus;
(ii) vacuole moves towards the surface of the epithelium which bears the cilia;
(iii) secretion of mucus across the surface of the epithelium;
(iv) process restarts.

secondary oocytes to the site of fertilization, and the zygote and developing embryo to the site of implantation.

Pseudoepithelia may be glandular (mucus secreting) as in the lining of the upper respiratory tract and in certain ducts of the male reproductive system.

Compound (or stratified) epithelia

This type of tissue consists of at least two or more layers of cells. Only the basal layer lies in contact with a basement membrane. Cells of the other layers are derived from this layer. Compound or stratified epithelia are found wherever mechanical stresses are present, for example at the surface of the skin. One of their homeostatic functions is to protect underlying tissues, but some produce secretions, for example those lining the mouth and the anus.

The naming of stratified epithelia is dependent upon the shape of the surface cells.

Stratified squamous epithelia

These epithelia are found wherever mechanical stresses are severe. The basal cells are cuboidal, or columnar, are in contact with the basement membrane, and are mitotically active. The new 'daughter' cells produced by mitosis go through a series of changes before attaining the squamous shape of the most superficial cells. These cells are sloughed off during times of friction. Locations of this type of epithelium are the lining of the mouth, tongue, oesophagus, and vagina, i.e. wet areas that are subjected to wear and tear.

Keratinized stratified squamous epithelia

This is a particular form of squamous epithelium in which the cells contain the waterproofing protein keratin. This enhances the barrier properties of the tissue, making it resistant to friction and aiding the prevention of

pathogenic invasion. The epidermis of the skin is of this type.

Stratified cuboidal epithelium

The function of this tissue is mainly protective. It is located in sweat glands, the pharynx, and the epiglottis.

Stratified columnar epithelia

The functions of this tissue are protection and secretion. It is located in the male urethra, and in the lactiferous ducts of the mammary glands.

Transitional epithelia

This is usually made of three or four layers of cells and is a tissue capable of being stretched. Prior to stretching it is of cuboidal shape, but when stretched the cells have a squamous appearance (Figure 4.4). Its expansion properties help prevent rupture of the organ in which it is found. An example of its location is the lining of the urinary bladder.

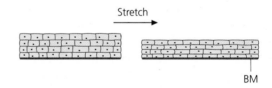

Figure 4.4 Transitional epithelium, side view. BM, basement membrane.

Pseudo-stratified epithelium

This tissue appears to be an epithelium of several layers of columnar or cuboidal cells. It is in fact a simple epithelium as all the cells have a direct contact with the basement membrane (Figure 4.5). Examples of location are the lining of the larger excretory ducts of

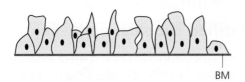

Figure 4.5 Pseudo–stratified epithelium, side view. BM, basement membrane.

many glands, and parts of the Eustachian tube which connects the middle ear with the pharynx.

Glandular epithelia

The homeostatic function of this type of epithelium is the secretion of various substances from glandular cells, which either cover a lining epithelium or lie deep to a covering epithelium. This production and secretion of substances requires energy expenditure, therefore such cells have a rich mitochondrial content. In addition, they usually have an abundance of endoplasmic reticulum and Golgi apparatus which are responsible for the production and packaging of the secretions. Glands are classified as either exocrine or endocrine; their embryological development is summarized in Figure 4.6.

Exocrine glands

Exocrine glands secrete their substances into ducts (either as simple or compound exocrine glands) or directly on to a free surface (unicellular exocrine glands, Figure 4.7). Secretions from exocrine glands that are of a watery constitution are referred to as serous secretions. In contrast mucus glands produce a viscous secretion (mucous secretions).

Most glands in the body are exocrine, including:

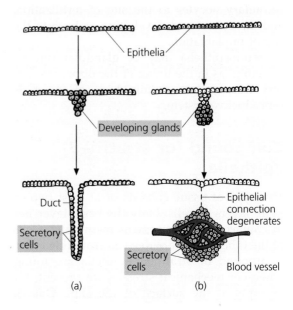

Figure 4.6 Development of (a) exocrine and (b) endocrine glands.

1   Sweat glands. Their homeostatic function is to secrete sweat or perspiration to cool the skin. Sweat also contains excretory products such as urea (Chapter 17).

2   Digestive glands. Their homeostatic function is one of catabolism of food materials, which provides blood, and hence body cells, with their nutrient requirements (Chapter 7).

3   Ceruminous glands. Their homeostatic function is to act as an external defence mechanism. They secrete earwax (or cerumen) which adheres to atmospheric dust particles and microbes which have entered the outer ear canal, thus preventing their entry into the delicate organs of the inner ear (Chapter 14).

4   Lachrymal glands. Their homeostatic functions are to moisturize and cleanse the surface of the eye by secreting tears, thus acting as an external defence mechanism (Chapters 10 and 14).

Exocrine glands are classified according to the complexity of their ducts, for example

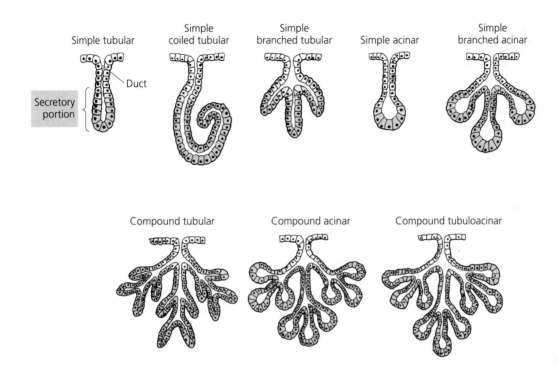

Figure 4.7 Structural types of multicellular exocrine glands. The secretory portions of the glands are indicated in purple. The blue areas represent the ducts of the glands.

simple or compound glands, the shape of their secretory structure, for example simple or compound tubular (Figure 4.7), or how the gland releases its secretion (Figure 4.8a–c). Mode of secretion is referred to as holocrine, apocrine, or merocrine:

HOLOCRINE GLANDS (HOLOS = ENTIRE)

Figure 4.8a illustrates that the secretion from these glands occurs after the entire cell has become packed with secretions causing them finally to lyse or burst, thus releasing these secretions. Future secretions from this tissue depends upon the lysed cell being replaced by the mitotic division of stem cells. The skin's sebaceous (oil) gland cells are examples of a holocrine tissue.

APOCRINE GLANDS (APO- = OFF)

Figure 4.8b illustrates how the secretory products accumulate at the margin of the cell's membrane. This portion (together with the surrounding cytoplasm) pinches off from the rest of the cell to form the secretion. Further secretions require a period of anabolic reconstruction of the secretory products. Mammary (lactiferous) glands are examples of an apocrine tissue.

MEROCRINE (MEROS = PART)

As Figure 4.8c illustrates, these cells merely provide their secretory products in vesicles which are then exocytosed. Salivary glands are examples of merocrine tissue.

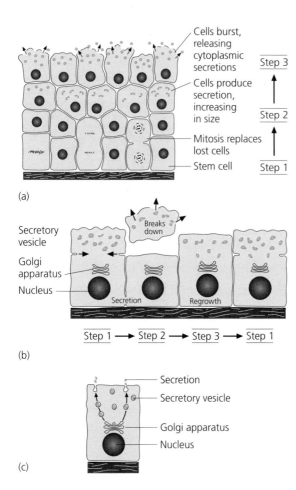

(a)

(b)

(c)

Figure 4.8 Mechanism of glandular secretion. (a) Holocrine secretion occurs when superficial gland cells break apart. (b) Apocrine secretion involves the loss of cytoplasm. Inclusions, secretory vesicles, and other cytoplasmic components may be shed in the process. (c) In merocrine secretion, secretory vesicles are discharged at the surface of the gland cell through exocytosis.

Endocrine glands

Endocrine glands do not have ducts and are sometimes referred to as 'ductless glands'. These glands secrete their products (i.e. hormones) directly into the circulatory system, which takes them to a site of action in their target tissues. The endocrine system, together with the nervous system, coordinates all bodily activities in order to provide overall homeo-

static functions. The main endocrine glands are considered in Chapter 15.

Mixed glands

Mixed glands contain a mixture of exocrine and endocrine glandular tissue. The pancreas is such a gland, secreting a variety of hormones (Chapter 15) from its endocrine glandular tissue and a host of digestive enzymes (Chapter 7) from its exocrine tissue.

CONNECTIVE TISSUES

Connective tissues are the most common tissue type in the body. The general homeostatic functions of connective tissues are:

1 Protection for the delicate organs which they surround.

2 Provision of a structural framework for the body.

3 Supporting and binding of other interconnecting tissue types within organs.

4 Transportation of substances from one region to another.

5 Internal defence mechanism against potential pathogenic invaders.

6 Storage of energy reserves.

The binding and supportive connective tissues are highly vascular. An exception is cartilaginous connective tissues, which are avascular (a- = absence), and as a consequence repair is not perfect following damage. These various tissues have distinct diverse appearances, but all have three common characteristics. That is, they all possess a fluid, jelly-like or solid ground substance called a matrix, various cell types which are responsible for secretion of the matrix, and various proteinaceous fibres.

Connective tissues can be subdivided into the 'true' connective tissues, and those which are specialized for particular functions (Figure 4.9).

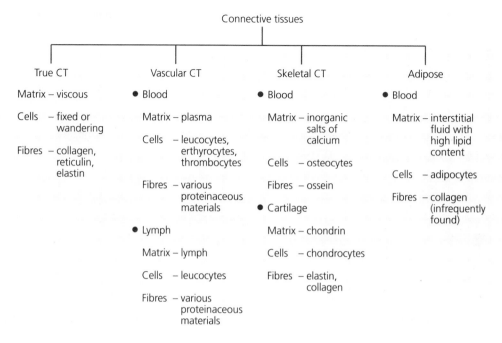

Figure 4.9 Connective tissue (CT) classification.

True (proper) connective tissues

These contain a viscous matrix and two types of cells:

1 Fixed (immobile) cells. Some of these cells have homeostatic repair functions (e.g. stem cells, or those called fibroblasts or fibrocytes), whereas others have homeostatic defence functions (e.g. macrophages), or storage functions (e.g. adipocytes, melanocytes).

2 Wandering cells. These include cells of various properties. Mobile defence cells (e.g. macrophages or mast cells) go to sites of injury. These cells produce and release substances such as histamine and heparin at the site which have local circulatory effects. T- and B-lymphocytes are wandering cells responsible for the cellular and humoral immune responses (Chapter 10).

Three different kinds of proteinaceous fibres are associated with connective tissues.

Collagen fibres are long straight, stiff, and strong and give the tissue tensile strength. Reticular fibres, made of reticulin, are interwoven between the collagen fibres, adding flexibility to the properties provided by the collagen. Elastic fibres, made of elastin, are branched and stretchable and give the tissue some elastic properties.

True connective tissues are of four types (Figure 4.10).

White fibrous tissue

This tissue may be termed dense collagen tissue because of the large numbers of these closely packed fibres. There is less matrix associated with this tissue when compared with loose connective tissue.

The fibres are produced by types of fibrocytes located between the fibres and are usually arranged in parallel bundles. The tissue appears white or silvery and is tough but pliable. It is located in tendons, which attach muscles to bone, and in ligaments, which strengthen joints between bones.

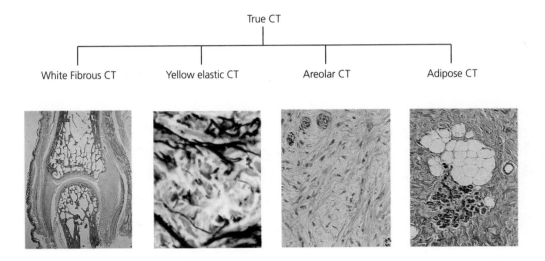

Figure 4.10 True (proper) connective tissue (CT) classification.

Less frequently the fibres are arranged in an irregular fashion. These tissues form the fascia of muscles, the dermis of the skin, the periosteum (external lining) of bone, and the supportive capsules around organs such as the kidneys, testes, etc.

Yellow elastic tissue

This connective tissue is composed of elastin fibres produced by another type of fibrocyte. These fibres make a loose branching network, and are capable of stretching and returning to their original position. Much more matrix is present than in white fibrous tissue.

Examples of location are in those ligaments which must provide more elasticity than collagenous ligaments, in the trachea, bronchial tubes, true vocal cords, and the lungs themselves, and in the walls of arteries.

Loose areolar connective tissue

This tissue contains the three different types of connective tissue fibres – collagen, elastin and reticulin – and thus has the properties of all three. Cell types present depend upon location but include macrophages, plasma cells (antibody-producing cells, derived from B-lymphocytes), melanocytes (melanin-producing cells), and adipocytes (fat-storing cells). Consequently this tissue has defence, protective and energy storage homeostatic functions.

Loose connective tissue is found throughout the body. Examples are the mucus membranes, the outer layers of blood vessels and nerves, the choroid layer of the eye, the covering of muscles, the mesenteries of the gut, and the subcutaneous layer of the skin.

The collagen fibres of the subcutaneous layer of the skin firmly fix the skin to the muscle underneath, although the elastin fibres allow some stretching of the skin and allow the skin to recoil immediately whilst the reticulin fibres add flexibility. A thick viscous matrix of hyaluronic acid is present and the enzyme hyaluronidase (which catabolizes hyaluronic acid) may be added to hypodermic injections, as this changes the constitution of the matrix into a water consistency and so aids the transportation of drugs, lessens tension and so eases the pain of injection. Some bacteria, macrophages, and sperm cells also utilize this enzyme to increase their penetrative capacity.

Cartilage

Hyaline cartilage   Yellow elastic cartilage   White fibrous cartilage

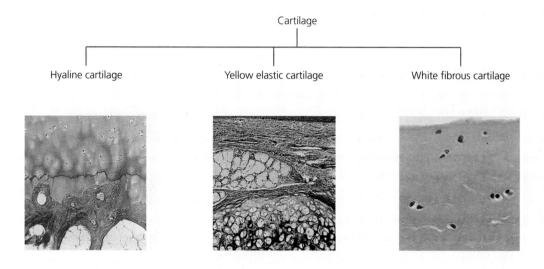

Figure 4.11 Classification of skeletal connective tissues: cartilage.

Adipose connective tissue

This tissue is concerned with the storage of fat and contains large fat-containing cells, or adipocytes, but has little matrix and few fibres. It is located subcutaneously (as the fat of the skin), around vital organs such as the kidneys, at the base and the surface of the heart, and in the marrow of long bones. The homeostatic functions of this tissue are the storage and provision of energy (mobilized fatty acids can be utilized by the mitochondria of most cells), insulation to reduce heat loss, and to protect organs against injury.

Suction lipectomy, or liposuction, is the removal of subcutaneous fat (lipo = fat; ectomy = removal of) from certain areas of the body, such as the buttocks, thighs, etc. This treatment only results in temporary removal of fat, however, and is not used to treat obesity. It is usually performed for cosmetic reasons.

Skeletal connective tissue

This tissue is of two types: cartilage and bone.

Cartilage

Cartilage contains a large amount of solid but flexible matrix made from a particular protein, called chondrin, which is secreted from cells (which are therefore called chondrocytes). Each cell is found inside a tiny space, or lacuna. When the cartilage grows it does so by two processes:

1 Interstitial (endogenous) growth. This type of growth involves a rapid increase in the number of chondrocytes, which gradually move away from each other by producing more chondrin between the cells, bringing about expansion within itself, hence its name.

2 Appositional (exogenous) growth. This growth follows interstitial growth, and commences in childhood and continues throughout life. The growth results from an increase in activity of the inner layer of the membrane covering the cartilage called the perichondrium. Fibroblast cells divide, and some differentiate into chondrocytes. Matrix

is then added and so this type of growth is responsible for an increase in the width of the cartilage.

There are three types of cartilage (Figure 4.11):

1 Hyaline cartilage. This tissue is referred to as 'gristle' and, although it is tough, it is also flexible due to the presence of many collagen fibres. Examples of location are the cartilaginous connection between the ribs and the sternum, the articular surface in synovial joints between bones, the respiratory passageways including the trachea, larynx, bronchi, and bronchial tubes, and most of the embryonic skeleton. The main homeostatic function for such a tissue is that of support.

2 Yellow elasto-cartilage. This is a resilient and flexible tissue due to the presence of many elastin fibres. Examples of location include the outer ear (pinna), the end of the nose, the supporting tissue of the vocal cords, and the epiglottis.

3 White fibro-cartilage. An abundance of collagen fibres gives this tissue its white appearance, and there is little matrix present. Examples of location are tendons, the intervertebral discs of the vertebral column, the pubic symphysis between the pubic bones of the pelvis, and part of the Eustachian tube from the middle ear to the pharynx.

Bone (osseous) connective tissue

Bone is a tough and rigid tissue. The mature cells are called osteocytes, and the protein fibres present (called ossein) are similar to collagen, which is also present in bone. The matrix is made up of inorganic salts of calcium (mostly calcium carbonate and phosphate) and these give bone its hardness. The salts make up about 65% of bone and 70% of tooth dentine, making this substance the hardest component of living tissue. The combination of calcium, ossein and collagen make bone strong but flexible, and this is necessary in order to resist forces which may shatter bones. Calcium on its own would make bones very brittle and less resistant to such forces.

BONE FORMATION AND STRUCTURE

Embryos have a cartilaginous skeleton. The conversion to bone is termed ossification. By birth the human skeleton is about 50% bone, but within 2 years this has increased to about 65% bone and 35% cartilage, and it remains about this level in adults. Ossification is carried out by specialized bone cells called osteoblasts. These cells enter the cartilage and start to lay down layers of bony matrix around themselves.

Eventually the matrix builds up into a solid mass of bone called compact bone. This solidity would make some bones, such as the long bones of the arms and the legs, too heavy to move easily. In such cases, some of the bone is removed internally by specialized osteocytes called osteoclasts, and these produce spaces of various sizes, making bones lighter and hence more mobile. Such bone is called spongy bone or cancellous tissue (Figure 4.12). The spaces in this type of bone are filled with bone marrow, a tissue which is responsible for the production of blood cells (Chapter 8).

The part of bone at which active growth takes place is called the epiphysis. In long bones, growth takes place at either end in discs of cartilage called the epiphyseal plates. Osteoblasts remain active in these plates until about 20 years of age when the maximum size of bone has been reached. Each bone is surrounded by a layer of white fibrous connective tissue called the periosteum: the tendons of muscles merge into this. The heads of bone are covered with hyaline cartilage, which forms a synovial joint with adjoining bones. Internally, the long bone is composed of a layer of compact bone surrounding areas of spongy bone. The shaft of a long bone contains a large marrow cavity.

Bones are living tissues even when fully grown but the osteocytes in compact bone become trapped inside small cavities, or lacunae, within the hard matrix. These lacunae

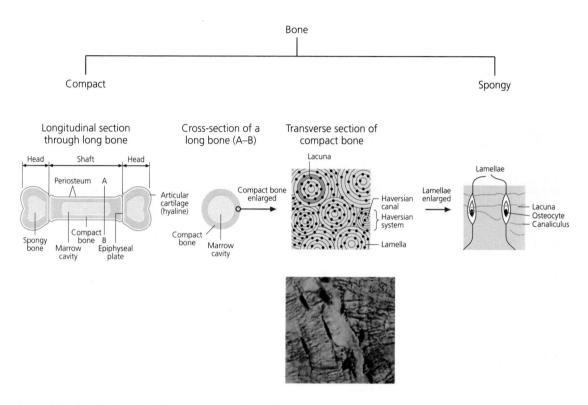

Figure 4.12 Classification of skeletal connective tissues: bone.

are arranged into concentric cylinders called Haversian systems with layers (lamellae) of bone in between them, and nutritional support is dependent upon the presence of a canal (Haversian canal) running along the centre of the cylinder, which contains an artery, a vein, a lymphatic vessel and a nerve. Subdivision of the canals into smaller branches called canaliculi provide for individual osteocytes within their lacunae. The structure of bone is considered in Figure 4.12 and in more detail in Chapter 16.

Vascular connective tissues

These are the liquid connective tissues of blood and lymph. The matrices are plasma and lymph respectively and so the main constituent is water. The fluids have a similar composition, which is not surprising since lymph originates mainly from plasma (via capillary exchange, Chapter 9).

A variety of cell types is present in blood including erythrocytes, leucocytes, and thrombocytes and their immature counterparts. Leucocytes are present in lymph tissue but erythrocytes and thrombocytes are absent, unless there has been some damage to blood vessels.

The 'fibres' of blood and lymph are of various dissolved proteinaceous materials (e.g. prothrombin, fibrinogen, albumin, and globulins). The structural and homeostatic details of blood and lymph are considered in Chapters 8 and 10 respectively.

NERVOUS TISSUE

This complex tissue contains two main types of cells: neurons and neuroglial cells. The details of the structures of these two types of cell, and their

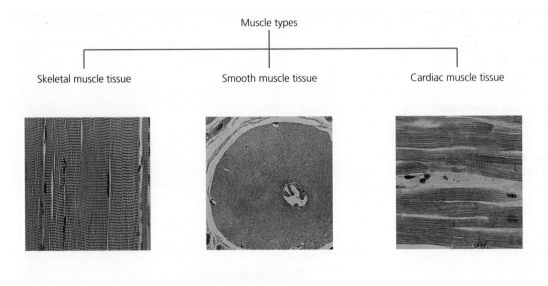

Figure 4.13 Classification of muscle types.

homeostatic functions, are considered in Chapter 13 and only a brief mention is made here.

Neurons

Neurons are the structural and functional cells of the nervous system. They are highly specialized for:

1 Receiving environmental stimuli and converting this information into an electrical impulse. These cells are called sensory or afferent neurons.

2 Conducting the impulse to other neurons (sensory and relay neurons).

3 Conducting impulses to effector organs in order to promote a response (efferent neurons).

Neuroglia

The specialized homeostatic functions of neuroglial cells are to protect and support neurons. These cells are often the site of nervous system tumours.

MUSCLE TISSUE

Muscle tissue can be subdivided into three types according to appearance and/or location: (1) skeletal, or striated, muscle, (2) smooth muscle, and (3) cardiac muscle (Figure 4.13). These tissues consist of specialized contractile cells which, when activated, are able to promote tissue movement. Their homeostatic functions are therefore to provide movement and maintain posture of the body (skeletal muscle tissue), and to promote the movement of substances throughout various tubes and cavities of the body (smooth and cardiac muscle). Skeletal muscle tissue is also important in the maintenance of body temperature during cold conditions, since heat production is a byproduct of muscle contraction during physical activity and shivering.

Skeletal (striated, striped, or voluntary) muscle tissue

The alternative names of this tissue are used in relation to its location (i.e. attached to the skeletal system), its microscopic appearance (it appears striated or striped), and the degree of conscious (voluntary) control that can be exerted. The tissue consists of very large cylindrical cells (or fibres), held together by loose connective tissue. The collagen fibres surrounding these cells merge to form tendons which are the means of attachment to bones. The tendons conduct the force of contraction and provide the energy to change the position of the bone. Muscle contraction is promoted by activation of associated nerve cells.

Skeletal muscle fibres may be up to 30 cm in length, and each one contains many nuclei; a muscle 'cell' is a functional syncytium of numerous cells which have combined to form a single unit. The fibres lie parallel to each other in the tissue, and their contraction results in a shortening of the entire muscle. Each muscle fibre is surrounded by its plasma membrane (in muscle cells this is called the sarcolemma), which encloses its cytoplasm (sarcoplasm). The contractile elements within the fibre are proteinaceous myofibrils known as myosin and actin (sometimes referred to as the thick and thin filaments respectively). It is the arrangement of these filaments which is responsible for giving the muscle tissue a 'striped' appearance. Further details of fibre anatomy, and the contractile process, are given in Chapter 16.

Smooth (non-striped, unstriated or involuntary) muscle tissue

The alternative names of this tissue illustrate its appearance (unstriated, unstriped), and its unconscious control (involuntary). This type of muscle tissue is located in the walls of blood and lymph vessels, in the tubes of the gastrointestinal tract, and throughout other involuntary controlled organ systems. Unlike skeletal muscle tissue, smooth muscle cells are individual and are therefore much smaller than skeletal muscle fibres. They have a spindle shape and are uninucleated. Contractile filaments are arranged in a less organized fashion than in

skeletal muscle cells, hence the lack of striations. Contraction of smooth muscle is stimulated by activation of associated nerve cells, or by certain hormones.

Cardiac (heart) muscle tissue

As its name indicates, this is a specialized type of muscle found only in the heart. The cells are uninucleated, but they possess striations, and are connected together via specialized conduction plates of tissue called intercalated discs. These discs are responsible for conducting the force and stimulus for contraction between cardiac cells, giving this tissue myogenic activity (Chapter 9).

The contractile machinery of cardiac muscle is the same as for the other muscle types. Cardiac muscle does not, however, require nervous innervation or hormones to stimulate it, as the heart has its own 'pacemaker' stimulatory tissue, although the activity of the 'pacemaker' cells is influenced by the autonomic innervation of the heart and by the hormone adrenaline. Cardiac muscle is under involuntary control but it can be voluntarily modified via conscious influences on the autonomic nervous system. However, voluntary modification is limited and cannot actually stop the contractility. A more detailed discussion of cardiac muscle tissue is provided in Chapter 9.

EPITHELIAL MEMBRANES

Epithelial membranes are not to be confused with epithelial tissue: they are a combination of an epithelium and its underlying connective tissue. They can be subdivided into three types: serous membranes, mucous membranes, and cutaneous membranes. Synovial membranes are also found in the body, around skeletal joints, but these are not epithelial membranes as they have no epithelia. They are composed of loose connective tissue, elastic fibres, and fat. Synovial joints are considered in detail in Chapter 16.

Serous membranes (or serosa)

These membranes cover the surface of organs and consist of a loose connective tissue and a layer of mesothelium, which is an epithelial layer of cells similar to simple squamous epithelium. They are single membranous structures but fold back on themselves, leaving a small space between the 'outer' and 'inner' portions; they therefore appear histologically as a double membrane. The inner, or visceral, membrane covers the surface of an organ, and the outer or parietal layer attaches it to the wall of the cavity in which the organ lies (for example the visceral/parietal pleurae around the lungs and the visceral/parietal pericardia around the heart). The peritoneum is the largest serous membrane in the body and lines the abdominal and pelvic organs, and body wall.

Mucous membranes (or mucosa)

Unlike serosal membranes, these line cavities which open directly to the exterior, that is the digestive, respiratory and reproductive tracts. The mucosa has an epithelial layer which secretes mucus. The homeostatic functions of mucus are to prevent cavities from drying out, to act (in the respiratory tract) as an external defence mechanism by preventing dust and potential pathogenic organisms from passing down the airways to the delicate respiratory surfaces, and to moisten and lubricate food in the digestive tract so as to ease the passage through the tract and to aid the processes of digestion and absorption.

The structure of the membrane varies according to location and function. For example, in the oesophagus and the anal canal the epithelial layer is of the stratified type as there is much wear and tear. In the intestine a simple columnar epithelium aids the absorption of nutrients.

Cutaneous membrane (skin)

This membrane has a complex structure involving a variety of tissues. Its anatomy and function are considered in detail in Chapter 17.

Homeostasis at tissue level: wound healing

The homeostatic functions of tissue repair, regeneration, and replacement are necessary following tissue injury and/or tissue death in order to maintain the numbers of cells within their homeostatic limits, and also to maintain cellular, tissue, organ, and organ system homeostatic functions.

Tissues can be divided into three categories according to their repair capabilities. Labile tissues, such as the skin, undergo mitosis throughout life and therefore have excellent repair capabilities. Stable tissues, such as the liver, normally exhibit little mitotic activity during adult life but are capable of increasing division if they are damaged. Although such tissues may heal, their complex architecture may not regenerate and they may not necessarily be restored to full function. Permanent tissues such as the brain and skeletal muscle also exhibit little mitotic activity during adult life, but they are so complex that little repair other than scarring can be achieved following injury.

The restoration of tissue following injury involves two processes: first the area is isolated via inflammation and the damaged area is cleansed by removing debris and potential pathogens, and this is followed by repair, regeneration, or replacement of the damaged or dead tissue cells.

INFLAMMATION

Inflammation is an accumulation of interstitial fluid within the damaged area, and this is promoted by an increased blood capillary permeability in response to substances such as histamine and bradykinin released from the site of injury. Proteins will enter the wound from the plasma, as will also various phago-cytic (= 'eating') white blood cells such as macrophages. The latter dispose of damaged tissue, foreign material, and any micro-organisms. This process is facilitated by the presence in the exudate of other white cell components of the immune system called lymphocytes. The protein fibrinogen, and other clotting factors, will also pass into the site of injury from the blood plasma, and a fibrin 'clot' will form which helps to adhere the surfaces of the wound together. The process of inflammation is summarized in Table 4.1, and further details are given in Chapter 10.

REPAIR AND REGENERATION I: SKIN REPAIR AS AN ILLUSTRATION OF WOUND HEALING

Wound healing does not, of course, only apply to the skin, though the skin is more susceptible to damage than are underlying tissues. The healing process following injury to the skin is a good illustration of the basic processes of healing.

The healing of superficial wounds to the epidermal layer of the skin alone, for example after mild abrasion, is a relatively straightforward process. Any damage to the basal layer of cells (the epidermis is a stratified squamous epithelium) is repaired by the migration of basal cells from the periphery of the wound across the exposed surface of the dermal layer. The migrating cells are replaced in the periphery by cell division of others.

Why cells should begin to migrate is not completely understood. It is thought that the loss of contact between a cell and those surrounding it promotes the movement, that is 'contact inhibition' is removed (Figure 4.14a). Movement stops when the cell is once more surrounded by others, although these must be of the same 'type' (cancer cells, for example, appear to lose contact inhibition).

Once the migrated cells have formed a new basal layer they will divide and new epidermal strata will be formed. Any scab over the wound will slough away, and the new epidermis will become toughened by the production of the protein keratin. The whole process will normally take place over 24–48 hours after injury.

Deep wound healing of the skin is more complicated and protracted as this will involve dermal, and perhaps even subcutaneous, repair. Inflammation will occur and this is important as an initial phase. A meshwork of fibrin strands produced by the clotting process help to support the regenerating tissue (Figure 4.14b).

Cell migration occurs, forming a thin covering over the wound. Other cells within the wound site transform into connective tissue cells (fibrocytes), possibly in response to substances produced by the macrophages which penetrated the wound during the inflammatory response. The fibrocytes migrate throughout the fibrin network and begin to secrete collagen which, if the wound is extreme, will form the basis of a scar. This phase is called the migratory phase.

Maintenance of cell proliferation in and around the wound site requires metabolic support, particularly the provision of oxygen, substrates (especially amino acids), warmth, vitamins (particularly B-complex, C and E) and minerals (especially zinc). Dietary provision will support wound healing, but healing can only progress efficiently if a blood supply is established.

Table 4.1 A summary of the inflammatory response

Event	Primary effect	Secondary effect	Functional significance
Step 1: Injury disrupts homeostasis	Chemical damage with or without homeostasis	Triggers change in interstitial fluids	inflammatory response
Step 2: Chemical change in interstitial fluids	Mast cells release histamine and heparin	Dilation of vessels, increase in blood flow and vessel permeability	Area becomes red, swollen, and warm
Step 3: Increased blood flow and vessel permeability	Increased oxygen, nutrients; fewer toxins, wastes	Slower spread of inflammation; abnormal chemicals appear in the bloodstream	Increases metabolic activity of phagocytic and repair cells
Step 4a: Increased permeability of vessels	Leakage of fibrinogen from plasma	Clot formation	Encloses area, slows the spread of inflammation or infection
Step 4b: Abnormal chemicals appear in bloodstream	Stimulates plasma cells (B lymphocytes)	Production of antibodies	Helps destroy or inactivate invading micro-organisms or foreign toxins
	Free macrophages and microphages attracted to area	Migration of cells into inflammation site	Removes cell debris, toxins, and micro-organisms
Step 5: Reduction in tissue concentrations of debris, toxins, micro-organisms	Histamine and heparin release by mast cells stops	Reduction of inflammation	Return to homeostasis

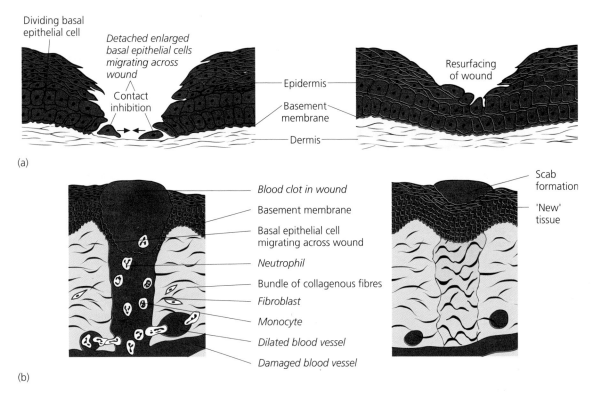

Figure 4.14 Epidermal wound healing. (a) Division of basal cells and migration across superficial wound. (b) Resurfacing of deep wound.

Cardiovascular efficiency is essential in the repair processes in order to maintain the substrate delivery to the wound site necessary to support the mitotic activity that provides replacement cells. Capillary 'buds' develop from the periphery of the wound and grow into the site at about 0.5 mm/day. Substances produced by cells within the wound, possibly by macrophages or fibrocytes, may promote this process. The filling of the wound with tissue during this phase is usually referred to as granulation and is illustrated in Figure 4.14b.

The importance of an adequate blood supply in granulation is illustrated by the slow rate of healing induced by circulatory deficiencies in conditions such as diabetes mellitus. Granulation is also slowed in the elderly, partly because of reduced cardiovascular efficiency, but also because rates of cell division and cell metabolism decline with age.

In the maturation phase the fibrocytes begin to disappear, collagen fibres become more organized and fibrin is removed by the action of plasmin.

REPAIR AND REGENERATION II: HEALING OF INJURIES TO CARTILAGE AND BONE

Cartilage

It was noted earlier that cartilage is avascular, i.e. the cells, or chondrocytes, depend upon the diffusion of substrates from surrounding tissue, and through the matrix, for their nutrition. Damaged cartilage is therefore slow to heal and severely damaged cartilage can result in chondrocyte death, resulting in the cartilaginous material not being replaced.

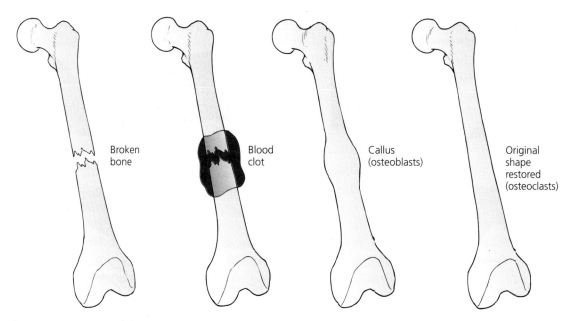

Figure 4.15 Bone remodelling.

Fibrocytes deposit collagen, causing a change in the properties of these severely damaged elastic tissue areas. Damaged cartilage of the extremities, such as that of the nose or ears, may eventually require cosmetic surgery.

Bone

Unlike cartilage, bone is constantly being remodelled and complete repair can occur even when severely damaged. When a bone is broken, blood vessels are torn around the break and the resultant blood clot is invaded by osteocytes from the broken bone (fibrocytes within the periosteum covering of the bone may also transform into osteocytes). These cells behave as osteoblasts and begin to deposit a new bony matrix around themselves. They eventually produce a solid mass of bone, called a callus, over the damaged area. The osteocytes now behave as osteoclast cells, removing any excess bone matrix to restore the original shape of the bone (Figure 4.15).

Examples of homeostatic disturbance

Any disorder results in, or is caused by, a disturbed tissue function. Many examples are provided in other chapters and this section will only consider the signs of a disturbance in the healing process.

Pus

Pus is a mixture of living and dead cells from the body, and may also include living and dead microbial cells. In addition, it consists of cell debris such as proteinaceous fibres and bacterial toxins.

Abscess

This is pus enclosed within a tissue space. Abscesses are formed as a result of trauma, bacterial infection, and toxin accumulation as a consequence of failure of the body's natural homeostatic controls to remove the stressor (for example, bacteria) involved. The repair process will only proceed once the causative stressors are removed.

Inflammation of an abscess increases the pressure within it, and this may result in a rupture of the abscess, spreading the contents to the surrounding healthy tissue cells. Although potentially detrimental to a wider tissue area, rupture of an abscess releases the built-up pressure and can be looked upon as bringing about drainage. For a surface abscess in the skin, drainage removes the abscess contents from the body and can be considered as being advantageous. Deep abscesses may require surgical incision to encourage drainage.

Cyst

Cysts are abscesses which are not eliminated. In time they become fibrotic and encapsulated and are really evidential signs that one's homeostatic defence processes have failed. If large enough, or in a particularly sensitive position, cysts can become troublesome and necessitate surgical removal.

Scar

Scars consist mainly of a fibrous meshwork and may be the end result of an abscess, or are observed when injured tissue fails to regenerate completely. They provide mechanical strength to the previously weakened tissue. The disadvantage is that scar tissue loses the 'normal' function of the tissue it is replacing, and so can lead to dysfunction of vital organs if a large enough area is affected. If this is the case, then overall homeostatic functions of the body are at risk because of the interdependency between organs and organ system functions.

Summary

1 Tissues perform specialized homeostatic functions essential for the maintenance of overall body homeostasis.

2 There are four principal tissues, namely epithelial, connective, nervous, and muscle tissues. Membranes are composites of epithelial and connective tissue.

3 The principal tissues are classified according to:

(a) the number of cell layers they possess;

(b) their structure;

(c) their function.

4 The 'principle' of complementary structure and function predestines the tissue's location. Epithelial tissues, for example, may possess specialized structures such as microvilli which increase their surface area – these are present in areas concerned with absorption.

5 Glandular epithelia may be simple or multicellular, and their secretions are defined as apocrine, holocrine and merocrine according to how they are released from the cell.

6 Connective tissues possess cells and their products, i.e. fibres and a matrix. They are classified according to the fibre distribution (loose or dense), and usually by the type of fibre they possess (elastin, reticulin, and collagen). The exception is adipose connective tissue which is named after its specialized fat storage cells – adipocytes.

7 Skeletal connective tissues are either cartilaginous or bony tissues. Cartilage cells (chondrocytes) produce a chondrin matrix. Cartilage is classified in the same way as connective tissue according to the number and type of fibres they possess.

8 Bone cells (osteocytes) produce the specialized fibres (ossein) which provide flexibility to this tissue; and its matrix which is hard due to the presence of calcium salts.

9 Bone is highly vascularized and is capable of complete repair even after severe damage, unlike the avascular cartilaginous tissue.

10 Blood and lymph are specialized vascular connective tissues which have a fluid matrix.

11 Neural tissues are adapted for electrochemical transmission. The cells are classified as to whether they:

(a) respond to environmental changes (stimuli) – these are receptors;

(b) conduct impulses to the central nervous system – these are sensory or afferent neurons;

(c) conduct impulses between neurons within the central nervous system – these are relay neurons;

(d) are responsible for the passage of the impulse away from the central nervous system towards effector organs which bring about a response – these are called motor or efferent neurons. Other nerve cells are called neuroglial cells and these provide support for the neurons.

12 Muscle tissues (skeletal, smooth and cardiac) are adapted for contraction and are therefore essential for the homeostatic processes involving tissue movement. Classification depends upon their appearance, their location, and the degree of voluntary control the individual has over its contraction.

13 Membranes are either serous, mucous, cutaneous, or synovial, the latter membrane being the only one which does not contain an epithelium and so is not an epithelial membrane.

14 Inflammation is a homeostatic control mechanism which initiates the repair of damaged or injured tissue areas.

15 The second stage of wound healing involves cell migration from the periphery of the wound. Cells include fibrocytes which produce a collagen matrix and this provides a structural framework (with fibrin clots) for the support of regenerated cells and blood vessels. This latter is referred to as granulation and is followed by a maturational phase when the structural architecture of the damaged tissue is reformed and excess collagen and fibrin is dissolved.

16 Abscesses, cysts, and scars are signs that the homeostatic mechanisms involved in inflammation and tissue regeneration have failed.

Review Questions

1 Name the principal tissues found in the human body.

2 How are epithelial tissues classified?

3 How are connective tissues classified? List the different types.

4 Where would you expect to find the following tissues;
(a) simple cubical epithelium with microvilli;
(b) simple squamous epithelium;
(c) pseudo-stratified epithelium;
(d) transitional epithelium;
(e) hyaline cartilage;
(f) spongy bone;
(g) yellow elastic tissue;
(h) white fibrous connective tissue.

5 Described the location and function of the following connective tissues:
(a) areolar,
(b) adipose,
(c) elastic,
(d) reticular,
(e) hyaline,
(f) osseous,
(g) blood,
(h) lymph.

6 What is the link between loose, dense, areolar, and collagenous connective tissues?

7 How do apocrine, merocrine, and holocrine glands differ from one another?

8 Distinguish between the following:
(a) serous and mucous membranes;
(b) exocrine and endocrine tissue;
(c) ligaments and tendons;
(d) striped and unstriped muscle tissue;
(e) neurons and neuroglia cells.

9 What are the main steps involved in tissue repair?

10 What conditions affect tissue repair?

5 Intracellular and extracellular fluids

Introduction: relation of body fluids to cellular homeostasis

Overview of the chemistry of water and electrolytes

Details of body fluid physiology

Introduction to water and electrolyte homeostasis

Role of body fluids in homeostasis

Examples of homeostatic control system failure and principles of correction

Summary

Review questions

Introduction: relation of body fluids to cellular homeostasis

Cellular processes can be looked upon as being those of chemical breakdown and of chemical synthesis. These enzymatically controlled metabolic reactions ultimately determine how a cell functions and it was described in Chapter 3 how cells require a wide variety of different substrate chemicals. If the countless reactions which occur from moment to moment are to progress efficiently, it is important that the general environment in which those reactions are taking place is maintained as constant as possible, or perhaps is allowed to change in a controlled way. Water is the environment in which metabolic reactions occur in all forms of life. Dissolved in that water will be a variety of substances but mineral salts are amongst the most abundant. This chapter describes the principal mineral contents of body fluids and their role in cellular function, and introduces the ways in which those contents are regulated.

Overview of the chemistry of water and electrolytes

CHEMICAL PROPERTIES OF WATER

Because of its abundance in everyday life, water is commonly regarded as being chemically inert and as a simple space-filler in organisms. In fact, the electrical polarization of water molecules (see Chapter 3) makes water a versatile solvent of salts and of other polarized substances such as sugars and alcohol. Non-polarized substances such as fats and oils are not soluble in water.

SALTS AND ELECTROLYTES

Salts are chemicals which dissociate into component ions (electrolytes) when dissolved in water (see Chapter 3). These components are classified according to the charge they carry. If the charge is positive the ion is called a cation, if negative it is an anion. Typically a salt consists of a cation and an anion held together by a chemical bond (note: as with magnetism, like charges repel, opposite charges attract). Our diets contain a variety of salts and not surprisingly our bodies also contain a wide range of them, some of which are undissolved, for example the calcium salts found in bone and teeth.

The concentrations of ions dissolved in our body fluids must be closely controlled because the ions are physiologically active. The concentrations of different ions relative to each other may be very different, however. The most abundant ions in our body fluids are sodium (symbol Na^+), potassium (K^+) and chloride (Cl^-) but even those which are considerably less abundant, for example hydrogen ions (H^+), have physiological actions.

Some ions, such as those of zinc (Zn^{2+}) and aluminium (Al^{3+}), are found in such low concentrations that they are referred to as 'trace' elements. Their presence is essential, however, for certain enzymes to function normally. In excess they may be extremely toxic. Regulation of the concentrations of 'trace' ions is little understood, and this chapter will concentrate on the more abundant ions present in body fluids.

Acids, bases and buffers

An acid is a chemical which produces hydrogen ions on dissolving in water. For example, hydrogen chloride gas (HCl) will dissociate in water to hydrogen and chloride ions:

$$HCl \rightleftharpoons H^+ + Cl^-$$
Acid　　　　　Hydrogen　　　Chloride ions

In this example the dissolved gas has produced hydrochloric acid. Although the reaction is reversible, that is the ions will recombine to form hydrogen chloride, the tendency to dissociate again is such that at any given moment in time the solution will be comprised almost entirely of hydrogen and chloride ions. This tendency of hydrochloric acid to be fully dissociated makes it a 'strong' acid. In contrast, some acids do not dissociate very easily. For example, if carbon dioxide is combined with water, carbonic acid is produced:

$$CO_2 + H_2O \rightleftharpoons H_2CO_3 \rightleftharpoons H^+ + HCO_3^-$$
Carbon　Water　　Carbonic　Hydrogen Bicarbonate
dioxide　　　　　acid

Again the reaction is reversible but in this example will tend toward the undissociated form: this is a 'weak' acid. Nevertheless hydrogen ions will be present and it is these, for example, which give the familiar tang to fizzy (i.e. carbonated) drinks.

Carbon dioxide is a major product of cellular metabolism and by combining with water will form carbonic acid and thus produce hydrogen ions. Being a gas, carbon dioxide is considered a 'volatile' source of hydrogen ions. More hydrogen ions are also produced from other metabolic sources such as amino acid catabolism (a 'non-volatile' source).

Hydrogen ions are extremely reactive and one of their most detrimental actions in biological systems is to combine with proteins, including enzymes, thus altering cellular function and disturbing homeostasis. In order to avoid the major cellular dysfunction which would result from the presence of too many hydrogen ions, their concentration must be homeostatically regulated (see Chapter 12 for details). One regulatory mechanism involves the 'buffering' of hydrogen ions so that they are effectively removed from solution. Chemical bases are substances which will combine with hydrogen ions to form undissociated molecules. The interacting acid and base is called a buffer system.

In the above example, the bicarbonate ions produced when carbonic acid dissociates will be bases. Thus, if a solution contains sufficient bicarbonate ions any addition of hydrogen ions will promote the reaction to form undissociated carbonic acid and as a result few of the added hydrogen ions will remain free in the solution (see Figure 5.1). In the other example given above, chloride ions produced when hydrochloric acid dissociates will also be bases. These, however, will be ineffective as buffers because of the tendency for hydrochloric acid always to be dissociated: as soon as hydrogen ions combine with chloride the resultant acid immediately dissociates again and so the added hydrogen ions will remain free. Clearly, buffers may be bases, but not all bases can act as buffers. Important buffers in body fluids include bicarbonate ions, phosphate ions, and some proteins (including haemoglobin).

The concentration of ions in solutions are given using the units of millimoles per litre (see Appendix A). Hydrogen ion concentration may also be given this way, but conventionally the concentration of these ions is measured using a pH meter. pH (which is the –logarithm

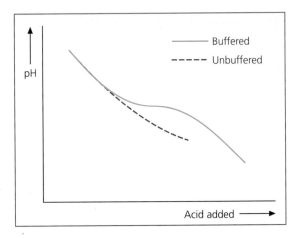

Figure 5.1 Influence on pH of adding acid (i.e. hydrogen ions) to either a solution which is unbuffered (------) or to one which contains a buffer chemical (—). Note the plateau region where pH is held almost constant by the buffer.

of the H^+ concentration) is a scale from 1 to 14 in which a value of 7 is neutral. Thus, the pH scale for the measurement of acidity/alkalinity looks like this:

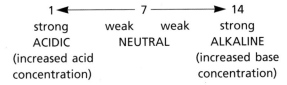

The neutral point relates to a situation when hydrogen and alkali ions are equal and is the pH of pure water (remember H_2O dissociates very weakly into H^+ and OH^- ions). At a pH of 7 a solution contains 10^{-7} moles of hydrogen ions per litre (i.e. 0.000 0001 mol/l, or 0.0001 mmol/l). Acids have a pH value of less than 7. For example hydrochloric acid with a pH of 3 will contain 10^{-3} (or 0.001) moles of hydrogen ions per litre (= 1 mmol/l; 10 000 times more than water at pH 7). Similarly an alkaline solution with a pH greater than 7 will have a lower concentration of hydrogen ions than water. For example a solution of sodium bicarbonate with a pH of 10 will contain 10^{-10} (or 0.000 000 0001) moles of hydrogen ions per litre (0.000 0001 mmol/l; 1000 times less than that of water). Note that decreased pH values reflect an increased hydrogen ion concentration, and vice versa.

By preventing an increase in hydrogen ion concentration, buffers keep the pH of a solution almost constant (see Figure 5.1) over its effective range. Note, though, that the continued addition of hydrogen ions will, by combining with the buffer, eventually deplete the solution of the buffering base chemical. At this point the buffering capacity of the solution is exceeded and the pH will start to decrease as hydrogen ions begin to remain free in solution. The addition of more buffer will help to prevent this and is the basis of one of the homeostatic mechanisms which come into play when the hydrogen concentration of body fluids is chronically disturbed (see Chapter 12).

OSMOTIC PRESSURE

In Chapter 2 it was described how water can move from one compartment to another by a process of osmosis. Movement across a selectively permeable membrane, such as a cell membrane, will occur if the solution on one side of the membrane has a higher osmotic pressure than the solution on the other side. The osmotic pressure may result from a single type of solute, but in body fluids results from numerous different kinds of solute, including various ions and substances such as glucose, proteins and urea. Individually, these substances will have osmotic effects of differing magnitude since the effect is dependent upon the concentration of the ion or molecule. Thus the osmotic pressure of a solution is determined by the net effect that its solutes exert. The osmotic pressure of a solution is usually given as the solution's osmolality and is measured by the effects solutes have on depressing the freezing point of water (see Appendix A). Note, though, that the osmolality gives no information as to the types of solute present or of their individual concentrations.

Details of body fluid physiology

BODY FLUID COMPARTMENTS

Our bodies contain some 40–45 litres of water (Figure 5.2). Approximately 25 litres of this is found inside our cells (as the intracellular fluid), and the remaining 18 litres or so comprises the extracellular fluid (extra- = outside). The extracellular fluid is subdivided into the interstitial or tissue fluid (the component which bathes our cells; approximately 12 litres), the blood plasma (approximately 3 litres; blood cells come under the intracellular compartment) and the transcellular fluids (trans- = across; so called because these specialized fluids are secreted by epithelia; 1–3 litres). All of our body fluids contain ions of various types. The most abundant are those of sodium, potassium, chloride, bicarbonate, phosphate, and calcium and the distributions and physiological activities of these ions are discussed in the next sections.

Extracellular fluids

Plasma and interstitial fluid

The ionic compositions of plasma and interstitial fluid are almost identical (Table 5.1). This is because the two fluids are continuous at the level of blood capillaries. Cellular function requires substances to be transported to and from the cells but, close though they may be, capillary blood vessels remain separated from

Table 5.1 Concentrations of main ionic constituents of intracellular and extracellular fluids

Constituent	Extracellular fluid		Intracellular fluid
	Plasma (mmol/l)	Interstitial fluid (mmol/l)	Skeletal muscle cell (mmol/l)
Cations			
Sodium Na$^+$	142	145*	12
Potassium K$^+$	4.3	4.4	150
Calcium Ca^{2+}	1.2†	1.2†	4
Anions			
Chloride Cl$^-$	104	117*	4
Bicarbonate HCO$_3^-$	24	27*	12
Phosphate HPO$_4^{2-}$, H$_2$PO$_3^-$	2	2	40
Proteins (g)	70	approx. 0	25
pH	7.4	7.4	7.0

* Slight differences from plasma result from negative charge on plasma proteins.
† Ionized calcium. Total calcium concentration in plasma is about twice this (see text).

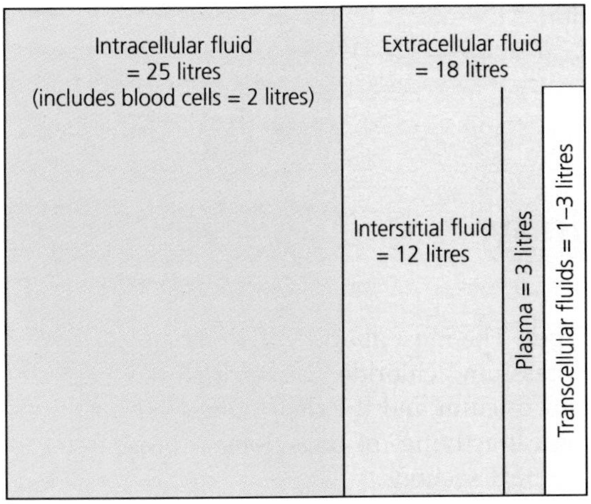

Figure 5.2 Body fluid compartments. Strictly speaking, transcellular fluids are part of the extracellular compartment. They are, however, separated from plasma by a layer of cells (an epithelium) and so have compositions different from that of plasma and interstitial fluid.

the cells by the interstitial fluid. Reliance on simple diffusion to allow adequate exchange of substances between cells and plasma clearly would not be efficient. A better system is one in which the substances are actually carried to the vicinity of cell membranes and this is achieved by passage of water, with its dissolved solutes, out of the plasma into the interstitium, and then back into the plasma again. One requirement for this dynamic process is that capillaries are highly permeable to water and solutes. The permeability is not so great, however, that large molecules such as proteins will enter the interstitium in significant amounts. The main difference between the composition of plasma and interstitial fluid, therefore, is that plasma has a considerably higher protein concentration.

The most abundant ions in the extracellular fluid are those of sodium and chloride. Their abundance relative to other ions means that they are the major contributors to the osmotic pressure of the fluid. Potassium ions are present in relatively low concentrations but variations in the concentration can have dire consequences for the function of excitable cells such as nerve and muscle cells (see below).

About half the calcium present in the extracellular fluid is chemically bound to proteins. Being bound and un-ionized, this component

Table 5.2 Mean ionic composition of some transcellular fluids

Fluid	Na^+ (mmol/l)	K^+ (mmol/l)	Cl^- (mmol/l)	HCO_3^- (mmol/l)	pH
Saliva	33	20	34	0	6.6
Gastric juice	60	9	84	0	3.0
Bile	149	5	101	45	8.0
Pancreatic juice	141	5	77	92	7.7
Cerebrospinal fluid	141	3	127	23	7.5
Sweat	45	5	58	0	5.2

will not directly influence cell function. That component which is dissolved in the fluid, and therefore ionized, is present in relatively low concentration but can profoundly alter the function of excitable cells should that concentration change. Many calcium salts have a relatively low solubility in water, illustrated by the deposits found in kettles and central heating systems of houses in 'hard' water areas. In plasma and interstitial fluid the concentration of calcium ions and associated ions, such as those of phosphate (HPO_4^{2-}), is close to that at which the salts will start to precipitate out of solution. Close regulation of the concentrations of these ions is therefore also desirable to prevent deposits occurring in the circulatory system.

The pH of blood averages 7.4, that is it is slightly alkaline (with a H^+ concentration of about 0.0004 mmol/l) largely because hydrogen ions produced by metabolism are buffered by the blood. Proteins, especially haemoglobin in red blood cells, have a role in this (Chapter 12) but the concentration of bicarbonate in plasma and in interstitial fluid is also extremely important. As can be seen in Table 5.1 the concentration of bicarbonate ions is relatively high, though nowhere near that of sodium or chloride. Phosphate ions are another buffer chemical in the extracellular fluid but the concentrations of this in plasma and interstitial fluid are very low (see previous paragraph).

Transcellular fluids

The transcellular fluids are separated from blood plasma by a continuous layer of cells (i.e.

by an epithelium) and are produced as secretions of those cells. They include the specialized fluids found in our brain and spinal cord (cerebrospinal fluid), in parts of our stomach (gastric fluid), and in our eyes (intraocular fluid), and also secretions such as saliva, pancreatic and intestinal juices, semen, cervical fluid and sweat. The total volume of transcellular fluid is variable, particularly because of changes in the secretion of gut fluids, but on average amounts to some 1–3 litres.

The composition of transcellular fluids may be kept near constant, as in the cerebrospinal fluid, or may vary according to the circumstances at the time, as in gastric fluid. One aspect they all have in common, however, is that their composition is different from that of the blood plasma and the interstitial fluid (compare Tables 5.1 and 5.2). This is because they are secreted by cells which exert some control on the composition of the secretion.

Intracellular fluids

Since cells have widely differing functions it is not surprising that there is some variation in the composition of the intracellular fluid, depending upon which tissue is studied. Some generalizations can be made, however, and the composition of fluid from muscle cells, as shown in Table 5.1, gives a general impression.

Intracellular fluids and extracellular fluids are of course separated by the cell membrane which is not fully permeable to solutes. Indeed, the permeability to many solutes is 'selective' and one consequence of this selectivity is that intracellular fluids have a very different composition from that of the interstitial fluid which bathes the cells. The situation is complicated by the presence in cell membranes of ion-transporting processes such as the sodium/potassium exchange pump (Chapter 2). This pump actively transports sodium ions from the intracellular fluid and releases them into the extracellular fluid whilst potassium is transported in the opposite direction. As a consequence, intracellular fluids contain high concentrations of potassium but relatively low concentrations of sodium (Table 5.1). In general terms this is the opposite situation to that found in the extracellular fluids.

Maintenance of the concentration gradients for sodium and potassium across cell membranes is essential for the function of nerve and muscle cells, but is also important for other aspects of cell membrane function, for example the transport of nutrients (see below).

Calcium ions take part in many reactions within the cell, for example by acting as cofactors which aid the actions of certain enzymes. It may seem surprising therefore that intracellular concentrations of calcium ions are similar or even lower than they are outside the cell (Table 5.1). The availability of calcium ions, however, is a factor in the control of many reactions, for example in muscle contraction (see Chapter 16 for details), and a large proportion of the calcium content of a cell will be bound to proteins and released as required. The total calcium content (ionized + bound) of cells, therefore, may be considerable.

Since metabolic processes generate hydrogen ions it is important that buffer chemicals are also present in intracellular fluid to prevent the resultant disruption of cell function. Phosphate ions and proteins are the main buffers within cells. Phosphate is abundant within cells, not only as a buffer, but as an integral part of cellular metabolic processes. For example, phosphate-based compounds such as ATP act as energy transporters within the cell. Bicarbonate ion concentration is considerably lower than that found in extracellular fluids.

MOVEMENT OF WATER AND SOLUTES WITHIN AND BETWEEN COMPARTMENTS

Within compartments

Fluid compartments are not static and water, with its constituents, is constantly on the move. Within the intracellular compartment this is achieved by 'cytoplasmic streaming'. This flowing of the fluid helps to move substances around the cell, a process which will be more efficient than if diffusion alone was the only mechanism. Within the extracellular compartment fluid movement is a process of bulk flow and also an exchange between the blood plasma and the interstitial fluid.

Bulk flow

As the term implies, bulk flow is the movement of material *en masse* from one point to another. Obvious examples are the peristaltic movement of gut contents through the digestive tract, and the flow of blood through the circulatory system. The rate of perfusion of tissues with blood is determined by the pressure gradient available to drive the movement, the volume of blood available and the diameter of the blood vessels. As with cytoplasmic streaming, bulk flow provides the means of transporting substances from one point to another in the shortest possible time, only on a larger scale.

Exchange between the plasma and interstitium

The exchange of fluid and solutes between the plasma and the interstitial fluid is essential since reliance on diffusion alone to transfer substances from the plasma through the interstitial fluid to the cells would be too slow to sustain normal cell function. The exchange of fluid occurs in tissues at capillary level, where blood vessels come into the proximity of cells. Capillary exchange occurs as a result of:

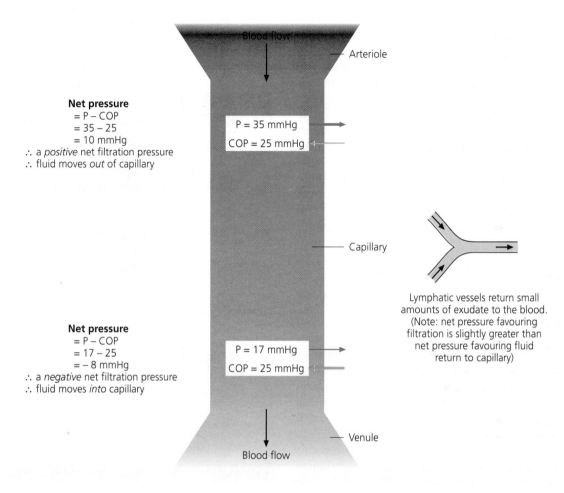

Net pressure
= P – COP
= 35 – 25
= 10 mmHg
∴ a *positive* net filtration pressure
∴ fluid moves *out* of capillary

P = 35 mmHg
COP = 25 mmHg

Arteriole

Blood flow

Capillary

Lymphatic vessels return small
amounts of exudate to the blood.
(Note: net pressure favouring
filtration is slightly greater than
net pressure favouring fluid
return to capillary)

Net pressure
= P – COP
= 17 – 25
= – 8 mmHg
∴ a *negative* net filtration pressure
∴ fluid moves *into* capillary

P = 17 mmHg
COP = 25 mmHg

Venule

Blood flow

Figure 5.3 Fluid exchange between plasma and interstitial fluid across the capillary wall. The net movement of fluid into or out of the capillary will depend upon the difference between the pressure favouring movement out (the hydrostatic pressure, P) and the pressure favouring movement in (the colloid osmotic pressure due to plasma proteins, COP).

1 having a capillary endothelium which is fully permeable to water and most solutes, although not to most macromolecules such as proteins; and

2 the interplay of physical forces that promote such movements.

The forces involved in capillary exchange are illustrated in Figure 5.3. Basically, the relatively high hydrostatic pressure within the capillary tends to force fluid out into the interstitium, and this force is opposed by the osmotic pressure (called colloid osmotic pressure or oncotic pressure) due to the plasma proteins retained in the capillary. At the arterial end of the capillary the net pressure favours movement of water out of the blood vessel. The hydrostatic pressure diminishes along the capillary, however, as a result of the resistance to flow provided by the vessel and the fluid loss from it. A point will therefore be reached when the colloid osmotic pressure exceeds the hydrostatic pressure, and so water (and solutes) will now be drawn back into the vessel from the interstitium. As a result there is virtually no difference in the volume of blood entering and leaving the tissue. The processes involved highlight the importance of plasma proteins, especially albumins, in maintaining blood volume and hence systemic blood pressure.

In practice, small quantities of protein do penetrate the interstitium and this slight alteration in the balance of forces acting across the capillary endothelium results in a small net loss of fluid from the plasma. These proteins, and the excess fluid, are returned to the circulatory system via the lymphatic system (Chapter 10).

Between intracellular and extracellular compartments

The regulation of intracellular fluid composition, and the transfer of nutrients and metabolites between the intracellular and extracellular fluids, is dependent upon the maintenance of extracellular fluid composition and also upon the functions of the cell membrane. Cell membrane physiology has already been discussed in a previous chapter (Chapter 2). In brief, cell membranes are selectively permeable to solutes and, although lipid-soluble substances such as urea cross the lipid membrane with little difficulty (provided a concentration gradient is present), it is generally the case that water-soluble substances do not and rapid movements of such solutes across cell membranes require the presence of carrier proteins or 'channels' (= pores) through the membrane.

On the other hand, the chemical properties of water, and the small physical size of water molecules, enable it to cross cell membranes relatively easily and this will occur if an osmotic gradient exists across the membrane. Thus, although intracellular and extracellular fluid compositions are very different, the total osmotic concentration is usually the same. One consequence of this is that if the osmotic pressure of the extracellular fluid increases as a result of dehydration, this will osmotically remove water out of cells and result in cellular dehydration also. This disrupts cell function as enzymes require a constant intracellular environment in which to function.

THE PHYSIOLOGICAL ACTIONS OF WATER AND ELECTROLYTES

Water

As noted previously, water is the solvent in which most of the chemical reactions that comprise metabolism take place. The concentrations of solutes dissolved in that water are largely dependent upon the rate of addition and removal of those solutes. It is also the case, however, that changes in the amount of water present will alter the concentrations of substances dissolved in it either by dilution or by concentration, and will also alter the volume of fluid compartments. For example, dehydration will increase the osmotic concentration of our body fluids and if the rehydration response is inadequate cell function may begin to deteriorate as the intracellular environment changes.

Sodium and chloride (Na$^+$; Cl$^-$)

Sodium and chloride ions are the main electrolytic determinants of the osmotic pressure of body fluids and changes in sodium chloride concentration will result in a change in the osmotic pressure of the fluid. Since osmolality is the parameter which is monitored to detect any changes in water balance (see 'Principles of regulation of body fluids'), a change in sodium content will normally stimulate a change in hydration so that the osmotic pressure is returned to normal. Sodium is present in highest concentrations in the plasma and interstitial fluids and any change in sodium (and resultant water) content will therefore primarily affect these compartments.

In addition to determining the osmolality and volumes of extracellular fluid, sodium ions also influence cell membrane processes. In particular, the sodium concentration gradient across cell membranes drives the carriage of substances such as glucose and amino acids into the cells. In order to do this sodium and, say, glucose both combine with a protein carrier molecule in the cell membrane (see Chapter 2).

Chloride ions (with other anions) are important in maintaining electrical neutrality, or electrical gradients, across cell membranes. In doing so they may influence the movement of positive charged ions, which will be attracted by them. This effect is particularly important in the central nervous system where chloride ions may influence the electrical charge which is found across the membranes of neurons to the extent that the stimulation of that cell is prevented (i.e. it can inhibit transmission across the gaps or synapses between adjacent nerve cells – Chapter 13).

Potassium (K+)

The concentration gradient for potassium across cell membranes is mainly responsible for the resting membrane potential of cells. This is the electrical status of the cell membrane and changes in its value (in millivolts) above the minimum required to activate nerve and muscle cells (i.e. above the 'threshold') are responsible for the carriage of electrical activity along nerve cells, and for initiating the contractile mechanism of muscle cells (Chapters 13 and 16). Variations in the potassium gradient will slightly change the membrane potential, making it approach or deviate further from the threshold value. For example, an increase in extracellular potassium concentration makes the potential approach the threshold and this makes the membrane easier to stimulate. If the concentration continues to rise, however, the membrane's electrical properties will not return to normal and the cell will be incapable of being stimulated again. Similarly a decrease in extracellular potassium concentration causes the membrane potential to deviate further from the threshold, thus making the

cell more difficult, perhaps impossible, to stimulate using physiological stimuli.

Calcium (Ca^{2+})

The threshold membrane potential at which excitable cells are stimulated is influenced by the calcium ion concentration of extracellular fluids. Thus a reduction in calcium ion concentration reduces the threshold with the result that the cell is more easily stimulated.

Calcium ions also have important intracellular actions. Various hormones stimulate the release of calcium ions from the membranes of their target cells and these ions then promote the actions of enzymes (i.e. they are second messengers – Chapter 15). In muscle cells the ions are necessary for the contractile process (Chapter 16).

Bicarbonate and phosphate (HCO$_3^-$; HPO$_4^{2-}$)

As discussed early in this chapter, bicarbonate and phosphate ions are important buffer chemicals in body fluids and changes in their concentration will affect the efficiency at which hydrogen ions are buffered. Cellular enzymes operate at an optimum pH and the pH of body fluids is kept at or close to this value. An excess or deficiency of buffer chemicals will therefore affect enzyme efficiency by altering the concentration of hydrogen ions present (i.e. the pH). In view of their relative concentrations, bicarbonate ions are more important than phosphate ions as buffers of the extracellular fluid. The reverse is the case for intracellular fluids.

Intracellular phosphate ions also play an essential role in energy production and utilization, for example in the interconversion of adenosine diphosphate (ADP) and adenosine triphosphate (ATP).

Phosphate ions, when combined with calcium ions, form the main mineral component of bone. There is therefore a continual process of release and uptake of phosphate to and from the extracellular fluid as bone is formed and resorbed.

Introduction to water and electrolyte homeostasis

BALANCE

From the preceding discussion it is clear that body fluids contain many different kinds of ions, some positively charged, others negative, the concentrations of which must be maintained nearly constant in order to maintain normal cellular function. Ions are continually added to our body fluids through our diets, and are continually lost from them by excretion in urine and sweat. In order to regulate the ionic contents of our body fluids the rate of addition and the rate of excretion must be kept equal, i.e. we must remain in a state of ionic balance. The homeostatic regulation of water and electrolyte balance is shown diagrammatically in Figure 5.4.

Most of the ions ingested in our foods are absorbed by the gut and this is the case whether we are deficient in them or not. Our diets normally contain more than adequate amounts of ions and the ionic constitution of our body fluids is mainly determined by the rate at which they are excreted, especially in the urine. Thus a typical daily balance chart for sodium may look like this:

Sodium input:	Sodium output:
Food 200	Faeces + sweat 20
	Urine 180
TOTAL 200 mmol/day (= approx. 9 g/day)	TOTAL 200 mmol/day

Note: individual values will vary with diet.

In addition to solute addition or removal, the concentration of substances dissolved in the body fluids, and the fluid volumes, will also be influenced by our state of hydration. We therefore maintain a state of water balance in which output from the body is matched to input. Water is lost from the body via a number of routes: urine, expiration, sweat, faeces. In temperate climates most will be lost via urine

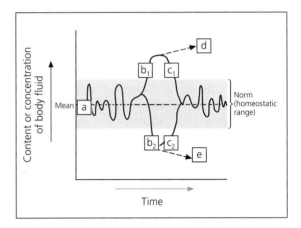

Figure 5.4 Water and electrolyte balance: homeostatic regulation of water or electrolyte content of body fluids.
a, Mean water or electrolyte content necessary for optimal cell function (i.e. balance).
b_1, increased water or electrolyte content due to increased addition to fluids *or* reduced excretion (i.e. input > output).
b_2, decreased water or electrolyte content (i.e. output > input).
c_1, c_2, restoration of optimal content by adjustment to input or to output (usually output by adjusting excretion).
d, excessive increase in water or electrolyte content due to inadequate excretory response (i.e. intake remains > output), leading to cell dysfunction.
e, excessive decrease in water or electrolyte content due to excessive excretion, or inadequate intake (i.e. intake remains < output), leading to cell dysfunction.

and expiration. Sweat can form a significant route during hot weather, however, as evaporation is used to promote heat loss from the body and the volume of sweat can amount to some 4.5 litres per day, depending upon environmental temperature and the amount of physical work being performed. Water intake is mainly via water drunk as part of our diet and from food (even the driest of food has some water content). Some of the water added to our body fluids is also generated as a product of metabolic reactions. A daily water balance chart for someone in a temperate climate might look like the following:

Water input:		Water output:	
Drink	1500	Urine	1400
Food	800	Evaporation:	
Metabolic		Lungs	500
production	200	Skin	400
		Faeces	200
TOTAL 2500 ml/day		TOTAL 2500 ml/day	

Note: values will vary with diet and environmental conditions.

Water lost via sweat and respiration is termed 'insensible' loss and the volume is largely unaffected by our state of hydration. During dehydration water balance is mainly achieved by the stimulation to drink more and by reducing urinary losses ('sensible' excretion).

GENERAL PRINCIPLES OF REGULATION OF BODY FLUIDS

Much of the regulation of water and electrolyte balance involves changing the rate of excretion appropriate to the input. Since most excretion occurs via the urine, details of fluid and electrolyte homeostasis are provided in Chapter 12; this section introduces the means by which disturbances are detected in relation to the physiological actions of water and electrolytes mentioned previously.

Fluctuations in body fluid composition are more likely to occur in those fluids which exchange substances with our external environment, in other words the extracellular fluid (Figure 5.5), and the homeostatic mechanisms which regulate body fluid composition are stimulated by such changes. The detection of change involves receptor cells and it is more precise to consider the regulatory responses to changes in extracellular fluid composition as being stimulated by the effects that such changes have on the membrane function and/or the intracellular composition of these specialized cells.

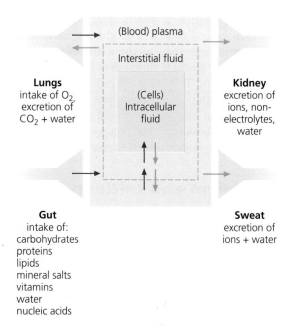

Figure 5.5 Schematic diagram of exchanges between fluid compartments and the external environment. Note that the composition of blood plasma (+ interstitial fluid) is most susceptible to the intake and excretion of solute and water, and also that the intracellular fluid will be indirectly influenced by those changes.

Water

Changes in the osmotic pressure of plasma and interstitial fluid as a consequence of overhydration or dehydration will cause the movement of water by osmosis into or out of cells. This stimulates receptor cells (called 'osmoreceptors' – see Chapter 12) to initiate rapid changes in water intake by influencing our perception of thirst, and in urine production, which results in the restoration of water balance. Renal responses are hormonally mediated via the hypothalamic posterior pituitary gland axis.

Sodium

It has previously been noted that changes in sodium balance result in changes in the osmotic pressure of fluids, and consequently disturb water balance. The change in volume will apply primarily to the extracellular fluid since most sodium ions are found in that compartment. This will include a change in blood volume and the renal excretion of sodium (and water) is altered when such a change is detected. The response is largely mediated by hormones (Chapter 12).

Potassium and calcium

Changes in potassium and calcium ion concentrations can have profound effects on excitable cells. It is not surprising, therefore, that the concentration of these ions in plasma are monitored directly: by the adrenal gland (cortex) and the parathyroid glands respectively (see Chapter 15). Responses include changes in the excretion of potassium in urine,

and changes in the mobilization of calcium from bone, its uptake from the gut and its excretion in the urine.

Hydrogen

Hydrogen ion concentration must be regulated very closely and is directly monitored. One of the sources of hydrogen ions is from carbon dioxide and changes in carbon dioxide excretion via the lungs, promoted by alterations in blood pH, is one way in which their concentration can be regulated. Alternatively, an increase in the hydrogen ion concentration of blood passing through the kidneys promotes their urinary excretion. By a related mechanism the kidney may also alter the buffering capacity of plasma by changing the excretion of buffers, especially bicarbonate ions.

Role of body fluids in homeostasis

Body fluids and their constituents are integral components of our general physiology. In Chapter 1 it was described how normal physiological function requires an integration of processes at all levels of organization. Operating within this is the homeostatic regulation of parameters which could have profound effects on cellular and ultimately bodily function, should their values change in an uncontrolled fashion. The constituents of body fluids must be considered as some of those parameters whereby a change in their concen-

trations will influence the chemical processes occurring within cells and cell membranes. The changes in cell function arising from these effects will be widespread, ultimately altering tissue and organ functions throughout the body. In addition the disruption of nerve cell function will affect the way in which various systemic functions are integrated. In doing so the control of those other parameters normally regulated by those systems, for example cardiac output and blood pressure, will also change, thus compounding the consequences.

Examples of homeostatic control system failure and principles of correction

This chapter has discussed the role of body fluids in physiological function and the importance of regulating their composition to maintain cellular and systemic homeostasis. There are numerous examples of how failure to regulate fluid volume and composition results in ill-health. Some are provided in other chapters and only examples of fluid overload/depletion are included here.

Oedema

This is an accumulation of fluid in the interstitial compartment possibly, but not necessarily, at the expense of plasma volume. Oedema is the consequence of a disturbance in the capillary exchange of fluids and may result from a number of causes:

1 Elevated capillary hydrostatic pressure as a consequence either of arteriolar vasodilatation, as occurs in inflammation, or the dilatation of blood vessels during hot weather, or of increased venous pressure, as occurs in congestive heart failure, or in gravity-induced venous pooling.

2 Decreased colloid osmotic pressure (due to hypoproteinaemia; hypo- = lower than normal; -aemia = blood) as a consequence either of loss of plasma proteins via the urine, of reduced synthesis of plasma proteins, as occurs in various liver conditions or in malnutrition, or of plasma dilution resulting from fluid overload.

3 Blocked drainage of interstitial fluid by lymphatic vessels, perhaps caused by a tumour or by parasitic organisms.

Oedema may form peripherally, either locally or generalized, which though unpleasant is not usually life threatening, or in the abdomen (peritoneal oedema, or ascites) or in the lungs (pulmonary oedema) where it impairs gas exchange.

Although treatment must aim to correct the underlying cause, some relief may be provided in many cases by utilizing gravity to reduce capillary hydrostatic pressure. This may simply involve sitting the individual up, but could also require tilting the bed or suspending limbs, depending upon the site of the oedema. Extracellular fluid volume might also be reduced by the use of diuretic drugs to promote urinary sodium and water excretion. Alternatively, treatment may be aimed at restoring normal plasma protein concentration by the infusion of plasma concentrates, or albumin.

Dehydration and overhydration

Dehydration results in a concentration of the intracellular fluid and a reduction in cell volume. Obvious signs are a dry oral mucosa and 'hollowing' of tissue around the eyes. If oral rehydration is not possible then intravenous therapy must be applied. Caution must be taken, however, since cells do have some capacity to produce inert organic solutes which harmlessly raise the osmotic concentration of the intracellular fluid thus reducing the severity of water loss to the extracellular fluid. If rehydration is applied too quickly, without allowing for the time required for cells to remove these solutes, there is a danger of causing too rapid an influx of water into the cells, thus causing overhydration. Overhydration, as distinct from oedema, results in dilution of intracellular fluids and an increase in cell volume. Dehydration and overhydration affect the function of all cells, but symptoms of neurological dysfunction are initially the most noticeable with individuals experiencing headaches or if the imbalance is more severe, lethargy, personality changes, mental confusion, or even coma and death.

Summary

1 Body fluids are subdivided into the extracellular and intracellular compartments.

2 The extracellular fluid is comprised of blood plasma, the interstitial fluid and transcellular fluids. Transcellular fluids are secreted by specialized epithelia and therefore have a different ionic composition from that of the rest of the extracellular fluid.

3 Intracellular fluids and the interstitial fluid are separated by the cell membrane and have different ionic compositions.

4 Normal cell function, appropriate for the tissue in which it is found, requires the rigorous regulation of all the processes which take place. Ions play a central role in determining cell function and part of homeostatic regulation requires a control of the intracellular ionic environment.

5 The intracellular environment, and cellular volume, are largely regulated by the control of extracellular fluid composition and also by the maintenance of cell membrane functions. The regulation of extracellular fluid composition and volume helps to stabilize cell membrane activities, and is also necessary to ensure that chemical processes occurring in this fluid also progress efficiently.

6 An important aspect of water and ionic regulation is that a balance between input and output (excretion) is maintained and much of the regulatory process involves the control of urinary excretion of ions and water.

7 Disturbances in fluid and electrolyte balance are commonplace, both in day-to-day living (relatively minor since diets and homeostatic changes in renal function rapidly correct the imbalance) and clinically (potentially severe).

Review Questions

1 Define:
(a) metabolism;
(b) catabolism;
(c) anabolism.

2 Distinguish between an anion and a cation.

3 List the most abundant anions and cations in the human body.

4 Differentiate between acid and alkali solutions, using your knowledge of the pH scale.

5 Discuss the biological importance of buffers.

6 Define osmotic pressure, hydrostatic pressure and oncotic or colloidal pressures with reference to capillary exchange.

7 Distinguish between intracellular and extracellular fluids.

8 Discuss the biological importance of having different concentrations of electrolytes in intracellular and extracellular fluids.

9 What are transcellular fluids?

10 Discuss the biological importance of having:
(a) fully permeable endothelial membranes;
(b) cellular selective permeable membranes.

11 List the entry and exit routes for the main electrolytes of the body.

12 List the entry and exit routes for water.

13 Distinguish between 'insensible' and 'sensible' excretion with reference to water losses from the body.

14 List the physiological actions of the following:
(a) water;
(b) sodium;
(c) chloride;
(d) potassium;
(e) calcium.

15 List the possible physiological cause of the homeostatic imbalances:
(a) oedema;
(b) dehydration.

Nutrition

6

Introduction: relation of nutrition to cellular homeostasis

Overview of dietary constituents

Regulation of nutrient intake

Role of nutrition in homeostasis

Examples of homeostatic control system failure and principles of correction

Summary

Review questions

Introduction: relation of nutrition to cellular homeostasis

A German philosopher, Ludwig Feuerbach (1804–1872), once quipped

> 'Man ist was man isst' ('one is what one eats').

From a biological viewpoint this play on words is not far from the truth in the sense that our diet provides all the chemicals that are necessary for the production of cell structures, for cell metabolism and for the body fluids within and outside cells.

Nutrition and cell structures

Cells are complex structures but basically consist of chemical molecules, especially macromolecules, such as proteins, carbohydrates, nucleic acids and lipids, combined together as membranes and other structures. These molecules are synthesized using energy provided by cellular respiration, particularly the breakdown of glucose. The substrates for the construction of cellular structures come from our diet.

Nutrition and metabolic needs

The mass of chemical reactions occurring within cellular structures, and cytoplasm, that are essential to maintain intracellular homeostasis will also involve a variety of molecules many of which will be synthesized by the cell itself.

Chemical processes within the cell are catalysed by enzymes, the synthesis of which is determined by the cell's genetic complement. Metabolic processes can only continue, however, if the necessary substrates are available, and also if chemicals necessary to promote enzyme activity (i.e. nutrient cofactors – usually vitamins or minerals) are present. Ultimately these substances must be obtained from the diet.

Nutrition and body fluids

Body fluids provide the environment in which metabolic reactions take place and contain various ions which directly or indirectly influence cell functions (Chapter 5). Not surprisingly the ionic concentrations inside and outside cells are homeostatically controlled and losses of minerals and water from the body must be replenished from the diet.

Cell function, then, is dependent upon the provision of chemicals from our diet. The necessity of maintaining a balance between provision and utilization (i.e. nutritional homeostasis) is illustrated in Figure 6.1a.

The metabolic substrates required by cells may not be eaten in a form suitable for utilization by our cells and our foods must therefore initially be 'digested' using enzymes to release the smaller molecular subunits of which they are composed (e.g. proteins to amino acids). These processes will be described in Chapter 7. Other nutrients such as vitamins, water, and minerals are already in a usable form and will be absorbed directly from food materials in the gut. The aims of this chapter are to describe the constituents of our diet, their necessity for normal function, how dietary needs relate to stages of our lifespan, and to outline how dietary intakes are regulated.

The study of diets is a discipline in its own right and readers are referred to the many dietetic texts that are available. Readers are also referred to Chapter 3 of this text for details of the chemistry of carbohydrates, proteins, and fats.

Overview of dietary constituents

Our diets contain a variety of constituents:

1　Carbohydrates (other than 'fibre');

2　Proteins;

3　Lipids (or fats);

4　Energy (not a chemical but considered a dietary constituent);

5　Fibre (mainly forms of carbohydrate);

6　Vitamins;

7　Minerals;

8　Nucleic acids;

9　Water.

All constituents are necessary for the maintenance of growth and health. In terms of bulk, however, most of our food intake consists of carbohydrate, protein, and fats. The main dietary sources of nutrients, and their functions, are outlined in the next section. Recommendations regarding the daily intake of each nutrient vary according to age or pregnancy, and also with life-style, and accordingly these are considered separately in a later section.

SOURCES AND FUNCTIONS OF DIETARY CONSTITUENTS

Carbohydrates

Carbohydrates are widespread in nature. Almost all are polysaccharides (poly- = many; saccharide = sugar), that is they are macromolecules consisting of large numbers of simple sugars, or monosaccharides (mono- = single) bonded together. Some, though, are found as smaller molecules, consisting of perhaps only two or three monosaccharides combined together, called di- or trisaccharides respectively. Others are present in our foods as the simple sugars themselves. Common carbohydrates found in our diet are shown in Table 6.1.

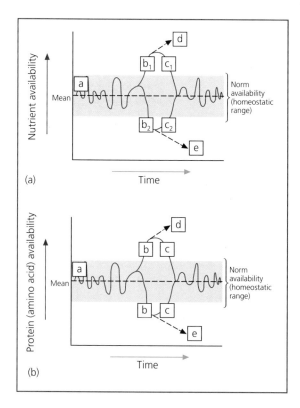

Figure 6.1 Outline of the homeostatic regulation of nutrient availability to cells. (a) General schema.
a, 'balance' state in which nutrient supply is equal to nutrient utilization and excretion.
b, increased (b_1) or decreased (b_2) nutrient levels in tissue due to supply and utilization/excretion being unequal.
c, increased nutrient utilization (c_1) or nutrient intake/mobilization (c_2).
d, excessive nutrient intake or inadequate utilization/excretion leading to disordered state (e.g. obesity, hypercholesterolaemia).
e, nutrient deficiency, or excessive utilization/excretion leading to disordered state (e.g. poor growth rate, anaemia, hypoglycaemia).
(b) Protein.
a, 'protein balance' (i.e. protein availability is equal to amino acid utilization.
b, increased amino acid availability or inappropriately decreased amino acid 'pool'.
c, increased amino acid utilization or increased protein intake/amino acid mobilization.
d, excessive amino acid availability leading to disordered state (e.g. of phenylalanine in phenylketonuria).
e, amino acid deficiency leading to disordered state (e.g. in starvation, anorexia, uncontrolled diabetes, kwashiorkor).

Carbohydrates are important energy stores in organisms – as starch or sucrose in plants and as glycogen in animals. The glycogen content of animal tissues is generally low, however, and most of our dietary carbohydrate is derived from plant tissues. The polysaccharides ingested must be capable of being digested to their simpler components, however, if they are to be useful, and there are some from plants which do not provide nutrition. For example, our digestive glandular epithelium does not produce the enzyme cellulase (-ase = enzyme) and so cellulose (-ose = sugar) from the cell walls of plants cannot be digested. Such polysaccharides provide dietary 'fibre' (see below).

Starch consists of chains of glucose molecules bonded together (see Chapter 3) and comprises about 60% of the carbohydrate in our diet. It is found in large quantities in the stems, roots, tubers and seeds of plants. Glycogen also consists of numbers of glucose molecules bonded together and both starch and glycogen, with smaller dietary saccharides (such as the disaccharides sucrose from sugar cane and sugar beet, and lactose from milk), are digested to their simple sugar constituents (Table 6.1). Other nutritious carbohydrates ingested may already be in the forms of monosaccharides, for example glucose syrups prepared from starch and fructose from fruits and vegetables.

As monosaccharides, sugars can be absorbed from the gut and utilized. Much of these will be used to provide energy or will be converted to glycogen for storage (Chapter 3). Some will also enter synthetic processes to produce molecules such as glycoproteins (i.e. a protein molecule with an attached glucose molecule), or glycerol (a constituent of triglyceride fats). A diet becoming deficient in carbohydrate will result in the mobilization of glucose from glycogen stores, and the synthesis of novel glucose molecules from amino acids and glycerol by a process called gluconeogenesis. Continued carbohydrate deficiency will place a greater emphasis on fatty acid and amino acid catabolism as sources of energy.

Table 6.1 Common carbohydrate constituents (excluding fibre) of a Western diet

Carbohydrate class	Examples	Source	Products
Polysaccharides	Starch	Plant tissues	Digested to glucose
	Glycogen	Animal tissues, esp. liver	Digested to glucose
Disaccharides	Sucrose	Sugar cane/beet	Digested to glucose + fructose
	Maltose	'Malted' foods (from starch)	Digested to glucose
	Lactose	Milk	Digested to glucose + galactose
Monosaccharides	Glucose	Fruits, honey, vegetables	Absorbed + utilized as glucose
	Fructose	Fruits, honey, vegetables	Absorbed + utilized as fructose
	Galactose	Digestion product of lactose	Converted to glucose in liver
Sugar alcohols	Sorbitol	Fruits + manufactured from glucose	Converted to fructose in liver
	Inositol	Cereal brans + manufactured from glucose	Inositol is inert

In dietary terms sucrose obtained from plant sources is called an 'extrinsic' sugar because it is not a component of cell walls (Figure 6.2). The complex of sugars found in honey, and also the lactose in milk, are also extrinsic sugars. In addition to these carbohydrates, though, our foods will also contain those which do form important structural components of cells. These are intrinsic sugars and include fructose and glucose found in fruits.

Proteins

Proteins are major constituents of cellular structures, they form enzymes, plasma proteins, and also hormones, antibodies and other cellular secretions. They are substances containing carbon, hydrogen, and oxygen and also nitrogen and usually sulphur. In fact, dietary proteins are our main source of nitrogen.

Proteins are macromolecules that are mainly comprised of combinations of up to 20 different amino acids. Each amino acid differs slightly in chemical structure from the others, and digestion of proteins in the gut releases the constituent amino acids, which can then be absorbed and utilized. Some amino acids can actually be synthesized in the liver from other

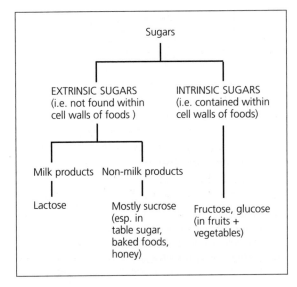

Figure 6.2 Classification of dietary sugars. Note that non–milk extrinsic sugars are a major cause of dental caries. Only 10% of energy intake should come from these sugars. Also, breast–fed infants obtain about 60% of their energy from lactose alone.

amino acids by a process called transamination but 10 cannot be made in sufficient quantities, if at all, and these are called the 'essential' amino acids, which must be provided in our diets. They are:

Arginine	Methionine
Histidine	Phenylalanine
Isoleucine	Threonine
Leucine	Tryptophan
Lysine	Valine

When amino acids are broken down (catabolized) further in cells, the nitrogen within them cannot be re-used. In fact it is excreted from the body as part of urea produced by the process of deamination. To maintain nitrogen homeostasis its intake (as protein) must therefore be equal to these losses (see Figure 6.1b) and so protein intakes must be relatively high.

Protein foods may be in the form of animal or vegetable protein. From a nutritional viewpoint these differ in their essential amino acid contents: most animal proteins have all the essential amino acids and are 'complete' proteins, but vegetable proteins may not contain adequate amounts of all the essential amino acids. For example, beans are deficient in those amino acids, such as cysteine, which contain sulphur, but wheat is a rich source of these. Similarly, wheat is deficient in the amino acid lysine, but some beans are rich in this. Wheat and beans therefore contain 'complementary proteins' in that, if eaten together, they will provide adequate amounts of these particular amino acids.

In an average Western diet about a third of dietary protein comes from plant sources and two-thirds from animal sources. Main animal sources are meat and fish (i.e. from muscle) and dairy products (mainly from milk). The main plant sources are seeds including cereals, peas, beans, and nuts. Root vegetables are usually deficient in protein, though potatoes contain significant amounts. Green vegetables are not a rich source of protein.

Lipids (fats)

Dietary fats are more correctly termed lipids. They are important energy sources and contain over twice as much energy per gram as carbohydrate, and even the thinnest person will have some fat stores. In addition to providing energy, lipids are also used to make cell membranes (see Chapter 2) and hormones (e.g. steroids, Chapter 15) and they are also essential to transport fat-soluble vitamins into the body (Chapter 7).

A typical dietary lipid is called a triglyceride because it consists of three fatty acids combined with a glycerol molecule (see Chapter 3). Other forms are diglycerides (with two fatty acids), monoglycerides (with one fatty acid) and phospholipids (two fatty acids and a third molecule containing phosphate). Cholesterol is another type of lipid which is found in animal fat and has a very different structure from these other lipids. It is the precursor to important molecules such as steroid hormones and is a component of cell membranes. It can be synthesized in the liver from saturated fatty acids and, therefore, a large dietary intake is not essential and may even be harmful if the excess is not utilized; cholesterol deposits in blood vessels are implicated in cardiovascular disease. Plasma concentrations of cholesterol above 5.2 mmol/l are associated with an increased risk of disease.

There are about 40 different naturally occurring fatty acids which differ in two main ways. First, they differ in the number of carbon atoms which form the 'backbone' to the molecule, for example 'long-chain' fatty acids have 14–25 carbon atoms. Second, they differ in the saturation of the carbon atoms with hydrogen atoms (see Chapter 3). Dietary fats containing high levels of polyunsaturated fatty acids, but low levels of saturated fatty acids, appear to have a role in reducing the risk of heart disease.

Of the variety of polyunsaturated fatty acids, only three are considered essential for life. These are long-chain fatty acids called linoleic acid, linolenic acid and arachidonic acid. It is most important that we obtain linoleic acid from our diets since the other two can be synthesized by the liver (note that this is different from the situation of essential amino acids, all of which must be present in the diet). Foods vary in their content of linoleic acid; sunflower oil, corn oil, nuts, and wheat germ are rich sources.

Beef, lamb, and pork are rich sources of fats, even when visible fat is removed. The white meat of poultry is low in fat but duck and goose may contain as much fat as beef. Animal fats may be saturated or unsaturated and the cholesterol content varies: egg yolk and dairy fats are high in cholesterol. Fat in fresh fish varies according to species. Thus, cod and haddock have low fat contents whilst that of mackerel is quite high. The fat in fish is usually unsaturated, however, and the cholesterol content is normally low.

Most vegetable fats are polyunsaturated except olive oil (which is monounsaturated) and palm and coconut oils (which are saturated). Plants do not synthesize cholesterol.

How much fat is required from our diets is unclear and recommendations in terms of grams per day cannot be made. Rather, recommendations are usually related to energy needs, and expressed as a proportion of the total energy intake.

Energy (calories)

Energy is required by the body to maintain basal metabolic activities and to sustain an increase in those activities when necessary. The amount of energy required by an individual is therefore dependent upon two factors: the basal metabolic rate (or BMR) and the physical activity level (or PAL).

As the name implies, basal metabolic rate is the overall energy utilization when the body is totally at rest and no additional influences such as a recent meal or recent exercise are imposed. The BMR is slightly higher when we are awake as brain metabolism is increased. If allowance is made for body size, which varies with sex and age, the BMR is remarkably similar between individuals.

Physical activity level is a factor used to convert the BMR to an energy intake recommendation, i.e.

BMR × PAL = estimated average requirement for energy

(Note: the estimated average requirement standard, and reference values for PAL, are explained in the next section.)

The energy content of foods is still usually given in calories, which are units of heat energy and not measures of how good food tastes!

By definition:

1 calorie is the amount of heat required to raise the temperature of 1 gram of water (i.e. 1 ml) by 1°C.

Caloric values of foods are usually quoted in kilocalories (ie. 1 kcal= 1000 calories). Thus, 1 kcal of heat will raise the temperature of 1 kg of water (i.e. 1 litre) by 1°C.

The caloric value represents the energy incorporated into chemical bonds that is released during metabolism. For example, 1 g of carbohydrate produces 4.1 kcal during metabolism and 1 g of fat produces 9.2 kcal. Clearly fats are a richer source of energy, weight for weight, than are carbohydrates and form the main energy store in animals. On the other hand most cellular energy is derived from carbohydrate metabolism, hence there is a greater dietary requirement for carbohydrate than fats.

The unit 'calorie' has recently been superseded by the 'joule'. This is because heat is only one form of energy and so a calorie must be considered a derived unit and not an empirical unit of energy, which the joule is. One calorie is equivalent to 4.2 joules (i.e. 1 kcal = 4.2 kJ).

Fibre

Dietary fibre is that carbohydrate (mainly) component of ingested plant material which cannot be fully digested, and includes cellulose, hemicellulose, pectin, and gum. Strictly speaking, fibre is not a nutrient but it is nevertheless an important dietary constituent.

Fibre is not digested in the conventional way, but some fibre dissolves in water and is partially broken down in the colon by bacteria, producing gas, water, and short-chain fatty

Table 6.2 Fat-soluble vitamins

	Source	Storage in body	Homeostatic functions	Effects of deficiency	Effects of excess
A	Liver, green leafy vegetables. Synthesized in gut from B-carotene	In liver	Maintain epithelia Provide visual pigment Bone/teeth growth	Atrophy of epithelia, e.g. dry skin + cornea, increased susceptibility to respiratory/urinary/digestive tract infection, skin sores 'Night blindness' Slow bone/tooth growth	Anorexia, dry skin, sparse hair, raised intracranial pressure in children. Blurred vision, enlarged liver in adults
D	Synthesized as provitamin D_3 in skin using UV light. Also in fish liver, fish oils, egg yolk, milk	Slight at most	Absorption of calcium + phosphate from gut	Demineralization of bone (rickets in children, osteomalacia in adults)	Excess calcium absorption from gut. Calcium deposition in soft tissues
E	Nuts, wheatgerm, seed oils, green leafy vegetables	In liver, adipose tissue + muscle	Inhibits catabolism of membrane lipids. Promotes wound healing + neural function	Abnormal organelle/plasma membranes. Oxidation of poly-unsaturated fatty acids	Toxic build-up unlikely
K	Produced by intestinal bacteria. Also in spinach, cauliflower, cabbage + liver	In liver + spleen	Synthesis of blood clotting factors	Delayed blood clotting	Haemolysis + increased bilirubin in blood in children. Otherwise toxic build-up unlikely

acids (note that these latter are not components of the original carbohydrate molecule, but are produced from the carbohydrate by the gut bacteria). These kinds of fibre are called 'soluble' fibre and include hemicellulose, pectin, and gum. Dry beans, oat bran, and cabbage-type vegetables are rich sources of soluble fibre.

When uncooked, 'insoluble' fibre such as cellulose will not dissolve in water or fats and is largely unchanged in the gut. Cereal bran is an important source of insoluble fibre.

Fibre is thought to have a number of beneficial effects. For example, fibre in the colon will absorb water and help to increase the water content of faecal stools, thus making them easier to pass. Fibre also seems to promote peristaltic contractions of the gut (see Chapter 7) and so reduces the time required for faecal matter to pass through the gut. This reduces the time available for micro-organisms to produce a substance called deoxycholate, a known carcinogen, from bile salts secreted into the gut from the gall bladder, and it is thought that dietary fibre helps to reduce the risk of bowel cancer.

Fibre also interferes with the absorption from our gut of minerals, fats, and bile salts. This is not usually detrimental and may even be beneficial. For example, soluble fibre interferes

Table 6.3 Water-soluble vitamins

	Source	Storage in body	Homeostatic functions	Effects of deficiency	Effects of excess
B₁ (thiamin)	Whole grain, eggs, pork, liver, yeast	Not stored	Coenzyme in carbohydrate metabolism. Essential for acetylcholine (neurotransmitter) synthesis.	Build-up of pyruvic/ lactic acids. Energy deficient. Partial paralysis of digestive tract/skeletal muscle (beri-beri). Degeneration of myelin sheath (polyneuritis)	Toxic build-up unlikely
B₂ (riboflavin)	Small quantities produced by gut bacteria. Also in yeast, liver, beef, lamb, eggs, whole grain, peas, peanuts	Not stored	Component of coenzymes in carbohydrate + protein metabolism, esp. in eye, blood, skin, intestinal mucosa	Blurred vision, cataracts. Lesions of intestinal mucosa. Dermatitis. Anaemia	Toxic build-up unlikely
B₃ (niacin or nicotinamide)	Yeast, meats, liver, fish, whole grain, peas, beans. Also synthesized from amino acid tryptophan	Not stored	Component of coenzyme NAD in intracellular respiration. Assists breakdown of cholesterol	Hard, rough, blackish skin. Dermatitis, diarrhoea (pellagra). Psychological disturbance	Burning sensation in hands/face, cardiac arrhythmias, increased glycogen utilization
B₆ (pyridoxine)	Salmon, yeast, tomatoes, maize, spinach, whole grain, liver, yoghourt. Some synthesized by gut bacteria	In liver and muscle	Coenzyme in fat and amino acid metabolism	Dermatosis of eye, nose, mouth. Nausea. Retarded growth	Toxic build-up unlikely
B₁₂ (cyanocobalamin)	Liver, kidney, milk, eggs, cheese, meats. Not found in vegetables. Requires intrinsic factor from stomach for absorption	In liver	Coenzyme for haemoglobin synthesis. Also amino acid metabolism	Pernicious anaemia. Nerve axon degeneration	Toxic build-up unlikely
Folate (folic acid, folacin)	Synthesized by gut bacteria. Also in green leafy vegetables and liver	Not stored	Synthesis of nucleotides. Red/white blood cell production	Macrocytic anaemia due to abnormally large red blood cells	Toxic build-up unlikely
Pantothenic acid	Liver, kidney, yeast, cereals, green vegetables	In liver + kidney	Constituent of coenzyme A in carbohydrate metabolism, gluconeogenesis and steroid synthesis	Fatigue. Muscle spasms. Lack of some steroid hormones	Toxic build-up unlikely
Biotin	Synthesized by gut bacteria. Also yeast, liver, egg, yolk, kidney	Not stored	Component of coenzymes for pyruvic acid utilization in cellular respiration	Mental depression. Muscular pain. Dermatitis. Fatigue. Nausea	Toxic build-up unlikely
C (ascorbic acid)	Citrus fruits, tomatoes, green vegetables	A little in plasma	Promotes protein metabolism. Promotes formation of connective tissue. Detoxifier. Promotes wound healing	Retardation of growth. Poor connective tissue repair/growth (scurvy) including swollen gums, tooth loosening, fragile blood vessels. Poor wound healing	Not toxic. Note: no evidence for effect to prevent infection

with the absorption of fatty acids and of bile salts, which are produced from cholesterol, leading to a greater cholesterol and fatty acid utilization in the body. Consequently fibre may help to reduce blood lipid concentrations.

Vitamins

The presence of some vitamins is essential for certain enzyme-catalysed reactions to proceed but, although indispensable, they are required in only minute amounts. The name 'vitamin' is a shortened version of 'vitamine', i.e. an amine vital for life. It is now known that not all vitamins are of this type of chemical; they are a diverse group of substances.

Thirteen vitamins are known to be essential for life although others may eventually be recognized. Most were originally named according to the order of their discovery, but vitamin 'B' was then found to consist of a group of substances each with individual actions. Numbers (e.g. B_1, B_2) were introduced but some were subsequently found to have existing names (e.g. vitamin B_3 = nicotinic acid). Others were later found not to be true vitamins at all and were deleted from the series (e.g. there is no vitamin B_4). Vitamin nomenclature is therefore confusing.

Vitamins are usually classified according to whether they are soluble in water or fat. Thus, vitamins A, D, E, and K are classed as fat-soluble vitamins, whilst vitamins of the 'B' complex and vitamin C are classed as water-soluble vitamins.

As shown in Tables 6.2 and 6.3 vitamins have a wide range of functions and are found in a variety of foodstuffs. Limited amounts of some of the vitamins we eat are actually stored in the body, for example fat-soluble vitamins are stored in fat (adipose) tissue and in the liver. The stores are not normally extensive, although excessive intake of these vitamins can raise stores to toxic levels. Thus, excess vitamin D promotes excessive uptake of calcium from the gut with the consequence that the mineral

begins to be deposited in soft tissues, and excess vitamin A can cause liver damage. Such large build-ups of vitamins are unlikely from normal dietary intakes but are possible if vitamin preparations are taken. Vitamin deficiencies, rather than excesses, are more likely to occur but are avoidable with a balanced diet.

Little of the water-soluble vitamins is stored, with the exception of vitamin B_{12}. The liver contains sufficient of this vitamin for a 2–3 year supply!

Minerals

Mineral salts are present in the tissue fluids of plants and animals and have various physiological functions (see Chapter 5 and Table 6.4). Some are 'trace' elements in that only minute quantities are required from our diets.

Minerals are generally not stored to any degree. Important exceptions are calcium, phosphorus, fluoride, iron, and iodine. Most calcium and phosphorus in the body is found in bone and teeth from which some can be released, as a homeostatic control mechanism, into the body fluids if calcium ion concentration falls below normal. In extreme conditions this loss of calcium may cause significant demineralization, resulting in a weakening of bone called osteomalacia. Fluoride is also a component of bone and teeth. Iron is necessary for the synthesis of haemoglobin and is stored in the liver and spleen. Iodine is a component of thyroid hormones and is concentrated in the thyroid gland.

The body content of many minerals is under physiological control (see Chapter 5). Others, particularly stored minerals, can build up and become toxic in excess. Using the above examples of stored minerals, excessive iodine has toxic effects on the thyroid gland (causing thyrotoxicosis) whilst excessive iron is a major cause of poisoning in young children. Excessive fluoride causes mottled teeth and porous, brittle bones.

Table 6.4 Dietary sources of selected minerals, and their functions

Mineral	Source	Function	Effects of deficiency
Calcium	Milk, egg yolk, shellfish, green leafy vegetables	Formation of bones/teeth. Blood clotting, muscle contraction. Muscle/nerve action potentials. Endo- and exocytosis. Cell division	Loss of bone density, e.g. osteomalacia/ rickets
Phosphorus	Milk, meat, fish, poultry, nuts	Formation of bones/teeth. Buffer chemical. Muscle contraction/nerve activity. Component of ATP, DNA, RNA + many enzymes	Deficiency rare
Potassium	Widespread. 'Lo-salt'	Action potential of muscle/nerve cells	Neuromuscular depression
Sodium	Widespread. Table salt	Major osmotic solute of extracellular fluids. Action potential of muscle/nerve cells	Hypovolaemia
Chlorine (chloride)	Non-processed foods. Usually found with sodium, e.g. table salt	Involved in acid–base balance. Major osmotic solute of extracellular fluids. Formation of gastric acid	Deficiency usually occurs with sodium
Magnesium	Beans, peanuts, bananas	Constituent of many coenzymes. Role in bone formation and muscle/nerve cell functions	Muscle weakness. Convulsions. Hypertension
Trace minerals Iron	Widespread but esp. meats, liver, beans, fruits, nuts, legumes	Component of haemoglobin. Component of chemicals involved in cell respiration	Anaemia
Iodine (iodide)	Seafood, cod-liver oil, iodized table salt	Component of thyroid hormones	Thyroid hormone deficiency (induces thyroid goitre)
Fluorine (fluoride)	Tea, coffee, fluoridated water	Component of bones/teeth	Decreased bone/teeth density
Zinc	Widespread but esp. meats	Component of some enzymes. Promotes normal growth, spermatogenesis. Involved in taste and appetite	Dermatitis. Growth retardation. Diarrhoea
Copper	Eggs, wholewheat flour, liver, fish, spinach	Haemoglobin synthesis. Component of some enzymes or acts as cofactor	Retarded growth. Cerebral degeneration
Chromium	Yeast, beer, beef	Involved in insulin synthesis. Maintains HDL concentrations in plasma	Rare – suggestion involved with diabetes

Nucleic acids

Nucleic acids, that is DNA and RNA, are macro-molecular components of cells and must be synthesized by our cells during cell division and during replication respectively (see Chapter 2). The components of nucleic acids include nitrogenous bases, phosphates, and pentose or ribose sugars and these are obtained from the nucleic acids ingested in our diets following their digestion and absorption in the gut.

Water

Some 60% of our body weight (range 50–70% depending upon the proportion of fat) results from water which is distributed in a precise and regulated way (see Chapter 5) and deter-mines the volumes and, to a certain extent, the solute concentrations of the various body fluids. Water is also a component of many metabolic reactions.

Water is constantly lost from the body and must be replenished from our diets. Most water is ingested in the fluids we drink but even the driest of foods contain a significant amount of water. For example, cereal grains are comprised of 10% water by weight.

RECOMMENDED DAILY INTAKES OF NUTRIENTS

Nutrient intake supports the metabolic processes occurring within cells. Apart from water, most of our body (and that of other organisms) is comprised of protein, carbohy-drate, and lipids and most of our food intake will also be these three classes of nutrient. This does not detract, however, from the impor-tance of other nutrients and health organiza-tions make recommendations regarding the intake of almost all nutrients. Recommended intakes are calculated from their rates of utilization, storage, or excretion and are contin-ually under review.

The aim of nutrition standards is to ensure that everyone in the country or group receives sufficient amounts of each nutrient. The standard used is under continual review and in the past has included recommended daily intake (RDI) values (1969) and the revised recommended daily amount (RDA) values (1979). The difficulty with setting standards, though, is that there are individual differences in metabolic needs and also in the rates at which nutrients are absorbed from the gut. Thus, someone who absorbs a nutrient at half the rate of another individual must eat twice as much to obtain the same amount. The 1969 and 1979 reference values do not adequately allow for individual variations and, accordingly, a number of indices (collectively called dietary reference values; DRVs) have since been devel-oped. Readers are referred to a publication by the UK Department of Health (1991) for more details.

The need for nutrients varies during our lifespan according to age, stage of develop-ment, and life-style. The remainder of this section will outline the changes in nutrient requirement related to development using estimated average requirements (EARs), as recommended by the UK Department of Health. EARs are estimates of the age require-ment for food energy or a nutrient. As can be seen in Figure 6.3, however, many people will need more than this average and many will need less.

ESTIMATED AVERAGE REQUIREMENTS OF ENERGY AND NUTRIENTS

Nutrient requirements change during growth and development, with age, and during pregnancy and lactation. For easy reference most of the changes in protein, energy, vitamin, and mineral requirements are presented in Tables 6.5 -6.7. EARs for carbohy-drate and fat intakes have not been set by the

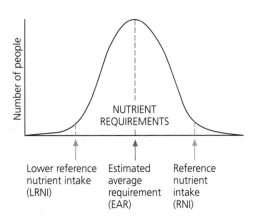

Figure 6.3 Relationship between various nutrient reference values. Note that estimated average requirement data will not be applicable to all people; some will have a lower requirement, others higher.

UK Department of Health, since intakes are related to energy needs.

The main reasons for variations in nutrient needs during the lifespan are explained below.

Newborn to infant

There are two nutritional considerations during this period of life: the requirements of the nursing mother, and those of the baby, who is entirely dependent at this time.

Human milk is highly varied in composition, and changes even between feeds. In general, 100 g of breast milk provides about 290 kJ (70 kcal) of energy (Table 6.8). The average woman produces 700 ml of milk per day and so the energy cost to the mother during lactation will be of the order of 2000 kJ (or 2 MJ; 500 kcal) per day. Some of this energy is supplied from

Table 6.5 Estimated average requirements for protein and energy intake

Age	Protein g/day		Energy kcal/day (MJ/day)	
			male	*female*
0–3 m	–		545 (2.28)	515 (2.16)
4–6 m	10.6		690 (2.89)	645 (2.69)
7–9 m	11.0		825 (3.44)	765 (3.20)
10–12 m	11.2		920 (3.85)	865 (3.61)
1–3 y	11.7		1230 (5.15)	1165 (4.86)
4–6 y	14.8		1715 (7.16)	1545 (6.46)
7–10 y	22.8		1970 (8.24)	1740 (7.28)
	male	*female*		
11–14 y	33.8	33.1	2220 (9.27)	1845 (7.92)
15–18 y	46.1	37.1	2755 (11.51)	2110 (8.83)
19–49 y	44.4	36.0	2550 (10.60)	1940 (8.10)
50–59 y	42.6	37.2	2550 (10.60)	1900 (8.00)
60–64 y	42.6	37.2	2380 (9.93)	1900 (7.99)
65–74 y	42.6	37.2	2330 (9.71)	1900 (7.96)
74+ y	42.6	37.2	2100 (8.77)	1810 (7.61)
Addition to pre-pregnancy value:				
Pregnancy	+6			+200 (+0.8)
Lactation	+8–11		up to 1 m	+450 (+1.9)
			1–2 m	+530 (+2.2)
			2–3 m	+570 (+2.4)

Values for energy intake in adults of 19+ years assumes low activity levels with a physical activity level of 1.4.

Table 6.6 Estimated average requirements for vitamins (amounts per day)

Age	A (µg retinol equivalent)	B₁* (mg/1000 kcal)	B₂ (mg)	B₃* (mg/1000 kcal)	B₆† (µg/g protein)	B₁₂ (µg)	Folate (µg)	Pantothenic (mg)	Biotin (µg)	C (mg)	D (µg)	E (mg)	K (µg/kg body wt)
0–1 y	250	0.23	0.3	↑	6–10	0.25–0.35	40	No EAR set.	No EAR set.	15	<10	<4 but related	0.5–1 adequate
1–3 y	300	0.30	0.5			0.40	50			15	provided	to	
4–6 y	300	0.30	0.6	5.5	13	0.70	75	7–10 adequate →	10–200 adequate →	20	exposure	fatty	
7–10 y	350	0.30	0.8	↓		0.80	110			20	to sun →	acid intake →	
	♂ ♀		♂ ♀										
11–14 y	400 400	0.30	1.0 0.9			1.00	150			22			
15–50+ y	500 400	0.31	1.0 0.9			1.25	150			25			

Addition to pre-pregnancy intake:

	A	B₁*	B₂	B₃*	B₆†	B₁₂	Folate	Pantothenic	Biotin	C	D	E	K
Pregnancy	+100	Related to inc. energy require-ment	+0.3	Related to inc. energy require-ment	No extra	No extra	+100	As above	As above	+10	10 is adequate	4 adequate	As above
Lactation	+350		+0.5	No extra needed	No extra needed	+0.5	+60	At least as above	As above	+30	10 is adequate	4 adequate	As above

Note: EARs for B₆ and B₁₂ increase during the 1st year, hence range is given.
*Values are related to energy intake.
†Values are related to protein intake.

Table 6.7 Estimated average requirement for selected minerals (daily amounts)

Age (years)	Calcium (mg)	Phosphorus (mg)	Sodium* (mg)	Potassium* (mg)	Iron (mg)	Zinc (mg)	Magnesium (mg)	Copper† (µg)	Iodine* (µg)
0–1	400	310	140–350	400–800	1.3–6.0†	3.3–3.8‡	40–60‡	<0.3	40–60
1–3	275	215	200–500	450–800	5.3	3.8	65	<0.4	40–70
4–6	350	270	280–700	600–1100	4.7	5.0	90	<0.6	50–100
7–10	425	325	350–1200	950–2000	6.7	5.4	150	<0.7	55–110
	♂ ♀	♂ ♀			♂ ♀	♂ ♀	♂ ♀		
11–14	750 625	580 480	460–1600	1600–3100	8.7 11.4	7.0 7.0	230 230	<0.8	65–130
15–18	750 625	580 480	575–1600	2000–3500	8.7 11.4	7.3 5.5	250 250	<1.0	70–140
19+	525 525	400 400	575–1600	2000–3500	6.7 11.4	7.3 5.5	200 250	<1.2	70–140
50+					6.7 6.7				

Addition to pre-pregnancy values:

	Calcium (mg)	Phosphorus (mg)	Sodium* (mg)	Potassium* (mg)	Iron (mg)	Zinc (mg)	Magnesium (mg)	Copper† (µg)	Iodine* (µg)
Pregnancy	No extra necessary	No extra necessary	Extra not established	Extra not established	No extra	No extra	No extra	No extra	No extra
Lactation	+500	+425	Extra not established	Extra not established	See text	+6	+50	+0.3	No extra

Note that chloride intake is likely to be equivalent to that of sodium, and that the ratio between calcium and phosphorus intake should be between 1.2:4 and 2.2:1 especially in infants.

*EARs are unclear so lower and upper intake limits are shown.
†EAR is unclear. Upper limit only is shown.
‡Requirement changes during 1st year of life. Range is shown.

Tbale 6.8 Comparison between the composition of breast milk and cows' milk

	Carbohydrate g/100 ml (lactose g/100 ml)	Protein g/100 ml (% casein)	Fat g/100 ml	Energy kcal/100 ml (kJ/100 ml)	Vitamin D µg/100 ml	Vitamin B₂ (Riboflavin) µg/100 ml	Vitamin B₃ (Nicotinic acid) µg/100 ml
Breast milk	7.3 (7.0)	0.8 (40%)	4.2	70 (293)	0.8	30	220
Cows' milk	5.0 (4.8)	3.5 (80%)	3.5	66 (275)	0.15	190	80

fat deposits stored by the mother during pregnancy but much must be supplied by the mother's diet. The energy costs will also increase with time as the growth of the baby accelerates. In proportionate terms the energy needs of the baby during the first 6 months of life are higher than at any other time of life (see Figure 6.4).

The infant will double his birth weight during the first year of life and nutritional requirements will change periodically. Provision of all nutrients remains important in order to sustain normal growth and development. Particularly important nutrients during this time are protein (for growth), iron (for blood), vitamin D (to promote calcium uptake by the gut) calcium, and fluoride (for bone and teeth development, even before teeth have erupted).

If breast-feeding the nursing mother must increase her intake of protein and most minerals. The dietary needs for iron usually increase only after the first 5–6 months as the baby's stores are quite high at birth.

Not all infants are breast-fed initially and infant formulas are commercially treated to modify their composition. Although nutritionally adequate, these formulas will be deficient in other constituents of breast milk, such as antibodies.

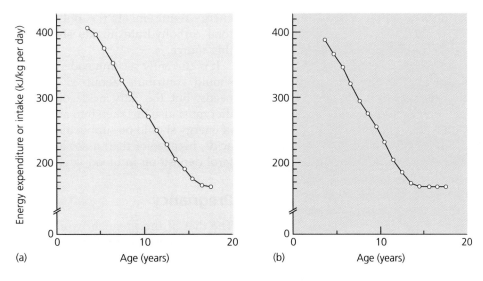

Figure 6.4 Energy requirement, standardized for body weight, in (a) boys and (b) girls up to the age of 18 years.

Substitution of cows' milk for breast milk is not recommended. For example, there is less lactose in cows' milk, and the protein of cows' milk, mainly casein, is harder to digest (although human milk also contains some casein; Table 6.8). The absorption of iron from breast milk is also considerably more efficient than from cows' milk, and the latter also contains more sodium, which places a greater demand on the infants' kidneys to excrete the load. In addition, the free amino acids contained in breast milk are also beneficial as there are more 'essential' dietary amino acids for infants than adults (12 versus 10). The vitamin content of cows' milk is also very different from that of breast milk, and the baby may also respond to allergens present.

Babies are developmentally unready for solid food until about 4 months of age. In particular they have difficulty in moving food to the back of the mouth for swallowing and they have difficulty digesting cereals. Delay in weaning runs the risk of inducing protein deficiency as the growth of the baby accelerates.

Growing child, adolescent, and young adult

Growth during childhood is steady up to about 10 years of age when rates accelerate as the child enters puberty. These are therefore critical periods for nutrition and recommended intakes of nutrients increase sharply. Energy requirements relative to body size are therefore higher in children and adolescents than in adults (see Figure 6.4) in order to support the rate of growth and the high levels of physical activity exhibited by this group. Mineral and vitamin requirements increase accordingly.

Adults – 23–50 years

Growth effectively ends between the ages of 19–22 and nutrition then largely becomes a case of maintenance. In Western societies many people are more at risk of overnutrition than undernutrition.

Energy requirements are particularly influenced by levels of physical activity. For example, an adult who partakes in little physical activity at work or during leisure time will have a physical activity level (PAL) of 1.4. Thus, if the BMR is 7300 kJ per day (= 1740 kcal per day):

EAR = 7300 × 1.4 = 10200 kJ (2430 kcal) per day

For men with high levels of activity, PAL will be 1.9. Thus,

EAR = 7300 × 1.9 = 13900 kJ (3300 kcal) per day

PAL values are slightly higher for men than women. Thus, with moderate activity levels PAL is 1.6 for women and 1.7 for men, and with high levels of activity PAL is 1.8 for women and 1.9 for men.

Although carbohydrates form the main source of energy the ideal proportion of carbohydrate, relative to fats and protein, remains the subject of debate. On average, dietary protein provides about 15% of our energy needs and, on this basis, it is currently considered that carbohydrates should comprise about 50% of our energy intake. Since non-milk extrinsic sugars, such as sucrose, promote dental caries, it is considered that only 10% of energy requirements (i.e. only about a fifth of total carbohydrate intake) should come from this source.

It is currently recommended that dietary fats should contribute about 35% of our energy needs, but the fatty acid composition of the diet must also be taken into account. Only 10% of energy should be supplied by saturated fatty acids, because of their association with cholesterol deposition in blood vessels.

Pregnancy

The diet of the pregnant woman must clearly support the increased tissue mass produced by an increased uterus size, the fetus and placenta, an expanded blood volume, and extra fat deposits, and also maintain the increased metabolic activity related to that increased mass. Studies have shown, however, that food intake is only observed to increase in the third trimester which suggests that additional energy intake (0.8 MJ/day; 200 kcal/day) is most important during that period.

Tissue growth requires protein, minerals, and vitamins. For some minerals and vitamins an increased intake during pregnancy is probably unnecessary as the efficiency at which they are absorbed across the gut of the mother is increased and adequately supplies the extra needs.

Adults – 50–75 years

The ageing process is most noticeable after about the age of 50 when physical activity may decline, basal metabolism diminishes, digestive activity is reduced, secretions (e.g. of saliva) are less pronounced, perceptions of taste and smell change and life-styles alter. Nutrient requirements are generally the same as at 30 years old, however, except that less energy is needed.

Adults – 75+ years

Most people over 75 years of age show a decrease in activity levels compared with a 50–60 year-old, although there is a wide variation. Basal metabolic rate is appreciably decreased above 75 years of age. Food requirements generally diminish, but there is a risk that the low food intakes observed in inactive elderly people may not provide adequate nutrients for health.

Regulation of nutrient intake

'Hunger' is the perception that we should ingest some food, whereas 'appetite' largely determines how much we eat. Appetite normally equates with the energy needs of the body and body weight generally remains fairly constant over long periods even though food intake may vary. 'Satiety' is the feeling that the amount of food ingested is enough, that is, the appetite has been satisfied. The consequences of lesions indicate that the hypothalamus (see Chapter 13) contains areas which alter food intake when stimulated. Their role in hunger and satiety are discussed in the next chapter. The mechanisms that promote hunger induce a relatively rapid response, and the regulation of body weight over a period of years represents an as yet unidentified homeostatic process.

Thirst centres are also present in the hypothalamus and respond to changes in an increased osmotic pressure of blood plasma arising as a consequence of dehydration. Sodium depletion, which promotes a reduction in blood volume (see Chapter 5), also induces a 'salt' appetite in which salty foods are eaten in preference and this also seems to involve the hypothalamus.

Regulation of the intake of many individual nutrients such as vitamins is coarse and imprecise. As noted above, hunger arises as a need for energy and the requirement of other nutrients is secondary to this, which emphasizes the need for a balanced diet to ensure deficiencies of specific nutrients do not occur.

Although neural centres have been identified which modulate our feelings of hunger, there are clearly a variety of social aspects to eating including cultural customs and diets, media-induced food 'fads' and reducing diets to remove excess fat after the homeostatic regulation of body weight has failed!

Role of nutrition in homeostasis

The adequate provision of nutrients is a prerequisite for cell function. Deficiencies will therefore affect cells and systems throughout the body, the effects becoming exacerbated as systemic integration is disrupted. Examples are given in the next section.

Some nutrients have highly specific functions and deficiencies of these will initially disrupt those functions. For example, iron is essential for the synthesis of haemoglobin, the pigment required for oxygen transportation by blood, and iron deficiency results in anaemia which reduces the maximum volume of oxygen that blood can carry. If severe enough the anaemia will cause general tissue hypoxia (hypo- = less than normal; -oxia = oxygen), the effects of which will be particularly noticeable in 'active' tissues (nervous and muscle), resulting in fatigue and apathy.

Examples of homeostatic control system failure and principles of correction

The main control exerted on nutritional intake is via appetite, which is linked to the energy needs of the body. Malnutrition (mal- = disordered) arises as a consequence of a failure to satisfy the appetite, of a failure to recognize satiety, or of an unbalanced diet which is lacking in, or contains excessive amounts of one or more nutrients.

Principles of correction are aimed at either reversing the deficiencies or excesses by improving diet, or by correcting any sociopsychological disturbance involved.

EXCESSIVE NUTRIENT INTAKE

Bulimia and obesity

These are conditions in which food volume in excess of body requirements is eaten. This usually arises from sociopsychological disturbances, although there is also some evidence for an inherited propensity to obesity.

Bulimia is a condition whereby an individual impulsively consumes a large amount of food in a short space of time. Self-induced vomiting, or even laxative abuse, is then used in an attempt to prevent weight gain or perhaps promote weight loss. Many bulimics have a normal body weight or are only slightly overweight.

Obesity is a condition in which body weight is at least 20% above the 'ideal'. Excess weight is a consequence of excessive fat deposits and results from a prolonged intake of energy in excess of body requirements. One theory, still unproven, regarding the difficulty of people to reverse obesity is that appetite is elevated after a while and this maintains a high food intake.

Correction of bulimia and obesity generally requires an understanding of the psychological cause of the disturbed physiological homeostasis.

Hypercholesterolaemia

Hypercholesterolaemia (hyper- = excess; aemia = of blood) may be an inherited familial condition, but can also arise from excessive intake of saturated fats (which may be converted to cholesterol) and cholesterol (Figure 6.5).

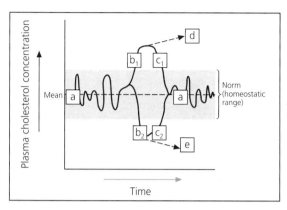

Figure 6.5 Maintenance of plasma cholesterol within an 'ideal' range. Note that cholesterol is only partially regulated in that a high dietary intake will result in a persistently high concentration, regardless of utilization.
a, Fluctuations of plasma cholesterol within an 'ideal'range – cholesterol derived from dietary lipids and synthesis by liver sufficient for needs.
b_1, elevated plasma cholesterol into 'risk' zone (i.e. concentration > 5.2 mmol/l) usually due to excessive dietary intake of saturated fats.
b_2, cholesterol deficiency due to inadequate intake *or* inadequate liver synthesis.
c_1, decline in cholesterol concentration as a consequence of utilization exceeding intake/synthesis.
c_2, increased cholesterol due to hepatic synthesis exceeding utilization.
d, excessive cholesterol as a consequence of *either* maintenance of a diet rich in saturated fat *or* inadequate metabolism (an inherited trait), increasing the risk of atheroma and cardiovascular disease.
e, inadequate cholesterol concentration due to inadequate intake or synthesis, leading to deficient utilization (e.g. steroid hormone deficiency).

Although an important lipid, evidence indicates that cholesterol in excess promotes its deposition in blood vessels and is an important factor in the development of heart disease. A high dietary intake is unnecessary to provide for the body's needs, since cholesterol can be synthesized in the liver.

INADEQUATE NUTRIENT INTAKE

Inadequate intake can relate to insufficient volume of food, as in starvation or anorexia nervosa, or to diets deficient in specific nutrients.

Starvation and anorexia nervosa

These are conditions characterized by an emaciated state as, faced with inadequate energy intake, fat stores and then body protein (especially muscle) are mobilized to provide cells with substrates for respiration. Both produce complex symptoms arising from general nutrient deficiency.

Anorexia nervosa is a complex sociophysiological disturbance, usually in adolescent women, which appears to arise from concern regarding changes in body weight during puberty. Hunger and appetite are suppressed, although individuals may resort to laxative abuse, enemas and self-induced vomiting. Bulimic episodes may occur.

Specific nutrient deficiency
Protein deficiency

Kwashiorkor is an example of protein deficiency, and is particularly observed in children since they need relatively large intakes to maintain normal growth. Kwashiorkor has a complex array of symptoms some of which have also been related to inadequate vitamin and mineral intake. Muscle wasting, growth failure, and a general 'failure to thrive' are characteristic. A deficiency in plasma protein concentration (hypoproteinaemia) has been suggested to be a contributory factor in the development of oedema (see Chapter 5).

Kwashiorkor relates to protein deficiency but deficiencies in specific amino acids are also possible. Vegetarians are particularly at risk unless 'complementary proteins' are included in the diet.

Vitamin and mineral deficiencies

The effects of these have already been outlined in Tables 6.2–6.4.

References

Department of Health (1991) *Dietary reference values: a guide.* London: HMSO.

Summary

1 A variety of nutrients are essential to life.

2 In terms of bulk, carbohydrates, proteins, and lipids are the main constituents of our foods and are essential for growth, tissue renewal and energy production. Their efficient utilization also depends upon adequate dietary provision of vitamins and minerals.

3 The kinds of foods we eat contain different amounts of the various nutrients and so it is essential that a 'balanced' diet is consumed.

4 How much of each nutrient or nutrient class must be consumed for 'health' is subject to continuing debate and recommendations change periodically.

5 Requirements are related to stages of development, in particular to body size, growth rate, and physical activity.

6 The physiological control of food intake appears to be coarse and seems related to our energy status. Thirst and salt appetite are also apparent during water and sodium deficiency, respectively.

7 Long-term control of body weight seems to be present but is little understood. The mechanism appears to be easy to overcome, as evidenced by the sociopsychological aspects of eating which can cause obesity or weight loss.

Review Questions

1 Discuss the use of molecular building-blocks in the human body.

2 Distinguish between the following members of the carbohydrate family:
(a) polysaccharides;
(b) disaccharides;
(c) monosaccharides.

3 Give examples of the above members of the carbohydrate family and their associated functions and suggested food sources.

4 Compare and contrast the structure of carbohydrates with that of fats.

5 What is the difference between saturated and unsaturated fats? Of what importance is this to human health?

6 How is the structure of a protein related to its function?

7 Distinguish between animal and vegetable proteins, giving examples of each.

8 Define:
(a) basal metabolic rate (BMR);
(b) physical activity level (PAL).

9 What is the calorific valve of fats, carbohydrate and proteins?

10 Why is fibre considered to be an important dietary constituent but not a nutrient?

11 What is the relationship of vitamins to coenzymes?

12 Distinguish between fat-soluble and water-soluble vitamins.

13 What are trace elements?

14 Discuss why the estimated average requirements of energy varies with the following developmental stages:
(a) newborn to infant;
(b) growing child;
(c) adolescent;
(d) post-retirement.

The digestive system

7

Introduction: relation of the digestive system to cellular homeostasis

Overview of the anatomy and physiology of the digestive system

Details of the physiology of the digestive system

Examples of homeostatic failure and principles of correction

Summary

Review questions

Introduction: relation of the digestive system to cellular homeostasis

The digestive system aids the correct functioning of the cell by ensuring that the body is provided with the 'normal' requirements of molecules necessary to maintain cellular metabolism at a rate compatible with life. The importance of a balanced diet was discussed in Chapter 6 and it was emphasized that one's consumable nutrients consist of a diversity of molecular compounds. The bulk of the diet is provided by three main classes of food: carbohydrates, lipids, and proteins. These are usually consumed as large and insoluble molecular complexes, and must be reduced in size, and made soluble, before they can be absorbed into blood, transported to their site of action, and utilized in cellular metabolism, for growth, repair of component parts, production of energy, etc.

The breaking down and increase in solubility of ingested molecules is termed digestion. In addition to the three main classes of food, dietary constituents must also include water, vitamins, and minerals. These micromolecules are already 'soluble' and are small enough to

be absorbed into blood, hence their digestion is unnecessary.

This chapter is concerned with describing how food intake is regulated, the process of digestion, and the liver's role in determining the fate of the majority of these end products of digestion.

REGULATION OF FOOD INTAKE

Many areas of the brain have been identified as having a role in feeding and satiety. However, the most important area is the hypothalamus, which has two centres involved in the regulation of food intake:

1 Hunger (feeding) centre.

2 Satiety (cessation of feeding) centre.

The hunger centre is constantly active unless it is inhibited by input from the satiety centre. There are many theories as to the regulatory factors associated with food intake. The 'glucostat' theory suggests that feeding is initiated by low levels of plasma glucose which stimulate the hunger centre activity and depress the inhibitory action of the satiety centre. Conversely, a high plasma glucose concentration results in inhibition of hunger centre activity and thus stops feeding. The same reasoning has been put forward with reference to plasma levels of amino acids, the difference being that the amino acid responses appear less effective than the glucose responses. Lipids have also been indicated as important factors; this theory suggests that the rate of feeding decreases as the volume of adipose tissue increases. It could be argued that it is unlikely to be as simple as this, since this theory cannot satisfactorily explain the occurrence of obesity!

The 'body temperature' theory attempts to explain why it is that we tend to eat more in winter, linking this with the colder environmental temperatures which result in a lowering of the body temperature and a stimulation of the hunger centre. The reverse reasoning is given to explain why we tend to eat less in hot summer months. This theory may partly explain why we tend to gain a little weight in the winter months, but many other contributory factors are also important.

The above factors may influence food intake, but the theory which has received most recognition in controlling food intake, and the cessation of intake, is the gastrointestinal 'stretch receptor' theory (Figure 7.1). This suggests that distension of the stomach and duodenum by the presence of food stimulates stretch receptors in these organs above their 'normal' or baseline firing range. These receptors send sensory (afferent) impulses to the hypothalamic satiety centre, which in turn inhibits hunger centre activity bringing about cessation of food intake. Conversely, if the degree of stretching falls below the baseline firing rate then the afferent information is not sufficient to stimulate the satiety centre output. Thus, the inhibition to the hunger centre is removed with the result that feeding is promoted.

Overview of the anatomy and physiology of the digestive system

The anatomy and physiology of the digestive system evolved to convert consumed food into a form which can be used by the cell. The conversion can be divided into five principal physiological processes:

1 Ingestion (eating). The process of taking food into the mouth.

2 Digestion. The physical and chemical breakdown of food; both processes are necessary to render food into a state for the third process of absorption.

3 Absorption. The passage of the end products of digestion from the digestive tract into the transporting (cardiovascular and lymphatic) systems, which distribute these metabolites to the cells that require them.

4 Assimilation. The liver's homeostatically controlled utilization of these molecular substances in order to keep blood levels optimal for cellular metabolism.

5 Defecation (egestion). The elimination of indigestible substances, such as fibre, certain excretory products (for example, bile salts and bile pigments), and unabsorbed substances (for example, some water and electrolytes) from the body.

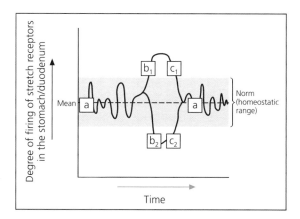

Figure 7.1 The regulation of food intake.
a, 'normal' level of firing of stretch receptors. Stimulus *not* enough to stimulate satiety centre and the degree of hunger centre output is *not* sufficient to seek food.
b_1, increased rate of firing of stretch receptors, above their baseline level, resulting in afferent (sensory) input to the satiety centre. This centre inhibits the hunger centre's output and so causes the cessation of food intake.
b_2, decreased rate of firing of stretch receptors below their baseline level, resulting in a decrease in afferent fibre input to the satiety centre (i.e. insufficient to stimulate it), thus stimulating the hunger centre activity, causing the individual to seek food.
c, restoration of 'normal' stretch receptor activity by appropriate changes in satiety (c_1) and hunger (c_2) centre activity.

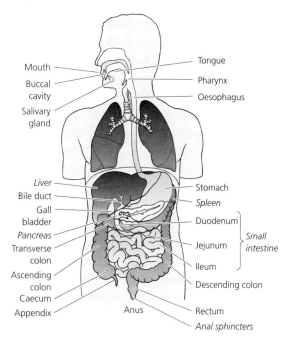

Figure 7.2 Human alimentary canal.

The digestive system, as illustrated by Figure 7.2, is adapted to perform these physiological functions. Thus regional anatomical differentiation can be identified that facilitates the performance of specialized functions. In particular, the structure of the mouth is suited to the chewing and moisturizing of food, and swallowing. The stomach provides a large distensible region for food holding, for the 'sterilization' of food, and for the commencement of protein digestion. Beyond the stomach the gut consists of the small and large intestines. The small intestine continues the digestive process and is supported by the release of enzymes from the pancreas, and of bile. Distal parts of the small intestine are particularly concerned with the absorption of food products. Many of the products are rapidly assimilated by the liver. The large intestine also exhibits limited absorptive activities. Its main role is to consolidate undigested remains into semi-solid faecal masses. A flora of bacteria present within the large intestine also contributes to the digestive process by promoting further breakdown of undigested material.

Exposure to pathogens is a potential problem because the tract is in contact with the external environment but lymphatic 'patches' throughout the tract help to remove infectious agents. Furthermore, the marked pH changes observed throughout the tract provide another external defence mechanism to potential pathogenic invaders. However, if the invaders survive these mechanisms and gain entry into the blood then our internal defence mechanisms are activated in an attempt to destroy these organisms.

The major regions of the gastrointestinal tract are separated from one another either by circular rings, or sphincters, of involuntary muscle fibres (for example, the pyloric sphincter separates the stomach from the small intestine), or by a valve-like structure (for example,

Table 7.1 The main organs and accessory organs of the digestive system

Main organs	Accessory organs
Mouth	Lips, teeth, tongue, salivary glands, palate
Pharynx	
Oesophagus	
Stomach	
Small intestine	Pancreas, gall bladder, liver
Large intestine	

the ileocaecal valve, which separates the terminal part of the small intestine from the first part of the large intestine). The functional significance of these structures is to aid a unidirectional movement of food along the tract, and to provide a means of control over that movement.

The organs of the digestive system can be divided into two groups (Table 7.1):

1 The main organs of the alimentary or gastrointestinal tract, i.e. the stomach, intestines, etc.

2 The accessory digestive organs, i.e. the pancreas, liver, etc.

The alimentary tract is a continuous tube approximately 10 metres in length extending from the mouth to the anus. The accessory organs associated with the digestive system (except the tongue) are positioned outside the digestive tract and are involved in the production and release of various digestive secretions. The glandular part of the lining epithelium also produces secretions, which are transported along ducts to their site of action. Most secretions contain enzymes necessary for chemical digestion (the exception is bile). For this process to operate efficiently, however, physical churning and maceration of foodstuffs must also occur and processes of both physical and chemical digestion can be identified throughout the tract.

The remainder of this chapter discusses each individual region and its associated physical and chemical digestive processes. First, though, it is important that the reader becomes familiar with the types of cell and membranes found in the alimentary canal. Reference to Chapter 4 may be useful whilst reading this section.

GENERAL HISTOLOGY OF THE GASTROINTESTINAL TRACT

The gut has a complex histological structure and various epithelial and muscular layers can be identified. Figure 7.3 illustrates the generalized histological appearance of the gastrointestinal tact. The tract has four principal layers or coats, called tunicae: (1) the mucosa, (2) the submucosa, (3) the muscularis externa, and (4) the serosa.

Mucosa

The mucosa is a mucous membrane which forms the inner lining of the tract. The function of mucus is to lubricate the food to ease its passage. This membrane has two layers.

The inner glandular epithelial membrane

This is the layer exposed to the lumen and, thus, the contents of the digestive tract. It is a non-keratinized glandular simple epithelium (throughout most of the tract), and hence it is adapted for secreting watery digestive juices. Most of the digestive glands develop from this inner membrane. It is also involved in absorption and thus has adaptations for this process

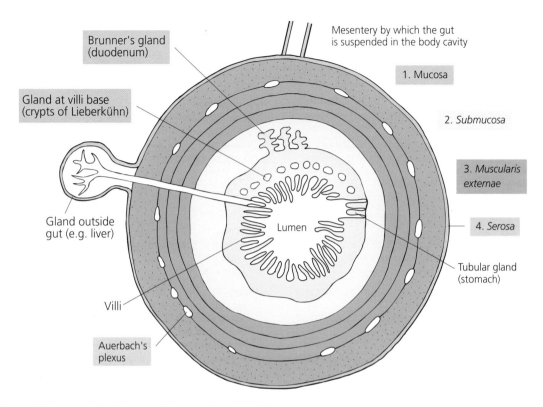

Figure 7.3 A generalized diagram of the structure of the human gut.

in appropriate areas. The oesophagus and anal canal require the additional protection of a stratified, or layered, epithelium as they are exposed to much wear and tear. The epithelium is derived from embryonic endoderm, with the exception of the epithelia lining the anal canal and parts of the mouth cavity, which is of ectodermal origin.

The outer membrane or lamina propria

This is a loose connective tissue which supports the glandular epithelium. It accommodates digestive glands, blood and lymph vessels, providing nutritive and defence functions to the glandular epithelial layer. The propria is attached to a smooth layer of muscle called the muscularis mucosa. This muscle's fibres are subjected to a sustained tonic state of contrac-

tion and are responsible for the folded appearance of the digestive and absorptive surfaces.

Submucosa

The submucosa is a highly vascularized and innervated layer (the nerve cells form a meshwork called the Meissner's plexus), and also contains a large amount of collagen fibres, and elastic fibres. It functions to control the tract's secretory activities and to bind the mucosa to the third coat, the muscularis externa.

Muscularis externa

In most regions the muscularis externa consists of an outer sheet of longitudinally arranged smooth muscle fibres and an inner sheet of

Table 7.2 Regional histological features of the alimentary canal

Oesophagus

Folded mucosa
Stratified squamous epithelia
Thick muscularis mucosa
Some glands are present
Absence of serosa
Thickest muscularis externa. Upper third is voluntary,
    mid-third a mixture of voluntary/involuntary and the
    latter third is involuntary
Papillae project into the epithelium

Stomach

Large mucosal folds – rugae
Thick muscular wall
Numerous gastric pits
An abundance of exocrine glands in the lamina propria
Parietal cells in the fundus
Oblique layer in the muscularis externae
No villi, no goblet cells

Small intestine

Duodenum
    An abundance of villi compared with jejunum and
        ileum; villi are short, leaf-shaped
    Two types of epithelial cells
    Goblet cells
    Intestinal folds – plicae
    Brunner's glands
    Crypts of lieberkühn

Jejunum
    As for duodenum except:
        taller plicae
        villi tongue-shaped

Ileum
    As for duodenum except:
        fewer or no plicae
        finger-shaped villi
    Aggregates of lymph nodules – Peyer's patches

Large intestine

Appendix
    Lymphatic tissue, with lymphocytes between the
        crypts
    Narrow lumen

Colon
    No villi
    Long tubular glands
    Few goblet cells
    Thin muscularis externa consisting of three muscular
        bands – taeniae (giving this region a pouched
        appearance)
    Large lumen
    Peyer patches project into submucosa

Rectum
    As for colon, except:
        no taeniae
        thick muscularis externae
    Stratified epthelium near the retroanal junction.
    Longest glands

circularly arranged muscle fibres. A meshwork of nerves, called Auerbach's plexus, lies between these sheets of muscle fibres and is responsible for coordinating their activity. Contraction of these fibres generates the specialized movements of the gastrointestinal tract which function to move the food along the tract and in doing so aid the mixing of its contents and, therefore, facilitate the digestive process.

Serosa

The serosa is part of a serous membrane (Chapter 4). It is an areolar connective tissue known as the visceral peritoneum as it is attached to the surface of the digestive organs.

Its counterpart, the parietal peritoneum (not a part of the gut serosa), lines the wall of the abdominal cavity. The fluid-filled space between these serous membranes, called the peritoneal cavity, provides a protective cushioning of the gut during digestion and upon changes in intra-abdominal pressure associated with breathing movements. An extension of the peritoneum forms the mesenteries of the gut. These are outward folds of the serous coat of the small intestine, and bind this organ to the posterior abdominal wall. The mesenteries accommodate the blood vessels, lymphatics, and neurons which supply this region.

The regional adaptations of the membranes in the gut are summarized in Table 7.2.

Details of the physiology of the digestive system

Digestion is the sum total of all the processes involved in breaking down consumable food from complex insoluble macromolecules to simple soluble molecules, so that these substances can be readily absorbed into the blood for carriage to cells which utilize them. There are two processes involved in this break-down:

1 Physical (mechanical) digestion. This involves a variety of structural components of the digestive tract which mechanically reduce the size of the ingested food particle; Figure 7.4a illustrates this process. The function of physical digestion is to increase the surface area of the food particles to aid chemical digestion.

2 Chemical digestion. This involves the break-down of chemical bonds within molecules too large to be absorbed into the blood. Enzymes speed up (i.e. catalyse) this catabolism by promoting hydrolysis of the molecules, that is, breakdown using water. Hydrolysis results in a hydrogen group being added to one of the products of catabolism and a hydroxyl group to the other (Figure 7.4b). The Figure also shows that heat is given off as a result of this process and so the actions of digestive enzymes also contribute to the thermoregulation of cells and extracellular fluid.

Physical and chemical digestion occur simultaneously. For convenience, however, the processes will be described individually for each anatomical region of the gut. Pancreatic and liver functions will also be separately described,

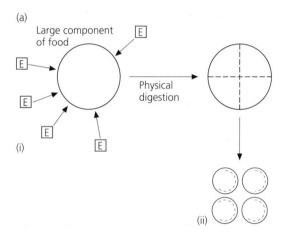

Figure 7.4 (a) Physical digestion, an aid to chemical digestion. (i) Before physical digestion the enzymatic action is limited to the area surrounding the food component: E, enzymes. (ii) After physical digestion a greater surface area is now available (------) for enzymatic action. Note: physical and chemical digestion occur simultaneously. Physical digestion merely makes chemical digestion more efficient by increasing the available surface area for enzymatic attack. (b) Hydrolysis of (i) peptides and (ii) disaccharides. Under enzyme catalysis, a water molecule is added to the two residues as shown, breaking the covalent bond holding the residues together.

Table 7.3 Homeostatic functions of saliva components

Salivary components	Homeostatic roles
Water	Dissolves food for the appreciation of taste. Vital for digestion (catabolic hydrolysis) and to provide the necessary aqueous medium for the enzyme's maximum catalysing efficiency
Bicarbonates and phosphates	Buffering action keeps the pH within its homeostatic range (6.35–6.85), essential for enzymatic action. pH changes to slightly alkaline during chewing, this is important for maximizing the catalysing effects of salivary amylase and also this pH destroys the enzyme systems of acid-liking bacteria
Amylase	Initiates carbohydrate digestion via catalysing catabolic hydrolysis
Lysozymes and antibodies	Destroys bacteria, hence prevents infection
Mucin	Forms soluble mucus in the presence of water. This has a lubricating and moisturizing action
Urea	Excretory products of amino acid metabolism
Chloride	Being a cofactor, it aids salivary amylase

but it should be remembered that integration of regional functions determines the final outcome of the digestive/assimilative processes.

THE MOUTH, PHARYNX AND OESOPHAGUS

The mouth

The mouth (oral or buccal) cavity is the opening of the alimentary canal which aids ingestion. This is the only region which is surrounded by bony skeletal structures, i.e. the upper and lower jaws, or the maxilla and mandible respectively. The muscles associated with these bones are responsible for controlling the overall size of the mouth. The opening is guarded by the muscular lips, or labia, and the roof of the buccal cavity is formed by the hard and soft palates, the latter tapering backwards, forming a projection called the uvula. The cheeks form the sides of the mouth, with the tongue forming the floor. The jaws support the cavity and contain the sockets which accommodate the teeth. The mouth is lined with a mucous stratified epithelial membrane, reflecting the wear and tear associated with this area.

Salivation

Water makes up 90–95% of saliva the remaining 5–10% being dissolved solutes. These include:

1 Ions, such as bicarbonates (HCO_3^-), chlorides (Cl^-), phosphates (PO_4^{2-}), sodium (Na^+), and potassium (K^+).

2 The enzyme salivary amylase.

3 Lysozymes.

4 Organic substances, such as urea, albumins, and globulins (especially gammaglobulins or antibodies, in particular immunoglobulin A).

5 Mucin derived from mucus-secreting cells.

Each component has a homeostatic role, as illustrated in Table 7.3.

Saliva production varies between 1 and 1.5 litres per day. Most is produced from three

3 Sublingual glands. These are the smallest of the paired glands and are responsible for about 5% of the daily total. Their cells are mainly mucus-secreting cells and are responsible for producing a very viscous secretion, with little enzyme present. These glands are positioned under the tongue and have several (Rivinus's) ducts which open on to the floor of the mouth.

The submandibular and sublingual glands are responsible for the spray of saliva which sometimes flows out when one yawns.

Other salivary glands are also present over the palate, tongue, and upon the inner side of the lips. They respond to mechanical stimulation from the presence of food in the mouth, rather than neural activity to the gland.

CONTROL OF SALIVATION

Saliva production by the paired glands is mainly controlled via parasympathetic neurons originating in the brainstem. There is always a constant flow of saliva in moderate amounts, because it has homeostatic functions other than its role in digestion (Table 7.3) including aiding speech via its lubricating action.

These glands cease to secrete in states of dehydration as part of the homeostatic conservation of body water. As a result the mouth becomes dry and this stimulates the sensation of thirst, another homeostatic function, so that one seeks out liquid intake to restore body fluid volumes to within their homeostatic ranges. Sympathetic nerve stimulation during the stress response (Chapter 22) is also responsible for producing a sense of dryness and results in the secretion of a thick viscous saliva. Excessive salivation occurs in response to the swallowing of irritant chemicals, or during nausea. This is presumably a defence response to dilute the irritant or to stimulate its removal via vomiting.

An increase in the basal level of saliva secretion (and also that of stomach secretions) occurs with the sight, smell, and touch of food, together with the sound of food preparation, or the anticipation of food intake. This is known as 'Pavlovian' conditioning after the Russian

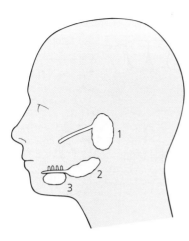

Figure 7.5 Human salivary glands: 1, parotid glands (Stenson's duct); 2, submandibular glands (Wharton's duct); 3, sublingual glands.

main pairs of salivary glands (Figure 7.5) whose ducts open into the buccal cavity on either side of the internal surface of the mouth. These are the (1) parotid, (2) submandibular, and (3) sublingual glands. Saliva secretion from these glands is largely controlled by the autonomic nervous system.

1 Parotid glands. These are the largest salivary glands. Despite this they are only responsible for approximately 25% of the daily secretion. Their cells are specialized for contributing to the watery and enzyme-rich component of saliva. They are positioned just below, and in front of, the ears, and their ducts (called Stenson's ducts) open at a point opposite the second upper molar teeth.

2 Submandibular glands. These glands are positioned under the base of the tongue in the posterior aspects of the mouth. Their ducts (called Wharton's ducts) extend centrally along the floor of the mouth opening behind the lower central incisors. They are responsible for approximately 70% of the daily production. Their cells are specialized to function in a similar way to the parotid cells, but they also secrete mucus and so produce a more viscous secretion.

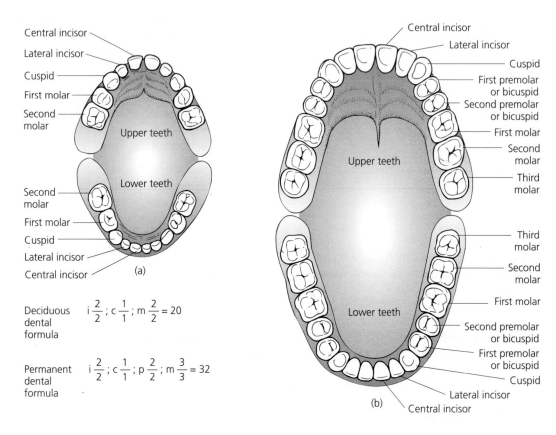

Figure 7.6 Dentitions and dental formulae. (a) Deciduous dentition. (b) Permanent dentition. Dental formulae include the number of teeth associated with one–half of either lower or upper jaw.

$$i\frac{2}{2} \; ; c\frac{1}{1} \; ; m\frac{2}{2} = 20$$ Deciduous dental formula

$$i\frac{2}{2} \; ; c\frac{1}{1} \; ; p\frac{2}{2} \; ; m\frac{3}{3} = 32$$ Permanent dental formula

psychologist who first described the principle. The stimuli increase salivary flow as a result of conditioned reflexes set up from our association areas and memory regions of the brain (Chapter 13). Such psychophysiological responses are important as they allow the mouth to lubricate food and commence chemical breakdown as soon as it enters. The presence of ingested food stimulates an even greater salivary flow, by stimulating taste buds on the tongue and other regions in the mouth. Any object rolled on the tongue has the same effect. Once the food is swallowed a large flow continues which cleanses the mouth, 'washing' the teeth and diluting food residues.

The tongue

The tongue is an accessory organ of the digestive system. Its extrinsic muscles are important in moving this structure from side to side and in and out, whereas the intrinsic muscles are responsible for changing its shape. The superior surface and the sides of the tongue contain projections called papillae, including the filiform, fungiform and circumvallate papillae. The latter two papillae are associated with taste as they contain the taste buds; the details of taste are discussed in Chapter 14.

Tongue movements alter the shape and volume of the mouth cavity and these are, of course, also vital in forming speech.

Teeth

Individuals develop two sets of teeth throughout the lifespan (Figure 7.6).

1 Milk (or deciduous) teeth. There are 20 milk or 'baby' teeth. The first ones erupt at approximately 6 months, and this is usually followed by the eruption of one pair per month. The deciduous teeth are lost at between 6 and 12 years of age.

2 Permanent teeth. There are 32 teeth in the permanent dentition and these generally replace the milk teeth as they are shed. Permanent molars do not have analogous milk teeth. The first permanent molars appear at approximately 6 years, the second at 12 years and the third (if they develop at all) molars, or the 'wisdom' teeth, appear after the age of 18 years. The latter may be a source of pressure and pain as the relative size of the jaw recedes with age. If this is the case they must be surgically removed.

Physical digestion in the mouth – mastication (chewing)

Physical digestion reduces the size of the food particles to aid the chemical processes involved in digestion. It involves the action of the jaw muscles, the teeth, and the tongue. The size of the mouth opening, together with the biting action of the teeth, are responsible for determining the size of the food particle ingested. Mouth opening is voluntarily controlled by powerful jaw muscles and the size of this opening is restricted by the perimeter of the muscular lips and the joint between mandible and cranium. The incisors, or biting teeth, mainly control the size of the particle we take in (that is, if the whole particle cannot be ingested!). The canines are used to a limited extent for tearing and shearing of fleshy meat from its bone, although as man's diet and

social eating habits have changed these teeth have become less important in ingestion and they have become much less prominent in modern man.

Once inside the mouth, the premolars and molars crush and grind the food particles, reducing their size. This is controlled by the jaw muscles and the mechanical process is termed mastication. Also important in this chewing process is the involuntary movement of the tongue, which moves food particles around the oral cavity and in doing so produces friction between the particles and structures that they rub against; the particle is fragmented as a result. Simultaneous with this physical breakdown is the mixing and lubrication of food with saliva. Saliva also contains the enzyme amylase and this initiates the chemical breakdown of carbohydrate within the food.

Chemical digestion in the mouth

The chemical breakdown of insoluble macromolecules in food begins in the mouth. Salivary amylase, previously known as ptyalin, initiates the breakdown of the carbohydrate starch (amylose = starch) by breaking down the bonds between the monosaccharide subunits from which starch is constructed (Figure 7.7a).

Most dietary carbohydrates are in the form of polysaccharides (Chapter 6). In theory, amylase is capable of converting starch into the disaccharide maltose, which consists of two glucose molecules joined together. However, this takes time. In practice the food is in the presence of amylase for only 15–30 minutes: food is usually in the stomach within 4–6 seconds of eating it, but remains for a while in areas of the stomach in which gastric acid is not present. Eventually the food is passed to acidic areas of the stomach where the acidity denatures or inactivates the amylase and so this stage of carbohydrate digestion ceases. Thus, the carbohydrate components of the food at this point are starch macromolecules, which have not been in contact with amylase

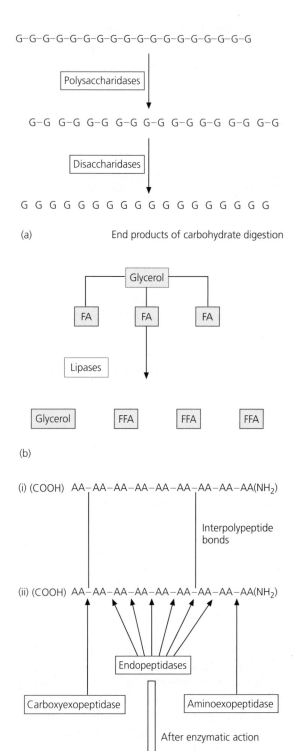

(a)   End products of carbohydrate digestion

(b)

(c)

molecules: dextrins (intermediate breakdown products between starch and the disaccharide maltose), and to a small extent maltose itself. No other foods are broken down in the mouth or on the food's journey to the stomach.

As a result of these physical and chemical processes, the food leaving the mouth is reduced to a soft, flexible 'ball', or bolus, that is easily swallowed.

The pharynx and oesophagus

The pharynx, or throat, is a cone-shaped cavity, approximately 12 cm long. It is subdivided into:

1 The nasopharynx (area behind the nasal passageways). This is concerned with the flow of air through the respiratory pathways.

2 The common pharynx or oropharynx (this contains the tonsils on its lateral walls). Anterior to this is the mouth.

3 The laryngeal pharynx (around the larynx). This bifurcates into the larynx and oesophagus.

The oesophagus is a collapsible muscular tube approximately 25 cm long, running from the pharynx to the stomach, anterior to the thoracic vertebrae, but behind the trachea. The oesophagus penetrates the diaphragm before

Figure 7.7 Digestive enzymes. (a) The mode of action of carbohydrases. (b) The mode of action of lipases on a triglyceride (most dietary fats are in the triglyceride form). (c) The mode of action of proteases. (i) + (ii) = polypeptide chains (protein molecules consist of two or more polypeptide chains). G, monosaccharide (e.g. glucose); FA, fatty acid; FFA, free fatty acid; AA, amino acid; (COOH)AA, carboxylic acid terminal amino acid; (NH_2)AA, amino terminal amino acid; endopeptidases, enzymes which catabolize the bonds between amino acids other than the terminal bonds;carboxyexopeptidases, enzymes involved in breaking the terminal peptide bond associated with the amino acid in which its carboxyl acid group is exposed; aminoexopeptidases, enzymes involved in breaking the terminal peptide bond associated with the amino acid in which its amine group is exposed.

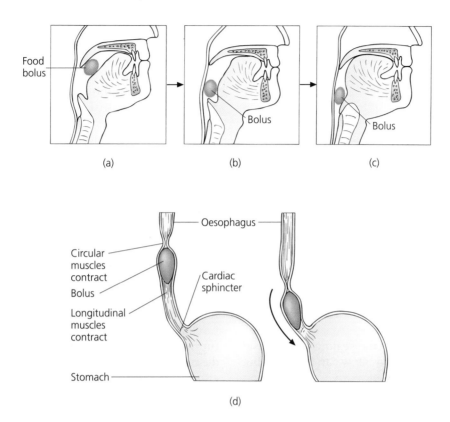

Figure 7.8 Deglutition: (a) voluntary stage (the tongue rises against the palate); (b) and (c) involuntary pharyngeal stage (nasal and laryngeal passages sealed off); (d) oesophageal stage (peristaltic motion and entry to the stomach).

entering the stomach via the oesophageal hiatus, or cardiac sphincter.

Both pharynx and oesophagus are lined with a stratified non-keratinized mucosal membrane (Chapter 4), as these regions are associated with a great deal of wear and tear during the passage of food.

The swallowing process

The swallowing of food, called deglutition, is aided by the moist consistency of the bolus of food resulting from the presence of saliva and mucus secreted from the lining of the mouth and oesophagus. In addition, the absence of cartilage from the posterior surface of the trachea helps to reduce friction as the food passes down the oesophagus. This is because the anterior surface of the upper section of the oesophagus lies against the posterior surface of the trachea; the presence of cartilage would make swallowing extremely uncomfortable.

The swallowing process involves a triad of responses illustrated by Figure 7.8a–d:

1 The voluntary stage. The tongue voluntarily moves the bolus of food to the back of the mouth, and then into the oropharynx. This involves the tongue rising, and pushing itself against the soft palate (Figure 7.8a).

2 The involuntary pharyngeal stage. This begins with the bolus stimulating receptors in the oropharyngeal region, resulting in an involuntary swallowing reflex. Sensory (afferent) impulses ascend to the deglutition (swallowing) centre of the medulla and lower pons of the brainstem. Parasympathetic motor (efferent) output causes the soft palate, and its extension the uvula, to move upwards, thus sealing off the nasal passageways and preventing food from entering the nasal cavity (Figure 7.8b). Parasympathetic motor impulses also cause the larynx to move upwards, sealing off the opening of the larynx, called the glottis, with the epiglottis (Figure 7.8c), and widening the space between the laryngeal pharynx and oesophagus; this aids the passage of the bolus. Once food has moved into the oesophagus, breathing is resumed with the opening of the respiratory pathway. Occasionally, when we drink liquids very quickly the sealing of the nasal passageways is too slow and the drink passes into them. Alternatively, food particles may be swallowed so fast that the sealing of the glottis is incomplete and food becomes lodged at the top of the larynx, stimulating the coughing reflex and expelling the irritant particles from the larynx.

3 The oesophageal stage. Once the bolus has entered the oesophagus specialized muscular movements called peristalsis are responsible for its transport to the stomach. Although the main function of peristalsis is to propel the food along the tube, it is inevitable that there will be friction between food boli and the oesophageal surfaces as they 'rub' against each other and this will aid physical digestion to a limited extent. Peristaltic movement of food occurs throughout the gastrointestinal tract, from the oesophagus to the final elimination via the anal canal.

The medulla of the brainstem controls the events in the first part of the oesophagus via parasympathetic motor impulses and may influence gut movements in other sections of the tract. A myenteric plexus of nerve cells is capable of generating peristaltic movements in the absence of extrinsic stimulation, however. Figure 7.8d illustrates the peristaltic process: circular muscle fibres contract immediately behind the bolus, which constricts the oesophagus in this region and forces the bolus downwards. Longitudinal fibres immediately in front of the bolus simultaneously contract, shortening and expanding the diameter of the section, allowing the forward propulsion of the bolus. The coordinated action of these muscular movements provides the appearance of a continuous wave of contraction. Swallowing also promotes the relaxation of the normally contracted cardiac sphincter and allows passage of the bolus into the stomach.

The duration of swallowing depends upon the consistency of the food (fluid-like foods travel quicker) and the body's position (upright body positions facilitate a more rapid descent). Taking these extremes into consideration, the time for the passage of boli from entering and leaving the oesophagus ranges from 1 to 8 seconds.

Table 7.4 summarizes the regulation of mouth and oesophageal function.

THE STOMACH

The stomach is a 'J'-shaped muscular organ, located immediately below the diaphragm on the left side of the abdominal cavity. Its size and shape varies according to content (the stomach's folds, or rugae, disappear when the stomach is distended), and according to which part of the respiratory cycle the person is experiencing. That is, upon inspiration the diaphragm is pulled down, and this slightly displaces the stomach downwards. With expiration the stomach extends upwards. The opening from the oesophagus, and the exit into the first region of the small intestine, are guarded by the cardiac and pyloric sphincter

Table 7.4 Regulation of the alimentary canal's activities

Region	Functional activity	Regulator of function
Mouth	Opening via jaw muscular movement	Mainly by the trigeminal nerve, but also the facial nerve
	Taste	Glossopharyngeal nerve – sensory to posterior third of tongue – and facial nerve – sensory to anterior two-thirds of the tongue
	Mastication	Trigeminal nerve
	Tongue movements	Facial nerve
	Salivary flow	Facial nerve (submandibular and sublingual glands), glossopharyngeal nerve (parotid glands)
Swallowing reflex	Upward movement of soft palate	Facial nerve
	Movement of the epiglottis over the larynx	Vagus nerve
	Oesophageal peristalsis	Facial nerve and mesenteric/Auerbach's plexus
Stomach	Entry via relaxation of the cardiac spincter	Innervated by vagus nerve
	Churning	Innervated by vagus nerve
	Gastric juice secretion	Innervated by vagus nerve. Actions of gastrin (gastric and duodenal)
	Exit via the relaxation of the pyloric sphincter	Innervated by vagus nerve
Small intestine	Peristalsic segmentation	Vagus nerve
	Pancreatic juice secretion	Cholecystokinin-pancreozymin (CCK-PZ) and secretin
	Bile secretion from the gall bladder	CCK-PZ
	Succus entericus secretion	Vagus nerve
Large intestine	Entry from the small intestine through the ileocaecal valve	Gastrocolic reflex controlled by vagus nerve
	Peristalsis	Vagus and pelvic nerves
	Exit via: 1 Relaxtion (opening) of the internal sphincter	Pelvic nerve
	2 Relaxation (opening) of the external sphincter	Voluntary controlled

muscles respectively. These are normally contracted, thus preventing passage of stomach contents. The stomach is held in position by the mesenteries of the peritoneum. Figure 7.9a illustrates the four main regions of the stomach which are:

1 The cardiac region. This surrounds the cardiac sphincter muscle.

2 The fundic region. This is the elevated rounded part around, and to the left of, the cardiac portion.

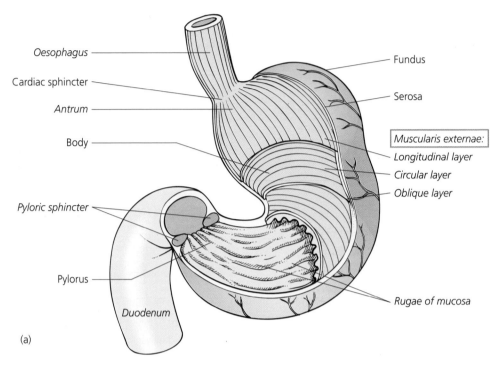

(a)

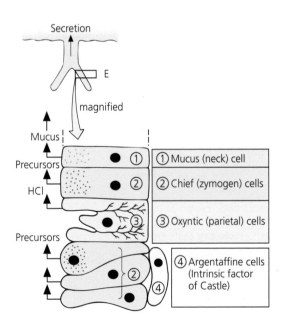

Figure 7.9 (a) The human stomach. (b) The gastric (tubular) gland.

3 The body region. This occupies most of the stomach and lies between the fundic and pyloric parts.

4 The pyloric region. This is the most inferior part of the stomach, lying superior to the pyloric sphincter.

Entry of food

The cardiac sphincter relaxes and the sphincter opens when food is present in the lower oesophagus, allowing entry of boli into the stomach. Simultaneously the pyloric sphincter, which guards the exit from the stomach, contracts so that food cannot pass immediately into the small intestine without first undergoing gastric digestion.

Physical digestion in the stomach

The stomach 'churns' food, using a mechanism peculiar to this organ. A three-dimensional muscular movement is brought about by the presence of an additional oblique muscular layer (Figure 7.9a). This movement provides a greater physical breaking down of food boli which have entered this region, and a thorough mixing of food with the stomach's chemicals, or gastric juice, thus facilitating chemical digestion.

There is regional variation in the peristalsis movements of the stomach: the fundic region exhibits only a few peristaltic waves as this is the 'storage' area of the stomach, whereby food is not mixed with gastric secretions (and so salivary amylase continues to work here), but the waves of contraction beginning in the body of the stomach become more vigorous in the inferior regions, becoming very forceful in the pylorus region. These latter waves of contraction allow liquidized foods a more rapid exit from the stomach should the pyloric sphincter relax. Contraction of the sphincter, however, seals off the exit from the stomach, resulting in the temporary backward movement of the food within the pylorus, producing a more efficient mixing of the gastric content.

Chemical digestion in the stomach

The stomach's secretion is called gastric juice, and is produced from the compound tubular glands of the gastric pits at approximately 2–3 l/day. The main function of this secretion is the conversion of the semi-solid boli of food into a semi-liquid chyme. In addition, the gastric juice contains a protease enzyme which initiates protein breakdown.

Each gastric gland possesses four types of specialized secretory cells (Figure 7.9b), which secrete separate components of the gastric juice. These cells are called mucus cells, chief cells, oxyntic cells and argentaffine cells.

Mucus (or neck) cells

Mucus cells are located mainly in the neck of the gland and secrete the mucus part of the juice. Mucus adheres to the gastric mucosal surface, and its importance is in the prevention of autodigestion of the stomach wall by the hydrochloric acid and proteolytic enzymes present in gastric juice.

Chief (zymogen) cells

Chief cells produce two enzyme precursors (inactive enzymes), pepsinogen and prorennin, which are activated by the acidic gastric juice to pepsin and rennin, respectively. Both enzymes accelerate protein digestion. Pepsin converts proteins into polypeptides (long chains of amino acids); it is an endopeptidase enzyme and so breaks the peptide bonds in places other than at the terminal peptide positions (see Figure 7.7c). Rennin converts the soluble protein of milk into an insoluble form, in order to retain it in the stomach for longer periods, so that pepsin can have its proteolytic effects. Rennin is only produced in appreciable amounts in infants as their diet is largely milk. Gastric lipase is another enzyme that is secreted into the gastric juice of infants, and this breaks down butterfat molecules in milk. It requires a pH of 5–6 for its actions, however, and so has a limited role in the adult stomach where pH values are generally lower. Adults rely on lipases secreted into the small intestine to digest lipids.

Pepsin is responsible for between 10 and 15% of all protein digestion, the rest occurring in the small intestine.

Oxyntic (parietal) cells

These cells contain intracellular channels, called canaliculi, in which hydrochloric acid is produced. The initial chemical reactions leading to hydrochloric acid production occur in the cytoplasm, but the final reactions occur in the channels away from the cytoplasm. The acid in gastric juice has the following functions:

1   Activation of the precursor enzymes.

2   Provision of the optimal pH (pH 2–3) for the action of pepsin (and rennin).

3   Inactivation of salivary amylase.

4   Bactericidal. HCl denatures the pH-dependent enzyme systems of alkali-liking bacteria present in the ingested food.

5 Dissolve splinters of bone which may have been swallowed.

Argentaffine cells

Argentaffine cells are small and fairly uncommon and are responsible for producing the intrinsic factor of Castle. This chemical is essential for the carriage of vitamin B_{12} through the stomach, and for its absorption by the small intestine. People without this factor exhibit the homeostatic imbalance of pernicious anaemia (Chapter 8).

A fifth cell type is also present in the gastric mucosa. These are specialized endocrine cells that secrete the hormone gastrin which stimulates a greater flow of gastric juice. It is released when food is present in the stomach.

Exit of food

The pyloric sphincter is usually partially open when food is present in the stomach, thus allowing liquid material to pass through very quickly. However, chyme is only semi-liquid and requires the sphincter to be completely open to allow the passage of large quantities per unit time.

Regulation of gastric functions

The secretion of gastric juice is usually related to the presence, or anticipation, of food. There are three phases which are responsible for controlling the secretion of gastric juice. These are referred to as (1) the cephalic phase, (2) the gastric phase, and (3) the intestinal phase.

The cephalic stage

This stage involves parasympathetic nerve stimulation of the stomach via the vagus nerve and is a conditioned association reflex that occurs when we smell, see, or taste food, i.e. it is preparatory for the arrival of food. It is responsible for inducing contractions of stomach muscle, which bring about churning, and an increased rate of gastric juice secretion.

Gastric phase

The presence of food in the pyloric region of the stomach results in the release of the hormone gastrin, and this aids gastric motility (muscular movement) and stimulates the increased secretion of gastric juice.

Intestinal phase

Once food comes into contact with the mucosa of the first region of the small intestine, called the duodenum, a variety of hormones (e.g. cholecystokinin-pancreozymin, or CCK-PZ, gastric inhibitory peptide, or GIP, and secretin) are released. Most of these inhibit gastric motility and gastric secretion and so delay gastric emptying. This allows more time for digestion in the duodenum, particularly of lipids. In addition, these hormones help prevent homeostatic imbalances, such as gastric ulcers occurring in the stomach as a result of excessive gastric acid secretion in the absence of food. Conversely, duodenal gastrin may also be released when the chyme is rich in proteins and polypeptides. This is identical to the stomach's gastrin and so promotes protein digestion of food remaining in the stomach.

THE SMALL INTESTINE, PANCREAS AND GALL BLADDER

General features of the small intestine

The small intestine extends from the pyloric sphincter to the ileocaecal valve located at the junction with the large intestine. It is approximately 6.5 metres in length, having a diameter of 2.5 cm. The small intestine is a coiled structure occupying a large part of the abdominal cavity. It is suspended at the posterior by the mesenteries which carry the blood and

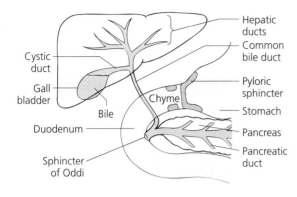

Figure 7.10 Relationship between the stomach, liver, and pancreas.

lymphatic vessels and nerves that support this area. The small intestine is the main area of digestion and absorption and is anatomically divided into three distinct regions (see Figure 7.2) as follows.

Duodenum

This is the shortest section, extending from the pyloric sphincter for approximately 25 cm. It forms a loop inferior to the stomach, and encloses the body of the pancreas. The united ducts from the gall bladder and the pancreas empty into the duodenum via the sphincter of Oddi (Figure 7.10).

Jejunum

This is approximately 2.7 metres in length extending from the duodenum to the final part of the small intestine, or the ileum. The duodenum and jejunum are both mainly concerned with digestion.

Ileum

This is approximately 3.6 metres in length and connects the small intestine with the large intestine, or caecum, via the ileocaecal valve. It is the main area of absorption.

The mucosal epithelium of the small intestine has circular folds, or plicae, projecting from which are finger-like projections called villi. The villi bear further projections called microvilli. These folds and projections increase the surface area available for digestion of the chyme and also for the process of absorption of the products of digestion. At the base of the villi are intestinal glands called crypts of Lieberkühn and these are responsible for secreting the intestinal juice. Brunner's glands are also present in the duodenal submucosa, and these produce an alkaline mucus secretion which, together with pancreatic and bile salts, neutralize the acidic chyme as it enters the duodenum from the stomach. The pH actually becomes slightly alkaline and this is conducive to the optimal functioning of intestinal enzymes. Mucus protects the intestinal wall from autodigestion by the multiple enzymes secreted into the intestine, particularly the proteases.

The pancreas

The pancreas is a triangular or oblong shaped organ. Its head lies within the loop of duodenum and the whole structure positions itself horizontally to the stomach (Figure 7.10). The pancreas is approximately 12–15 cm in length and 2.5 cm thick. Histologically it contains both exocrine and endocrine secretory cells.

Exocrine or digestive (acinar) cells

These cells are responsible for secreting precursor and active digestive enzymes into the duodenum via the pancreatic duct. Other cells produce the bicarbonate-rich, alkaline fluid into which the enzymes are secreted before being released into the duodenum.

Endocrine cells (islets of Langerhans)

These include:

1 Alpha-cells. These produce the hormone glucagon.

2 Beta-cells. These produce the hormone insulin.

3 Delta-cells. These produce the hormone somatostatin.

All three hormones are important in blood sugar regulation: insulin lowers blood glucose (it is a hypoglycaemic agent), whereas glucagon raises the blood glucose level (it is a hyperglycaemic agent). Somatostatin has a paracrine role, and inhibits insulin and glucagon secretion from beta- and alpha-cells in the locality when the blood glucose concentration is within its homeostatic range.

The pancreas is referred to as a mixed gland since it has both endocrine and exocrine tissue. Its exocrine roles are described below and the endocrine roles are considered in more detail in Chapter 15.

The gall bladder

This pear-shaped organ is approximately 7–9 cm in length and is attached to the undersurface of the liver. Its function is to store and concentrate bile and to secrete it into the bile ducts which unite with the pancreatic duct and enter the duodenum via the sphincter of Oddi (Figure 7.10). Bile is synthesized within the liver.

Physical digestion in the small intestine

The principal movement within the small intestine is called segmentation and is illustrated by Figure 7.11a–c. This mechanism involves a series of isolated contractions in alternating, localized positions. The contractions of circular muscle fibres constrict the tube, segmenting the food chyme into smaller masses. Next the muscle fibres within the individual segments contract, with the result that further smaller masses are produced. Then as the muscle fibres relax the larger segments are reformed. The overall results are that food particles are mechanically broken into smaller particles, and there is a thorough mixing of the food with digestive juices.

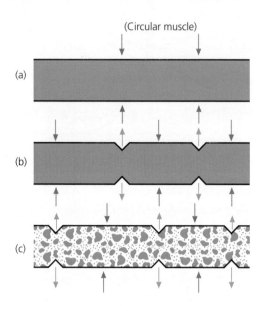

Figure 7.11 Segmentation: (a) semi–liquid chyme in one mass; (b) chyme segmented via isolated contraction of circular muscle fibres; (c) chyme segmented further as other areas contract. Note: relaxation occurs as an inevitable consequence of contraction.

Segmentation stops periodically and a wave of peristalsis moves the food further along the intestine. This movement also contributes to the physical breakdown of food as friction occurs between the food and the intestinal wall. Peristaltic movement is weaker in this region compared with the oesophagus and stomach, and so food is retained in the small intestine for longer periods of time, reflecting the time required for digestion to be completed.

Bile

Bile is a yellow-green alkaline (pH 7.6–8.6) fluid. Approximately 80–100 ml bile are produced by the liver daily, and are transported to the gall bladder by the hepatic and cystic ducts (Figure 7.10). Bile is stored and concentrated in this organ until it is required in the small intestine. Bile is mainly a watery secretion; other components include bile salts, bile pigments, cholesterol, lecithin, mucus, and several types of ion. It has two principal functions as follows.

Physical digestion by bile

Bile is frequently not recognized as being involved in 'mechanical' digestion because it is a chemical secretion. Bile salts (sodium taurocholate and sodium glycocholate) and lecithin, however, are responsible for emulsification, i.e. the reduction of large globules of fat (lipids exist as globules, in a watery intestinal chyme solution) into small droplets. Thus, this process falls more under the broad heading of physical breakdown, since there are no enzymes involved. The increased surface area produced by emulsification aids the actions of digestive enzymes (lipases) to catalyse the chemical breakdown of lipids. The emulsification process is rather like pouring cooking oil into water. As the large globule of oil enters the water it disperses into smaller fat droplets, increasing the total surface area.

After bile salts have performed their digestive function, they are then involved in another homeostatic function by aiding the absorption of long-chain fatty acids (see later). Most of the salts are reabsorbed in the process and recycled by the liver into bile. A further homeostatic function of bile salts is to contribute to the alkaline medium within the intestine, which buffers the acidic chyme and produces a pH at which intestinal enzymes operate with maximum efficiency.

Excretory function of bile

The bile pigments, bilirubin (rubin = red) and biliverdin (verdi = green), are produced by the liver from the breakdown of haemoglobin released when aged erythrocytes are destroyed. The liver removes the iron and protein (globin) part of haemoglobin; these are then homeostatically recycled (see later). The remaining parts of haemoglobin comprise the bile pigments, the principal one being bilirubin. When the bile is secreted into the intestine, this pigment is converted into urobilinogen and stercobilin. The former is absorbed into blood and then transported to the kidneys where it becomes responsible for the yellow colorization of urine, whereas the latter remains in the intestine and is responsible for colouring the faeces. These components of faeces and urine are genuine excretory products as they have been involved in cellular metabolism (which differentiates them from the indigestible material present in faeces).

Chemical digestion in the small intestine

Chyme entering the small intestine consists of a mixture of nutrients (Table 7.5). These include:

1 Members of the carbohydrate family. These consist of various polysaccharides, arising from partially digested starches. Some disaccharides, such as maltose, may be present, reflecting some success on the part of salivary amylase activity. In addition, depending upon what food was consumed, other disaccharides may be present such as lactose (milk sugar) and sucrose (cane or table sugar). The monsaccharides glucose, fructose (fruit sugar) and galactose (grape sugar) may also have been taken in.

2 Fats are not digested up to this point and enter the small intestine in their consumed chemical form, consisting mainly of triglycerides.

3 Polypeptides are present as a result of the proteolytic actions of gastric pepsin.

4 Vitamins, minerals, and water. These nutrients, together with monosaccharide molecules, are not digested because they are small enough to be absorbed across the gut wall. The rest of the components of chyme must be chemically digested and the small

Table 7.5 Action of the enzymes of the human alimentary tract

Enzyme	Site of secretion	Site of action	Substrate acted upon	Products of action
Salivary amylase	Mouth	Mouth	Starch	Disaccharides (few), dextrins (mainly)
Pepsinogen→pepsin	Stomach	Stomach	Proteins	Polypeptides
Pancreatic amylase	Pancreas	Small intestine	Starch	Disaccharides (maltase)
Enterokinase	Small intestine	Small intestine	Trypsinogen	Trypsin
Trypsinogen→trypsin	Pancreas	Small intestine	Polypeptides/chymotrypsinogen	Peptides/chymotrypsin
Chymotrypsinogen→chymotrypsin	Pancreas	Small intestine	Polypeptides	Peptides
Carboxypeptidases	Pancreas	Small intestine	Peptides	Smaller peptides (oligopeptides)
Aminopeptidases	Pancreas	Small intestine	Peptides	Smaller peptides (oligopeptides)
Lipase	Pancreas	Small intestine	Triglycerides	Diglycerides, monoglycerides, fatty acids, glycerol
Nucleases	Pancreas	Small intestine	Nucleic acids	Nucleotides
Disaccharidases (maltase, sucrase, lactase)	Small intestine	Small intestine	Disaccharides (maltose, sucrose, lactose)	Monosaccharides (glucose, fructose, galactose)
Peptidases	Small intestine	Small intestine	Oligopeptides	Amino acids
Nucleotidases	Small intestine	Small intestine	Nucleotides	Nucleosides, phosphoric acid
Nucleosidases	Small intestine	Small intestine	Nucleosides	Sugars, purines, pyrimidines

intestine initiates and completes these processes via secretions of the pancreas and the intestinal mucosa.

Digestive secretions of the pancreas

Approximately 1200–1500 ml of pancreatic juice are produced and secreted daily. Water is again the main constituent of this clear, colour-less secretion. Other constituents include:

1 Pancreatic salts. The most common salt is sodium bicarbonate. These salts contribute to the alkalinity (pH 7.1–8.2) of pancreatic juice. The neutralizing effect of this juice, of bile salts and of intestinal secretions on gastric acid as it enters the duodenum has already been described.

2 'Protein' digesting enzymes (i.e. proteases) but more accurately called polypeptidases or polypeptide digesting enzymes. Pancreatic juice contains two endopepti-dases (i.e. enzymes which act on peptide bonds within the protein molecule), called trypsin and chymotrypsin. Figure 7.12 illus-trates how both are secreted into the duode-num as the precursors trypsinogen and chymotrypsinogen respectively. These are rapidly activated within the duodenum. Trypsinogen is activated by an enzyme called enterokinase that is secreted from the duodenal mucosa. Once trypsin is produced, this activates a further conversion of trypsinogen into trypsin (an example of a positive feedback response) and also converts chymotrypsinogen into its active form, chymotrypsin. Being endopeptidases they break down large polypeptide fragments into smaller and smaller subunits called peptides (see Figure 7.7c).

  A further role of trypsin is the activation of another pancreatic precursor, called procarboxypolypeptidase. Once activated, this operates as an exopeptidase (an enzyme which acts on peptide bonds at the end of a

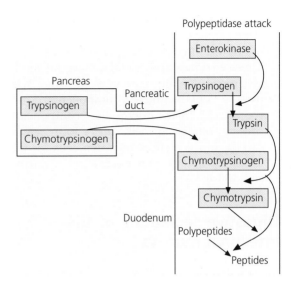

Figure 7.12 Action of trypsin/chymotrypsin (endopeptidases).

protein molecule), breaking down the termi-nal peptide bond and exposing the carboxylic acid part of the amino acid molecule (see Figure 7.7c). Exopeptidases gradually remove terminal amino acids one at a time from the ends of the chain until a dipeptide is formed (two amino acids connected by a peptide bond).

3 Carbohydrate digesting enzyme, or pancre-atic amylase. This active enzyme breaks down remaining polysaccharides into the disaccharide sugar maltose (Table 7.5).

4 Fat digesting enzyme, or pancreatic lipase. This enzyme, together with intestinal lipase, detaches fatty acids from glycerol one at a time (triglyceride fat molecules consist of three fatty acids attached to a glycerol molecule; Chapter 3). A mixture of the following may therefore be found in the duodenum: triglycerides, diglycerides, monoglyceride, glycerol, and free fatty acids (Figure 7.7b). Lipases continue their break-down actions until all the fatty acids are removed from the ingested lipids.

5 Nucleic acid digesting enzymes, or nucle-ases. These include ribonucleases, which act

on RNA, deoxyribonucleases, which act on DNA, and nucleosidases and nucleotidases, which act on DNA fragments (Table 7.5). These enzymes are essential since all foods consumed are of cellular origin and will usually contain nuclear components. Thus we must break down the components present, rendering them into a form which can be utilized within our own cells for the synthesis of our own nucleic acids during cell division.

Digestive secretions of the intestinal mucosa

Intestinal juice, called succus entericus, is a clear yellow alkaline (pH 7.6) fluid produced at a rate of 2–3 l/day from Brunner's glands in the duodenum and from the crypts of Lieberkühn in the ileum. The juice is mostly of a watery constitution, but includes a variety of digestive enzymes (summarized in Table 7.5). These enzymes are concerned with the final chemical breakdown of ingested foods. These include:

1 'Protein' digesting enzymes, more correctly termed peptidases. A variety of dipeptidases are present in intestinal juice. These enzymes are responsible for breaking down dipeptides into individual amino acids respectively. At this point protein digestion is complete and the end products of protein digestion, amino acids, can now be absorbed into the circulation.

2 Carbohydrate digesting enzymes, or disaccharidases. This group includes three enzymes which are responsible for digesting disaccharides (molecules of two simple sugar units) into their constituent monosaccharides. The enzymes are named after the disaccharide which they break down. Thus, maltase catabolizes the disaccharide maltose into its two constituent glucose molecules, lactase converts lactose into glucose and its other monosaccharide component galactose, and sucrase converts sucrose into glucose

and fructose. Carbohydrate digestion is now complete and monosaccharides can be absorbed into blood.

3 Fat digesting enzymes, or lipases. These operate in the same way as pancreatic lipases, i.e. they cleave fatty acids from glycerol. The breakdown products of fats are now absorbed into the blood and lymphatic circulations.

4 Intestinal nucleases have also been identified and share the catabolic functions with pancreatic nucleases; they break down nucleic acids within the food chyme.

Regulation of the functions of the small intestine

The control of intestinal motility and secretions is mainly hormonal. However, parasympathetic neurons (via vagus, splanchnic, and pelvic nerves) also play a part. The presence of food, and the resultant mechanical stimulation of the intestinal walls by food, causes a release of a variety of hormones. The main ones are as follows:

1 Secretin. This hormone is released in response to the presence of an acidic chyme in the duodenum (having entered from the stomach) and it causes the release of an alkali-rich pancreatic juice in order to buffer this acidity.

2 Cholecystokinin-pancreozymin (CCK-PZ). This hormone was once thought to be two separate hormones, hence its complex name. It stimulates the release of bile from the gall bladder (once called the cholecystic gland, hence cholecystokinin) and an enzyme rich pancreatic juice (hence pancreozymin). The stimulus for its release is a nutrient-rich chyme in the duodenum, in particular the presence of fats (note the role of bile in fat digestion).

3 Motilin. This hormone is responsible for stimulating a more forceful contraction of the intestinal muscles. It is thought to have

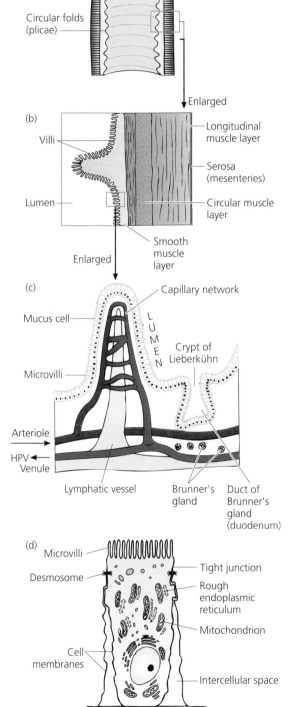

(a)
Circular folds (plicae)

Enlarged

(b)
Villi
Lumen
Enlarged

Longitudinal muscle layer
Serosa (mesenteries)
Circular muscle layer
Smooth muscle layer

(c)
Mucus cell
Microvilli
Arteriole
HPV
Venule
Lymphatic vessel

Capillary network
L U M E N
Crypt of Lieberkühn
Brunner's gland
Duct of Brunner's gland (duodenum)

(d)
Microvilli
Desmosome
Cell membranes

Tight junction
Rough endoplasmic reticulum
Mitochondrion
Intercellular space

a role to promote a greater movement of food along the tract, particularly in the small intestine.

4 The secretion of intestinal 'juice' is thought to result from the mechanical contact of food with the intestinal mucosa. The exact mechanism of release, whether it be hormonally or neurally controlled, is uncertain. The intestine is a rich source of putative hormones, i.e. substances with demonstrable action but which have yet to be accepted as genuine chemical messengers.

ABSORPTION

Absorption is the process whereby the end products of digestion (i.e. monosaccharides, amino acids, fatty acids, glycerol), and the ingested 'soluble' substances which do not need to be broken down (vitamins, minerals, water, and consumed monosaccharides), are transported from the lumen of the alimentary tract into the body's transporting systems. Most are absorbed directly into blood, although some end products, such as long-chain fatty acids, are absorbed into the lymphatic circulation. The ileum accounts for 90% of absorption and is anatomically adapted for this process (Figure 7.13a–d). Adaptations include:

1 A large surface area. The ileum is very long (approximately 6.5 metres), and the surface area of its lining is increased by many circular folds (plicae) and the finger-like projections, villi, and microvilli.

2 A very thin absorptive epithelium. The ileum's mucosal membrane is a simple columnar epithelium. This is constantly being damaged and worn away, and so cells must be mitotically active (especially at the bases of the villi) in order to replace the cell loss.

Figure 7.13 Villi: (a) longitudinal section of duodenum showing circular folds; (b) vertical section through one circular fold; (c) vertical section through one villus; (d) enlarged intestinal cell.

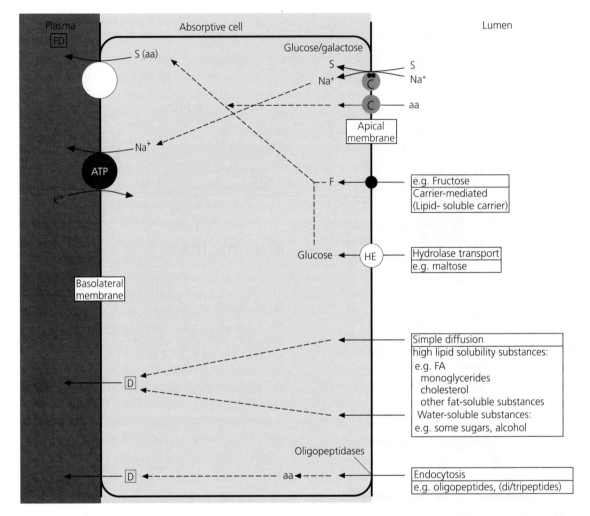

Figure 7.14 The transport mechanism of absorption in the ileum: aa, amino acid; C, carrier; D, diffusion; FA, fatty acid; FD, facilitated diffusion; S, sugar; HE, hydrolysing enzyme.

3 An extensive blood and lymphatic supply to the villi.

4 A small extracellular space between the absorptive cell and the blood capillaries and lymphatic vessels.

5 The walls of the blood and lymphatic vessels consist of a squamous (i.e. thin) endothelium.

The remaining 10% of the end products of digestion are absorbed by the mouth, stomach, and large intestine. Oral absorption is clinically useful. For example, the drug glyceryl trinitrate (GTN), used to treat angina, is absorbed sublingually (under the tongue), providing a quick entry to the blood. The result is a rapid dilatation of coronary blood vessels, leading to an improved delivery of arterial oxygen to the cardiac muscle and so removing the ischaemic anginal pain. Substances absorbed by the stomach include glucose, salts, a little water, and vitamin B_{12}. Alcohol is mainly absorbed in the small intestine (80%), but the remainder is absorbed by the stomach, hence its rapid effects. A large intake of a protein-containing meal decreases the rate of alcohol absorption from the stomach. Absorption by the large intestine, particularly the colon, is mainly that of water, although most of this is absorbed by the ileum.

Nutrient absorption in the ileum

Absorption of materials occurs specifically through the epithelial membranes of villi. The process depends upon mechanisms involving facilitated and passive diffusion, osmosis, active transport, and pinocytosis. These mechanisms were discussed in Chapter 2 and it is advised at this point that the reader should re-familiarize him/herself with these processes. Figure 7.14 summarizes the main processes involved in absorption.

There are two stages in the absorption process. First, the nutrient components must enter the luminal side (the apical membrane) of the epithelial cell and this involves a variety of different mechanisms, described below. Second, the materials must leave via the lamina propria (or basolateral membrane) surface of the mucosal epithelial cell into the blood capillaries and central lymphatics, or lacteals. This mainly relies on passive diffusion.

MONOSACCHARIDE ABSORPTION

Fructose is transported into the epithelial cell by carrier-mediated facilitated diffusion, whereas glucose and galactose molecules are cotransported with sodium. Glucose and sodium share the same carrier protein, which contains two specific receptor sites, one for glucose, the other for sodium, and both need to be occupied before transport can take place. Monosaccharide absorption is completed by the terminal part of the ileum.

AMINO ACID ABSORPTION

This occurs mainly in the duodenum and the jejunum. Cotransport with sodium is again the mechanism involved. Occasionally, dipeptides and tripeptides are absorbed into epithelial cells by pinocytosis and the final stages of their digestion occur within those cells.

FATTY ACID ABSORPTION

There are two mechanisms concerned with fatty acid absorption depending upon the length of the fatty acid chain. Short-chain fatty acids (i.e. those with fewer than 10–12 carbon atoms), pass into the epithelial cell and thence out into the circulation by simple diffusion because of their high lipid solubility. This accounts for approximately 20% of fat transported. Most dietary fats, however, contain long-chain fatty acids (those with more than 12 carbons atoms) and these must combine with fat-soluble vitamins (A, D, E, and K), glycerol, monoglycerides, and bile salts to form a micelle-like structure which is pinocytosed into the epithelial cell (Figure 7.15). Once inside the cell, the micelle breaks down into its component parts. The bile salts and fat-soluble vitamins diffuse into blood, whereas the free fatty acids are combined with glycerol and monoglycerides to form triglycerides. Thus, the initial digestion of dietary fats is simply to facilitate the formation of this micelle so that fats, fat-soluble vitamins, and bile salts could collectively pass over the apical membrane of the epithelial cell.

Within the epithelial cell the triglycerides next become coated with a lipoprotein coat to form water-soluble structures called chylomicrons. These diffuse into the lacteals of a villus and are then transported into the thoracic lymphatic duct which drains into the circulation at the junction of the left subclavian and left jugular veins in the neck (Chapter 10). Finally, they arrive at the liver through the hepatic artery. Cells which metabolize these substances contain lipoproteases, to break down the coat of the chylomicron, and triglyceridases, to release individual fatty acids.

WATER-SOLUBLE VITAMINS (C AND B COMPLEXES)

These are absorbed by diffusion, although for vitamin B_{12} absorption conjugation with the stomach's intrinsic factor of Castle is necessary.

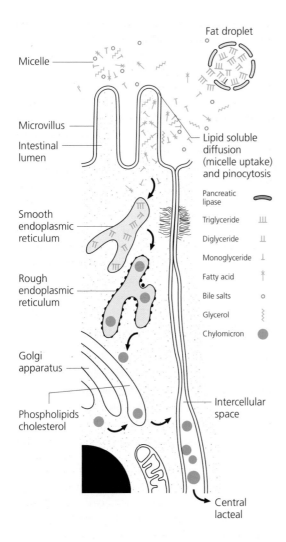

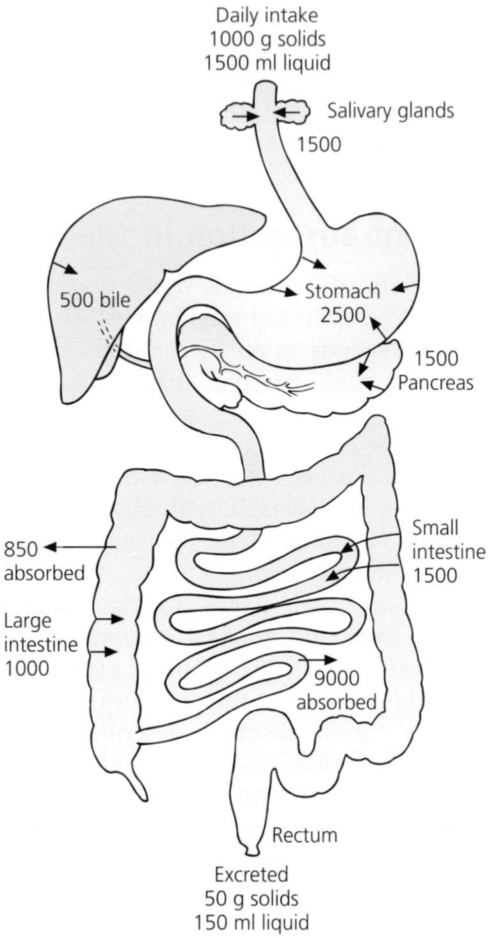

Figure 7.15 Transport of lipids from intestinal lumen through absorptive cells and into the interstitial space. Products of triglyceride digestion – monoglycerides, fatty acids, and glycerol – form micelles with the bile salts in solution. They enter the absorptive cell by pinocytosis across the microvillous membrane. Within the cell the products accumulate in the smooth endoplasmic reticulum, from which they are passed to the rough endoplasmic reticulum. There, they are resynthesized into triglycerides and, together with a smaller amount of phospholipids and cholesterol, are stored in the Golgi apparatus as chylomicrons – droplets about 150 nm diameter. These then leave the basolateral portions of the cell by exocytosis.

Figure 7.16 Water fluxes in the human alimentary canal, in millilitres. Figures vary with the condition and size of the subject.

WATER

Approximately 9 litres of water a day is absorbed. This is comprised of 1–2 litres from an ingested source (this varies depending upon thirst and social habits), and the remainder is from the accumulation of gastrointestinal secretions. As Figure 7.16 illustrates, the main area of absorption is the small intestine which absorbs some 8–8.5 litres; the remainder is absorbed in the colon of the large intestine in order to consolidate the faeces. The absorption

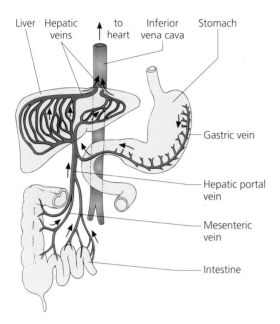

Figure 7.17 The hepatic portal system. Blood is carried directly from the stomach and intestines to the liver via the mesenteric, gastric, and hepatic portal veins. Hepatic veins then convey it to the heart by way of the inferior vena cava.

of water into ileal epithelial cells, and then into the blood capillaries lining the villi, is via osmosis, and is promoted by the absorption of electrolytes and digested foods.

ELECTROLYTES

These are absorbed from gastrointestinal secretions and from ingested components, and help to maintain electrolyte homeostasis. In addition to active transport, electrolytes can also move in and out of cells by diffusion. Negatively charged ions (anions), such as chloride, iodide and nitrates, passively follow positive ions (cations), such as sodium. Parathyroid hormone (PTH) and, in particular, vitamin D are important in regulating the active transport of calcium from the gut (Chapters 12 and 15). Iron, magnesium, phosphate and potassium absorption is dependent upon active transport methods.

Absorbed products pass via capillaries into venules which drain from the intestinal wall into larger veins. These then link up with veins from other areas of absorption (stomach and colon) to form the hepatic portal vein. This large vessel carries the end products of digestion directly to the liver (Figure 7.17). All the absorbed components take this route except long chain fatty acids, which pass to the liver via the hepatic artery after being drained into the lymphatic system as previously mentioned. The liver assimilates the products and has a role in the homeostatic control of the blood concentrations of some components. Some products of digestion, or products of liver synthesis, are then transported in blood to the specific cells of the body which require them to sustain their intracellular homeostatic processes.

THE LARGE INTESTINE

General features of the large intestine

The large intestine extends from the ileocaecal valve to the external sphincter muscle of the anus and is approximately 1.5–2 metres in length. It has a wider diameter (approximately 6.5 cm) than the small intestine, hence its name. The longitudinal muscle layer forms three bands, called taeniae, which are maintained in a tonic state of contraction, giving this part of the intestine a 'pouched' appearance. Structurally the large intestine has four main areas: the caecum, the colon, rectum, and anal canal.

Caecum

This is the first pouch. Inferiorly, it leads to a blind ending tube of lymphatic tissue called the appendix.

Colon

This initially consists of the ascending colon, which is superior to the caecum on the right abdominal side. The ascending colon passes vertically to the transverse colon, which lies just under the inferior surface of the liver. This extends across the abdominal cavity until it becomes the descending colon on the left side of the abdomen. After descending, the colon becomes the sigmoid colon, which projects to become the third principal part, the rectum.

Rectum

This is approximately 16–20 cm long and lies anterior to the sacrum and coccyx bones. Its terminal 2–3 cm becomes the fourth principal part, the anal canal.

Anal canal

This area is richly supplied with arteries and veins, its opening to the exterior is called the anus and is regulated by two sphincter muscles; the internal one is involuntarily controlled, whereas the external sphincter is under voluntary control.

Homeostatic functions

Homeostatic functions of the large intestine include:

1 Storage of indigestible food until it is eliminated from the body.

2 Secretion of mucus, which ensures lubrication of the faeces and eases the elimination process. Mucus also contributes to the alkaline pH of this region, because it contains HCO_3^- ions.

3 Absorption of most of the remaining water, electrolytes, and some vitamins. The amount of water absorbed depends upon the length of time that the residue of food remains in the colon. Of this residue 70% is eliminated within 72 hours of ingestion, the remainder may stay in the colon for a week or longer. The longer it stays there the more water will be absorbed.

4 Vitamins K and some of the B complexes (B_1, B_2, and folic acid) are produced by symbiotic bacteria within the colon. The small amounts of vitamin synthesized are not nutritionally significant, unless the individual has a diet which is deficient in these vital nutrients, in which case this may be regarded as a crude homeostatic mechanism for the maintenance of these vitamins in blood. The small amount of vitamin B_{12} produced is also insignificant as the vitamin is absorbed only in the small intestine, thus any in the colon is eliminated.

Colonic bacteria also ferment any remaining carbohydrates, releasing gases (carbon dioxide, hydrogen, and methane) which contribute to flatulence. The amount of flatulence varies depending upon the amount and type of food consumed. For example baked beans, onions, etc. increase the rate of fermentation and so lead to an increased flatulence. Bacteria also metabolize any remaining proteins and fatty acids in the gut, and convert bilirubin into urobilinogen and stercobilirubin, which are responsible for the characteristic colour of the urine and faeces respectively. Sluggish colonic movement is more conducive to bacterial growth, and these bacteria are potentially pathogenic if released in other areas of the body. For example, if released into the abdominal cavity they may cause inflammation of the peritoneum, called peritonitis. Long-term antibiotic therapy results in a loss of these symbiotic bacteria and encourages the colonization of this area with other potentially pathogenic antibiotic-resistant bacteria.

5 Consolidation of faeces. The caecum and ascending colon continue to absorb water, and the semi-liquid chyme is converted to a semi-solid faeces. Components of the faeces include some water, inorganic salts, bacteria and components of bacterial decomposition, alimentary canal cells which have sloughed off, indigestible remains (cellulose and vegetable fibres, known as roughage or fibre), small amounts of the end products of digestion which have not yet been absorbed, and excretory products (bile salts, bile pigments and mucus).

6 Defecation. Rectal distension as a consequence of the accumulation of faecal matter stimulates rectal wall receptors which send sensory (afferent) neuronal input to the sacral region of the spinal cord. This results in parasympathetic motor output to the rectum and anal canal, thus completing the reflex arc. Simultaneously, impulses pass via the spinal cord to the cerebral cortex, so that we can voluntarily inhibit defecation if necessary.

Defecation results from longitudinal muscle contraction which causes a reduction in length of the rectum, thus increasing the pressure within it. This increased pressure, together with voluntary contractions of diaphragmatic and abdominal muscles, forces the internal sphincter open and the faeces are expelled through the anus via the voluntarily relaxed external anal sphincter muscle (which is usually in a state of tonic contraction; this voluntary control is learnt through one's potty training). The degree of rectal muscle contraction and 'straining' required depends upon the consistency of the faeces.

The gastrocolonic reflex is an important stimulus for defecation. This reflex occurs two to three times daily, usually following meals, and increases peristaltic wave activity to move food along the colon. This is more noticeable after breakfast, because it is eaten when the stomach is empty. The gastrocolonic reflex results in an increased contraction of the terminal ileum, relaxing the ileocaecal valve and stimulating colonic peristalsis. This reflex, therefore, allows filling of the colon, and as a consequence, a mass movement of food residue occurs. The subject becomes aware of this only when the faeces enter the rectum.

THE LIVER

The liver is the largest gland in the body. The bulk of the liver occupies the right upper quadrant, or hypochondrium, of the abdominal cavity under cover of the lower ribs, which function to protect it. On the left side of the abdomen the liver lies superior to the upper part of the stomach. Above the liver is the diaphragm, anterior to it is the anterior abdominal wall and below it are the stomach, gall bladder, bile ducts, duodenum, right colonic flexure of the colon, the right kidney, and adrenal glands (see Figure 7.2).

The liver is responsible for approximately 55% of the total weight at birth and is largely responsible for the protruberant abdomen of infancy. As growth rate slows during childhood there is a corresponding decline in metabolism and, as a result, the liver becomes proportionately smaller and in the adult represents approximately 2.5% of the body weight. The liver is soft, and is extremely red due to its rich blood supply (approximately one-fifth of the liver weight is blood). Lacerations of the liver are dangerous as the individual bleeds profusely and such injuries are difficult to repair.

Anatomy

The liver is almost entirely covered by peritoneum. It has two main lobes – a large right and a smaller left lobe – separated from each other by ligaments. The right lobe is associated with two further lobes called the inferior quadrate and posterior caudate. The hepatic portal vein from the gastrointestinal tract enters the liver on its lower surface, and subdivides into smaller and smaller vessels, which finally enter an anastomosing system of smaller blood spaces, or sinusoids.

The lobes of the liver are composed of microscopic structural and functional units known as the liver lobules (Figure 7.18a). Each lobule is surrounded by a hexagonal capsule of connective tissue, called Glisson's capsule. Internally each lobule consists of chains, or cords of cells referred to as hepatocytes. Cords are arranged radially around a central vein. Between the cords are found the blood and bile sinusoids, which are equivalent to the circulatory capillaries of other tissues and allow an exchange of substances between hepatocytes, blood, and bile channels.

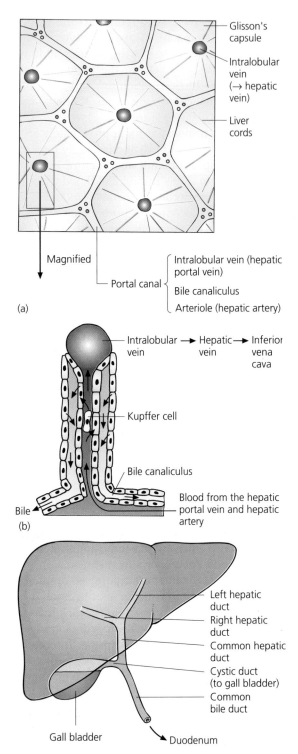

(a)

Magnified

Portal canal
- Intralobular vein (hepatic portal vein)
- Bile canaliculus
- Arteriole (hepatic artery)

Glisson's capsule

Intralobular vein (→ hepatic vein)

Liver cords

(b)

Intralobular vein → Hepatic vein → Inferior vena cava

Kupffer cell

Bile canaliculus

Bile

Blood from the hepatic portal vein and hepatic artery

Left hepatic duct
Right hepatic duct
Common hepatic duct
Cystic duct (to gall bladder)
Common bile duct

Gall bladder

Duodenum

Figure 7.18 (a) Magnified view of several liver lobules. (b) Magnified view of one liver cord. (c) Bile ducts.

The blood sinusoids carry hepatic arterial (from an interlobular arteriole) and hepatic portal (from interlobular veins) blood from the edge of each corner of the hexagonal capsule to the central vein. Of the hepatic circulation, 80% of the blood is from the portal vein and 20% is from the hepatic artery, and so these sinusoids contain a mixture of oxygen-rich arterial blood and nutrient-rich (portal) venous blood. Oxygen, nutrients, and certain poisons, such as alcohol, are extracted by the hepatocytes for assimilation or detoxification (see below). Also present within the sinusoids are reticuloendothelial, or Kupffer cells, which destroy aged erythrocytes, leucocytes, and bacteria. Sinusoidal blood drains into the intralobular, or central vein, which is a tributary of the hepatic vein that drains blood from the liver into the inferior vena cava and thence to the heart.

Bile channels are concerned with the transport of bile produced from the hepatocytes lining them. Flow of bile is in the opposite direction to that of blood, and so flows towards one of the small bile channels, or bile canaliculi, present at the corners of the hexagonal capsule (Figure 7.18b).

Thus, the corners of each liver lobule contain branches of the hepatic artery, the hepatic portal vein, and a bile canaliculus. This collection of vessels is sometimes referred to as a hepatic triad. The latter drain into the right and left hepatic ducts which then form the common hepatic duct, and this transports the bile into the gall bladder via the cystic duct (Figure 7.18c). Bile is stored and concentrated in this bladder until it is required by the duodenum. Bile production and the regulation of its release was discussed earlier in this chapter.

Homeostatic roles of the liver

The liver is an extremely important homeostatic organ. It is vital in the intermediate metabolism of many end products of digestion and has a homeostatic role as an assimilatory organ. It also has an exocrine role in the secretion of bile, which is conveyed to the gall bladder. The liver's homeostatic functions are as follows.

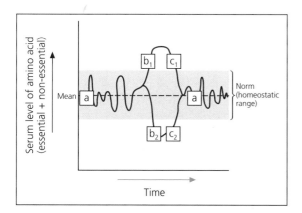

Figure 7.19 The liver's utilization of the end products of globin breakdown.
a, Homeostatic pool of serum amino acids (aa; essential and non–essential).
b_1, aa above their homeostatic range as a result of post–absorption of a protein–rich meal (and/or excessive haemolysis (breakdown) of erythrocytes).
b_2, aa below their homeostatic range due to insufficient dietary protein.
c_1, restoration of (i) serum non–essential aa levels via deamination of the excess into urea (ornithine cycle) and energy (glycolysis and Krebs cycle).
c_2, increased non–essential aa via transaminating excess of some aa into those below their homeostatic range and/or proteolytic breakdown and/or increased dietary intake; (ii) increased essential aa via increased dietary intake.

Assimilation

The liver is part of the reticuloendothelial system which is involved in breaking down worn-out erythrocytes (Chapter 8) and removing the useful components of haemoglobin. For example, iron is extracted and used to maintain its homeostatic range within blood, in order to support the metabolic reactions that require it, such as the production of 'new' erythrocytes to replace homeostatically the loss of 'old' ones. The globin part of the haemoglobin molecule is catabolized into its constituent amino acids which are added to the essential and non-essential amino acid 'pool' within blood to help maintain their individual homeostatic values. If some of the non-essential amino acids are already within their homeostatic range, then these can be converted, or transaminated, into other non-essential amino acids if

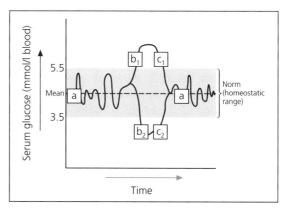

Figure 7.20 The liver's role in blood glucose regulation.
a, Normal blood glucose level.
b_1, elevation post–absorption of a meal.
b_2, decreased glucose levels due to greater cellular uptake for increased metabolism.
c_1, glucose in excess of its homeostatic range taken into hepatocytes and skeletal muscle cells mediated by insulin's effects. Consequently, intracellular levels rise and this is used in cellular respiration and in promoting a glucose store in the form of glycogen (glycogenesis). If glycogen stores are full, the excess glucose is converted into fat (lipogenesis) within to fat stores throughout the body.
c_2, depressed glucose levels in blood are corrected by measures such as glycogenolysis (i.e. convert glycogen to glucose). If levels remain low, lipolysis and proteolysis (fat and protein breakdown respectively) occurs. The latter occurs only in severe starvation states. c_2 events mediated by glucagon, somatomedin, adrenaline, noradrenaline, thyroxine, and sympathetic nervous system, which act to increase glucose availability.

necessary (Figure 7.19). Conversely, if these amino acids are already within their homeostatic range, the excess may be broken down, or deaminated, into urea by the ornithine cycle of reactions (some of the urea is excreted) and also is converted into glucose-like compounds which are metabolized to form energy via glycolysis and Krebs' cycle (Chapter 6).

Excess glucose molecules are taken from sinusoids into the hepatocytes to maintain blood glucose concentrations homeostatically (Figure 7.20). As a consequence of this uptake, the intracellular glucose within the hepatocytes may rise above its homeostatic range, and thus the excess must be removed. Some of the excess is used in cellular respiration in order to sustain normal metabolic processes, the remainder is anabolized into the storage component glycogen by a process called glycogenesis. If there is still intracellular excess of glucose when the cell stores of glycogen are full, then this excess is converted into fat by a process called lipogenesis. Note that these mechanisms are reversible, so that when blood glucose concentrations are low the glucose stores (first glycogen, then fats) are converted back to glucose in order homeostatically to raise the blood glucose level.

The fat-soluble vitamins (A, D, E, and K), together with the minerals iron (Fe) and copper (Cu) are stored by hepatocytes when the absorption of a meal produces blood levels in excess of their individual homeostatic ranges. Excess water-soluble vitamins (C and B complexes), together with water and other minerals, pass through the sinusoids, except for that which is taken into hepatocytes for their metabolic needs, as the liver cannot store them, transfer them into other substances, or destroy them. These excesses are then removed by the body's excretory organs in order to maintain their individual homeostatic levels (Figure 7.21).

Excess fatty acids and glycerol are converted into glucose only if hypoglycaemia is present and the individual has inadequate glycogen stores. Otherwise, these substances pass through the liver to the storage regions of the body, i.e. the adipose tissues.

Secretory functions

The liver secretes bile salts, which are important in the emulsification process and in the absorption of fats, phospholipids, and lipoproteins. The anticoagulant heparin, and the plasma proteins, are also synthesized by the liver.

Detoxification/deactivation functions

The liver contains detoxifying enzymes which are responsible for transforming poisons such as alcohol into harmless substances. Similarly, ammonia produced when excess amino acids

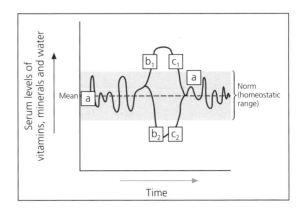

Figure 7.21 The liver's role in vitamin, mineral, and water regulation.
a, Normal levels of vitamins, minerals, and water pre-absorption.
b_1, increased levels of vitamins, minerals, and water above their homeostatic range (HR), following dietary intake.
b_2, decreased levels of vitamins, minerals, and water below their HR as these nutrients are used in metabolism.
c_1, excess fat–soluble vitamins (A, D, E, and K), minerals (iron and copper) are stored in hepatocytes. Excess water–soluble vitamins (C and B complexes), minerals and water pass through the liver to the excretory organs in order to restore their HR.
c_2, corrective measures to restore these nutrients to within their serum HR, i.e. the liver releases its stores of fat–soluble vitamins and iron, copper. Water–soluble vitamins, other minerals, and water must be consumed in the diet to restore their HR.

are deaminated to provide energy is converted into urea. Moderate amounts of urea are harmless to the body, and the excess is easily excreted by the kidneys and the sweat glands. Various hormones are also deactivated by the liver, thus reducing their blood concentrations and hence physiological activities.

Storage functions

In addition to the storage of the various nutrients, the liver also stores some poisons that cannot be catabolized and excreted (for example, DDT).

Other functions

Because liver cells have hundreds of enzymes, it is responsible for at least as many important homeostatic functions some of which remain to be identified. For example, the liver, together with the kidneys, is involved in the activation of vitamin D, and it indirectly contributes to the regulation of blood pressure by synthesizing angiotensinogen, the precursor of the hormone angiotensin. The liver's role in cholesterol metabolism is discussed in Chapter 6.

Heat production

As a result of the liver being involved in a large number of metabolic reactions, it is inevitable that many of these give off heat. Thus, the liver is an important contributor to thermoregulation.

Examples of homeostatic failure and principles of correction

A person's nutritional status can be compared with scientific tables of 'ideal' weight for height and build or can be explored more specifically. This section is mainly concerned with the common regional problems associated with the alimentary canal, starting at the mouth and terminating at the anus. The development of endoscopes has aided the internal examination of body cavities. Endoscopy is a general term used to describe this visual inspection. Gastroscopy is a term which describes the inspection of the stomach. Specialized devices can be fitted to endoscopes and used to dilate or constrict parts of the gastrointestinal tract, to remove objects, such as gallstones, and to investigate lesions.

PROBLEMS ASSOCIATED WITH THE MOUTH, PHARYNX, AND OESOPHAGUS

Homeostatic imbalances arise because of disturbances in the ability to masticate or swallow food. In the mouth such disturbances can result from poor functioning of the mucous membranes, teeth, gums, tongue, or salivary glands. Common problems affecting pharyngeal or oesophageal function are tonsilitis and hiatus hernia, but other relatively common conditions also affect these regions, for example, abscess and oesophageal diverticulosis.

Mucous membranes

These membranes are normally of a shiny red appearance; however, a common problem with people who are frequently distressed, or who have a poor state of health, is the presence of small greyish-white mouth ulcers. These are often painful and as a result may interfere with eating. Local mild antiseptics (e.g. TCP) usually aid their healing.

Teeth and gums

A general homeostatic problem associated with teeth is the accumulation of plaque which may lead to inflammation of the gums (gingivitis), dental decay and carie formation, leading to loss of teeth. Prevention is necessary and involves avoidance of foods which have a greater tendency for plaque formation, and adequate oral hygiene.

Tongue

The visual appearance of the tongue is of concern to many people, but the following are only cosmetically displeasing as they are considered quite 'normal':

1 Furring, common in mouth breathers.

2 Fissuring, common to the elderly population (this may be an indication of the wear and tear associated with the ageing process).

3 Sublingual vein varicosities.

However, there are many deviations from the tongue's normal moist pink appearance which are indicative of deficiency diseases, such as the pallor of anaemia, the smooth red appearance of pernicious anaemia, and the dry tongue of the dehydrated patient. The tongue may appear temporarily dry when an individual is anxious, nervous, or frightened, as sympathetic nervous system activity inhibits the flow of watery saliva and stimulates a viscous secretion. Tongue movements, particularly during swallowing, will be adversely affected as a consequence of certain neural lesions involving areas of the brain, especially of the brainstem, which regulate the movements, or of the cranial nerves which supply the tongue.

Superficial inflammation of the tongue, called glossitis (glossa = tongue), may be associated with inflammation of the mouth, generally referred to as stomatitis (stoma = mouth). Thus glossitis may arise from dental caries, gum infection, gastric disorders, excessive smoking and drinking, or membrane infections. Treatment varies with each case and an important part of treatment is allaying the patient's fear of cancer.

Salivary glands

Inflammation or infection of these glands cause electrolytes to become concentrated and may result in salivary stone formation, causing blockage of the glandular ducts, and so result in a swelling of the affected gland. Tumours of the nerve or the blood vessel supplying the glands (particularly the parotid glands) also give rise to painful swelling. 'Mumps' is an inflammation owing to a viral infection and an enlargement of the parotids, and this is accompanied by moderate fever, malaise, and a painful throat especially when swallowing.

Tonsillitis

Tonsillitis is an inflammation of the tonsils due to bacterial infection; this painful throat problem responds well to antibiotic therapy. If this condition is associated with swollen, red tonsils with spots of watery exudate, the condition should be treated carefully because of the risk of cardiac and respiratory problems due to infection of blood. Chronic tonsillitis requires surgical removal, as this condition is painful and is associated with general upset, fever, raised pulse, and often enlarged neck glands.

Hiatus hernia

Hiatus hernia occurs when part of the stomach herniates, or distends, through the oesophageal gap (hiatus) in the diaphragm. It is either congenital or results from an acquired weakness. Often there are no symptoms, but pain and 'heartburn' from the reflux of gastric acid can occur. Correction involves external manipulation of the herniated region back into the abdomen. If this is unsuccessful, then a simple and effective operation removes the problem.

PROBLEMS ASSOCIATED WITH THE STOMACH

There are many common disorders of the stomach, the symptoms of many of which are exacerbated by the high acidity of gastric juice. Disorders may arise because of localized inflammation (e.g. gastritis) and ulceration of the gastric mucosa is a relatively common disorder. Nausea and vomiting are frequently associated with stomach disorders.

Gastritis

Some drugs, such as aspirin, may cause cell damage. Thus prolonged aspirin ingestion can lead to gastric irritation (gastritis) and bleeding, and aspirin should never be administered to patients with lesions of the gastric mucosa or who suffer from indigestion (dyspepsia). Aspirin increases the permeability of cell membranes, resulting in a lower intracellular pH, and so affects enzyme systems. The subsequent cell damage may result in hypoxia and eventually necrotic areas of gastric mucosa, and can lead to the formation of an ulcer. Healing of the ulcer is made more difficult by the presence of gastric acid and by the autodigestive actions of proteolytic pepsin. Arthritic patients who are prescribed aspirin as an analgesic are given enteric-coated aspirin, the coat preventing its absorption from the stomach.

Mucus protects the lining of the stomach. It normally has a thickness of approximately 1 mm and hypersecretion occurs as a natural homeostatic protective mechanism in response to gastritis and in response to the presence of irritant chemicals, such as alcohol or microorganisms. Chronic gastritis is treated with a bland diet, avoidance of irritant foods and avoidance of anxiety which initiates gastric secretion when the stomach is 'empty'.

Peptic ulcers

Peptic ulcers are caused by gastric secretions but are not necessarily found only in the stomach; they are either gastric or duodenal and occasionally oesophageal in origin. The presence of ulcers is a sign of an homeostatic imbalance associated with either excessive secretion of gastric juice, reduced resistance of the gastric mucosa to the secretion, or the presence of a short stomach. Contributory causal factors are:

1 Hereditary tendency.

2 'Stress' or type 'A' personality.

3 Patients on steroids, as these decrease mucosal resistance.

4 In the duodenum pancreatic disease increases duodenal acidity because of the reduction in secretion of alkaline pancreatic juice.

Although both gastric and duodenal ulcers are classified as peptic ulcers, they have differing symptoms. For example, the pain of gastric ulcer comes soon after eating and is not relieved by eating more food, whereas duodenal ulcer pain comes approximately 2 hours following a meal, when food chyme exits the stomach, and is temporarily relieved by further eating.

Principles of correction are based upon eating an easily digestible meal, antacid preparations to neutralize the gastric acids or the use of other drugs to diminish gastric secretion and/or gastric motility.

Nausea

Nausea is an unpleasant sensation which may occur as a result of an emotional disturbance, unpleasant sights, smells, indigestion, gastritis, etc. Nausea may be accompanied by autonomic nervous stimulation, resulting in any of the following: pallor, sweating, a sudden secretion of saliva into the mouth, or an antiperistalsis from the pylorus to the cardiac region of the stomach.

Vomiting

This is forceful expulsion (regurgitation or antiperistalsis) of the contents of the gastrointestinal tract, usually preceded by nausea and salivation. Vomiting is a reflex resulting in the following:

1 A closure of the larynx via the epiglottis, sealing the glottis.

2 A closure of the nasal passageways in order to prevent the entrance of the vomitus.

3 Forceful contraction of the diaphragm and abdominal wall muscles.

4 A closure of the pyloric sphincter, which increases the stomach pressure, causing gastric regurgitation.

The responses are determined by neural output from the vomiting centre of the medulla of the brainstem. The centre sends efferent (motor) impulses to the above areas to initiate the act, in response to afferent (sensory) impulses from one (or more) of the following:

1 Gastrointestinal irritation by chemicals, micro-organisms or handling of the viscera during surgery, thus acting crudely as a 'protective' response to remove the initiating stressor.

2 Cerebral tumour or a raised intracranial pressure.

3 Higher cerebral centres in response to intense fear, anxiety, unpleasant smell, etc.

4 Impulses from the vestibular apparatus, or balance organ, of the ear, for instance in sea-sickness.

5 Some drugs, for example tartar emetics (emesis = vomiting). Thus, the principle of pharmacological correction is the use of anti-emetic drugs.

Examination of the products of the vomit, called the vomitus, is indicative of the associated aetiological factor. For example, the presence of blood indicates gastric ulceration, whereas the presence of undigested food could indicate an obstruction to the pyloric sphincter.

The consequence of vomiting, particularly if chronic, is to reduce nutrient uptake, and to change body fluid composition. There is a loss of fluid and electrolytes, and the loss of gastric acid can result in metabolic alkalosis, although chronic vomiting may induce a metabolic acidosis because the body utilizes body fats as an energy source, as a consequence of reduced carbohydrate intake. Weight loss and nutritional disturbances occur if vomiting is prolonged. In addition, inhalation of vomit and its consequences may also occur.

Principles of correction are varied depending upon aetiology, for example the avoidance of gastric irritants such as alcohol. Also the consequences may require correction, including fluid replacement and/or buffer therapy.

PROBLEMS ASSOCIATED WITH THE SMALL INTESTINE

Disorders of the small intestine commonly relate to disturbances in enzyme or mucus secretion, or in absorption. Since many digestive enzymes originate from the pancreas, pancreatic infections (pancreatitis) or blockage of ducts (as in cystic fibrosis) will disturb the digestive process. More commonly, disorders arise through surgical lesions or as a consequence of inflammation (gastroenteritis).

There is no appreciable difference in digestive and absorptive functions when quite a large amount (up to 50%) of the intestine is surgically removed. However, if only 25% or less remains, digestion and absorption is so reduced that the patient can only survive via parenteral feeding, that is, infusion of nutrients into a large vein.

Gastroenteritis

Gastroenteritis is an inflammation of both the stomach and the intestines, and is characterized by diarrhoea, vomiting, high temperature, and signs of dehydration. There are four main causes of gastroenteritis:

1 Infections, such as cholera and dysentery.

2 Metabolic and/or absorptive homeostatic imbalances, such as indigestion following excessive starch intake, diarrhoea following too much protein, and various conditions such as coeliac disease which exhibit in an inability to digest fat.

3 Emotional and nervous conditions, for example 'nervous diarrhoea'.

4 Various other causes, such as allergies or tumours, though the latter most commonly occur in the colon.

Principles of correction depend again on the aetiological factors, but generally food is withdrawn for a day or so, but drinking water is encouraged. Antibiotics and other drugs

Table 7.6 Causes of diarrhoea and constipation

Diarrhoea	Constipation
Foods rich in spices, fruits such as gooseberries, prunes, and alcohol	Deficiency in dietary fibre
Distress	Depression and dementia
Drugs, for example, antibiotics and laxatives	Drugs such as narcotic opiates (codeine, morphine, etc.), some antihypertensives (e.g. methyldopa), anticholinergics, and aluminium antacids
Neoplasms. Malignant growths may result in a change in bowel habit, such as alternating periods of diarrhoea and constipation	Neoplasms. Change in bowel habits brought about by intestinal growths can lead to alternating bouts of diarrhoea and constipation
Gastrointestinal inflammation, this increases peristaltic motions	Inactivity
Malabsorption syndrome	Weak pelvic floor musculature
Pathogenic infective organisms, such as *Salmonella*, usually as a result of ingestion of contaminated foods; other symptoms include abdominal pain and nausea	Dehydration

may not be given until the cause is established, since they may mask the cause of inflammation.

Diarrhoea

Diarrhoea usually occurs when intestinal movements are too rapid for adequate absorption of water, resulting in a large amount of water being eliminated. Other causes are disorders of nutrient absorption, for example, the effects of cholera toxin on electrolyte transport. Severe diarrhoea results in a large loss of water and electrolytes (particularly sodium and potassium bicarbonate), resulting in dehydration and electrolyte imbalance. Chronic diarrhoea produces hypokalaemia (low blood potassium) and the loss of alkaline digestive juices of the intestine may cause metabolic acidosis. Causes of diarrhoea are summarized in Table 7.6.

Principles of correction depend upon the cause. However, routine treatment of simple cases is usually based on kaolin or chalk mixtures which absorb toxins and allay intestinal irritation. Antibiotic therapy may also be used. Since there is fluid loss, sweetened drinks, with a little salt, are useful in restoring water and electrolyte balance. Severe diarrhoea may require intravenous infusion of a suitable solution (McVicar and Clancy, 1992).

PROBLEMS ASSOCIATED WITH THE LARGE INTESTINE

Disorders of the large intestine are relatively common and include inflammation which may be localized as in appendicitis, ulcerative colitis, and diverticulitis. Rectal function disturbance as a result of blood vessel congestion (haemorrhoids) is also relatively common.

Appendicitis

Inflammation or abscess formation occurs if the opening to the appendix is blocked by a hard mass of faeces. The inflammation may cause the enlarged appendix to burst, producing inflammation of the peritoneum (peritonitis) as the faecal matter penetrates and irritates the abdominal cavity. Correction of the problem is essential and involves surgical removal of the appendix.

Ulcerative colitis

The cause of ulcerative colitis is unknown. The acute illness is associated with fever, severe diarrhoea, passage of blood, weight loss, etc. It becomes chronic with remissions and relapses. Local complications include abscesses, a risk of carcinoma, and perforation.

Principles of correction involve fluid and nutrient replacement, management of diarrhoea, antibiotics, and steroidal therapy. Persistent severe disease, or when the risk of carcinoma is high, may require surgical intervention, such as removal of part or all of the colon, called colectomy, or externalization of the ileum, called ileostomy, which bypasses the colon.

Diverticulosis and diverticulitis

Diverticulosis occurs when a small protrusion of the mucous membrane bulges out through a weak part of the bowel's muscular wall. Although the causes of diverticuli are unknown, diverticulosis tends to occur in the older person with a long history of constipation and is associated with a low fibre diet. The diverticula are usually numerous and become filled with stagnant faecal matter, which may cause infection and inflammation of the surrounding tissue. Acute diverticulitis, that is inflammation of the diverticuli, may proceed to abscess formation or peritonitis and requires prompt surgical treatment. Chronic diverticulosis requires investigation to exclude the possibility of other conditions. X-ray and barium enema will show evidence of these pocket-like diverticulae. If the condition is extensive, or long standing, and perhaps giving rise to symptoms of obstruction, it is often best dealt with by removing the affected area of the bowel.

Haemorrhoids (piles)

Haemorrhoids are dilated, enlarged, and often inflamed venous plexuses of the rectum and anal canal. External piles are dilatations of the inferior rectal plexuses. They originate in the anal canal and in many cases present with no symptoms, except an occasional burning sensation when a constipated motion is passed. Internal piles are dilatations of the superior/middle rectal plexuses and occur in the part of the bowel and anal canal which is covered with mucous membrane. They may remain in the anal orifice and only on occasion produce slight and intermittent bleeding, or fleshy masses of faeces may be passed, and can cause considerable amounts of pain, bleeding, and itching. Extreme pain is associated with a dilated vein becoming thrombosed and inflamed. Most cases are due to constipation and straining at stool. Thus, a diet high in fibre is a good preventive measure as stools are bulkier and of a softer consistency, which thus allows an easier passage through the intestine. Piles are also common in pregnancy due to the rise in intra-abdominal pressure, which can cause venous engorgement by compressing the gut.

If the bowel is kept open with an appropriate diet and bland laxatives, then small piles usually subside. For more serious cases, an injection of an irritant fluid into the haemorrhoids may be necessary, causing scarring and obstruction to the distended vein. Surgical closure is seldom necessary. Avoidance of constipation is an important preventive measure.

The most widely used principle of correction for 'bleeding piles' that consistently cause severe pain is by ligation of the pile. This cuts off the blood supply and, in a few days, the pile dries-up and falls off. Infra-red photocoagulation, using high-energy light beams, may also be used to coagulate the haemorrhoids.

Constipation

Constipation refers to a failure or difficulty with the passage of hard stools. It is the opposite of diarrhoea in that the faeces are hard due to the absorption of most of the water, usually as a consequence of food residues remaining in the colon for long periods of time, for example when there is little fibre in the diet. Faeces become difficult and often painful to eliminate. Abdominal distension may become evident because of food retention. In addition, halitosis, a furred tongue, headache, irritability, and flatulence may also occur. The passage of hard stool may also result in haemorrhoid development. Causes of constipation are summarized in Table 7.6.

Everyone at some time in their lives experiences either diarrhoea or constipation, and one should not be overconcerned about this. However, if either condition becomes a chronic problem then this is usually indicative of some underlying pathology, such as bowel obstruction or poor bowel motility as a consequence of chronic hypokalaemia (e.g. with certain diuretic drug therapies), chronic hypercalcaemia (e.g. with PTH-secreting tumours), analgesics such as morphine, or spinal cord lesions. The principles of correction of constipation involve the use of mild laxatives that induce defecation, and treatment of the underlying pathology.

Faecal incontinence

Defecation is a reflex response to rectal distension. Faecal incontinence is an inappropriate emptying of the bowel, and may result from any of the following:

1 Severe fluid diarrhoea. This is because the sphincters are adapted to retain semi-solids or solid material and are inefficient at retaining fluids.

2 Fluid leakage around an impacted mass of hard faeces.

3 Profuse fluid discharge from some kind of rectal growths.

Faecal incontinence is more common in the elderly. This group of the population also have a greater risk of cerebrovascular accidents ('strokes'), following a sharp rise in blood pressure associated with elimination, especially during constipation. The elderly also commonly exhibit deterioration of cerebral and spinal cord functions, which may result in defecation as soon as rectal distension occurs.

Principles of correction vary and sometimes rehabilitation through education removes the problem for some people. For others the problem is incurable and, as a result, management may involve the use of incontinence pads and rubber sheeting.

PROBLEMS ASSOCIATED WITH THE LIVER AND GALL BLADDER

Disorders of the liver influence utilization of the products of digestion, but also may directly influence the digestive process if bile production is compromised. The consequences of gallstones, hepatitis, and cirrhosis are noted here. Jaundice, as a symptom of these disorders, is discussed in Chapter 8.

Gallstones

The production of stone-like concretions of the gall bladder is a result of either:

1 Inadequate bile salts or lecithin in the bile, which results in multiple-faceted stones composed of calcium and bile pigments.

2 Excessive cholesterol, resulting in its precipitation out of solution and crystallization. These cholesterol crystals coalesce and are responsible for 95% of all gallstones. As these gallstones increase in size they may be responsible for minimal, intermittent, or complete obstruction to the flow of bile from

the gall bladder into the duct system. The more common situation is partial obstruction to the outlet from the gall bladder, resulting in a heartburn pain or discomfort (biliary colic) after eating. If the stone becomes mobile and lodges itself there is intense pain and fever, with jaundice also appearing in due course. Complete obstruction of the flow may even be fatal. Correction involves administering gallstone dissolving drugs, surgery, or fragmentation of stones using high-frequency sound waves.

Hepatitis

Hepatitis is an inflammation of the liver that may arise as a result of poisoning from various drugs or, more commonly, from viral infection, of which there are three types:

1 Hepatitis A (infectious hepatitis). This tends to occur as local outbreaks and is transmitted by the faecal–oral route, i.e. faecal contamination of food, clothing, etc., with the virus. An attack usually starts with the appearance of jaundice and bile-coloured urine, following signs of toxaemia, loss of appetite, and fever. It does not cause lasting liver damage and most people recover in 4–6 weeks.

2 Hepatitis B (serum hepatitis). This virus may be transmitted through contaminated syringes and transfusion equipment or via other body secretions such as tears, saliva, and semen. The virus may produce chronic liver inflammation, which can persist throughout one's lifetime. It is a hazard which must be considered during blood transfusion, renal dialysis, and in transplant surgery. Infected patients are also at an increased risk of cirrhosis (see below). Even when recovery is complete patients can remain carriers of the virus.

3 Non-A, non-B hepatitis. This cannot be traced to the A or B viruses. Clinically, it is similar to hepatitis B and is often transmitted through blood transfusion. Some texts refer to this as hepatitis C.

The principles of control involve the use of gammaglobulins (antibodies) in order to prevent, or treat, the infective hepatitis.

Cirrhosis

Cirrhosis refers to an irreversibly distorted or scarred liver, resulting from chronic progressive inflammation caused by a parasitic infection, or more commonly by certain toxic chemicals (particularly alcohol) that destroy the liver cells. The scarred tissue impairs liver function as the normal functional liver cells are replaced by fibrosed or adiposed connective tissue cells. This impaired function frequently results in jaundice and other complications arise, such as congestion of the hepatic portal vein and abdominal oedema, uncontrolled bleeding, and an increased sensitivity to drugs.

Control primarily involves preventing further damage by the avoidance of alcohol intake, and by taking vitamin supplements to ensure optimal tissue repair and function.

Reference

McVicar, A. and Clancy, J. (1992) Which infusate do I need? Physiological basis of fluid therapy. *Professional Nurse* **7**(9), 586–591.

Summary

1 Providing that a balanced diet is ingested, the digestive system ensures that cells receive the nutrients (metabolites) necessary for their correct functioning (metabolism).

2 Digestion is breakdown of food; it involves physical processes (mainly provided by specialized gut movements), and chemical processes (i.e. hydrolysis, catalysed by specific enzymatic actions).

3 Hydrolysis converts insoluble macromolecules into soluble micromolecules which can be absorbed into blood.

4 The digestive system consists of an alimentary canal and several accessory organs.

5 Various regions of the canal are adapted to perform specialized functions:
   (a) The mouth is adapted to receive food, initiate digestive processes, and perform a limited amount of absorption. It also serves as the organ of speech.
   (b) The salivary glands secrete saliva which moistens food, helps bind food particles together, initiates carbohydrate digestion, makes taste possible and helps cleanse the mouth and teeth.
   (c) The pharynx and oesophagus act as passageways for boli of food.
   (d) The stomach receives boli of food, mixes it with gastric juice, initiates protein digestion, performs limited absorption duties, and passes chyme into the small intestine.
   (e) The small intestine receives secretions from the pancreas and the gall bladder, completes digestion of food, absorbs most of the end products of digestion, and transports the indigestible remains to the large intestine.
   (f) The large intestine absorbs water and electrolytes, and stores and expels the faeces.
   (g) The pancreas is a mixed gland. Its exocrine secretion, pancreatic juice, contains many enzymes which, together with intestinal juice and bile components, complete the digestive process.
   (h) The gall bladder receives bile from the liver, and stores and concentrates it until it is required by the small intestine. Bile is involved in emulsification.
   (i) The liver assimilates most of the absorbed nutrients in order to prevent nutrients becoming in excess of their homeostatic ranges within blood, and to synthesize other vital biochemicals.

6 Food is moved through the alimentary canal principally by peristalsis.

7 Homeostatic imbalances can result from malnutrition (insufficient intake of nutrients, or from an overindulgence of nutrients), or from a bowel disturbance involving digestive, absorptive, assimilative, and/or eliminative processes.

Review Questions

1 Define chemical and physical digestion.

2 Describe the general histological features associated with the wall of the alimentary canal.

3 List the effects of parasympathetic and sympathetic innervation on digestive actions.

4 What are the digestive functions of the mouth?

5 Describe the mechanisms involved in:
(a) the swallowing reflex,
(b) the gastrocolic reflex, and
(c) the defecation reflex.

6 How are the various types of teeth adapted to provide specialized functions?

7 Name the major salivary glands.

8 Describe the chemical and physical digestive processes of the stomach.

9 What is chyme?

10 Describe the valvular functions of the stomach.

11 Which hormones stimulate the release of pancreatic juice?

12 Describe the function of the gall bladder.

13 How does bile contribute to physical digestion?

14 List the enzymes associated with pancreatic and intestinal juices.

15 Discuss the importance of pH variation in the alimentary canal.

16 How does segmentation differ from peristalsis?

17 List the end products of digestion and describe how each is absorbed from the gut and taken to the liver.

18 Describe the assimilative roles of the liver.

19 Name a homeostatic failure associated with each region of the gut.

20 Suggest the principles of correction associated with the failures you have named in Question 19.

The cardiovascular system I: Blood

8

Introduction: role of blood in cellular homeostasis

Overview of the composition of blood

Details of the composition and physiology of blood

Homeostatic failures and principles of correction

Summary

Review questions

Introduction: role of blood in cellular homeostasis

The circulating blood acts as an intermediary between the external environment (outside the body) and the internal environment (tissue fluid and cells). Figure 8.1 illustrates the constant interchange between body fluids and the external environment that is necessary for the maintenance of extracellular and intracellular homeostasis. The importance of blood as an intermediary tissue (together with lymph) cannot be overemphasized, since any area of the body deprived of the contents of circulating blood will be subjected to functional impairment, resulting in tissue death within a matter of minutes if the circulation is not restored.

The development of the transportation fluids blood and lymph was necessary as an evolutionary adaptation to life as a complex multicellular organism. As cells became specialized there was a decline in the ability of individual cells to exist independently. A number of homeostatic functions can therefore be ascribed to blood and the circulatory system.

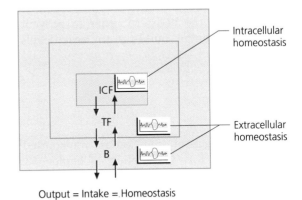

Output = Intake = Homeostasis

Figure 8.1 The interchange between external and internal environments in order to maintain homeostasis. Component intake must match component output in order to achieve extracellular and thus intracellular homeostasis. B, blood; TF, tissue fluid; ICF, intracellular fluid.

Respiratory gases

The blood transports oxygen from the lungs to cells for the process of cellular respiration. Carbon dioxide (CO_2) is produced by cellular respiration, and the excess (i.e. level above its intracellular homeostatic range) must be removed from the cell to prevent potential intracellular imbalance. Cellular CO_2 diffuses into blood which transports it for its excretion, mainly via the lungs. The removal of CO_2 from the blood is necessary to prevent homeostatic imbalances also occurring in this body fluid (see Chapters 5 and 11).

Metabolic wastes

These are generally considered to be substances that cannot be metabolized by cells but also include physiologically useful substances which are present in excess of their homeostatic range but which cannot be stored, destroyed, or transferred into other useful metabolites. The blood transports these substances to the excretory organs for their removal from the body, in order to prevent their consequential build-up to toxic levels (Chapter 12).

Nutrients

The end products of digestion are transported to the liver for assimilation (Chapter 7). Nutrients from storage areas, for example adipose tissue and muscles, are transported to cells requiring them for their own metabolic processes.

Regulatory materials

Enzymes and hormones are taken from their sites of production to their specific target cells.

pH and electrolyte composition

Buffer chemicals in blood contribute to the homeostatic regulation of body fluid pH and, to some extent, to the electrolyte composition of the extracellular fluids. Intracellular buffers are important in regulating the pH and electrolyte composition of intracellular fluids. pH regulation is essential for the optimum functioning of enzymes, and hence metabolism, within these compartments (see Chapter 5).

Thermoregulation

Heat generated by metabolism must be liberated by cells in order to prevent intracellular metabolic imbalances occurring due to the ineffective operation of enzymatic action, since enzymes operate within a narrow temperature range. The absorption of heat by blood may cause blood temperature to rise above its homeostatic range, for example, when cellular metabolism is high, as in strenuous exercise. The excess heat is distributed to the skin surface where it is dissipated by the evaporation of sweat (Chapter 17). Alternatively, heat may be redistributed to areas of the body which require warming, because their regional temperatures have fallen below their homeostatic ranges.

Haemostasis (the maintenance of a constant blood volume)

Blood clotting helps preserve body fluid homeostasis by restricting fluid loss through damaged vessels or injury sites. This helps prevent excessive loss of extracellular fluids, which could seriously affect blood pressure and cardiovascular function.

Cellular defence mechanisms

White blood cells and antibodies found in blood are instrumental in defending the body against pathogens and their toxic secretions. These processes are described in more detail in Chapter 10. The blood also transports toxic substances to the liver and kidneys, where they are detoxified and excreted respectively.

As blood is in constant interaction with tissues, its functions will clearly overlap with those of various tissues and organs. Many of these roles, such as pH regulation, temperature regulation, and gas transport have been described elsewhere in the appropriate chapters. Blood is a tissue in its own right, however, and its cellular components and capacity to be transformed from a 'liquid' to a semi-solid clot will be described in this chapter.

Overview of the composition of blood

The volume of blood circulating in the cardio-vascular system averages 5–6 litres in males and 4–5 litres in females and so accounts for approximately 8% of the total body weight of the individual. Blood appears to be a homogeneous dark red viscous liquid which, if left to stand for a few minutes, normally clots or solidifies. Subsequent microscopic investigation reveals, however, that blood is in fact a heterogeneous mixture of various cell types, suspended in a fluid compartment called plasma. Plasma and red blood cells account for about 55% and 44% of a blood sample respectively. The remaining 1% consists of white blood cells and platelets (Figure 8.2).

PLASMA

The body contains some 2.5–3 litres of plasma, a pale yellow fluid, 90% of which is water. The remaining constituents of this heterogeneous material include:

1 Plasma proteins (albumins, globulins, fibrinogen, and prothrombin).

2 Regulatory proteins (enzymes and hormones).

3 Various other organic substances, including nutrients such as glucose, amino acids, fatty acids and glycerol, and waste products of metabolism such as urea and creatinine.

4 Inorganic substances (electrolytes).

These components are responsible for giving plasma a greater density and viscosity than water. The dissolved proteins make this fluid sticky, cohesive, and resistant to flow.

BLOOD CELLS

The cellular components of blood are:

1 Red blood cells, or erythrocytes. Their main homeostatic function is the transportation of respiratory gases to and from cells. The presence of surface molecules, or antigens, on the erythrocyte membrane, together with certain plasma antibodies, determine an individual's blood group.

2 White blood cells, or leucocytes. These cells are important components of one's immune system and are concerned with defending the body against pathogenic invaders and their toxins.

3 Platelets, or thrombocytes. These cells are of fundamental importance in blood clotting. Their homeostatic role is in haemostasis, i.e. they prevent blood loss, and thus help maintain body fluid balance following injury.

Blood production or haemopoiesis occurs in three stages according to the individual's stage of growth and development. These stages are called the mesoblastic, hepatosplenic and myeloid stages.

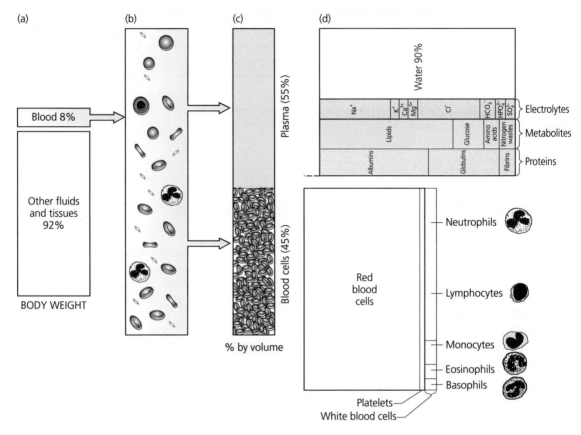

Figure 8.2 The homeostatic composition of body fluids and in particular blood. (a) Body fluids. (b) Whole blood. (c) Centrifuged blood. (d) Separate components of blood.

The mesoblastic stage

The first cells to produce blood cells originate from the mesoderm cell layer of the embryo (Chapter 18), and migrate to the yolk sac, where they form 'blood islands'. These islets of cells become hollow tubes which secrete a plasma-like fluid from their walls. Proliferation of cells lining these tubes form the early cells of the circulation; the nucleated cells (called megaloblasts of Ehrlich) contain the pigment haemoglobin and their sole purpose is to transport oxygen to the embryonic tissue cells. Blood production from these cells is sufficient for the first few weeks of embryonic life, but is inadequate to support further development.

The hepatosplenic stage

This phase of blood production begins at about 2 months of embryological life, and is necessary because the embryo/fetus is growing at a fast rate and its tissues require a correspondingly greater blood supply to sustain this activity. The liver and spleen become the main contributors of this enhanced blood production, although the thymus is also involved. The liver becomes the major haemopoietic site between 3 and 4 months, and continues to produce blood until the later stages of pregnancy.

The myeloid stage

The term 'myeloid' refers to the activities of blood precursor cells in bone marrow. The bone marrow becomes active in blood cell production from the fifth month onwards, establishing itself as the major haemopoietic organ of the fetus at about 7 months of age. Blood formation from this site continues throughout life. At birth, all the marrow is active and is called red active marrow, because, although it produces all blood cells, the extensive number of erythrocytes colour it red. As the infant grows, the active red marrow of the long bones is replaced by yellow inactive (or fatty, lymphoidal) marrow. The tibia and radius bones of the limbs are the first bones to lose this haemopoietic ability, followed by the femur and then the humerus. In the young adult, the active marrow is found in the flat bones, such as the cranium, ribs, sternum, pelvis, and in the vertebrae. The liver, spleen, and the yellow inactive marrow, are, however, capable of reverting back to their erythrocyte production functions when erythrocyte numbers are deficient in severe anaemias, and so act as homeostatic regulators.

The marrow's haemopoietic functions can be divided into erythropoiesis (red cell production), leucopoiesis (white cell production) and thrombopoiesis (platelet production). These processes will be discussed later.

Details of the composition and physiology of blood

PLASMA

Plasma forms approximately one-fifth of the total volume of extracellular fluid. Plasma and tissue fluids are very similar in composition, apart from the total amount of protein present. This is not surprising as the two are separated by the capillary vessel membrane and this is permeable to most substances. Tissue fluid is derived from plasma at the arterial side of the capillary beds and returns to the plasma at the venous side (Chapter 9). Despite the interchange of plasma and tissue fluid, there remain some differences in their composition. One of the most noticeable differences is in the concentration of the respiratory gases. Plasma has a higher concentration of oxygen, whilst tissue fluid has a higher concentration of carbon dioxide. As a result, oxygen diffuses from blood into tissue fluid, and carbon dioxide diffuses into the plasma. Diffusion, as discussed in Chapter 2, could be expected to result in a uniform distribution of the gases but this is not the case because cells are constantly removing and utilizing oxygen from tissue fluid, and supplying carbon dioxide to it, in order to maintain cell homeostasis. Thus, diffusion is a working concept to explain the movement of molecules down their concentration gradients.

Another notable difference between plasma and tissue fluid is the large presence of dissolved proteins in the plasma (70 g/l compared with the 20 g/l in tissue fluid). Plasma proteins are macromolecules that are too large to pass through pores in the capillary membranes, and thus generally do not pass into tissue fluid. Intracellular fluid has a different composition again that of plasma and tissue fluid because of the selectively permeable properties of cell membranes.

Plasma proteins

Plasma contains three principal types of proteins: albumins, globulins and fibrinogen. The latter is a protein involved in blood clotting and the plasma also contains various other proteins associated with clotting, for example a kind of globulin called prothrombin.

Albumins

Approximately 70% of the solutes found in plasma are proteins. Albumins comprise about 55–60% of this protein component and, thus, are important determinants of the viscosity of blood, i.e. the plasma proteins slow down the flow rate of blood. In addition, albumins osmotically draw water (and its dissolved components) from the exuded tissue fluid back into the venous side of the blood capillary. This maintains the blood volume and hence helps to maintain blood pressure. Albumins also have important transport functions. For example, they bind to calcium and bilirubin, thus maintaining the homeostatic concentration of these 'free' chemicals in body fluids (both are physiologically active only when unbound), and they bind to certain drugs, for example aspirin.

Although largely retained in plasma, some albumin is also found in the tissue fluid, albeit in small amounts, where it has similar properties to that in plasma itself.

Globulins

Globulins comprise about 33–38% of the plasma proteins. They are much larger molecules than those of the albumins and are subdivided into the following fractions:

1 Gammaglobulins. This group mainly consists of most of the known antibodies, and are concerned with protecting the body from pathogenic microbes, hence their alternative name immunoglobulins. Globulins are used as a basis of therapeutic administrations. For example, anti-tetanus injections consist of the antibody rich gammaglobulin fraction of horse serum.

2 Alphaglobulins. These globulins have several transport functions: they bind to smaller proteins, and certain electrolytes, and so prevent these substances from passing out in the urine.

3 Betaglobulins. These proteins also have several transport functions. Some contain specific metal-combining groups; for example, transferrin is a protein which transports iron, whereas others carry fat-soluble vitamins.

Fibrinogen and prothrombin

Prothrombin (a betaglobulin) together with fibrinogen act as precursors of the active clotting proteins, thrombin and fibrin. As with many plasma proteins, both are synthesized in the liver, and so their homeostatic in plasma levels will be affected in liver diseases.

Other generalized homeostatic functions of plasma proteins

In addition to the specific roles mentioned above, plasma proteins have other generalized roles. In the 'normal' slightly alkaline plasma, proteins exist as proteinate ions and are negatively charged. As ions they are capable of 'mopping-up' hydrogen ions when these are in excess of their homeostatic range, for example when the metabolic rate is increased. This important buffering action contributes to the homeostatic maintenance of blood pH, which is essential for optimum enzymatic activity.

Plasma proteins also act as a protein reservoir, i.e. plasma proteins can be utilized in times of chronic dietary protein deficiency. This may lead to protein depletion in the plasma (hypoproteinaemia), however, which has consequences for fluid distribution, etc.

Table 8.1 summarizes the homeostatic functions of plasma constituents.

Plasma is frequently the subject of clinical biochemical analysis as an indication of a person's state of health. Table 8.2 and Figure 8.3 indicate the homeostatic ranges of various organic and inorganic components within plasma and deviations from these values are indicative of one's fluctuating physiological condition or may be a sign of underlying

Table 8.1 Chemical composition, description, and homeostatic functions of plasma components

Component	Description	Homeostatic function
Water	Liquid portion of blood; constitutes approximately 90% of the plasma. Water is derived from absorption from the digestive tract and from cellular respiration	Transports organic and inorganic molecules, blood cells, and heat
Solutes		
Proteins	Constitutes approximately 7% of the plasma	
Albumins	Smallest plasma protein produced by the liver	Provides blood with viscosity, a factor related to the homeostatic regulation of blood pressure Exerts considerable osmotic pressure to maintain water balance between blood and tissues, hence, homeostatically regulates blood volume and thus blood pressure Binding functions Transports lipids
Globulins	Group to which antibodies belong	Gammaglobulins (antibodies) attack pathogenic organisms Include an important blood clotting precursor molecule (prothrombin) Important in transport of ions, hormones, and lipids
Fibrinogen	Produced by the liver	Homeostatic role in blood clotting, when it is converted into insoluble fibrin
Non-protein nitrogen-containing substances	Include urea, uric acid, creatinine, and ammonium salts	Byproducts of protein metabolism. These are excreted to prevent toxic build-up
Food substances	Products of digestion passed into blood for distribution to all body cells. Products include amino acids (from proteins), glucose (from carbohydrates), fatty acids, and glycerol (from fats) and vitamins	Used for: energy production; growth; repair and maintenance of cells
Regulatory substances	Enzymes and hormones	Enzymes catalyse chemical reactions to a rate which is compatible with life
Respiratory gases	Oxygen and carbon dioxide. These gases are also associated with haemoglobin or red blood cells	Hormones regulate metabolism Oxygen has a homeostatic role in cellular respiration (Krebs' cycle) Carbon dioxide is important in the regulation of pH of body fluids
Electrolytes	Inorganic salts of plasma. Cations include: Na^+, K^+, Ca^{2+} Anions include: Cl^-, HCO_3^-	Help to maintain: osmotic pressure; normal pH and physiological balance between tissues and blood[2]

Table 8.2 Normal homeostatic ranges of various organic and inorganic substances in plasma

		Concentration (homeostatic range)
Organic substance		
Glucose		
fasting		3.3–5.5 mmol/l
after a meal		≤ 10.0 mmol/l
2 hours after glucose		< 5.5mmol/l
Urea		2.7–8.5 mmol/l
Uric acid (urate)		150–580 µmol/l
Creatinine		40–110 µmol/l
Bilirubin		3–21 µmol/l
Aspartate aminotransferase (AST)		5–30 iu/l
Alanine aminotransferase (ALT)		5–30 iu/l
Hydroxybutyrate dehydrogenase (HBD)		150–325 iu/l
Creatine kinase		< 130 iu/l
Amylase (AMS)		150–340 iu/l
Alkaline phosphatase (ALP)		21–100 iu/l
Acid phosphatase (ACP)		< 8.2iu/l
Inorganic substances (ions)		
Sodium	Na^+	135–146 mmol/l
Potassium	K^+	3.5–5.2 mmol/l
Total calcium	Ca^{2+}	2.10–2.70 mmol/l
Chloride	Cl^-	98–108 mmol/l
Hydrogen carbonate	HCO_3^-	23–31 mmol/l
Phosphate	PO_4^{2-}	0.7–1.4 mmol/l

pathology. Thus, such levels are used as aids to diagnose specific disorders. Analysis of plasma components could be potentially difficult, as samples coagulate, or clot, within a matter of minutes after taking them. Thus, plasma analysis also involves the removal of the clotting proteins fibrinogen and prothrombin. The remaining plasma-like fluid is called serum.

CELLULAR COMPONENTS OF BLOOD

The cellular components of blood make up about 45% of whole blood (Figure 8.2c). The three principal cell types are classified as follows:

1 Erythrocytes (erythro- = red).

2 Leucocytes (leuco- = white). These contain two main groups, the granulocytes (subdivided into neutrophils, eosinophils, and basophils) and agranulocytes (subdivided into lymphocytes and the monocytes).

3 Thrombocytes (platelets).

Table 8.3 summarizes the homeostatic functions of blood cells.

Erythrocytes

Structure

Microscopically red cells appear as biconcave discs. Each cell has a doughnut shape, having a thick outer margin and a very thin middle region. Erythrocytes are approximately 7.2 µm in diameter, with a 2.2 µm thickness, its

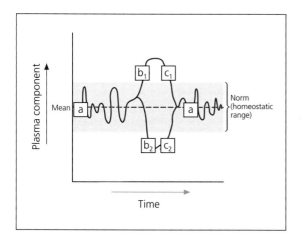

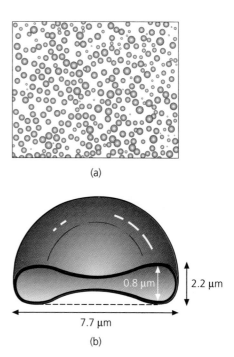

(a)

(b)

Figure 8.3 Clinical analysis of plasma components using homeostatic principles.

a, Homeostatic dynamism. Value fluctuating above and below the mean within the component's homeostatic range (see Table 8.2). The fluctuation is a result of the component entering and leaving the plasma. For example, some plasma components such as nutrients leave blood at the arterial side of the capillary bed, whilst others, such as metabolic wastes enter the blood at the arterial side of the capillary bed. Consequently the component's level fluctuates.

b_1, Plasma component in excess of its homeostatic range. The excess could be indicative of a clinical condition, e.g. the presence of the cardiac specific enzyme – creatine phosphokinase – above serum baseline level which occurs after a myocardial infarction (heart attack). Alternatively, the excess may be indicative of a 'normal' temporary change in the plasma level of the component (for example, an elevated glucose concentration – after absorption of a carbohydrate–rich meal.

b_2, A decrease in the component level below its homeostatic range. This again could be indicative of a clinical condition. For example, low levels of plasma proteins might be indicative of liver damage (as occurs in tissue fibrosis due to cirrhosis), since the hepatocytes produce plasma proteins and fibrosis impairs this synthesis. Alternatively, the low levels could be a 'normal' temporary change (e.g. hypoglycaemia, which occurs 1 hour post–absorption of a carbohydrate–rich meal due to the long durational effects of the hypoglycaemic agent insulin).

c_1 and c_2, Clinical intervention, or the body's normal negative homeostatic feedback mechanisms, which correct the temporary pathological and normal physiological homeostatic imbalances respectively.

Figure 8.4 The structure of erythrocytes. (a) When viewed in a standard blood smear, erythrocytes appear as two–dimensional doughnut–shaped objects. (b) In cross–section, erythrocytes appear as three–dimensional. The biconcavity produces a greater surface area for the process of gaseous exchange; ----- represents the smaller surface area of a spherical cell.

central portion narrowing to 0.8 μm (Figure 8.4). The biconcavity provides a large surface area with respect to volume (greater than a spherical-shaped cell), thus maximizing the

available membrane surface for the exchange of respiratory gases. This structural adaptation also gives these cells greater flexibility, enabling them to pass through capillaries which are even narrower than the diameter of the erythrocyte. The membrane, as with all cellular membranes, also contains various antigenic chemicals. Some of the blood cell antigens (or agglutinogens), namely A, B, and D (rhesus) types, are antigenic markers which determine an individual's blood group (described later).

The cytoplasm of the erythrocyte consists mainly of the red pigment haemoglobin, and the enzymes necessary for its function. This pigment accounts for approximately 95% of the intracellular protein and is responsible for approximately one-third of the cell's mass.

Table 8.3 Various types of blood cells. Reproduced from Craigwyle, M.B.L. (1975) *A Colour Atlas of Histology.* Wolfe Medical Publications Ltd, London.

Blood cell	Diameter (µm)	Number mm^3 (homeostatic range)	Differential white cell count	Homeostatic function
Leucocytes				
Granulocytes				
Neutrophil	9–12	3000–6750	60–65	Phagocytic – engulf pathogens or debris in tissues
Eosinophil	10–14	100–360	2–4	Phagocytic – engulf items in tissues that are labelled with antigens (combat allergies)
Basophil	8–10	25–90	0.5–1.0	Enter damaged tissue release histamine (combat allergies)
Agranulocytes				
Lymphocyte	6–12	1000–2700	20–35	Cells of the lymphatic provide defence against specific pathogens or toxins
Monocyte	10–15	150–170	3–8	Enters tissues and become free macrophages, engulf pathogens *or* debris
Erythocytes	7.0–7.7	4.2–6.2 million		Transportation of respiratory gases (particularly oxygen)
Thrombocytes	2–4	150000–400000		Blood clotting

A differential white cell count is taken by examining a stained blood smear, the values above represent the numbers of each type encountered in a sample of 100 leucocytes.

Table 8.4 illustrates the homeostatic values for erythrocyte number, volume, etc. The main functions of haemoglobin are the transportation of respiratory gases, and to help regulate blood pH, because when haemoglobin is not transporting respiratory gases it has a buffering action (Chapter 12).

Production and destruction of erythrocytes: a homeostatic process

Erythrocytes have a lifespan of about 120 days, when they are destroyed. Their produc-tion must match their loss, in order homeo-statically to control the number of red cells present, i.e. 5.4 million/mm^3, and 4.8 million/mm^3 for men and women respec-tively. The higher number in males is due to the need to transport more oxygen to support their greater metabolic rate. The haematocrit value represents the red cell mass relative to plasma and averages are 0.47 (or 47%) for males and 0.42 (42%) for females. This value is sometimes also referred to as the packed cell volume (PCV). Thus red cells account for nearly half the volume of whole blood. These values decrease in anaemia and increase in

Table 8.4 Erythrocytic homeostatic ranges

Measure	Homeostatic range
Erythrocytic count	Male 4.5–6.5 million/mm³ Female 4.5–5 million/mm³
Packed cell volume (PCV) (haematocrit)	Male 0.47 (47%) Female 0.42 (42%)
Haemoglobin (Hb)	Male 13–18 g/dl Female 11.5–16.6 g/dl

The higher erythrocytic count and haemoglobin levels in males reflect their higher metabolic rate

polycythaemia, which are discussed later in the chapter.

Approximately 1% of circulating red cells are replaced daily: this means that 3 million erythrocytes enter the circulation each second! All blood cells are thought to originate from a common stem cell called the haematocytoblast (Figure 8.5). These stem cells are themselves a result of cell specialization, since they are differentiated from other cells within the body once the particular genes for blood cell development are expressed. Once this initial specialization has taken place, producing the common stem cell, the cells divide mitotically and specialize further into either red cells, white cells, or platelets. This differentiation of the stem cell into blood cells is again by specific gene expression. Furthermore, once a cell has

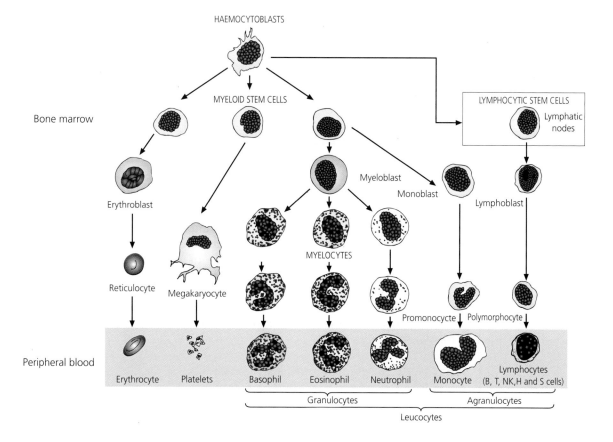

Figure 8.5 Haemopoiesis. The origin and differentiation of blood cells.

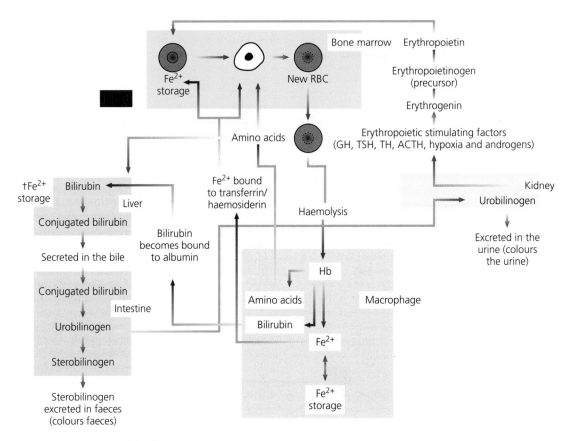

Figure 8.6 Production and destruction of erythrocytes: a homeostatic process. This diagram indicates the normal pathways for recycling the amino acids and iron content of old or damaged erythrocytes, and the pathway associated with red cell production. TSH, Thyroid stimulating hormone; ACTH, adrenocorticotropic hormone; GH, growth hormone; PN, pyrrol nuclei; RBC, red blood cell; * transamination (deamination if the amino acid pool is above the homeostatic range); † occurs if circulatory iron is in excess of its homeostatic range.

become specialized, it cannot be transformed into another cell (blood cell or otherwise).

ERYTHROCYTE PRODUCTION (ERYTHROPOIESIS)

Figure 8.5 diagrammatically simplifies the processes involved in erythropoiesis. The main characteristic changes for the development of a mature erythrocyte take about 1 week. During this time the cell gradually becomes smaller and smaller, the cell's nucleus 'ripens' with the loss of the nucleoli and the condensation of nuclear material, the cell cytoplasm 'ripens' due to the process of haemoglobinization, and some of the cytoplasmic organelles and partic-

ulates, for example the nucleus, mitochondria and ribosomes, are lost. Erythrocytes therefore cannot divide or produce proteins, and they are dependent upon anaerobic respiration for their ATP source. This form of respiration (as discussed in Chapter 3) produces much less energy from glucose catabolism. Thus, red cells come to the end of their lifespan when their ATP and enzyme levels fall below those necessary to maintain their homeostatic roles. Perhaps erythrocytic metabolism slows down so much that it becomes incompatible for the continued existence of that cell.

There are many factors that regulate the maturation process. These can be broadly

Table 8.5 Dietary components necessary for erythropoiesis

Dietary component	Homeostatic important in erythropoiesis
Protein	Synthesis of globin part of haemoglobin. Synthesis of other cellular proteins, including conjugated molecules, e.g. lipoproteins, glycoproteins
Iron	Contained in the haem part of haemoglobin
Vitamin B_{12} and folic acid	Synthesis of DNA
Vitamin C	Facilitates the absorption of iron by reducing ferric iron to ferrous iron. Important in normal folic acid metabolism
Vitamin B_6, riboflavin, and vitamin E	Important for normal erythropoiesis, since deficiency of these substances has been associated with anaemia
Copper and cobalt	Copper is essential for haemoglobin synthesis and cobalt is important in vitamin B_{12} synthesis in other organisms. Therefore, these trace elements may have a role in human erythropoiesis

divided into those which stimulate erythropoiesis (for example, hypoxia, and hypersecretion of the following metabolic hormones: thyroid stimulating hormone, thyroxine; adrenocorticotropic hormone, growth hormone and androgens), and those which inhibit erythropoiesis (for example an oxygen carrying capacity of the blood above or within its homeostatic range, and undersecretion of the above hormones).

The process of erythropoiesis is controlled by the release of the erythropoietic factor called erythrogenin from juxtaglomerular tissue of the kidney in response to hypoxia, etc. This factor converts a precursor protein in plasma, erythropoietinogen, into erythropoietin, which activates the erythropoietic tissues to increase red cell production and release them into the circulation (Figure 8.6). At sea level the atmospheric oxygen conditions are sufficient to meet the metabolic demands of humans and when erythrocyte production exceeds the homeostatic range (for example, values greater than 6.5 million/mm³ for men and 5 million/mm³ for women, Table 8.4), then production is inhibited because the secretion of erythrogenin is prevented. This is an example of a negative feedback mechanism. As time passes, the number of erythrocytes return

to their normal homeostatic levels, because cells are still being destroyed at their normal rate of breakdown. At this point (within the homeostatic range) production must begin again at a rate which matches that of destruction, in order to maintain the 'normal' levels. Thus, the levels of erythropoietin rise due to erythrogenin secretion and its activation of erythropoietinogen. Erythropoietin release is, therefore, tightly controlled within its 'normal' parameters. A change outside these parameters occurs, for example, when erythrocyte destruction becomes greater than production, resulting in low levels of erythrocytes, as is observed in haemolytic diseases.

Table 8.5 summarizes the dietary components essential for erythropoiesis to occur.

ERYTHROCYTE DESTRUCTION

When red cells are approximately 100–120 days old they are removed from the circulation by the reticuloendothelial system (i.e. the spleen, liver, subcutaneous tissue, and lymph nodes) and phagocytes ingest and destroy the aged erythrocytes. How these aged cells are recognized is still a mystery, but it is known that the spleen is involved. An enlarged spleen (called splenomegaly) is observed in conditions associated with abnormal red cells, for example in sickle cell anaemia.

Approximately 1% of red cells are removed and replaced daily. Haemoglobin undergoes an elaborate catabolism, which has evolved so that its most valuable components are conserved and re-utilized. The remainder are excreted in bile and in urine.

The structure of haemoglobin is discussed in detail in Chapter 11, and it is advisable for the reader to study that section before continuing.

The stages involved in the breakdown of haemoglobin (Figure 8.6) are as follows:

1 The haem molecule consists of four pyrrol nuclei, which form a porphyrin ring compound. A ferrous (Fe^{2+}) ion is found at the centre of each ring. Once ingested by macrophages, this ring is opened by the process of oxidation, forming a straight-chain molecule called choleglobin.

2 Iron and globin are now removed from choleglobin, converting it into bilirubin (red bile pigment). The iron and globin are useful substances, and are re-utilized by the body. Some of the iron is used for the resynthesis of haemoglobin and other iron-containing compounds, but if the iron released from the haemoglobin causes its availability to go above the homeostatic range, any excess is transferred into iron storage compounds, called ferritin and haemosiderin. Thus, an increased haemosiderin concentration (above its normal range) in the liver and the spleen is indicative of diseases in which there is excessive red cell breakdown. Iron is released from such stores when there is insufficient to meet metabolic needs. Very little iron is normally lost from the body, although significant amounts may be lost in women who experience heavy menstrual flow.

The globin molecule is hydrolysed into its constituent amino acids, which enter the amino acid metabolic 'pools'. If the constituent 'essential' amino acids (see Chapter 7) are already within their normal parameters, the excess may be deaminated; the product keto acids are used to produce energy, whereas the ammonia is excreted as urea. These amino acids cannot be stored or transferred into other amino acids, unlike the constituent 'non-essential' amino acids, which are transferred (transaminated) into other 'non-essential' amino acids, if these are below their homeostatic ranges; otherwise they are deaminated also.

3 Some bilirubin becomes tightly bound to albumin and this complex passes into the liver cells via a carrier-mediated mechanism. The free or unbound bilirubin, being lipid-soluble, passes into the liver cells with ease. The bound bilirubin complex within the liver cells is combined with glucuronic acid, forming a water-soluble complex known as conjugated bilirubin. Having been converted to a water-soluble form, the bilirubin–glucuronic acid complex can now be excreted. Together with other substances, such as bile salts, they form bile which is secreted from the liver via the hepatic ducts to the gall bladder, where it is stored and concentrated. From the gall bladder the bile is passed to the intestine where it aids the digestion of lipids (Chapter 7). Within the intestines, bilirubin is reduced to urobilinogen by bacterial action. Some urobilinogen is reabsorbed into the circulation and is re-utilized by the liver, although some is excreted in the urine, contributing to its colour. The urobilinogen remaining in the intestines is converted into stercobilinogen and is excreted in the faeces. This is oxidized upon exposure to the air into stercobilin which is responsible for faecal colour. In the gut of the neonate, bacterial cultures take time to establish and consequently the conjugated bilirubin is not converted but is excreted intact.

Leucocytes (white blood cells)

Structure

These cells are nucleated and do not contain haemoglobin. Leucocytes fall into two main groups: the granulocytes (i.e. neutrophils, eosinophils, and basophils) and the agranulocytes (i.e. lymphocytes and monocytes). The cytoplasm of granulocytes contains granules and the cell types are classified according to their reaction to staining techniques and to their size. All granulocytes possess a lobed nucleus, whereas agranulocytes have either spherical (lymphocytes) or kidney-shaped (monocytes) nuclei.

White cells are far less numerous than red cells and platelets, the average number being between 5000 and 9000/mm³. The range represents, however, quite a large variation in the number of leucocytes within individuals: the numbers even vary on an hour-to-hour basis (circadian rhythms of leucocyte production, Chapter 23), and with various accompanying 'physiological' and 'psychological' factors, such as exercise and emotions. A differential white cell count is taken by examining a stained blood smear, and the values obtained represent the number of each type of leucocyte encountered in a sample of 100 white cells. The homeostatic ranges and a summary of the homeostatic functions of leucocytes are included in Table 8.3.

Homeostatic functions of leucocytes

White cells are components of the immune system. As they circulate in blood vessels they are 'looking' for signs of pathogenic invasion in adjacent tissues. Leucocytes are chemically attracted to the site of inflammation by, for example, secretions of pathogens (toxins, etc.) and components of the inflammatory and immune responses. This chemotactic response attracts them to the invaders, damaged tissues and other white blood cells. The movement of the leucocytes across capillary membranes is called diapedesis (Chapter 10) and, in fact, most white cells are scattered throughout peripheral tissues, as there is no human tissue which is not susceptible to pathogenic invasion. In general, the mucous membranes and the skin are under constant threat, whereas deeper body tissues are less

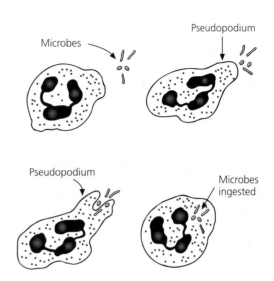

Figure 8.7 Phagocytic action of neutrophils.

threatened. Thus, white cells present in blood represent only a small fraction of the total population of leucocytes. The generalized homeostatic function of white cells is to protect the body by combating microbes using two processes; phagocytosis (Figure 8.7) and antibody production. The entire collection of leucocytes has the sole purpose of defending the body against pathogenic invasion, including the removal of toxins, wastes and abnormal or damaged cells.

Classification of leucocytes

GRANULOCYTES

Neutrophils Neutrophils account for the largest proportion (about 60–65%) of the circulating leucocyte population. Their name was selected because they are difficult to stain with either acid or basic dyes, but neutral dyes stain their granules purple. Neutrophils have a distinctive lobed nucleus, hence their alternative name polymorphonucleocytes (polymorph = many forms). They are between 9 and 14 μm in diameter and their granular components contain lysosomal enzymes and bactericidal compounds (Table 8.3). Neutrophils are very mobile and are the first cell type to arrive at a site of injury; they are the most active phagocytes in response to tissue destruction by bacteria. Large numbers of neutrophils are destroyed in any bacterial infection. These, together with dead bacterial cells and their contents, make the pus which occurs at the site. Some bacterial toxins act as fever-producing substances, or pyrogens, and it is thought that they activate neutrophils to produce further pyrogens which then cross the blood–brain barrier and affect the hypothalamic temperature-regulating centre. Increased numbers of neutrophils (called neutrophil leucocytosis) are observed in bacterial infection and inflammatory reactions associated with tissue cell death, for example cerebrovascular accidents (CVAs or strokes) and myocardial infarctions (MIs or heart attacks).

Eosinophils Eosinophils represent about 2–4% of the circulating white cells, and are generally only slightly larger than neutrophils. These cells have bilobed nuclei and easily take up acid dyes like eosin, hence their name (Table 8.3). Eosinophils are mobile and phagocytic, but not as phagocytic as neutrophils and monocytes. Eosinophils phagocytose bacteria more readily if the bacteria are coated with immunoglobulin antibodies, but these white cells also combat irritants that cause allergies. Thus, their numbers gradually increase in allergic reactions or in a parasitic infection. Their granules contain lytic enzymes and, by their involvement with IgE mediated immune responses, function to neutralize and limit the effects of inflammatory substances such as histamine and bradykinin. Eosinophils collect at the site of allergic reactions, for example in the respiratory mucous membranes in hay fever and asthma. Eosinophils and neutrophils are often called microphages, to avoid confusion with the larger phagocytes (macrophages) found in the blood and peripheral tissues.

Basophils Basophils account for approximately 0.5–1% of circulating blood cells. They are so called because their granules easily stain with basic dyes (Table 8.3). Basophils are also important in allergic reactions. They become

mast cells in inflamed tissue and secrete their granular contents (heparin, serotonin, and histamine) which exaggerate the inflammation response at this site.

Other chemicals released by activated basophils attract eosinophils and further basophils to the affected area. Basophils bind specific IgE antibodies (released in response to allergic irritants) to their surfaces, secretion and catabolism of basophil granules occurs upon subsequent exposure to the antigen, for which the bound IgE is specific. They release histamine and are also involved in hypersensitive reactions to allergens. Histamine is a vasodilator and therefore may cause a decrease in blood pressure, with a resultant increase in the heart rate. Itching and pain are also associated with hypersecretion of histamine.

AGRANULOCYTES

Lymphocytes These cells account for between 20 and 35% of the leucocyte population and most are found within the lymphatic system. Morphologically they are divided into large (10–15 μm) and small (8–10 μm) lymphocytes. The smaller cells are approximately the same size as red cells and their nucleus occupies most of the cytoplasm (Table 8.3). Functionally, lymphocytes are subdivided into T- and B-lymphocytes. These cells also have a number of subdivisions which are discussed in Chapter 10. To summarize, T-lymphocytes attack the antigenic microbes directly in the cellular immune response. B-lymphocytes differentiate into large 'plasma' cells characterized by the production of vast quantities of rough endoplasmic reticulum; these cells produce and secrete the proteinaceous antibodies (gammaglobulins) that attach to antigenic material in the humoral immune response. There is a high degree of specificity with regard to antibody–antigen binding. Once formed, the covered or bound antigen (i.e. microbe, or bacterial toxin) cannot come into contact with any other chemical in the body and, as a result, they are rendered harmless to body tissues. Antigen–antibody binding therefore helps combat infection and gives the body immunity to some diseases.

Monocytes Monocytes account for 3–8% of circulating leucocytes. These cells are easily recognizable under the microscope because of their large size (they are approximately 10–18 μm in diameter, nearly twice the size of a red cell) and distinctive kidney-shaped nuclei. These characteristics are illustrated in Table 8.3. There are a number of different categories of monocytes:

1 Free monocytes (macrophages). These cells are found outside the blood. They are extremely mobile, and so have an abundance of mitochondria. They arrive at the site of injury very quickly and are phagocytic. Macrophages release chemicals that attract other macrophages, fellow phagocytes and fibroblasts to the inflamed area (fibroblasts secrete a fibrous material which walls off the injured area). Macrophages and granulocytes respond to a diverse range of stimuli, unlike the lymphocytes which respond to specific antigens (microbes and their antigens).

2 Immobile (fixed) monocytes. These macrophages are found in most connective tissues, are slower to respond, and take longer to reach the site of invasion. Despite this they destroy more microbes, due to the vast quantities which enter the site of infection. Monocytes entering the infected tissues are called 'wandering' or 'scavenger' macrophages as they clean up the debris following an injury.

The monocytes that migrate into reticulendothelial tissues (bone marrow, spleen, liver and lymph nodes), develop into larger specialized cells, for example the liver's Kupffer cells. These survive for long periods of time, and are important in the destruction of aged erythrocytes.

Production and destruction of leucocytes: a homeostatic process

Leucopoiesis is the general term used for the production of all white cells. The process is subdivided and other terms are employed to describe specific leucocyte production and maturation. These include: granulopoiesis (granulocytes), lymphopoiesis (lymphocytes), and monopoiesis (monocytes).

Granulopoiesis occurs in the red active bone marrow and the development processes are characterized by the condensation and lobulation of the nucleus, loss of some organelles, such as the mitochondria, and the formation of cytoplasmic granules.

Although the homeostatic regulation of granulopoiesis has yet to be identified, it is known that the maturation process takes about 14 days. Approximately 50% of these newly formed mature cells adhere closely to the endothelial lining of blood vessels and are called marginating cells. The remaining granulocytes circulate in the blood. Within a matter of hours, however, some of these circulating cells enter the tissues requiring their services, and these are destined never to return to blood.

Agranulocytes, i.e. lymphocytes and monocytes, are also produced in the red bone marrow. Other areas, however, are also concerned with agranulopoiesis. For example, prior to birth and for a few months of neonatal life some lymphocytes (T-lymphocytes) are produced in the thymus gland, and later most lymphocytes (T- and B-lymphocytes) and monocytes are formed within the lymph nodes and other lymphatic tissue, such as the spleen and lymphoidal tissue associated with the gut (for example, the adenoids, tonsils, appendix, etc.; Chapter 10). The developmental processes are summarized in Figure 8.5.

The lifespan of a leucocyte is the shortest of all the cellular components of blood. Whilst red cells live for 100–120 days and platelets for 5–9 days, in a healthy body white cells will survive for only 4–5 days. Neutrophils have an even shorter lifespan, of approximately 12 hours or less, when they are actively phagocytosing bacteria, as the bacterial antigens interfere with metabolism and accelerate leukocyte death.

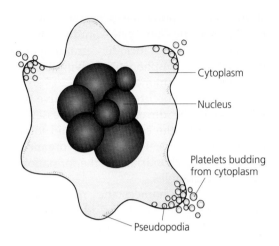

Cytoplasm

Nucleus

Platelets budding from cytoplasm

Pseudopodia

Figure 8.8 A megakaryocyte showing platelet budding.

Thrombocytes (platelets)

Structure

Thrombocytes are more numerous than leucocytes, but less numerous than erythrocytes; there are approximately 250 000/mm³. They form the smallest cellular component of blood, being only 2–4 μm in diameter. These cells do not have a nucleus and microscopically appear as a disc-shaped structure with a colourless cytoplasm. Their membranes are the site of many enzymatic reactions, and contain specific receptors for collagen and the hormones serotonin and adrenaline. Microfilaments can be observed in the cytoplasm composed of a contractile protein called platelet actomyosin (thrombosthenin). These function in the haemostatic process of clot retraction (described below). Thrombocytes possess numerous cytoplasmic granules which contain enzymes or factors that are released by exocytosis when platelets aggregate together and/or are lysed, as they are important in the homeostatic function of blood coagulation.

Production and destruction of thrombocytes: a homeostatic process

Thrombocytes are formed in the red marrow, lungs, and to some extent the spleen and liver,

by the fragmentation of very large cells called megakaryocytes (Figures 8.5 and 8.8). The rate of platelet production, a process called thrombopoiesis, is tightly regulated between the two interchangeable platelet 'pools' of the circulation and spleen. The feedback mechanism for thrombopoiesis and this interchange has yet to be identified. It must be stimulated, however, by a low platelet count (called thrombocytopenia). A platelet's lifespan is about 5–9 days, after which it is destroyed by specialized macrophages of the liver and spleen.

HAEMOSTASIS: A HOMEOSTATIC PROCESS

Haemostasis is the term used to describe the processes involved in arresting bleeding. Upon blood vessel damage three phases act to prevent further blood loss: (1) vascular, (2) platelet and (3) blood coagulation phases (Figure 8.9). These mechanisms are adequate as homeostatic controls in preventing blood loss if the damage is to small blood vessels. If large blood vessels are involved (resulting in mass haemorrhage), these mechanisms are inadequate, however, and, as with all homeostatic failures, there will be a need for clinical intervention to correct this imbalance.

Vascular phase

Damage to blood vessels causes the vessel's muscular wall (or tunica media) to contract immediately. This vasoconstrictive, vascular spasm decreases blood loss for up to 30 minutes, during which time other homeostatic mechanisms are initiated in the haemostatic response.

Platelet phase

The platelets that come into contact with the damaged vessel enlarge becoming irregular in shape. They become extremely sticky, adhering

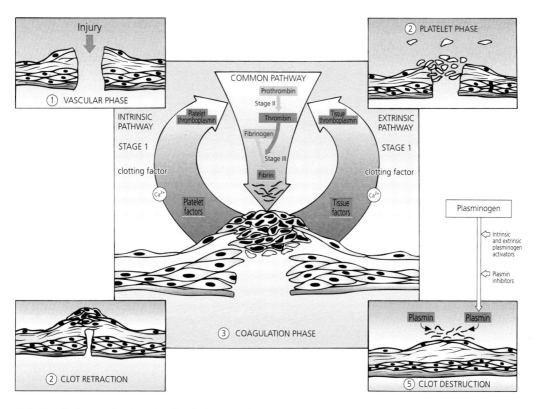

Figure 8.9 The clotting mechanism. Details of plasma and platelet clotting factors are discussed in the text and in Table 8.6. 1 Vascular phase. Vessels go into spasm in the damaged smooth muscle. This decreases blood flow. 2 Platelet phase. Thrombocytes aggregate, accumulate, and adhere to the damaged vessels, forming the platelet plug. 3 Coagulation phase. Activation of clotting and clot formation. 4 Clot retraction. Involves the contraction of the blood clot. 5 Clot destruction. Enzymatic (plasmin) destruction of the clot. + Stimulatory; – inhibition.

to the collagen fibres of the vessel wall. These thrombocytes secrete substances which activate more platelets, causing them to stick to the original ones. The aggregation and attachment of platelets forms a platelet 'plug', and forms almost immediately following the damage. The plug becomes strengthened by fibrin threads formed during the coagulation process and is extremely effective in preventing blood loss from small vessels.

Blood coagulation phase

Coagulation is a complicated metabolic pathway involving many interdependent enzymatically controlled reactions. Collectively these reactions are called the 'clotting cascade' and is a multiplicative process: proenzymes interact, and the conversion of one proenzyme creates an enzyme that activates a second proenzyme that activates a third proenzyme, and so on, in a chain reaction. There are many clotting factors involved (Table 8.6). These include plasma factors (numbered I to XIII), and platelet factors (Pf1 to Pf4). This cascade occurs rapidly once stimulated, and when blood is taken, or a vessel damaged, blood is quickly converted from its usual liquefied state into a gel-like clot. The process is initiated within 30 seconds of damage and completed after several minutes. The coagulation phase can be summarized as being a sequence of three stages:

Table 8.6 The homeostatic importance of coagulation factors

Coagulation factors	Homeostatic importance
Plasma coagulation factors	
I Fibrinogen•	Important factor in stage III of clotting, in which it is converted to fibrin
II Prothrombin*†	Important in stage II of clotting in which it is converted into thrombin
III Thromboplastin (thrombokinase)	In extrinsic pathway it is referred to as extrinsic thromboplastin; it is formed from tissue thromboplastin. In the intrinsic pathway it is referred as intrinsic thromboplastin; it is formed from platelet disintegration. Formation of thromboplastin signifies the end of stage I.
IV Calcium ions	Involved in all three stages of clotting. Removal of calcium or its binding in the plasma prevents coagulation
V Proaccelerin or labile factor	Required for stages I and II of both extrinsic and intrinsic pathways
VI No longer used in coagulation theory	
VII Serum prothrombin accelerator or stable factor	Required in stage I extrinsic pathway
V III Antihaemophilic factor	Required for stage I of intrinsic pathway. Deficiency causes classical haemophilia A
IX Christmas factor or plasma thromboplastin component	Required for stage I of intrinsic pathway. Deficiency caused haemophilia B
X Stuart factor or Stuart–Prower factor	Required for stages I and II of extrinsic and intrinsic pathways. Deficiency results in nose bleeds, bleeding into joints, or bleeding into soft tissues
XI Plasma thromboplastin antecedent	Required for stage I of intrinsic pathway. Deficiency results in haemophilia C
XII Hageman factor	Required for stage I of intrinsic pathway
XIII Fibrin stabilizing factor	Required for stage III of clotting
Platelet coagulation factors	
Platelet factor 1 – Pf1	Essentially same as plasma coagulation factor V
Platelet factor 2 – Pf2	Accelerates formation of thrombin in stage 1 intrinsic pathway and the conversion of fibrinogen to fibrin
Platelet factor 3 – Pf3	Required for stage I of intrinsic pathway
Platelet factor 4 – Pf4	Binds heparin, an anticoagulant during clotting

1 Stage I. The formation and the release of a collection of enzymes, collectively called 'thromboplastin' (or thrombokinase).

2 Stage II. Conversion of prothrombin into thrombin via the actions of thromboplastin.

3 Stage III. Conversion of the soluble protein fibrinogen into insoluble fibrin by the actions of thrombin; the fibrin then forms the threads of the clot.

The 'initiating' enzyme (thromboplastin) is released from damaged tissue cells, triggering the extrinsic coagulation pathway and/or by the lysis of platelets, which triggers the intrinsic coagulation pathway.

Extrinsic pathway

This pathway is initiated by the release of tissue factor (an enzyme) from damaged peripheral cells and/or damaged capillary endothelial cells. This enzyme together with certain plasma factors (IV, V, VII and X) forms extrinsic or tissue thromboplastin, which is equivalent to stage I of the clotting cascade. The second stage utilizes extrinsic thromboplastin to convert prothrombin into thrombin. The second stage is promoted with the conversion of fibrinogen into fibrin by the action of thrombin and plasma factors IV and XIII. Most steps in the extrinsic mechanism also require the presence of calcium ions.

Intrinsic pathway

This pathway is activated by a rough surface such as 'fatty' plaques or calcium deposits attached to the internal lining of the blood vessel. This stimulus removes the normal repulsion activities between platelets and endothelial cells lining the blood vessels, with the result that platelets adhere to the rough surface. The aggregation and clumping of platelets bring about their lysis, releasing platelet coagulation factors (Pf1–4) into the plasma. The clumping reaction is sometimes all that is necessary to plug lightly damaged areas.

Stage I of the intrinsic pathway involves four platelet factors (Pf1–4) and seven plasma factors (IV, V, VIII, IX, X, XI, XII) to form intrinsic thromboplastin. The second stage involves the conversion of prothrombin into thrombin by the thromboplastin. The third stage is the same for both intrinsic and extrinsic pathways. All stages of the intrinsic pathway require the presence of calcium ions.

Thrombin is a key chemical because of its involvement in the third stage and because it stimulates more platelets to adhere to one another, resulting in a further lysis of platelets and thus the consequential release of further platelet factors. The more thrombin that is released, therefore, the more platelet factors are released, resulting in a greater clot formation. This cyclical process is therefore a positive feedback mechanism and is a feature of the intrinsic pathway. It ensures continual platelet lysis until the clot is formed.

Once the fibrin meshwork has been formed the platelets and erythrocytes stick to its strands. The platelets contract with the result that the entire clot retracts, bringing the torn edges closer together and also stabilizing and consolidating the injury. The clot plugs the damaged vessel to prevent further blood loss and the retraction makes it easier for fibroblasts, smooth muscle cells, and endothelial cells to carry out their homeostatic repair functions. Once the area is repaired the clot is dissolved via the process of fibrinolysis, which involves tissue factors (intrinsic and extrinsic) that activate the precursor plasminogen into the catabolizing enzyme plasmin. The process is summarized in Figure 8.9.

BLOOD GROUPINGS

People can be classified into one of several blood groups depending on the presence, or absence, of particular genetically determined antigens, called agglutinogens or isoantigens, on the erythrocytic membrane, and on the presence or absence of genetically determined antibodies called agglutinins or isoantibodies, in an individual's plasma. There are over 35 blood groups world-wide (see Table 8.7 for some of the commoner ones) but, although these are of immense importance in forensic medicine, only the two principal blood group

Table 8.7 Red cell agglutinogens of the main blood groups

Blood group	Agglutinogens
ABO	A B *
Rhesus	D *
MNSs	M N S s
Lutheran	Lu^a Lu^b
Lewis	Le^a Le^b
Duffy	Fy^a Fy^b
Diego	Di^a Di^b
Kidd	Kj

* Includes subtypes not mentioned

systems, the ABO and Rhesus systems, are important clinically. This is because transfusion of an inappropriate type of blood can promote clumping, or agglutination, of red cells in the recipient.

ABO system

The ABO grouping is based upon two agglutinogens, symbolized as A and B. Erythrocytes have one, two or neither agglutinogen attached to their surfaces. Correspondingly, the plasma contains one, both, or neither corresponding agglutinins called anti-A (alpha, or a) or anti-B (beta, or b). These agglutinins are of the IgM type (Chapter 10) and appear at, or just after birth, and exist throughout life, although their production may decline or disappear during old age.

The four blood groups associated with the ABO system are groups A, B, AB, and O. Their frequencies exhibit ethnic variation but in England are 40%, 10% , 4%, and 46% respectively. People of group A have the A agglutinogen; those of group B have B agglutinogens; those of group AB have both A and B agglutinogens, and finally those of group O do not possess either agglutinogen (Figure 8.10a). If one follows the simple rule that the group is named after the agglutinogens present, then one can predict what plasma agglutinins (if any) will also be present. This is because there are only two agglutinins, anti-A and anti-B, and these interact with opposing agglutinogens A and B respectively. It is essential, therefore, to have different agglutinins and agglutinogens in order to prevent auto-cross-reactions which would cause agglutination and haemolysis as illustrated in Figure 8.10b. This reaction could be fatal if the clump of erythrocytes blocked a blood vessel to a vital organ such as the heart.

These principles are important when considering the essentials of successful blood transfusions. It is important to remember, though, that it is the effect of the recipient's plasma

(a)

Genotype	AA	AO	BB	BO	AB	OO
Blood group (phenotype)	A (43%)		B (8%)		AB (3%)	O (46%)

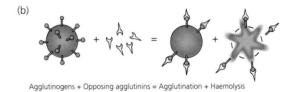

(b)

Agglutinogens + Opposing agglutinins = Agglutination + Haemolysis

Figure 8.10 (a) Blood grouping and frequencies within the United Kingdom. The blood group depends upon the presence of antigens (agglutinogens) on the surface of red cells. This is determined by alleles A, B, and O. The plasma contains antibodies (agglutinins) which will react with 'foreign' agglutinogens (i.e. a reaction takes place when the agglutinogens are of the same variety of agglutinins). See text for details. (b) Cross–reactions. Cross–reactions (incompatible transfusions) occur when the plasma's agglutinins (antibodies) encounter complementary erythrocytic agglutinogens (antigens). The result is extensive clumping (agglutination) of the affected red cells and subsequent haemolysis.

agglutinins on the donor's erythrocyte agglutinogens which may cause problems: the donor's plasma agglutinins are ignored, since they are soon diluted by the greater volume of fluid of the recipient. Thus, agglutination will occur whenever recipient agglutinins and donor agglutinogens of the same type are mixed. Such blood is said to be incompatible and Figure 8.10a illustrates which transfusion combinations can be successful. For example, blood group A can be transfused into its own blood group, but cannot be transfused into blood group B, since the recipient has the plasma anti-A agglutinins, and these would react against the donor's A agglutinogens. Group A can also be a donor to blood group AB since they do not possess either anti-A or anti-B. Group AB have been referred to as the 'universal recipients', as they can receive blood from any other blood group.

Blood groups A, B, and AB cannot be donors for blood group O. This is because O recipients have agglutinins anti-A and anti-B, and the A, B, and AB groups possess at least one agglutinogen. Conversely, group O individuals have been referred to as the 'universal donors', as they can give blood to any other blood group, since they do not have agglutinogens A or B on their surface and antibody–antigen reactions will not therefore be initiated. The use of the term 'universal' has fallen into disuse nowadays, however, since this term means all possible circumstances and takes no account of blood group systems other than the ABO. Usually blood of the same group within the ABO system will be used to prevent any possibility of mixing incompatible bloods.

Inheritance of the ABO blood groups

Before reading this section, the reader should be familiar with alleles and allelic variation, described in Chapter 20.

Chromosome 9 contains the alleles A, B, and O which determine one's blood group. Alleles A and B are codominant to each other and both are dominant to the recessive allele O. Thus, there are six genotypes which determine the four blood group phenotypes of the ABO system (Figure 8.10a). Blood group A is derived from homozygous dominant A (i.e. alleles AA) or heterozygous A (i.e. alleles AO) genotypes. Group B is derived from either the homozygous B (i.e. alleles BB) or the heterozygous B (i.e. alleles BO) genotypes. People of blood group AB have both alleles, A and B.

Finally, group O are homozygous for the O alleles, which are incapable of coding for agglutinogens.

Rhesus blood group and its inheritance

The rhesus system is so called because it was first identified in the rhesus monkey. People are classified as having either rhesus positive or rhesus negative blood; 85% of the UK population are rhesus positive, i.e. they possess the rhesus (D factor) agglutinogen on the erythrocytic surfaces. The remaining 15% of the population are rhesus negative, that is, they do not possess the rhesus agglutinogen. The presence of the agglutinogen is controlled by the rhesus (D) gene, found on chromosome 1. Thus, the possible genotypes responsible for determining one's rhesus status are: homozygous dominant (DD) and heterozygotes (Dd); these people will be rhesus positive and the homozygous recessive (dd) genotype which is not capable of coding for the rhesus agglutinogen; these people will be rhesus negative.

Unlike the ABO system, the plasma of rhesus negative people does not normally contain rhesus antibodies or agglutinins. However, transfusion of rhesus positive erythrocytes into a rhesus negative recipient may stimulate the humoral immune response in the recipient with the release of the anti-rhesus or, more commonly known, anti-D agglutinins that produce agglutination and haemolysis of the transfused cells. When considering transfusions, therefore, the rhesus factor must be taken into consideration in order to minimize the risks of incompatible transfusions and their fatal outcomes. At particular risk are rhesus positive fetuses being carried by rhesus negative mothers, as this may result in haemolytic disease of the newborn, which is discussed later.

Homeostatic failures and principles of correction

Haematology (the study of blood) involves estimating the number/values of cellular and non-cellular blood components and comparing these with the normal homeostatic ranges of specific components. The shape, or morphology, and size of the cellular components is investigated using a stained blood film. Bone marrow biopsies confirm a diagnosis suggested by clinical examination and blood investigations by providing information about the homeostatic status of haemopoiesis, the number of the respective cellular components, and the presence of atypical cells, as found in metastatic cancers and Hodgkin's disease.

Figure 8.11 represents a specimen laboratory slip used in clinical blood analysis.

Homeostatic disturbances of plasma composition have been considered in earlier chapters on metabolism, body fluids, and digestion and are

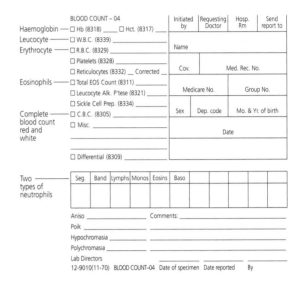

Figure 8.11 The laboratory slip requesting blood analysis.

Table 8.8 Plasma components for clinical use in redressing plasma component homeostasis*

Plasma component	Clinical homeostatic correction
Plasma protein fraction	Plasma replacement Blood volume expansion
Human albumin	Albumin replacement in hypoalbuminaemia, e.g. in nephrosis
Fresh frozen plasma	Clotting factor deficiencies, e.g. in liver disease.
Cryoprecipitate (factor VIII, fibrinogen)	Classical haemophilia (haemophilia A) Von Willebrand's disease Fibrinogen deficiency
Factor VIII concentrate and freeze-dried factor VIII	Classical haemophilia A
Factor IX concentrate	Christmas disease (haemophilia B)
Human immunoglobulin (Ig)	Hypogammaglobulinaemia, e.g. to produce passive immunity to viral diseases such as rubella (German measles)
Human specific globulin (specific antibodies)	To produce passive immunity to rare, life-threatening disease, e.g. tetanus.

* Apply principles shown in Figure 8.3.

discussed further in later chapters on respiration and immunity. Table 8.8 illustrates the use of plasma component therapy in re-establishing a patient's plasma homeostatic balance. This section is mainly concerned with homeostatic failures which involve the blood's cellular components and their principles of correction using the appropriate blood component therapy.

HOMEOSTATIC FAILURES AFFECTING THE ERYTHROCYTE POPULATION

Erythrocytic imbalances are due to a mismatch between erythrocyte production and destruction. In order to investigate such imbalances, a reticulocyte count is taken; those cells are precursors of erythrocytes and account for 0.5–1.5% of the erythrocyte population in blood. Reticulocyte counts of less than 0.5% of the total erythrocyte population indicate blood production cannot match the loss, and this occurs in pernicious anaemia, iron deficiency anaemia and during radiation therapy (Figure 8.12). Low reticulocyte counts may also be due to a deficiency of erythrogenin and/or erythropoietinogen and/or erythropoietin. If the count is above 1.5%, production is pathologically greater than destruction. This occurs in response to a number of different conditions including haemolytic anaemia, leukaemia, and metabolic carcinoma.

Measuring the packed cell volume (haematocrit) is another routine clinical test. Haematocrits of, for example, 0.15 (15%; low) and 0.65 (65%; high) reflect the homeostatic imbalances of severe anaemia and polycythaemia respectively.

Anaemia

Anaemia occurs when the number of erythrocytes, or the level of haemoglobin, is below the homeostatic range. Haemoglobin and erythrocytes are at first reduced equally, but as the bone marrow replaces erythrocyte loss, blood

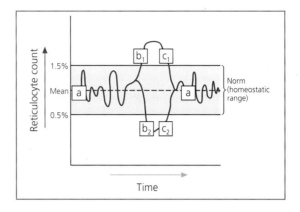

Figure 8.12 The homeostatic and clinical control of the number of erythrocytes (using a reticulocyte count as an indicator of the red cell number). The reticulocyte count is the percentage of reticulocytes within the total number of erythrocytes.

a, Normal homeostatic levels of reticulocytes – 'hunting about the mean'. This indicates that the erythrocytic homeostatic range is being achieved, i.e. red cell production rate matches destruction rate.

b_1, Reticulocyte count is beyond the homeostatic range (i.e. >1.5% of mature erythrocytes), indicating production is > destruction of red cells (resulting in polycythaemia). The excessive production can be considered a normal physiological reaction in response to altitude hypoxia, which results in hypersecretion of the hormone erythropoietin. Alternatively, the polycythaemia may be indicative of a pathological homeostatic imbalance, as experienced with cancers of erythropoietic sites and/or kidney cells, resulting in hypersecretion of erythrogenin.

b_2, Reticulocyte count is below the homeostatic range (0.5%), indicating production is < destruction. The low levels may be indicative of pathological homeostatic imbalances such as (i) anaemias (Table 8.9), (ii) liver or kidney diseases which cause hyposecretion of erythrogenin, resulting in less erythropoietin reaching the erythropoietic sites, (iii) conditions which cause a hyposecretion of the hormone precursor erythropoietinogen.

c_1, Clinical correction of pathological polycythaemias involves 'bleeding' therapy.

c_2, Clinical correction of red cell deficiency involves red cell infusions.

investigations may reveal an adequate number of red cells with abnormal low levels of pigment present. Anaemias are classified according to their causal factors, and are broadly divided into conditions which are a consequence of an increased blood loss and those which are due to a decreased blood production (Table 8.9).

Table 8.9 Classification of anaemia

Increased blood loss
    Haemorrhage – acute, e.g. accident
                   – chronic, e.g. menstruation
    Haemolysis   – intracellular cause, e.g. abnormal haemoglobin variant
                   – extracellular cause, e.g. bacteria

Decreased blood production
    Nutritional deficiency: e.g. iron, vitamin B_{12}, folic acid, protein
    Bone marrow failure – primary, e.g. congenital
                              – secondary, e.g. acquired (ionizing radiation)

Hereditary
    Sickle cell anaemia
    Thalassaemia

In general, irrespective of its type, anaemia affects all organ systems and is particularly characterized by signs and symptoms of oxygen shortage at peripheral tissues. These include a pallor of the skin, especially noticeable on the lips and eyelids, where the skin is thin, a feeling of tiredness and listlessness, a pulse which is full and soft, with both pulse and respiratory rates increasing unduly on slight exertion, a tendency for the ankles to swell due to peripheral oedema, and an appearance of central nervous system symptoms in severe anaemia, including tinnitis (ringing in the ears), headaches, spots before the eyes, fainting, and giddiness.

Minor signs aid differential diagnosis. For example, haemolytic anaemias often show the classical jaundice colorization due to the deposition of bile pigments in skin. However, standard laboratory tests based on the number, size and morphology of erythrocytes, and cellular haemoglobin content are required for accurate diagnosis. Obviously, it is important that the underlying cause is identified as this forms the basis of correction. For example, iron deficiency anaemia necessitates treating the patient with digestible iron salts (such as ferrous sulphate tablets), whilst simultaneously ensuring that the patient eats an adequate diet. Alternatively, severe anaemias may require blood transfusions, though this has the associated risk of fluid overload unless the anaemia was caused by acute haemorrhage.

Concentrated (packed) red cells are preferable to whole blood transfusions, in order to restore the oxygen carrying capacity of blood without greatly disturbing the blood volume. Washed red cells may be administered, in order to remove antigenic substances (such as some plasma proteins) attached to the erythrocytes. Frozen preparations may also be used because freezing lowers the leucocyte and thrombocyte content and also eliminates pathogenic organisms.

Polycythaemia

Blood with an increase of 2–3 million red cells per mm^3 above their normal homeostatic range are considered to be polycythaemic. The presence of excessive cells increases the blood's viscosity, slowing the flow rate to such an extent that there is an increased risk of intrinsic clotting and its potential consequences, such as ischaemic attacks and thrombotic infarctions. Polycythaemia occurs in dehydrated patients, as all body fluids are concentrated with the result that erythrocytes become relatively more numerous in any measured quantity of blood.

There are various pathological conditions of the heart, circulation, lungs, and bone marrow, which cause the body to manufacture extra erythrocytes, sometimes to twice the normal values, in order to carry sufficient quantities of oxygen to support metabolic demands. An increase in erythrocytes also occurs during prolonged hypoxia (a deficiency of oxygen in the tissues), when living at high altitudes. In such circumstances, polycythaemia is considered a homeostatic adaptation, whereby it becomes 'normal' and necessary to have a large number of cells as a compensatory mechanism for the low atmospheric oxygen levels. Polycythaemia therefore is not always pathological, but may be a consequence of the homeostatic set points being reset. Mountaineers and people living at 10 000–12 000 feet may have haematocrits as high as 0.65 (65%).

The causes of polycythaemia are largely unknown, but various hormones are known to affect the rate of erythropoiesis. Polycythaemia, therefore, may be a clinical sign of certain endocrine disorders, for example the hypersecretion of cortisol in Cushing's syndrome.

True polycythaemia is one of the very few diseases for which bleeding is still employed as a principle of correction of a homeostatic imbalance. Modern methods include the insertion of a wide-bore needle into a vein, and these have superseded the traditional methods of vein cutting, or application of blood-sucking leeches.

HOMEOSTATIC FAILURES AFFECTING THE LEUCOCYTE POPULATION

Leucocytosis and leucopenia

These are general terms used to indicate leucocytic levels above and below the homeostatic range. The suffixes -osis and -penia are used to indicate a specific leucocytic excess or deficiency respectively, for example, granulocytosis and granulocytopenia. A differential white cell count (a percentage of each cell in

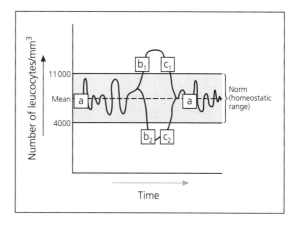

Figure 8.13 The homeostatic and clinical control of the number of leucocytes.

a, Homeostatic levels of the number of leucocytes, i.e. production rate = destruction rate.

b_1, Leucocytosis – white cells in excess of their homeostatic range (i.e. > 11 000 per µl). The excess can be a result of the homeostatic set–points being changed in response to altered states of health (such as pregnancy). The excess then can be considered quite a normal adaptation to changing metabolic demands. Alternatively, the excess may be an indication of a protective response to infection and/or some underlying pathology. A differential white cell count indicates which leucocytic imbalance is present. The differential white cell count is an important diagnostic aid (see Tables 8.10 and 8.11).

b_2, Leucopenia – white cells below the homeostatic range (i.e. < 4000 per µl). A leucopenia can be a lack of all white cells or as a result of inadequate levels of specific white cells (Table 8.10).

c_1, Clinical correction of the leucocytosis includes chemotherapy and radiotherapy. Bone marrow transplantation may be required for those patients experiencing very high–dose chemotherapy as this destroys all residual leucocytes.

c_2, Clinical correction of agranulocytosis includes removal of the aetiological factor (for example the rapid withdrawal of offending drugs such as sulphonamides and antihistamine), and by injections of hydrocortisone or adrenocorticotrophic hormone (ACTH). Granulocyte transfusions are still at the experimental stage, and are used when antibiotic therapy is ineffective in controlling severe infections in patients with bone marrow neutropenia.

100 leucocytes) confirms which specific white cell imbalance is present and is a diagnostic aid for certain clinical conditions. Figure 8.13 illustrates the homeostatic and clinical control of

Table 8.10 Classification of homeostatic imbalances of blood cells

| Blood cells | Homeostatic imbalances | |
	Excess	Deficiency
Leucocytes:		
general	Leucocytosis	Leucopenia
specific		
granulocytes	Neutrophilia ⎫ Basophilia ⎬ granulocytosis Eosinophilia ⎭	Neutropenia ⎫ Basopenia ⎬ agranulocytosis Eosinopenia ⎭
non-granulocytes	Lymphocytosis Monocytosis	Lymphopenia Monopenia
Erythrocytes	Polycythaemia	Anaemia
Thrombocytes	Thrombocytosis	Thrombocytopenia

Table 8.11 Types of leukaemia and the cells involved

Type of leukaemia	Cellular imbalance
Myeloid (myelocytic, myeloblastic)	Granulocytes
Lymphocytic (lymphoblastic)	Lymphocytes
Monocytic	Monocytes

Table 8.12 Typical results for a differential leucocyte count (numbers are percentage of total leucocyte population) on blood from a normal person and a patient with the homeostatic imbalance of leukaemia

Leucocytes	Normal person	Patient with chronic lymphatic leukaemia
Neutrophils	65	3
Monocytes	8	1
Lymphocytes	24	96
Eosinophils	2	–
Basophils	1	–

the leucocyte population. Table 8.10 refers to the classification of the homeostatic imbalances and how this can be used to aid clinical diagnosis. Slight temporary increases in leucocytes occur during the process of digestion and an increase of longer duration exists in pregnancy. The latter requires the homeostatic set-points to be changed to accommodate the altered metabolic requirements. In the majority of situations, however, a leucocytosis implies a normal protective reaction to a variety of pathological conditions especially in response to inflammation or infection. In any infection, a leucocytosis representing an increase from

9 000 to 15 000/ mm^3, is a good sign, indicating that white cells are responding to challenge. Conversely, no increase, or an inadequate increase, in leucocytes is an unfavourable sign. Once the infection subsides, the number of leucocytes return to the normal homeostatic parameters.

Leukaemia

This malignant disease or group of diseases is characterized by gross excessive activity of the leucopoietic organs (bone marrow, spleen, or lymph glands) and is frequently called 'cancer of the blood', because of the vast quantities of circulating leucocytes. These proliferating white cells crowd out other cells produced in the marrow, and so symptoms usually include a deficiency in red cells and platelets, i.e. anaemia and thrombocytopenia respectively. The causes of the leukaemias are largely unknown with only a few being identified. For example, some people have a genetic predisposition that is triggered by environmental factors, such as radiation and viruses. Leukaemias are classified according to the cell type involved (Table 8.11) and also according to their rate of development, i.e. acute and chronic leukaemias.

The most common cause of death from leukaemias is internal haemorrhaging, especially within the brain. Another frequent cause of death is uncontrolled infection owing to the lack of mature, or normal, leucocytes. Correction is aimed at removing this abnormal accumulation of white cells using radiotherapy and antileukaemic (cytotoxic) drugs. Partial or complete remission may be induced, with some lasting as long as 15 years. Table 8.12 compares the typical results of a differential white cell count of a normal individual, and a leukaemic patient. Bone marrow transplants are considered as a possible treatment for severe aplastic anaemias, acute leukaemias, infrequent congenital immune deficiency, and haemopoietic disorders. Although a transplant is the best chance of a cure for such patients, it is not without potential risks.

HOMEOSTATIC FAILURES OF THE CLOTTING MECHANISM (Figure 8.14)

Thrombocyte imbalances

Thrombocytosis is an abnormally high platelet count, and is a common sign of many diseases, including certain leukaemias, such as myeloid leukaemia. Thrombocytopenia is the commonest cause of haemostatic defects, however, as a consequence of a decreased blood platelet count to below 150 000/mm^3. Thrombocytopenia may be due to either a decrease in platelet production or an increased rate of

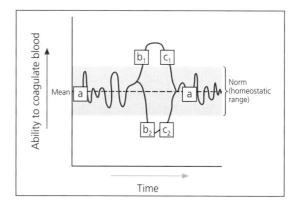

Figure 8.14 The homeostatic and clinical control of blood clotting.

a, Normal ability to coagulate blood, i.e. thrombocyte and clotting factors are within their homeostatic ranges.

b_1, An increased ability to clot the blood. This may be due to other homeostatic imbalances, e.g. hyperlipidaemia or hypercalcaemia, responsible for an increased tendency for atherosclerotic plaque and calcium deposit formation respectively. Both precipitate blood clotting. Alternatively, the increased clotting ability may be a result of a normal physiological homeostatic mechanism (haemostasis) which goes into operation when one damages a blood vessel.

b_2, Decreased ability to produce blood clots. This may be due to a homeostatic imbalance of the factors involved in blood clotting, e.g. hypocalcaemia, hypoprothrombinaemia, hypofibrinogenaemia, inadequate levels of vitamin K or factor VIII (haemophilia, etc.).

c_1, Clinical correction involves fibrolytic enzyme (streptokinase or urokinase) therapy.

c_2, Clinical correction of prolonged bouts of bleeding involves the administration of the deficient aetiological factors, e.g. factor VIII therapy in classical haemophilia A.

destruction. The latter may be a consequence of thrombocytes being crowded out of the bone marrow in certain bone diseases, such as certain leukaemias, pernicious anaemia or malignant tumours. X-irradiation, radioactive isotopes, cytotoxic drugs and other drugs, such as sulphonamides and phenylbutazone, may also reduce the thrombocyte concentration.

Thrombocytopenia is evident in various types of purpura, a condition characterized by small multiple haemorrhagic spots (petechiae), or as large blotchy areas on the skin and mucous membranes. Purpura is also a complication of other blood diseases, such as leukaemias and severe anaemias, and may also result from antibiotic and corticosteroid therapies.

Clotting factor imbalances

The cascade of enzymatic conversions during clotting means that a disorder which affects any individual clotting factor disrupts the whole clotting mechanism. Many clinical conditions can therefore result in clotting abnormalities, particularly those which disrupt calcium and vitamin K metabolism. Calcium ions are important in most of the cascade reactions, and so calcium imbalance has a direct effect on coagulation. Vitamin K is required for the synthesis of five clotting factors (including prothrombin) and its deficiency results in a breakdown of the common pathway. Deficiency can be due to either insufficient dietary intake, malabsorption problems, or its incorrect utilization. Dietary deficiencies are uncommon, as symbiotic colonic bacteria usually supply the individual with sufficient levels of this vitamin (Chapter 7). Deficiencies can occur, however, if these bacteria are interfered with, for example upon sterilizing treatments of the bowel. Malabsorption of vitamin K is the most common cause of depressed circulating levels. Being fat-soluble, this vitamin requires bile salts for its absorption, and so low circulating levels can occur in liver diseases, in prolonged

bilary tract obstruction and in any other disease which impairs fat absorption (for example, coeliac disease). Pancreatic disease and chronic diarrhoea may also be responsible for this vitamin's deficiency. Conversely, levels in excess of the homeostatic range of vitamin K or calcium may result in inappropiate clot formation, or thrombosis.

Increased fragility of capillary walls

Increased fragility of capillary walls results in bleeding (appearing as bruising under the skin), even when there is minimal damage. The main aetiological factors are thrombocytopenia, the use of certain pharmacological preparations (e.g. penicillin and aspirin), and autoimmune diseases.

The principles of correction involve treating the cause, but other measures include anti-inflammatory and immunosuppression therapy, removal of the spleen (splenectomy) and transfusions of preparations rich in thrombocytes.

Plaques

Hyperactivity of the clotting mechanism may result from a roughened or irregular surface within the cardiovascular system, causing platelet aggregation and/or lysis. In aggregation, platelets adhere to the roughened inner coat (tunica intima) of intact vessels, perhaps due to the presence of fatty streaks (precursors of atherosclerotic plaques, the lipid storage deposits found in the endothelial and smooth muscle cells), or endothelial calcium deposits. Both situations are inevitable consequences of the ageing process and may result in thrombosis.

Thrombosis

A clot is called a thrombus when it forms within an intact vessel (hence the term thrombosis). Once formed, the clot progressively enlarges, causing more and more of the lumen to become obliterated. This may progress until the clot severely impairs blood flow to the tissue's cells. If the oxygen supply is not restored, cells surrounding the area of the clot die (called necrosis) resulting in an infarction. Alternatively, a part of the clot may break off (dislodged thrombi are called emboli) and become lodged in small blood vessels producing ischaemic changes and infarction. The lungs are a common embolic site where the emboli will produce a pulmonary infarction. Emboli can also be produced as a result of platelet lysis.

Clotting can occur in the heart and arteries, but is more common in the veins, because blood flow is relatively slow-moving. The leg or pelvic veins are the most frequent site of venous thrombosis, and these carry a risk of subsequent pulmonary embolism. Venous thrombosis is promoted under various circumstances. For example, it can occur after childbirth, or following abdominal operations, and is one of the reasons for encouraging early mobility in surgical patients. Thrombosis may also result from blood conditions including: anaemia; infections; venous stagnation (as in varicose veins); prolonged bed-rest enforced by operation or illness; inflammation and degeneration of vessel wall. Venous stagnation may be prevented by limb exercises or, clinically, by application of an elastic stocking to the legs or by intermittent pneumatic compression of the limbs.

Common arterial clotting sites are the vessels of the heart leading to coronary thrombosis, and the brain's cerebral vessels, leading to a stroke. These, together with pulmonary infarctions, have high mortality rates. Deteriorating blood vessels in the elderly may promote thrombosis within the retinal artery, with the resultant loss of vision and/or thrombosis of leg arteries, resulting in gangrene of the foot.

Blood clotting is a continuous process in blood vessels, since roughened surfaces are constantly being formed (fatty streaks have been identified upon autopsies of children as young as 6 years old). However, coagulation is always homeostatically corrected by the body's own clot-preventing and clot-dissolving mechanisms, for example by the plasma factor plasmin.

The clinical correction of clotting hyperactivity involves administration of factors, called anticoagulants, which prevent clotting or factors which enhance thrombus dissolution.

Anticoagulation

Heparin, a fast-acting anticoagulant, is produced and secreted (within its homeostatic range) by the liver and inhibits the conversion of prothrombin to thrombin. However, blood vessel damage may cause the liver to reduce its secretion of heparin and so removes this inhibitor to the clotting process. Heparin administration is useful in preventing post-operative thrombosis and is vital for open heart surgery and other operations in order to prevent potentially fatal clot formation.

Prostacyclin, a type of prostaglandin (Chapter 15), is also an endogenous anticoagulant that is secreted from the lining of healthy vessels.

Vitamin K antagonists (e.g. warfarin, phenindione, dicoumarol) may be given to thrombosis-prone patients as a preventive measure. The drug operates by lowering the prothrombin concentration in plasma.

Various calcium-binding compounds may be added to sampled blood as anticoagulants (for example, EDTA – ethylenediaminetetra-acetic acid and ACD – acid citrate dextrose). These reduce the ionic calcium in plasma and so prevent the conversion of prothrombin into thrombin.

Thrombus dissolution

Thrombus dissolution therapy involves the administration of fibrolytic enzymes, called streptokinase and urokinase, which promote endogenous plasmin production. This is extremely effective at removing pulmonary, coronary arterial and deep vein clots.

Haemophilia

Haemophilia affects 0.01% of the population and is frequently referred to as the 'bleeding disease'. This is because haemophiliacs are at risk of excessive bleeding if accidental blood vessel damage occurs, or if they are subjected to factors which precipitate bleeding, such as overindulgence of alcohol or penicillin, as these may be responsible for producing internal haemorrhage.

Haemophiliacs lack the gene necessary for the production of specific clotting factors, or the gene is defective, or the gene is not expressed. These genes are on the X sex chromosome, and the condition predominantly occurs in males (see Chapter 20). Patients with this disorder are prone to repeated episodes of severe and prolonged bleeding at any site, particularly into muscles and joints with little evidence of trauma.

Haemophilia A

This is the most common haemophilia, and is associated with the absence of (or an abnormal) clotting factor VIII.

Haemophilia B

This is known as 'Christmas' disease and is a result of the inactivation of clotting factor IX (also known as Christmas factor).

For people who are prone to uncontrolled bleeding, clotting at a wound may be encouraged by applying thrombin, or a fibrin spray or a rough surface such as gauze. Longer term control involves administration of the deficient aetiological factor, for example factor VIII for the treatment of classical haemophilia A. Major injuries and operations require special measures, such as plasma transfusions and the administration of concentrated anti-haemophilic factors, in order to reduce or control the symptoms. The reader should refer to Figure 8.14 which illustrates the homeostatic and clinical control of blood clotting.

HOMEOSTATIC FAILURES OF THE PLASMA PROTEINS

Hyper- and hypogammaglobulinaemia

Hypergammaglobulinaemia is an excess of gammaglobulins and is indicative of chronic infection states, collagen diseases, and parasitic infections. Agammaglobulinaemia (few gammaglobulins) may occur as a congenital disease, and such patients are subjected to recurrent infection. Hyperfibrinogenaemia (excessive fibrinogen) occurs in pathological acute infections but also in pregnancy. Increased fibrinogen levels result in a faster 'erythrocyte sedimentation rate (ESR)' when a blood sample is allowed to stand for a while. Hypofibrinogenaemia (fibrinogen deficiency) and hypoprothrombinaemia (prothrombin deficiency) cause longer bleeding, or clotting times; the former occurs in liver diseases, such as cirrhosis, and can also cause problems in pregnancy.

Hypoalbuminaemia (albumin deficiency)

Hypoalbuminaemia occurs when there is damage to the glomerular capillaries of the kidneys, which results in quantities of albumin being filtered and passing out in the urine. Albumin synthesis by the liver is such that hypoalbuminaemia results only when there are large amounts of albumin lost from the body, or when inadequate dietary amino acid substrates prevent its synthesis. The condition, together with other hypoproteinaemias, causes a decrease in the plasma colloidal osmotic pressure, resulting in oedema of the tissue fluids. Such deficiencies in plasma proteins are caused by liver diseases, protein malnutrition, inflammation, and allergic reactions.

Correction involves replacement by plasma transfusions. Agglutination is avoided by infusing plasma minus any antibodies it may contain ('conditioned' plasma). Table 8.8 summarizes the clinical use of infused plasma components.

HOMEOSTATIC FAILURES CONCERNING BLOOD GROUPING

The problem concerning the availability of adequate supply of stored blood is being investigated by scientists, who are experimenting with the possibility of interconverting blood groups. Early attempts have been successful in converting blood group B into group O. In the future, such interconversions may abolish the problem of regional blood shortages.

HAEMOLYTIC DISEASE OF THE NEWBORN (HDNB)

Complications may occur if a rhesus negative mother bears a rhesus positive fetus. Genetically there is a 75% chance of this occurring, if the father is rhesus positive (Figure 8.15a).

Under normal circumstances in pregnancy there is no mixing of fetal and maternal bloods, although the two circulations are in very close proximity within the placental unit (Chapter 18). During childbirth, however, severe contractions of the uterus wall may squeeze some foetal rhesus positive erythrocytes into the maternal circulation (Figure 8.15b). The fetal agglutinins passed into the maternal circulation do not pose a risk to the mother, as the large maternal blood volume dilutes their effects many-fold. Maternal anti-D agglutinins are not produced in significant amounts against this 'antigenic insult' until after the delivery, and so the first infant is not affected. The agglutinins are gamma-immunoglobulins (Chapter 10), and are capable of crossing the placental membranes and entering the blood of subsequent fetuses. If a fetus is rhesus positive, the anti-D antibodies will cause a transfusion reaction, referred to as the haemolytic disease of the newborn (HDNB), or alternatively, erythroblastosis fetalis (since under these conditions immature red cells called erythroblasts enter the circulation from the bone marrow). This disease can be monitored *in utero* by amniocentesis, which assesses the bilirubin content of amniotic fluid, and by fetoscopy, which assesses fetal blood samples.

Without treatment such cases may result in stillbirths, or neonatal deaths soon after delivery, and premature delivery may be induced after 7–8 months of development. Prior to this, and in severe cases, the fetus can also be successfully treated by intrauterine transfusions. Neonates with HDNB have anaemia, coupled with jaundice. This is because:

1 the resultant rhesus antibody–antigen reactions cause excessive haemolysis (anaemia);

2 the metabolized pigment (now bilirubin) becomes deposited in the skin, mucous membranes and the eyes (jaundice).

Correction after birth depends upon the severity of the condition and may involve an exchange transfusion, whereby all the neonate's rhesus positive blood is replaced with rhesus negative blood. The transfused blood will eventually be replaced by the baby's own rhesus positive blood, by which time the signs and symptoms of anaemia and jaundice will have disappeared. Milder forms of jaundice may not require an exchange transfusion and principles of correction involve the application of artificial light. UV light converts the fat-soluble bilirubin into water-soluble biliverdin which is excreted in the urine.

If a risk of HDNB is known the potential problem is avoidable by rhesus immunization. This involves injecting rhesus negative mothers with anti-D immunoglobulins immediately after they have given birth to a rhesus positive child. This destroys any fetal cells which may have passed into the maternal blood before they have time to stimulate the mother's own immune response.

HDNB arises in only about 10% of cases mainly because the D carrying cells may be destroyed by the mother's own ABO agglutinins if the fetal blood is incompatible. If the child belongs to group A, for example, and the mother is group O, then her anti-A agglutinins haemolyse the fetal cells, regardless of the rhesus group. Many forms of HDNB exists, but

	Father	**Mother**
Parents' genotype:	DD	dd
Gametes:	D and D	d and d
Offspring genotype:	Dd Dd	Dd Dd
Offspring's blood group (phenotype):	Rh+ Rh+	Rh+ Rh+

	Father	**Mother**
Parents' genotype:	Dd	dd
Gametes:	D and d	d and d
Offspring genotype:	Dd Dd	dd dd
Offspring's blood group (phenotype):	Rh+ Rh+	Rh− Rh−

Figure 8.15 (a) The inheritance of rhesus positive offspring. There is a 75% chance of producing a rhesus positive (Rh+) child from a rhesus positive father and a rhesus negative (Rh−) mother, because the father could be homozygous dominant (DD) or heterozygous (Dd). Thus, both possibilities have to be taken into consideration when calculating the probability of producing a rhesus positive child from these two parental phenotypes. (b) Pregnancy and rhesus incompatibility.

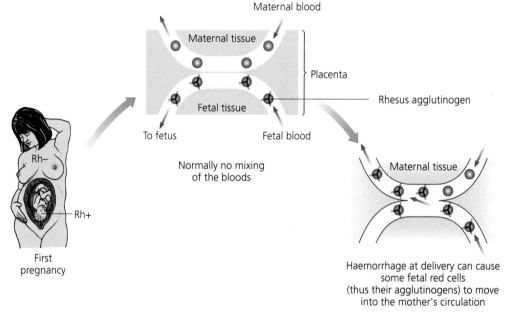

Maternal blood

Maternal tissue

Placenta

Fetal tissue

Rhesus agglutinogen

To fetus

Fetal blood

Normally no mixing of the bloods

Maternal tissue

Haemorrhage at delivery can cause some fetal red cells (thus their agglutinogens) to move into the mother's circulation

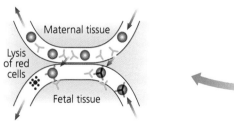

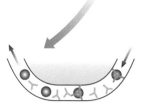

Rh−

Rh+

First pregnancy

Maternal tissue

Lysis of red cells

Fetal tissue

Second pregnancy.
Maternal agglutinins being of the IgG variety can pass over the selectively permeable placenta. This causes antibody–antigen complexing and its subsequent consequences (HDNB – see text for details)

Maternal agglutinin production in response to the above 'antigenic insult' most of them are so mild they remain undetected.

There is no equivalent haemolytic disease of the newborn with reference to the ABO system because the anti-A and anti-B antibodies are of the IgM type and so are too large to pass over the placental membranes.

Summary

1 Blood is the fluid which, under normal circumstances, is contained within the cardiovascular system. Its main components are plasma and erythrocytes.

2 Additional components found in smaller concentrations are other cellular elements – leucocytes and thrombocytes – and non-cellular materials which are dissolved in the plasma. The latter include organic substances (nutrients, enzyme, hormone, and urea, etc.) and inorganic substances (cationic and anionic electrolytes).

3 All components of blood must be maintained within their homeostatic parameters in order to:
(a) maintain blood volume (hence blood pressure);
(b) interchange vital materials to maintain intracellular homeostasis;
(c) combat pathogenic infection.

4 Deviations in the homeostatic ranges of blood constituents, together with the presence of abnormal constituents (e.g. cytoplasmic chemicals, such as cardiac-specific enzymes), make serum analysis one of the most important clinical diagnostic tools.

5 Different blood groups are associated with genetically determined differences in antigens on erythrocyte membranes and antibodies in blood serum.

6 The ABO and rhesus blood grouping systems are used to classify blood donated for transfusion.

7 Haemostasis (blood clotting) is a homeostatic mechanism which prevents the loss of blood when a blood vessel is damaged.

8 Thrombocytes (platelets) have an essential role in activating the enzymatically controlled clotting cascade.

Review Questions

1 What is the blood volume of a healthy adult female?

2 List seven functions of the circulating blood.

3 Describe the origin and functions of plasma proteins.

4 Name the cellular elements of blood.

5 Where are the plasma proteins produced?

6 Distinguish between the following: whole blood, serum, and plasma; neutrophils and eosinophils; agglutinogens and agglutinins; erythropoiesis and leucopoiesis.

7 Give a function for each of the following: plasmin; basophils; erythropoietin; fixed macrophages; megakaryocytes.

8 Define the following terms: anaemia; haematocrit; agglutination; proenzyme; haemostasis; polycythaemia; neutropenia; haemophilia.

9 Under what physiological conditions is erythropoietin released?

10 What is responsible for producing the homeostatic imbalance of sickle cell anaemia?

11 What happens when group O blood is transfused into type A recipient?

12 What accounts for the symptoms of the haemolytic disease of the newborn (HDNB), and how can this be prevented?

13 List the three stages of the clotting reaction.

14 Why does whole blood fail to clot when calcium ions are removed?

15 Describe the role of extrinsic and intrinsic thromboplastin.

16 How could an enzyme, such as streptokinase, assist in preventing unwanted clotting and removing clots already formed?

17 Suggest why the composition of blood is important for intracellular homeostasis.

18 Distinguish between the homeostatic failures of anaemia and polycythaemia.

19 Name the different stages of blood formation.

20 Describe the process of red blood cell breakdown.

The cardiovascular system II: Heart and circulation

9

Introduction: relation of the cardiovascular system to cellular homeostasis

Overview of the anatomy and physiology of the cardiovascular system I:
The heart

Overview of the anatomy and physiology of the cardiovascular system II:
Blood vessels and the circulation

Details of cardiac physiology

Details of circulatory physiology

Role of vascular system in systemic homeostasis

Examples of homeostatic control system failure and principles of correction

Summary

Review questions

Introduction: relation of the cardiovascular system to cellular homeostasis

The cardiovascular system consists of the heart and blood vessels of the body. The relation of this system to cellular homeostasis is that it delivers nutrients, oxygen, hormones, etc., to the cells of the body and removes 'waste' products of metabolism from them, so preventing toxicity. The cardiovascular system, however, requires the cooperative functioning of other systems in order to maintain blood composition and so preserve intracellular homeostasis (see Figure 1.1). The digestive and excretory organs are instrumental in maintaining the homeostatic constitution of blood, whilst the autonomic nervous system and endocrine system coordinate cardiovascular (and other system) functions. Each cooperative component is a homeostatic control system, and a disturbance in one results in malfunction of another as a consequence of the interdependency of organ system function as discussed in Chapter 1.

Cardiovascular function must be adaptable if adequate blood flow to the tissues is to be maintained during varying metabolic demands, such as when resting or exercising, since there is only a limited volume of blood available in the body. Blood may be directed to where it is needed most and away from the less active areas, but at all times there must be an adequate blood flow to the most vital organs (brain and heart) since these high priority tissues are particularly sensitive to reduced blood supply.

The cardiovascular system, therefore, provides the transport 'hardware' that keeps blood continuously circulating to fulfil intracellular homeostatic requirements. The heart (= cardio) is the transport system's pump; the delivery routes are the hollow blood vessels (= vascular) leading from, and eventually back to,

the heart (Figure 9.1). The blood is the transport medium. The essential principles underlying the homeostasis of blood composition were described in Chapter 8. This chapter describes:

1 Specific aspects of the heart including its size, location, functional anatomy, coronary circulation, conduction system and related electrocardiography, the cardiac cycle, and cardiac output.

2 The functional anatomy of the arterial, capillary, and venous systems, the routes of circulation and the homeostatic control of blood pressure.

3 Some common examples of cardiovascular homeostatic failures and their principles of correction.

Overview of the anatomy and physiology of the cardiovascular system I: the heart

The main role of the heart is to promote unidirectional flow of blood throughout the body, although it also produces a hormone (atrial natriuretic factor; Chapter 15). Flow of blood is promoted by the generation of a pressure gradient, and the pumping action of the heart is responsible for elevating blood pressure sufficiently to maintain an adequate blood supply to the tissues.

The volume of blood ejected from the heart by this pumping action must match the volume of blood entering the heart during the 'filling' phase of the pump cycle, otherwise the heart will become congested. This in turn relates to the physical activity being performed by the body; an increased activity reduces the time taken for blood to circulate around the body and so the heart must pump more blood per unit time. The heart, then, has to be versatile, with a variable pumping rate according to needs. The control of the heart is described in

a later section. This section outlines the basic structure and functioning of the heart in relation to the unidirectional flow of blood through it.

Heart size and location

Figure 9.2 illustrates that the heart is located obliquely (since the heart tips slightly to the left) between the lungs and is enclosed within the medial cavity of the thorax, called the mediastinum. It lies anterior to the vertebral column and posterior to the sternum. The heart weighs approximately 250–350 grams; its size is often compared to the person's closed fist to demonstrate the approximate dimensions. The heart's broad base, formed by the upper chambers, or atria, is approximately 9 cm wide, and projects superiorly and posteriorly, towards the right shoulder, extending some

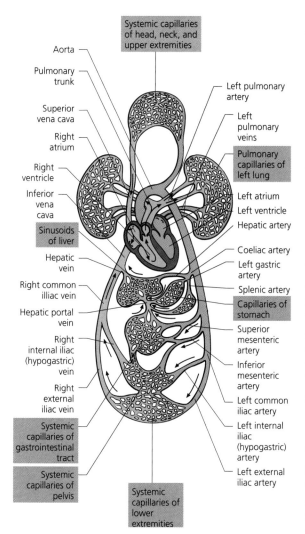

Figure 9.1 Circulatory routes: coloured arrows show systemic circulation; thick black arrows in the pulmonary blood vessels show pulmonary circulation; thin black arrows indicate hepatic portal circulation.

12–14 cm within the second or third intercostal space. The organ is fixed by vessels at its base, thus allowing its more pointed apex to move upwards on contraction. The apex, formed by the tip of the lower chambers, or ventricles, of the heart (particularly the left ventricle) is directed inferiorly and anteriorly, towards the left hip. It rests on the diaphragm, which separates the thoracic and abdominal regions

of the trunk. The apical heart beat, produced by contraction of the heart muscle, can be felt on the left side of the chest, about 8 cm from the sternum between the fifth and sixth intercostal spaces. Approximately two-thirds of the heart is located to the left of the sternum.

The upper border of the heart, formed by the atrial chambers, is where the great vessels, called the aorta, vena cavae, and pulmonary artery (see below), enter or leave the heart.

Functional anatomy of the heart

The heart is a four-chambered structure, enclosed within a supportive and protective membrane called the pericardium. The walls of the heart are mainly comprised of a specialized form of muscle called cardiac muscle. The chambers of the heart are separated by walls of tissue called septa, but communication between some of them is provided by valve structures.

Pericardium

The pericardium (peri = around) is a membranous sac of the fibroserous types (see Chapter 4) and is comprised of two layers: the fibrous and serous pericardium (Figure 9.3). The former is a tough dense connective tissue layer which protects the heart and anchors it to the diaphragm, great vessels, and sternum. Although the fibrous pericardium holds the heart in position, it is flexible enough to allow sufficient movement so that the heart can contract vigorously and rapidly when the need arises. The serous pericardium is a thinner, more delicate membrane which forms a double layer around the heart. The outer (or parietal) layer lines the inner surface of the fibrous pericardium. The inner, or visceral, layer (also called, the epicardium, meaning 'upon the heart') is attached to the muscle layer of the heart. Between these two serous layers is the pericardial cavity, which is a thin potential space containing a film of watery fluid. The

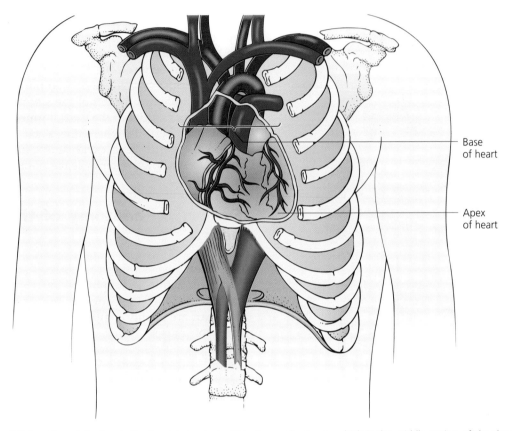

Figure 9.2 Location of the heart. The heart is located within the mediastinum, which is the middle region of the thoracic cavity.

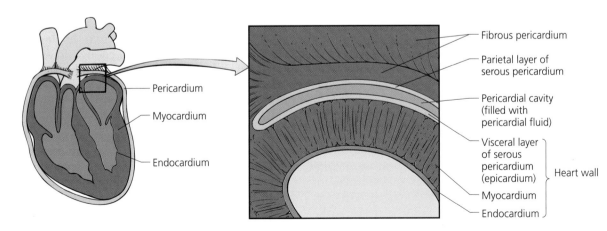

Figure 9.3 The pericardial layers and the heart wall.

tension produced by this film holds the two layers together. The fluid also prevents friction between the membranes when the heart contracts. A reduction in the amount of fluid occurs when the pericardium is inflamed (called pericarditis) and is often associated with pericardial friction rub which can be heard using a stethoscope.

Heart wall

The wall of the heart consists of three layers:

1 The epicardium (a component of the pericardial membrane, as discussed above);

2 The myocardium (myo- = muscle);

3 The endocardium (endo- = inner).
   (Figure 9.3)

MYOCARDIUM

The myocardium forms the bulk of the heart wall. Upon contraction it is responsible for pumping blood into the vessels of the circulatory system. The structure of cardiac muscle is discussed later but was also outlined in Chapter 4. The external surface of the myocardium is lined by epicardium, the internal surface by endocardium.

ENDOCARDIUM

The endocardium is a smooth glistening white sheet of squamous endothelium which rests on a thin sheet of connective tissue. Its smooth surface prevents activation of the blood cascade. It is continuous with the endothelial lining of blood vessels leaving and entering the heart and also covers the valves between the heart chambers.

Heart chambers

The heart's interior is divided into four hollow chambers which receive circulating blood. The two upper or superior chambers are called atria; (atrium, singular) and the two lower or inferior chambers are called ventricles (Figure 9.4). An internal partition divides the heart longitudinally and forms the interatrial and interventricular septa (septum, singular), which separate the atria and ventricles respectively. The interatrial septum possesses an oval depression, called the fossa ovalis, which corresponds to the location of the foramen ovale (foramen = window), an opening in the fetal heart (Chapter 18). Each atrium is separated from its respective ventricle by an atrioventricular valve.

The atria are the receiving chambers for blood returning to the heart from the circulation. They are small and thin-walled, since they only need to contract minimally to push the blood a short distance to the ventricles (very little pressure is generated within atria during their contraction). Flow into the ventricles is also encouraged by gravity. The ventricles are the discharging chambers and form the actual pumps of the heart; accordingly, ventricular walls are thicker than atrial walls since they must generate a greater pressure to promote adequate output. However, the muscular wall of the right ventricle is thinner than that of the left, since the right ventricular pump is responsible for circulating blood in the low-resistance pulmonary circulation of the lungs, whereas the left ventricular pump is responsible for circulating blood to the rest of the body and must generate a much higher pressure to maintain this.

Heart valves

Blood flow through the heart, and for that matter through the circulatory system, must be unidirectional if haemodynamic efficiency is to be maintained. Valves in the heart (and larger veins; discussed later) maintain this one-way flow.

There are four heart valves; the paired atrioventricular and semilunar valves (Figure 9.4). These open and close passively in response to differences in blood pressure on the two sides of the valve.

ATRIOVENTRICULAR (AV) VALVES

The AV valve between the right atrium and the right ventricle is often called the tricuspid valve, because it contains three cusps or flaps.

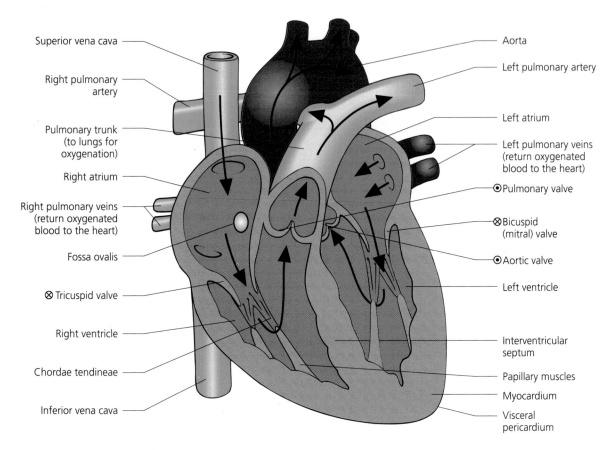

Figure 9.4 A frontal section of the heart: ⊗ atrioventricular (AV) valves (tricuspid and bicuspid); ⊙ semilunar valves (pulmonary and aortic).

Similarly the AV valve between left atrium and left ventricle is the bicuspid or mitral valve, because it consists of two cusps and also because of its resemblance to a bishop's mitre. The cusps are fibrous connective tissue covered with endocardium that extends from the chamber walls; their pointed ends project into the ventricles. White collagen fibres called the chordae tendineae, or 'heart strings', anchor the cusps to small papillary muscles within the ventricles.

The tendineae keep the valve flaps pointing in the direction of blood flow, so that the AV valve opens when blood is passed from atrium to ventricle upon atrial contraction. In this instance the papillary muscles relax, the chordae tendineae slacken, and allow the valves to open (Figure 9.5a). Upon ventricular contraction, however, blood is pumped out of the ventricle into an artery; any blood tending to pass back towards the atria drives the valve cusps upwards until they close the opening. Papillary muscles also contract, and this tightens the chordae tendineae and so prevents the flaps from inverting into the atria (Figure 9.5b).

SEMILUNAR VALVES

The semilunar valves are so called because of their half-moon shaped cusps. Aortic and pulmonary semilunar valves are located at the base of the large arteries, the aorta and pulmonary artery, which leave the left and right ventricle respectively. Their homeostatic role is to encourage unidirectional flow from ventricle to artery but their mechanism of

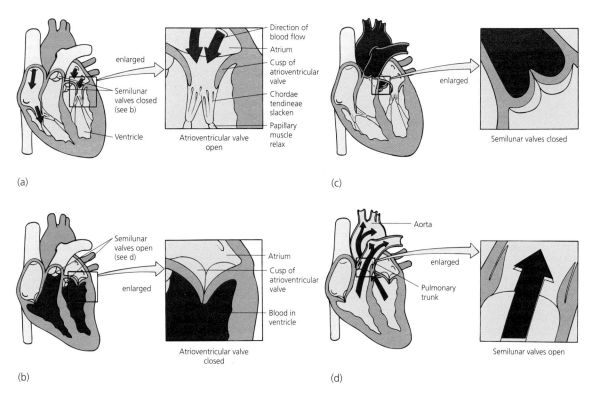

Figure 9.5 Heart and valvular action. (a) and (b) Operation of the atrioventricular valves of the heart. (a) Valves open when blood pressure exerted on the atrial side is greater than that exerted on the ventricular side. (b) Valves are forced closed when the ventricles contract and the intraventricular pressure rises, moving the blood upwards. (c) and (d) Operation of the semilunar valves. (c) During ventricular relaxation, the backward flowing blood in the aorta/pulmonary artery fills the valve cusp and closes the valves. (d) During ventricular contraction, the valves are open and their cusps flatten against their arterial walls.

action is different from that of the AV valves (Figure 9.5c,d)). Upon ventricle contraction the semilunar valves are forced open, and their cusps become flattened against the arterial wall as blood is ejected. Upon ventricular relaxation, pressure within the ventricle falls and blood is no longer propelled forward, but begins to flow backwards. This causes the cusps to close and this prevents backward flow into the ventricles.

Relationship of the heart sounds to heart pumping

When listening to the heart with a stethoscope, one does not hear the opening of the valves, since this is a relatively slow developing process which is silent. Valve closure is more sudden, however, and the sudden pressure differentials that develop across the valve produces vibrations of the valve and the surrounding fluid. The sounds given off travel in all directions through the chest. When ventricles first contract, the closure of the AV valves produces a long and booming sound since the vibration is low in pitch and is of relatively long duration. This is the first heart (or Korotkoff) sound and is described as 'lubb'. The second heart sound – 'dupp' – is caused by the closure of the semilunar valves at the beginning of ventricular relaxation. This sound is a relatively rapid 'snap' since valve closure is extremely fast, and thus the surroundings vibrate for a short period of time.

Damaged heart valves will impair cardiac function, although severe valvular deformity is required to cause serious impairment. Rheumatic fever, for example, can cause the cusps of the valve to stick together, thus narrowing their opening (a process called stenosis). Subsequent damage to the edges of the cusps impairs closure and backward flow occurs. The valve is now said to be incompetent. Although stenosis and incompetence coexist, often one predominates. Such valvular imbalances cause additional heart sounds known as murmurs, produced by the turbulence of blood flowing through the valve. In both instances the pumping efficiency of the heart declines and, as a consequence, the work load of the heart is increased. Ultimately, the heart becomes weakened, and this can cause heart failure. It is the mitral valve that is usually affected as pressure differentials developed by the left ventricle are greater than those across the tricuspid valve. Faulty valves can be replaced surgically with synthetic or animal (usually pig) heart valves.

Path of blood flow through the heart

The right atrium receives deoxygenated blood, i.e. blood which has given up some of its oxygen as it passes through tissues, from all parts of the body except the lungs. Blood enters the atrium via three vessels:

1 The superior vena cava which returns blood from structures above the heart (i.e. head, neck and arms).

2 The inferior vena cava which returns blood from structures below the heart (i.e. the trunk and legs).

3 The coronary sinus which collects blood from most of the vessels supplying the heart wall itself.

Relaxation of the atrium muscle enlarges the chamber and creates a suction pressure which draws blood into the right atrium (the

entrances of the above vessels are not guarded by valves). This atrium delivers blood to the right ventricle upon opening of the tricuspid valve. The right ventricle then pumps blood to the lungs via the pulmonary 'trunk' vessel through the opened pulmonary (semilunar) valve. The trunk divides into right and left pulmonary arteries which take the blood to the right and left lungs, respectively. Oxygenation of blood takes place in lung tissue, and the blood is transported to the left atrium via the four pulmonary veins (two from each lung). Blood flows into the left atrium upon atrial relaxation, which again creates a suction pressure. The blood then passes through the opened bicuspid valve into the left ventricle, which then pumps it into the aorta through the opened aortic (semilunar) valve. From here some blood passes into the first branch of the aorta, the coronary arteries, whilst the remainder is carried into the aortic arch, thoracic aorta, and abdominal aorta. Vessels branching from the aorta transport blood to all body parts to sustain intracellular homeostasis (Figure 9.1).

Coronary circulation

The heart chambers are continuously bathed with blood, and this provides nourishment to the endocardial cells. The myocardial and pericardial cells, however, are too far away to make diffusional movement of nutrients from this blood a practical means of supporting these cells. Nutrition is provided by a number of blood vessels which comprise the coronary circulation. Numerous vessels pierce the myocardium and carry blood to the vicinity of the myocardial and pericardial cells. This arrangement is essential since the oxygen consumption of the heart muscle is greater than that of any other tissue, because of its constant pumping action; at rest the oxygen consumption is 8 ml/100 g of heart tissue per minute. The supply of blood via the coronary circulation accounts for 1/20th of the total output from the heart, even though the heart represents only 1/200th of the body's weight. The main coronary vessels, the right and left coronary arteries, branch from the aorta just superior to the aortic valve. They lie on the heart's surface (the epicardium), encircling the heart in an atrioventricular groove (Figure 9.6a), and reminded early anatomists of a crown, or corona, hence the name of these vessels. Their branches and sub-branches penetrate deep into the cardiac muscle.

The right coronary arterial branches are:

1 The marginal artery. This supplies the lateral part of the right side of the heart, including the right atrium.

2 The posterior interventricular artery. This extends to the apex serving the posterior ventricular walls.

The left coronary arterial branches are:

1 The left anterior descending branch. This serves the interventricular septum and the anterior wall of both ventricles.

2 The circumflex branch. This supplies the left atrium and the posterior left ventricular wall.

Coronary vessels deliver most blood when the heart is relaxed. They are largely ineffective during ventricular contraction as they are compressed by the contracting myocardium, and their entrances from the aorta are partly blocked by the cusps of the opened aortic valve.

Having supplied the heart tissue, blood is collected from the left ventricle via the cardiac veins, which merge to form the coronary sinus. This empties into the posterior aspects of the right atrium. The sinus is comprised of the great cardiac vein, the middle cardiac vein, and the small cardiac vein (Figure 9.6b).

Blood from the right side of the heart is collected via the anterior cardiac vein which empties directly into the anterior aspects of the right atrium. Blood returning to the atrium will be deficient in oxygen. In fact, the blood has less oxygen than any other venous blood in the body since the active heart muscle extracts

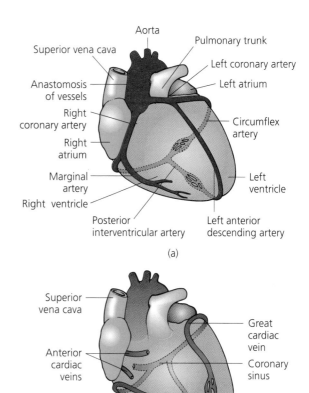

Figure 9.6 Coronary circulation. (a) Arterial supply. (b) Venous drainage.

more oxygen from the blood it receives than does other tissues.

Factors which influence coronary blood flow are:

1 The demand of cardiac muscle for oxygen. The removal of oxygen from the coronary circulation at rest is approximately three times greater than in normal circulation, and in times of increased oxygen demand (e.g. exercise) the additional oxygen required is supplied by an increased coronary blood flow. The change in blood flow is directly proportional to the oxygen requirements. The mechanism is intrinsic to the tissue (i.e. it is autoregulated by the tissue itself) but

the metabolic stimulus to provide the additional blood has yet to be identified.

2 Neural mechanisms. The autonomic nervous system indirectly affects coronary blood flow. Parasympathetic stimulation decreases the heart rate and slightly depresses myocardial contractility, resulting in a decreased cardiac oxygen consumption; therefore, coronary flow decreases. Conversely, sympathetic stimulation increases the heart rate and myocardial contractility, increases oxygen consumption, and, therefore, coronary flow is increased.

3 Aortic pressure. This is the principal factor which determines the rate of blood flow to the cardiac muscle, since the aortic pressure is produced by the heart itself. Any increase in aortic pressure generated by the contraction of the heart results in an increased coronary blood flow.

Conduction system

Before considering the conduction system of the heart, it is important that the reader understands the anatomy and functioning of cardiac muscle, and its differences from that of skeletal muscle (described in Chapter 16).

Myocardial muscle fibres have specialized anatomical features that reflect their unique function of pumping blood. Otherwise their structure is similar to skeletal muscle cells. Both are striated in appearance and their contractions are associated with the sliding filament mechanism (see Chapter 16 for details). Cardiac fibres, however, are small, fat, branched, and usually uninucleated, whereas skeletal muscle cells are taller, cylindrical, and are multinucleated. Adjacent cardiac cells are interconnected via intercalated discs and cross-bridges, unlike the independent skeletal muscle fibres. The intercalated discs contain anchoring structures called desmosomes that prevent separation of adjacent cells upon their contraction, and minute gap junctions which allow direct transmission of electrical depolarization across the whole heart.

The structure of cardiac muscle enables the entire myocardium to behave as a single unit or functional syncytium, but also ensures that the organ is contracted in different planes, unlike the linear contraction observed in skeletal muscle fibres.

Compared with skeletal muscle, myocardial cells also have more mitochondria, constituting 2% and 25% of the volume of these respective muscle fibres. This is because heart cells rely exclusively on aerobic respiration for their ATP synthesis, whereas skeletal fibres can also utilize anaerobic metabolism and still operate reasonably efficiently. Both muscle types use a variety of fuel molecules for respiration, although cardiac cells are more adaptable and can readily switch metabolic pathways to use whatever nutrient is available. The main problem associated with myocardial insufficiency, therefore, lies with a lack of oxygen and not of the fuel molecules.

The orderly and coordinated myocardial contraction, which produces an efficient emptying of the heart chambers, is controlled by an intrinsic regulatory mechanism – the cardiac conduction system. This is comprised of a number of patches, or nodes, and conducting fibres of specialized muscle tissue. They are called:

1 The sinoatrial node (SA node);

2 The atrioventricular node (AV node);

3 The atrioventricular bundle (AV bundle or bundle of His); comprising the left and right bundle branches;

4 The Purkinje fibres (Figure 9.7a).

The specialized myocardial cells of the nodes are self-excitatory, i.e. they spontaneously and rhythmically generate the electrical action potentials that result in their contraction. The resting rate of self-excitation of the SA node of an adult is faster than other members of the conducting system, hence it is called the pacemaker. The impulse which will eventually cause the heart to contract is therefore initiated within the SA node tissue located in the right

(a)

(b)

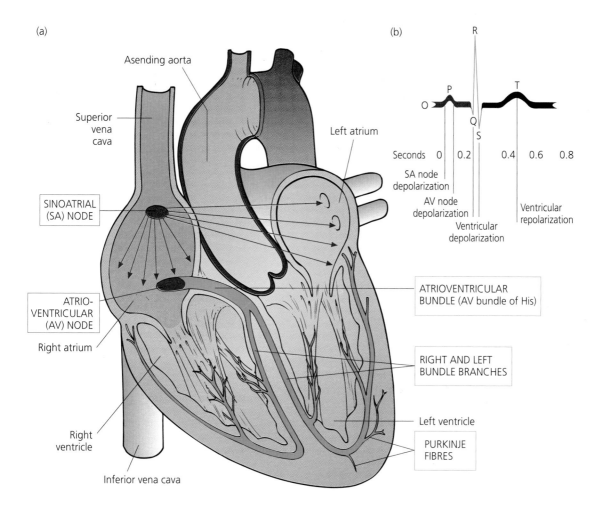

Figure 9.7 Conduction system of the heart and corresponding electrocardiogram. (a) Location of the nodes and bundles of the conduction system. Arrows indicate the flow of action potentials through the atria. (b) Normal electrocardiogram of a single heartbeat.

atrium, just below the opening of the superior vena cava. The impulse spreads from the SA node to atrial myocardial cells, causing their depolarization and subsequent contraction. It then enters the AV node located at the base of the interatrial septum. This is the last region of the atria to be depolarized; its slower conducting properties allow the atria time to empty their blood into the ventricles, before the ventricles begin their contraction. The atria therefore finish their contraction before the ventricles begin theirs and this facilitates unidirectional

blood flow. Once through the AV node, the impulse travels quickly through the rest of the conduction system, beginning with the bundle of His. This extends down to the heart apex as the right and left bundle branches, which distribute electrical impulses over the medial surfaces of the ventricles. Ventricular contraction is stimulated by the Purkinje fibres which emerge from the bundle branches and carry the impulses to the ventricular myocardial cells.

Although the rate of heart beat is determined by the intrinsic properties of the SA node, this may be altered by the autonomic nervous system, or by blood-borne hormones such as thyroxine and adrenaline. The SA node's ability to generate impulses in the absence of such external stimuli is referred to as autorhythmicity, and results from spontaneous changes in the permeability of cell membranes to potassium and sodium (see Chapter 13 for further details of action potentials). The gradual depolarization of the membrane reaches threshold, forming an action potential which is transmitted through the rest of the conducting system, resulting in myocardial contraction. Following the action potential, the SA node cell membranes return to their initial resting value and gradually depolarize again. This repetitive and self-excitatory mechanism causes the rhythmical and repetitive muscle contraction associated with heart activity. Although the SA node is the pacemaker, autorhythmicity is also displayed in other parts of the conduction system. For example, the AV node discharges at a rhythmical rate of 40–60 action potentials/min; the rest of the system discharges at a rate between 15 and 40 beats/min. In life these tissues rarely have the opportunity to generate action potentials because they have been depolarized by impulses from the SA node before they reach their own threshold levels. If, for some reason, the SA node is inactivated, the tissue with the next fastest autorhythmical rate (i.e. the AV node) takes over pacing.

The electrocardiogram (ECG)

The action potentials of myocardial cells are electrical changes that can be recorded as they move through the myocardium. This recording is known as the electrocardiogram. Furthermore, a comparison of the information obtained from surface electrodes placed at different sites on the chest wall and limbs enables one to check specific nodal, conducting, and contractile properties. The ECG is therefore useful in diagnosing abnormal cardiac rhythms (or arrhythmias) and in following the course of

recovery from myocardial damage as occurs in myocardial infarction, or heart attack.

The rhythm disturbances detected can indicate what course of action is necessary to re-establish homeostatic function. For example, in one type of arrhythmia (AV block), the ventricles fail to receive action potentials, causing them to beat independently of the atria. This problem is clinically corrected by the introduction of an artificial pacemaker.

The ECG recording varies according to the positioning of the monitoring electrodes or leads. Figure 9.7b illustrates the important features of an electrocardiogram as analysed with leads in one of the standard configurations. The three clearly recognizable events, or waves, normally accompanying each heart cycle are:

1 The first, a small P-wave upward deflection. This corresponds to atrial depolarization. The upward swing of the P-wave represents SA node depolarization; the downward deflection, AV node depolarization. A fraction of a second after the P-wave begins the atria contract (i.e. mechanical events follow electrical activity).

2 The second wave, the QRS complex, signifies ventricular depolarization. The complex begins as a downward deflection, continues as a large upright triangular wave and ends as a downward wave at its base. The relatively strong electrical signal reflects the comparatively larger mass of ventricular muscle compared with that of the atria.

3 The third wave, a smaller dome-shaped T-wave, is indicative of ventricular repolarization. There is no deflection corresponding to atrial repolarization, since it occurs during the ventricular depolarization period and the electrical event is hidden by the QRS complex.

ECG analysis involves measuring voltage changes (i.e. the relative heights of the wave deflection) and determining the duration and temporal relationships between the various components. That is, small electrical signals associated with specific waves may mean that the mass of heart muscle associated with that wave has decreased, for example small P-waves may represent atrial atrophy. Conversely, large electrical signals (large amount of depolarization) of specific waves may indicate heart muscle enlargement, for example larger than normal QRS complexes may indicate ventricular hypertrophy. The size and shape of the T-wave may be affected by any condition that slows ventricular repolarization (for example low energy reserves or poor coronary blood flow). The PQ interval (also called the PR interval because the Q deflection may not always be obvious) is the time between the start of atrial depolarization and the onset of ventricular depolarization. If this exceeds 0.2 seconds it may indicate damage along the conduction system or within the AV node. The QT interval, i.e. the period required for ventricles to undergo a single depolarization and repolarization cycle, approximates to the duration of a ventricular contraction. The interval may be extended by a conduction imbalance, poor coronary blood flow, or myocardial damage. Thus, the ECG is useful in diagnosing abnormal cardiac rhythms and conduction patterns. ECGs are also used to monitor fetal welfare.

Defects in the intrinsic conduction system cause arrhythmias. These are uncoordinated atrial and ventricular contractions, and may even lead to fibrillation, that is rapid and irregular contractions of the heart muscle. If the ventricles are fibrillating, they are useless as pumps and unless the heart is defibrillated quickly then circulation stops and brain death occurs. Defibrillation involves exposing the heart to strong electrical shocks which interrupt the chaotic twitching of the heart by depolarizing the entire myocardium, in the hope that the SA node will resume activities again and the normal (or sinus) rhythm is re-established.

Extrinsic innervation of the heart

Although external nerve stimulation is not required for heart contraction, the autonomic

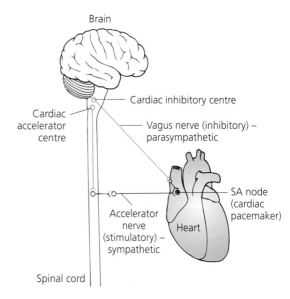

Figure 9.8 Neural pathways for controlling the heart rate.

nervous system modifies the activity of the intrinsic conduction system. The regulatory significance of this effect is discussed later. This section is concerned with the anatomy of the nerve supply to the heart. The general anatomy of the autonomic nervous system is outlined in Chapter 13.

The medulla oblongata of the brainstem (Chapter 13) contains two 'cardiac centres' which control autonomic nerve activity to the heart. The cardiac accelerator centre controls sympathetic nerve activity to the heart, whilst the cardiac inhibitory centre controls parasympathetic nerve activity to the heart (Figure 9.8).

Neurons from both centres innervate collection of nerve cells, or ganglia, within the heart wall, from which the neurons innervate the SA and AV nodes, and some of the heart muscle as well. Sympathetic stimulation (as occurs in exercise and in the stress response; Chapter 22) accelerates the heart rate, and increases the force of myocardial contraction. Conversely, parasympathetic stimulation decreases the heart rate, but has little or no effect on the force of myocardial contraction.

Overview of the anatomy and physiology of the cardio-vascular system II: blood vessels and the circulation

The regulation of cardiovascular function and the preservation of intracellular homeostasis involves an interaction between the cardiovascular system, circulatory components, tissue fluid and other organ systems mentioned in the introduction. Blood is transported in the systemic and pulmonary circulatory systems via a network of specialized vessels – arteries and arterioles transport blood away from the heart; capillaries exchange materials between blood and cells; venules and veins return blood to the heart. This section examines the structure and function of these vessels that constitute the vascular system.

Overview of blood vessels – structure and function

Blood vessel structure varies according to their function but all vessels, except capillaries, have the same basic structure (Figure 9.9a) of three distinctive layers, or tunicae (coats). These are (1) The tunica interna, (2) The tunica media, and (3) the tunica externa.

Tunica interna

The tunica interna, the innermost coat, consists of a single layer of flattened cells. This endothelial (endo- = inner) lining in vessels larger than 1 mm diameter is supported by connective tissue dominated by elastic fibres (Figure 9.9b,c). Capillaries are comprised of this layer only, with little or no elastic fibres, so as to aid the rapid exchange of water and solutes between the tissue fluid and blood plasma.

The tunica media

The tunica media, the middle coat, predominantly consists of smooth muscle fibres supported by a layer of collagen and elastin fibres.

The tunica externa

The tunica externa, the outer connective tissue sheath, principally consists of elastin and collagen fibres.

The relative thickness and fibre composition of each layer varies depending upon the vessel's function (Figure 9.9b,c). The middle layer shows the greatest variation. It is absent in capillaries, for example, but in large arteries close to the heart it is comprised mainly of elastin tissue.

In addition to elastic properties, arteries (especially the arterioles) have contractile functions due to their smooth muscle layer being innervated by the sympathetic nervous system. Contraction squeezes the wall around the vessel, a process called vasoconstriction, since the muscle fibres are arranged in rings around the vessel. Conversely, when sympathetic stimulation is suppressed, the smooth muscle fibres relax, causing the arterial lumen to increase in diameter, a process called vasodilation.

The arterial system

The characteristics of arteries are that they always transport blood away from the heart, and they usually carry oxygenated blood. The exceptions are the pulmonary arteries in the adult circulation, which carry deoxygenated blood from the right ventricle to the lungs, and the umbilical arteries in the fetal circulation, which carry deoxygenated blood from the fetus to the placenta.

Arteries are classified as elastic arteries, muscular arteries, and arterioles, according to size and function.

Elastic arteries

These large vessels have diameters of up to 25 mm. The aorta, pulmonary trunk, and their

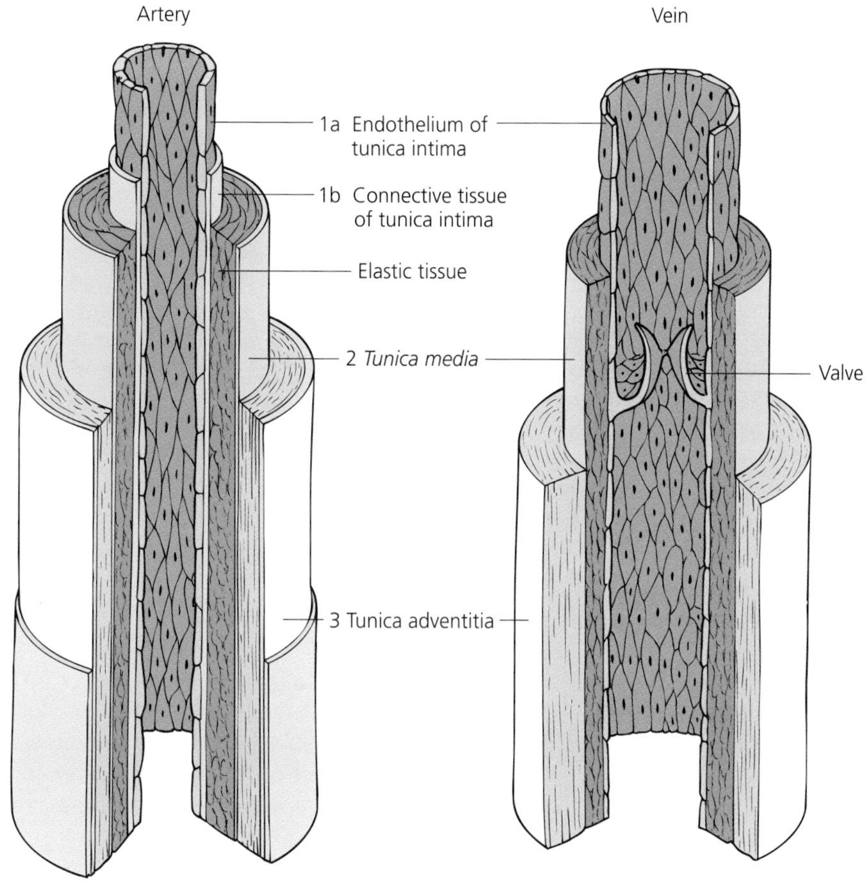

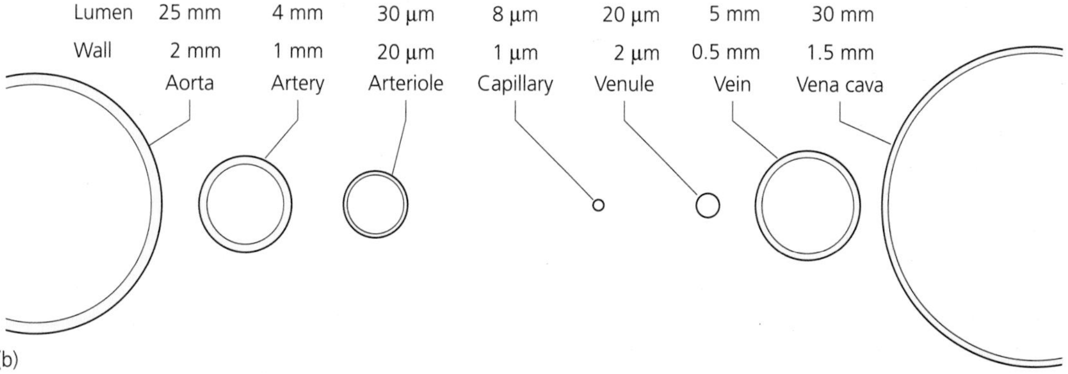

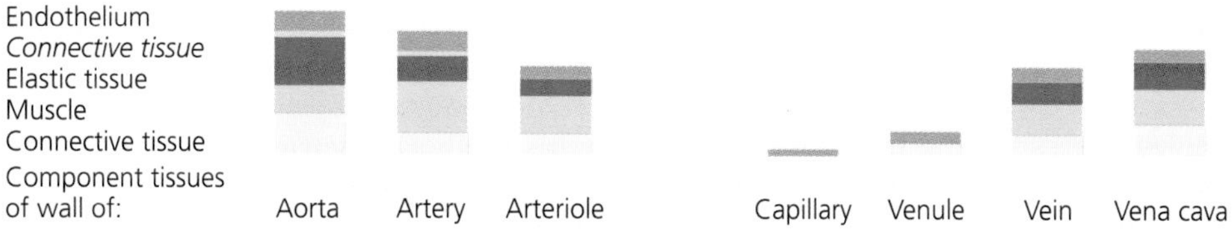

Figure 9.9 (a) Structure of blood vessels. (b) Variation in the thickness of the walls of blood vessels in the circulatory system. (c) Variations in components of the walls of the various blood vessels in the circulatory system.

major branches are elastic arteries. Their tunica media contains considerably more elastic fibres relative to smooth muscle and elastic fibres are also present in the other layers (Figure 9.9b,c). These fibres facilitate arterial stretching to accommodate the extra blood volume and pressure instigated by ventricular contraction, and arterial recoiling upon ventricular relaxation.

Consequently blood flows continuously even when the ventricles are filling during the relaxation period and output from the heart has momentarily ceased. In arteriosclerosis (i.e. a hardening of the arteries), the flow becomes more intermittent as the elastic properties decline. Despite their smooth muscle content elastic arteries have relatively ineffective vasoconstrictory powers.

Elastic arteries are the 'conduction arteries' since they conduct blood away from the heart to the muscular arteries.

Muscular (or distributing) arteries

Elastic arteries give rise to relatively more muscular arteries sometimes referred to as 'distributing arteries' because these medium-sized vessels of 1–4 mm diameter distribute blood to peripheral tissues. They are often named according to the tissue or part of the body that they supply (see Figure 9.15, for examples). The vessels have a thick tunica media which contains considerably more smooth muscle fibres relative to elastin fibres. They are therefore less distensible than elastic arteries, but are capable of greater vasoconstriction and vasodilation, adjusting blood flow to suit the needs of the structures supplied.

Arterioles

Arterioles are the smallest arteries, having an average diameter of 20–30 μm. They deliver blood to the capillary vessels within tissues. Those arterioles nearest to the muscular arteries have similar tunica components, whereas smaller arterioles change their characteristics. Those nearest the capillaries are comprised of an endothelial coat and an incomplete layer of

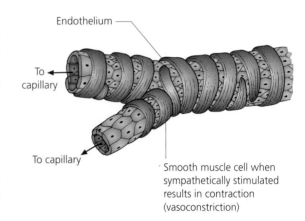

Figure 9.10 Structure of an arteriole.

smooth muscle; these muscle fibres enable the arteriolar diameter to be altered, and hence regulate blood flow through their dependent tissues. Relaxation of specialized regions called the precapillary sphincters (which consist of a few circular muscle fibres) close to the arteriolar–capillary junction may cause the capillary bed to become fully perfused with blood. Partial sphincter contraction reduces blood flow and total contraction causes capillary shutdown. Arteriolar and sphincter diameters are controlled by smooth muscle contraction induced extrinsically by the sympathetic nervous system, or intrinsically (called autoregulation) in response to changes in tissue fluid composition. An example of the latter is the central nervous system ischaemic response in which cerebral hypoxia causes dilatation of the cerebral arterioles.

Capillaries

Capillaries form that part of the circulation often referred to as the microcirculation, since they average only 8 μm or so in diameter. They are located close to almost all body cells, but their distribution varies according to the activity of the tissues they serve. For example, high activity sites, such as muscle, liver, kidney, lung, and nervous tissues have a rich distribution, whereas lower activity sites, such as tendons and ligaments, have a poor distribution. The skin's epidermis, the cornea of the eye, and cartilage tissue are devoid of capillaries and cells of these tissues have very low rates of metabolism.

A typical capillary consists of a tube of endothelial cells sitting on a basement membrane. In most regions this tube forms a complete lining with the endothelial cells being connected by tight junctions; these are referred to as continuous capillaries. Fenestrated capillaries are located in those few areas where extensive fluid exchange occurs, for example in the kidney glomeruli, and in the brain's choroid plexus. Discontinuous capillaries are located in the liver (sinusoids), bone marrow, and adrenal glands and form flattened irregular passageways which slow the blood flow through these tissues to maximize the period of absorption and secretion across the capillary walls (Figure 9.11a–c).

The prime homeostatic function of capillaries is to permit the exchange of metabolites and wastes between blood and tissue cells, and thus they are sometimes called the 'exchange' vessels. For efficient exchange it is necessary to have:

1 A short distance for substances to diffuse through. The structure and location of capillaries is admirably suited for exchange, since they comprise a single layer of cells that are in close proximity to tissue cells. The thick walls of arteries and veins present too great a barrier for this process to be efficient.

2 A large surface area. The total cross-sectional area of the capillaries throughout the body is many thousand times more than that of the aorta.

3 A steady but slow rate of blood flow. The capillary flow velocity is about 700 times lower than in the aorta because of the narrowness of these vessels.

Capillaries function as a part of interconnected networks known as a capillary plexus or capillary bed (Figure 9.12a). A single arteriole gives rise to dozens of capillaries that in

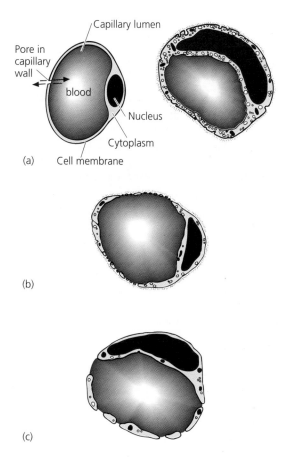

(a)

(b)

(c)

Figure 9.11 Various capillary types. (a) Continuous – connected by tight junctions (e.g. of location, muscles). (b) Fenestrated – allows external diffusion (e.g. of location, kidney glomeruli, brain choroid plexus). (c) Discontinuous – maximizes exchange of materials (e.g. of location, adrenal glands).

turn collect to form several venules. The capillary entrance is guarded by precapillary sphincters which control flow in a manner discussed earlier. Blood flow in arteries is of a pulsatile nature, related to the pulse in arterial blood pressure, but blood flow through capillaries between arterioles and venules is usually at a near constant rate. Within individual capillaries, however, it can be variable. Each precapillary sphincter's cycle of alternate contraction and relaxation occurs perhaps a dozen times

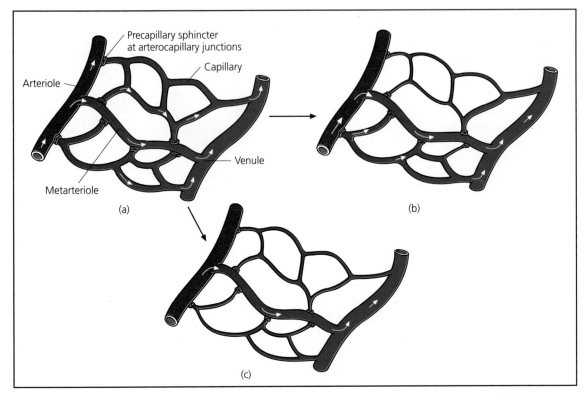

Figure 9.12 The organization of a capillary plexus. (a) Structure of a capillary plexus. (b) and (c) Two possible alterations in the pattern of flow through the capillary plexus as vasomotion occurs.

per minute. The activities of various sphincters within the tissue mean that blood may reach the venules by one route now, and by quite a different route later (Figure 9.12a–c).

Other mechanisms which modify circulatory supply to capillaries include:

1 Collateral circulation. Capillary networks may be supplied by more than one artery. These collaterals may fuse, called an arterial anastomosis, thus guaranteeing a reliable blood supply to tissues. Such vessels could be considered an evolutionary homeostatic adaptation since a blockage of one arterial supply to a capillary bed is compensated for by another route of supply.

2 Arteriovenous anastomoses (AV shunts). These vascular 'short circuits' result from a fusion of arterioles and venules, and are opened when the smooth muscle of arterioles contract, causing the capillary bed to be bypassed. Relaxation of this muscular component encourages flow through the capillary bed rather than through the anastomosis. Rates of blood flow through the low-resistance shunts can be very high and so they are found in tissues in which such rates are sometimes appropriate. In the skin, for example, they act as a thermoregulatory mechanism, by facilitating the conservation or loss of body heat (Chapter 17).

The venous system

The venous system is the collection or drainage system that takes blood from capillary beds (when blood has exchanged substances with tissue fluid) towards the heart (Figure 9.1). On route from the venous side of the capillary network, vessels increase their diameter, their walls thicken, and they progress from the smallest veins (called venules) to the largest veins (the vena cavae).

Venules

Capillaries merge forming venules which range from 8 to 100 µm in diameter. The smallest post-capillary venules consist almost entirely of a lining endothelium with a few surrounding fibroblast cells. They are, therefore, extremely porous. For example inflammatory substances and leucocytes (white blood cells) move easily through their walls from blood to the site of injury via the process of diapedisis (see Chapter 10). As venules approach veins, a sparse tunica media and tunica externa become apparent.

Veins

Venules merge to form veins, and these vessels have the three tunicae found in arteries (see Figure 9.9a). Their walls are thinner, however, particularly the tunica media, since they have less elastic tissue and smooth muscle. Their lumens are larger for a given external diameter (Figure 9.9a–c), and they offer lower resistance to blood flow. This is important because the pressure of blood within the venous circulation is low and provides little force to circulate blood. They are, however, still distensible enough to adapt to variations in volume or pressure of blood passing through them. In fact, the thin walls and large lumen mean that about two-thirds of the total blood volume is found within the venous system at any time, and this is why veins are referred to as the capacitance vessels or blood reservoirs (see Figure 9.13).

The following adaptations within this low pressure system aid the return of blood to the heart:

1 Large diameter lumens so that veins have little resistance to blood flow. The diameter

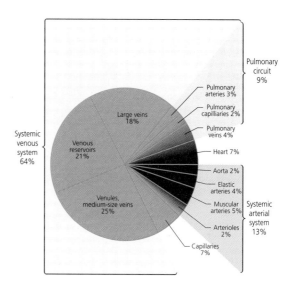

Figure 9.13 The distribution of blood within the circulatory system.

is influenced by the sympathetic nervous system, i.e. changes in sympathetic tone increase or decrease the pooling capacity of the vessel.

2 The presence of valves. These are internal folds of the endothelial lining of large veins and resemble the semilunar valves of the heart in structure and function. They are present in the deep veins of the limbs, and, since the upward flow of blood is opposed by gravity, these veins are compressed by surrounding skeletal muscles (skeletomuscular pumps) which ensure unidirectional flow (Figure 9.14a,b). Valvular damage occurs if the venous system is exposed to high pressure for long periods, as occurs in venous hypertension, pregnancy, obesity, and in people who stand for long extended periods. The incompetent valve causes a pooling of blood distal to the valve, and such varicose veins can become long and tortuous. Consequently oedema and varicose ulcers may develop (Figure 9.14c).

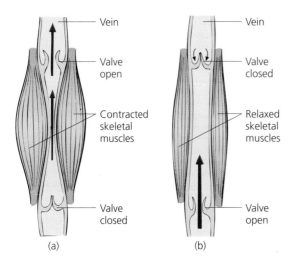

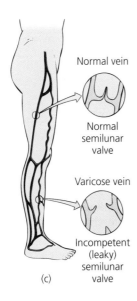

Figure 9.14 Operation of skeletomuscular pumps and vein valves in returning blood to the heart. (a) When skeletal muscles contract and press against the flexible veins, the valves proximal to the area of contraction are forced open and blood is propelled towards the heart. The valves distal to the point of contraction are closed by the back–flowing blood. (b) When skeletal muscles relax, the valves proximal to the muscle close to prevent backward flow, the distal valves open, creating an upward suction pressure and forcing blood upwards. (c) Varicose veins. Veins near the surface of the body (especially in the legs) may bulge and cause venous valves to leak. The enlarged vein is referred to as being varicose.

3 Large veins, such as the vena cavae, are responsive to pressure changes in the thoracic cavity as occurs during the respiratory cycle, thus assisting venous return to the heart by acting as a thoracoabdominal pump.

Venous sinuses

Venous sinuses, for example the coronary sinus mentioned earlier, are specialized flattened veins consisting of tunica intima supported by surrounding tissues rather than by other tunicae.

Blood reservoirs

As stated previously, two-thirds of the total blood volume normally is found at any time within the systemic veins, whereas arteries contain about 13%, pulmonary vessels 9%, the heart 7%, capillaries the remainder (Figure 9.13). Hence, the veins are known as the blood capacitance vessels or blood reservoirs, since they serve as storage depots for blood which can be moved quickly to other parts of the body if the need arises. For example, during strenuous exercise the vasomotor centre (vas = vessel; motor = excitatory nerve supply) of the medulla oblongata of the brainstem increases its sympathetic output to venous blood reservoirs, causing their vasoconstriction. This diverts blood away from these reservoirs and so increases the volume within the capillary beds of skeletal muscles, enabling the tissues to obtain more oxygen and nutrients and so manufacture ATP, the chemical of life necessary for the increased muscle contraction. Clinically, bleeding or haemorrhage causes a decrease in blood volume, and hence arterial blood pressure, and vasoconstriction of venous reservoirs acts as a homeostatic mechanism to compensate for the blood loss by redistributing blood and helping to raise the arterial pressure again.

Routes of circulation

The heart operates as a double pump, since it has left and right ventricular pumps that serve two distinctive circulatory circuits – the systemic circulation and the pulmonary circulation (Figure 9.1).

The systemic circulation routes oxygenated blood through a long loop circuit from the left ventricle of the heart (via the force created by the left ventricular pump), through the aorta and its branches to all body cells other than those of lung tissue. Blood is returned to the right atrium via the vena cavae and coronary sinus. The role of this circuit is to transport metabolites (e.g. oxygen, nutrients) to, and remove 'waste' products of metabolism (e.g. carbon dioxide) from, tissue cells.

The systemic circulation of the adult can be functionally subdivided according to the organs supplied: the coronary circulation (discussed earlier), the renal circulation (Chapter 12), the cerebral circulation (Chapter 13), the cutaneous circulation (Chapter 17), the skeletomuscular circulation (Chapter 16), the hepatoportal circulation, and pulmonary circulation.

The hepatoportal circulation consists of the hepatic artery, which supplies the liver with oxygenated blood, and the hepatic portal vein, which supplies nutrients directly from the digestive organs (this is deoxygenated blood). The hepatic vein drains blood from the liver into the inferior vena cava.

A 'portal' vein is one which carries blood from one capillary bed directly to another, without passing through the heart and being redistributed by arteries. There are a few such examples in the body (e.g. the vascular connection between the hypothalamus and the anterior pituitary gland; Chapter 15) but the hepatic portal vein is the largest. This vein receives blood from veins draining the stomach, intestines, and spleen (via the superior mesenteric vein and splenic vein), the pancreas (via the pancreatic vein and branches of the splenic vein), the colon (mainly via the inferior mesenteric vein) and the gall bladder (via the cystic vein).

The pulmonary circulation routes deoxygenated blood through a short loop circuit from the right ventricle of the heart (via the force created by the right ventricular pump) through the pulmonary trunk, which bifurcates into the left and right pulmonary arteries, taking blood to their respective lung. Within the lungs gaseous exchange occurs (Chapter 11) and a pair of pulmonary veins eventually merge from each lung, routing blood back into the heart's left atrium. These vessels are the only veins (in the adult) that carry oxygenated blood. The role of the pulmonary circuitry, therefore, is to transport deoxygenated blood to the lungs for oxygenation and carbon dioxide excretion.

BLOOD VESSEL NOMENCLATURE

Blood vessel nomenclature is complex and outside the intentions of this book. Accordingly, blood vessels are only named where appropriate, and chapters have only highlighted the important circulations and vessels associated with the homeostatic roles of particular organ systems. Suffice-to-say the name of a blood vessel usually gives a clue to its appearance and/or distribution (Figure 9.15a,b). Thus, if one becomes familiar with the major skeletomuscular and neural 'landmarks' there should be few surprises. The following, however, should be noted:

1 The peripheral distribution of arteries and veins on the left and right side are almost the same, except near the heart where large vessels (i.e. the vena cavae and pulmonary veins) connect to the atria and others (i.e. pulmonary trunk and aorta) connect to the ventricles.

2 A single vessel may change its name as it passes specific boundaries. The aorta, for example, is subdivided into the aortic arch, thoracic and abdominal aorta. This makes accurate anatomical descriptions possible where vessels extend to the periphery.

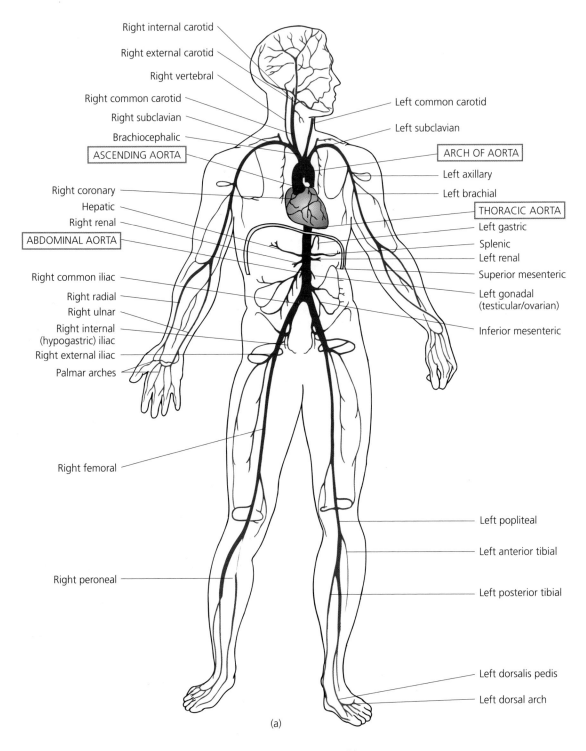

Right internal carotid
Right external carotid
Right vertebral
Right common carotid
Right subclavian
Brachiocephalic
ASCENDING AORTA

Left common carotid
Left subclavian
ARCH OF AORTA
Left axillary
Left brachial

Right coronary
Hepatic
Right renal
ABDOMINAL AORTA

THORACIC AORTA
Left gastric
Splenic
Left renal
Superior mesenteric
Left gonadal
(testicular/ovarian)
Inferior mesenteric

Right common iliac
Right radial
Right ulnar
Right internal
(hypogastric) iliac
Right external iliac
Palmar arches

Right femoral

Left popliteal

Left anterior tibial

Right peroneal

Left posterior tibial

Left dorsalis pedis
Left dorsal arch

(a)

Figure 9.15 Major blood vessels of the systemic circulation. (a) Arteries. (b) Veins.

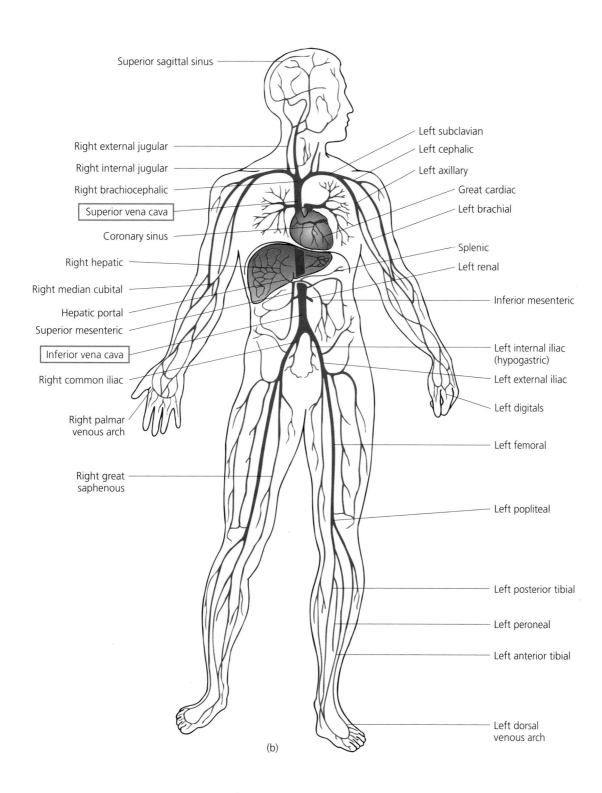

Superior sagittal sinus

Right external jugular

Right internal jugular

Right brachiocephalic

Superior vena cava

Coronary sinus

Right hepatic

Right median cubital

Hepatic portal

Superior mesenteric

Inferior vena cava

Right common iliac

Right palmar
venous arch

Right great
saphenous

Left subclavian

Left cephalic

Left axillary

Great cardiac

Left brachial

Splenic

Left renal

Inferior mesenteric

Left internal iliac
(hypogastric)

Left external iliac

Left digitals

Left femoral

Left popliteal

Left posterior tibial

Left peroneal

Left anterior tibial

Left dorsal
venous arch

(b)

Details of cardiac physiology

The heart is an extremely active organ, beating approximately 30 million times, and ejecting some 2.1 million litres of blood, per year. The previous section outlined the physiological basis for the coordinated contraction of the heart, the structure and function of blood vessels, and the specific routes of circulation. This section examines details of cardiac physiology associated with the events of each heart beat, the homeostatic control of cardiac output, and how cardiac parameters may be varied to meet changing peripheral demands.

CARDIAC CYCLE

The cardiac cycle represents the events associated with the flow of blood through the heart during one heart beat. Since the movement of blood is mainly achieved by alternate myocardial contraction and relaxation, the cycle employs the terms systole (i.e. contraction) and diastole (i.e. relaxation). Systolic contraction ejects blood from atria into adjacent ventricles, and from ventricles into the arterial trunks (i.e. pulmonary and aortic trunks). Diastolic relaxation is the period during which the heart chambers become filled with blood. Thus, the cardiac cycle is conveniently split into four phases: atrial and ventricular diastole, and atrial and ventricular systole. Since the sequence of events in the right and left sides of the heart are the same, we use the traditional approach of describing the cardiac cycle in terms of left-sided events (Figure 9.16). The main difference from the right-sided events is that the pressure generated by the left ventricle during systole is considerably higher than that generated by the right ventricle. This is because the total resistance to flow in the systemic circulation is greater than in the pulmonary circulation and so less pressure is required to promote circulation of the blood through the lungs; this is reflected by the relative thickness of the ventricular walls. Despite these pressure differences, the ventricles eject the same amount of blood with each contraction.

Our explanation of the cardiac cycle begins with the heart in total relaxation, when both atria and ventricles are relaxed, and it is mid-to-late diastole, i.e. the chambers are almost filled with blood.

Period of ventricular filling (mid–late diastole)

Pressure within the heart is low at this point, and so pulmonary venous blood flows passively into the left atrium. As blood enters, the atrial pressure becomes greater than ventricular pressure and consequently the atrioventricular (i.e. bicuspid) valve opens into the left ventricle and blood passes from the atrium to the ventricle throughout the diastolic period. The semilunar (i.e. aortic) valve is closed, since the pressure in the aorta is greater than the left ventricular pressure (Figure 9.16 – interval 1a). About 70–80% of the ventricular filling occurs during diastole. Towards the end of this period the tissue of the SA node spontaneously discharges and a wave of electrical excitation (i.e. a depolarization corresponding to the P-wave of the ECG), spreads throughout the atria; the subsequent atrial myocardial contraction, or atrial systole, accounts for the final 20–30% of ventricular filling (Figure 9.16 – interval 1b). The amount of blood within the ventricles at the end of ventricular diastole is called the ventricular end diastolic volume (VEDV). Atrial systole and ventricular diastole therefore occur simultaneously. Throughout diastole, the pressure in the aorta falls, since blood is moving throughout the systemic circuitry but is not being replenished by blood ejected from the left ventricle.

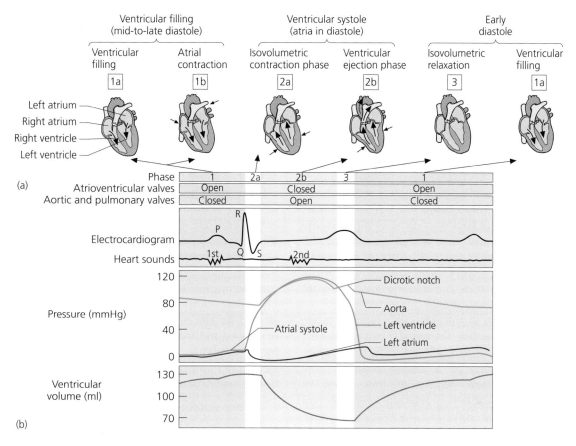

Figure 9.16 Summary of events occurring in the heart during the cardiac cycle. (a) Events in the left side of the heart. An ECG tracing is superimposed on the graph (top) so that pressure and volume changes can be related to electrical events occurring at any point. Time occurrence of heart sounds is also indicated. (b) Events of phases 1 through 3 of the cardiac cycle depicted in diagrammatic views of the heart.

Ventricular systole

Following contraction, the atria go into diastole and the wave of depolarization is passed from the AV node to the conduction system provided by the bundles of His, and then progresses throughout the Purkinje system. This need for ventricular systole to be slightly delayed after atrial systole highlights the importance of the electrical resistance provided by the AV node. Ventricular depolarization (corresponding to the QRS complex of the ECG) induces ventricular myocardial contraction, or ventricular systole. This causes the left ventricular pressure to rise sharply, closing the

atrioventricular (bicuspid) valve and preventing back flow into the left atrium. For a split second the ventricle is a completely sealed chamber, and this brief period is sometimes referred to as the isovolumetric ventricular contraction phase (Figure 9.16b – interval 2a) and is responsible for the rapid increase in the pressure within the ventricle. This phase ends as the ventricular pressure becomes greater than that in the aorta, when the semilunar (aortic) valve opens and ventricular ejection occurs (on the right side of the heart the right ventricle simultaneously ejects its blood into the pulmonary arterial trunk). The ejection is rapid initially, but then tapers off. The ejection of blood from the left ventricle (Figure 9.16b – interval 2b) causes the pressure in the aorta to reach approximately 120 mmHg. The left atrial pressure rises slowly throughout the ventricular ejection period, because of the continued flow of blood into it from the pulmonary veins.

Early diastole

During this brief phase (i.e. following the ECG T-wave), the ventricular myocardium relaxes, causing the left ventricular pressure to decrease to a value below the aortic pressure. This results in a backward flow of blood in the aortic trunk, and this causes closure of the semilunar (aortic) valve. Closure of the aortic valve causes a very brief rise in the aortic pressure known as the dicrotic notch (Figure 9.16a).

After closure of the semilunar (aortic) valve, the atrioventricular (bicuspid) valve remains closed for a split second, and thus, once again, the left ventricle is a sealed chamber; the ventricular blood volume at this phase of ventricular relaxation is referred to as the end systolic volume (ESV) and the relaxation phase as isovolumetric ventricular relaxation (Figure 9.16b – interval 3). Pressure within the ventricle falls sharply and this stage ends when the left atrial pressure rises (as a result of atrial filling) above the ventricular pressure, thus causing the atrioventricular valves to open and the ventricular filling phase begins once again. Atrial pressure falls to its lowest point and ventricular pressure begins to rise, completing the cycle.

At an average heart rate of 70 beats/min, each cardiac cycle takes about 0.8 seconds; atrial systole accounts for 0.1 second, ventricular systole 0.3 seconds, and the remaining 0.4 second is the period of total heart relaxation (diastole). There are two salient features to note about the cardiac cycle:

1 Blood flow through the heart is controlled entirely by pressure changes.

2 Blood flows along pressure gradients through the available opening, provided by the valves.

These pressure changes reflect the alternating systolic and diastolic periods, cause the opening and closing of the heart valves, and keep blood flowing in one direction.

CARDIODYNAMICS

Cardiodynamics investigates the movements of the heart and the forces generated by cardiac contraction. The stroke volume is the quantity of blood ejected into the systemic circulation with each left ventricular systole. Generally, this volume is directly related to the force of ventricular contraction, and, since the stroke volume may vary during beats, the total cardiac output is of great clinical interest.

Cardiac output is the quantity of blood ejected by the left ventricle each minute. It is expressed in litres per minute and is calculated by multiplying the stroke volume (volume ejected per contraction) by the number of heart beats (ventricular contractions) per minute; i.e.

Cardiac output (CO) = Stroke volume (SV) × Heart rate (HR)

The cardiac output, therefore, provides a useful indicator of ventricular homeostatic efficiency over a period of time. During 'normal' resting conditions the average heart rate is 70 beats/min, the stroke volume is 70 ml/beat, and so the cardiac output approximates to 5 l/min i.e.

CO = SV × HR = 70 × 70 = 4.9 l/min

Since the average adult blood volume is about 5 litres, the entire blood volume passes through the heart every minute. Cardiac output varies with the changing metabolic demands of the body, rising when the heart rate or stroke volume increases, falling when the heart rate or stroke volume decreases. The output can increase up to 25 l/min in a normal fit individual performing strenuous exercise, and up to 35 l/min in a well trained athlete. The increase above the resting cardiac output is termed the cardiac reserve. To understand how the cardiac output changes we need to examine its contributory factors. As a matter of convenience, the regulation of the heart rate and stroke volume will be considered separately, although alterations in cardiac output usually reflect changes in both aspects of cardiac function.

Regulation of the heart rate

The resting stroke volume under 'healthy' conditions tends to be relatively constant. However, when blood volume drops rapidly, for example following a haemorrhage, or when the heart is seriously weakened, as in myocardial infarction, the stroke volume declines and the cardiac output is maintained by an increased heart rate. Variations in the heart rate are induced by the influence of neural stimulation, and endocrine activity are induced chemically (see Chapter 22).

Neural mechanisms

The most important extrinsic influence affecting heart rate is that of the autonomic nervous system. The heart is innervated by both sympathetic and parasympathetic divisions (see Figure 9.8) via cardiac (or accelerator) and vagal nerves respectively. When sympathetically activated, as occurs with physical stressors (such as exercise) and certain emotional conditions, such as sexual arousal, the sympathetic neurons release noradrenaline at their cardiac synapses (at the SA node, AV node, and portions of the myocardium). This excitatory neurotransmitter increases the heart rate and the force of myocardial contraction. The latter prevents a decline of the stroke volume as would happen if only the heart rate was increased since the reduction of the diastolic period reduced the filling of the ventricle. By increasing the force of contraction the ventricle empties more efficiently and so maintains, or even increases, the stroke volume. Stimulants such as caffeine, nicotine, etc., have similar effects and when used in excessive amounts may increase the excitability to such a degree

that abnormal contractions, which could be considered as homeostatic imbalances, are observed. These are referred to as ectopic beats.

Conversely, the activation of the parasympathetic neurons in certain emotional conditions, such as severe depression, and/or in normal circumstances when stress thresholds are not achieved, release acetylcholine at their cardiac synapses. This inhibitory neurotransmitter hyperpolarizes the membrane of the sinoatrial cells by opening potassium channels, which stabilizes the membrane, reduces its rate of depolarization and so decreases the heart rate.

Both autonomic divisions are active under resting conditions, and so both acetylcholine and noradrenaline are normally released at the cardiac synapses. The predominant influence, however, is inhibitory, i.e. the parasympathetic nervous system (vagus nerve) exerts a 'vagal tone' or vagal brake' on the inherent rate of discharge of the SA node, which is about 100 beats/min, slowing the heart rate to 70–72 beats/min. Conversely, during exercise, the predominant influence is excitatory, and so sympathetic innervation dominates. The autonomic nervous system thus makes delicate adjustments in cardiovascular function to meet the demands of other systems.

The atrial (or Bainbridge) reflex

The atrial reflex involves a combination of intrinsic and neural (extrinsic) modifications of the heart rate which consequently affect the cardiac output. Intrinsically, an increased return of venous blood to the heart, observed when lying down or during exercise, stretches the right atrial wall. This causes a greater cardiac output because atrial stretch receptors respond by externally stimulating an increased sympathetic activity, thus causing the SA node cells to depolarize faster, and increasing the heart rate (by between 10 and 15%).

Endocrine control of the heart rate

Adrenaline secreted from the medulla of the adrenal gland by its sympathetic activation mimics the cardiac effects of the excitatory neurotransmitter noradrenaline, and so quickly enhances the heart rate and the force of myocardial contraction. Endocrine secretions of the thyroid gland (thyroxine), when released in large quantities, cause a slower, but more sustained rise in the heart rate. Endocrine secretions also enhance the cardiac effects of adrenaline and noradrenaline. Adrenaline and thyroxine are secreted in large quantities in Selye's general adaptation syndrome of stress (Chapter 22).

Intracellular and extracellular ionic homeostasis must be maintained for normal heart function, since some ionic imbalances which result from hormonal imbalances (Chapter 15) can interfere with cardiodynamics. Hypernatraemia (excess blood sodium) inhibits the transport of calcium into cardiac cells, by the membrane Na^+/Ca^{2+} exchange pump, thereby reducing contractility. Hyperkalaemia (excess blood potassium) lowers the cells' resting electrical potentials, which may result in cardiac excitation and increased heart rate, but in large excess prevents repolarization, and therefore restimulation of the membrane, leading to heart block and cardiac arrest. Hypokalaemia (insufficient blood potassium) produces a feeble heart beat thereby instigating life-threatening arrhythmias.

Other factors

Other factors which influence cardiac function are:

1 Age and gender;

2 Exercise;

3 Temperature;

4 Drugs.

AGE AND GENDER

The fetal resting heart rate of between 140 and 160 beats/min declines at birth and throughout life. The resting heart rate of an adult female is 72–80 beats/min and this is higher than that of an adult male (64–72 beats/min), reflecting gender differences in heart size and hence stroke volume.

EXERCISE

Sympathetic stimulation increases the heart rate during exercise. The resting heart rate of a trained athlete is, however, substantially lower than in a less physically fit individual (i.e. approximating between 40 and 60 beats/min), since the athlete has a well developed myocardium which is better equipped to pump more blood per contraction. Similarly, the heart rate necessary to maintain an increased cardiac output during exercise will also be lower in a trained athlete.

TEMPERATURE

A raised body temperature increases the heart rate by causing the SA and AV nodes to discharge more frequently. Conversely, a decrease in body temperature, such as that caused by prolonged exposure to a cold environment, depresses the heart rate.

DRUGS

Drugs which alter the heart rate are classified as positive chronotropic drugs (e.g. sympathetic agonists such as isoprenaline and adrenaline), and negative chronotropic (chronos = time) drugs (e.g. sympathetic antagonists including beta-blockers such as propranolol) which increase and decrease the heart rate respectively.

Homeostatic regulation of the stroke volume

The stroke volume represents the difference between:

1 The end diastolic volume (EDV), which is the amount of blood that collects in a ventricle during diastole or relaxation (left ventricular EDV is about 120 ml), and,

2 The end systolic volume (ESV), which is the amount of blood remaining in the ventricle after ventricular systole or contraction (left ventricular ESV is about 50 ml).

The resting stroke volume, therefore, approximates to 70 ml.

$$SV \text{ (ml/beat)} = EDV \text{ (120 ml)} - ESV \text{ (50 ml)}$$
$$= 70 \text{ ml/beat}$$

Consequently, a change in either the EDV and/or ESV will alter the stroke volume.

The end diastolic volume and the intrinsic regulation of stroke volume

The volume of blood within the ventricle at the end of diastole depends upon two interrelated factors:

1   The venous return, that is, the volume of blood entering the heart (and hence the ventricles) during ventricular diastole. This alters in response to changes in the cardiac output, the peripheral circulation, and other mechanisms which alter the rate of blood flow through the vena cavae.

2   The filling time, that is, the duration of ventricular diastole. This depends entirely on the heart rate. A slow heart rate provides a longer period of filling, hence a greater EDV, and a fast heart rate reduces ventricular filling.

The intrinsic control of stroke volume is illustrated by the responses of the heart to changes in venous return. If the venous return is suddenly increased, more blood flows into the heart and consequently the increased EDV stretches the myocardium further. This additional stretch of the muscle fibres promotes a more forceful contraction when the myocardium is stimulated and results in a greater volume being ejected. The 'more in – more out principle' is referred to as Starling's law of the heart. In this way venous return changes the ventricular EDV, and hence the stroke volume, and therefore cardiac output, since cardiac output = stroke volume × heart rate. Cardiac output and venous return will then remain in balance. Factors which alter the venous return are discussed later.

The end systolic volume and autonomic regulation of stroke volume

The stroke volume is also altered by autonomic-associated changes to volume of blood left in the ventricle after systole. Sympathetic neurons, as previously discussed, release noradrenaline when activated and also stimulate the secretion of adrenaline from the adrenal glands. These chemicals (classed as excitatory neurotransmitters and neuromodulators respectively) have two important effects on the heart:

1   The heart rate is increased causing shorter filling times (ie reduction of end diastolic volume).

2   The force and degree of myocardial contractility is enhanced. When stimulated the heart ejects more blood, consequently emptying the ventricle more efficiently and decreasing the ESV.

The interrelationship between the two factors is particularly noticeable during exercise when sympathetic activity is pronounced. Thus the increased venous return and the increased contractility of the heart act to produce a large increase in stroke volume (up to about 120 ml/beat). Reducing the end systolic volume might be expected to reduce the end diastolic volume as blood fills a more efficiently emptied ventricle. However, moderately increased heart rates during exercise actually cause the end diastolic volume to remain fairly normal due to the increased rate of venous return that is observed. However, heart rates above moderate levels reduce filling times, and decrease the end diastolic volume. Thus, stroke volume peaks at a heart rate of approximately 175 beats/min; further rises in heart rate are accompanied by a decrease in stroke volume. Conversely, parasympathetic neurons, via their inhibitory neurotransmitter acetylcholine decrease the heart rate, thereby contributing to the decreased cardiac output.

ASSESSING THE CARDIAC OUTPUT

Cardiac output can be assessed by direct or indirect means. Indirect methods may include measuring related variables, such as the urinary output. These variables are used to classify the cardiac output as being high, normal, or low. However, a more direct, and repeatable measurement such as thermodilution is required to monitor treatment accurately. Thermodilution involves inserting a triple lumen catheter, with a thermistor (temperature sensor) located at its tip, into a peripheral vein and advancing it to the right atrium. Subsequently, a bolus of cold saline of a known temperature is injected into the catheter. As the saline and right atrial blood mix, the temperature changes and this is sensed by a thermistor placed in the arterial system which records when the bolus passes its tip. The actual temperature recorded will depend upon the time taken for the bolus to reach this thermistor and the volume of blood into which the cold saline was dispersed. The data can then be used to calculate the cardiac output. Recent technology has largely superseded this method by using imaging techniques to assess the output. This methodology is non-invasive and also provides moment-to-moment evaluation of changes.

Details of circulatory physiology

From the previous section the reader should be aware that:

1 The heart is a muscular pump;

2 The arteries are the conduction and distribution vessels;

3 The arterioles are precapillary resistance vessels;

4 The capillaries are the exchange vessels;

5 The veins are the blood reservoirs and drainage vessels.

In order to understand how the supply of blood to a tissue is regulated in order to maintain cellular, tissue and organ system homeostatic processes, we need to consider three interrelated physical aspects of circulation: blood flow, blood pressure, and peripheral resistance. The latter two influence the rate of blood flow. Changes in cardiac output and peripheral resistance collectively determine how blood pressure is regulated.

BLOOD FLOW

Blood flow is the quantity of blood that passes through a vessel in a given period of time. Blood circulates in the systemic and pulmonary circuits, and the rate of flow is dependent upon two factors: arterial blood pressure and the peripheral resistance provided by blood vessels and blood viscosity.

The flow rate of any fluid is proportional to the pressure applied to that fluid. Thus fluid flows from high to low pressure regions and the greater the pressure differential, the faster the movement. Flow only continues, however, if the pressure exceeds the opposing forces of resistance. Therefore, the rate of flow is inversely proportional to the resistance since for a given pressure, the higher the resistance, the lower the flow rate,

$$\text{Blood Flow} = \frac{\text{Blood pressure differential}}{\text{Resistance to flow}}$$

The nature of the vessel's lining also influences blood flow. A smooth endothelial lining is associated with an even or lamina flow, whereas a roughened endothelium caused by calcium, fatty deposits, and/or thrombus formation, etc., causes irregular or turbulent flow. Lamina flow is silent, whereas turbulent flow may be heard using a stethoscope.

Initial pressure regulation occurs within the tissues themselves, since blood flow through capillaries is under local autoregulatory control. That is, if peripheral tissues become ischaemic, then local arteries and precapillary sphincters dilate and so increase blood flow and oxygen availability. The central nervous system ischaemic response is of particular note. It occurs immediately to minimize the period of cerebral ischaemia, as brain cells can be irreversibly damaged if deprived of oxygen for only a few minutes. Cells respond to ischaemic conditions by releasing carbon dioxide, lactic acid, adenosine, potassium and hydrogen ions, and other metabolites. These substances are responsible for the dilatation. Consequently, the increased blood flow to the tissues aids restoration of oxygen level to within its homeostatic range. This intrinsic mechanism is important for meeting the nutritional demands of active tissues, such as muscle, in times of strenuous exercise.

BLOOD PRESSURE

Blood circulates because the heart pump establishes pressure gradients. The highest average pressure, created by the left ventricular pump, is observed in the aortic arch prior to its coronary branches, where it approximates to 95 mmHg; the lowest average pressure is at the junction of the superior and inferior vena cavae, where it approximates to 3–5mmHg. Unless otherwise stated, the term 'blood pressure' refers to the pressure in the large arteries. The average pressure is most important since the left ventricle pumps blood in a pulsating manner and tissue flow generally varies accordingly. The

systemic arterial pressure in a resting young adult moves between about 120 mmHg and 80 mmHg. The higher value is observed following ejection of blood from the left ventricle during systole and so is called the systolic pressure. The lower value is that observed at the end of diastole and so is called the diastolic pressure. Figure 9.17 illustrates how blood pressure declines unevenly throughout the cardiovascular system. The difference between the blood pressure at the base of the aortic arch and the right atrium represents the circulatory pressure. Bearing in mind the relatively small pressures of the venous system, arterial pressure approximates to the circulatory pressure.

PERIPHERAL RESISTANCE

Resistance refers to the impedance or opposition to blood flow created by the amount of friction the blood encounters as it passes through the vessels. Peripheral resistance is the generally used term since most friction is encountered in the peripheral circulation. Resistance is related to:

1 Blood viscosity;

2 The length of blood vessels;

3 The diameter of blood vessels.

The viscosity or stickiness of blood is created by the ratio of blood cells and solutes to fluid molecules within blood. Homeostatic imbalances, such as polycythaemia, dehydration, and hyperproteinaemia, increase blood viscosity, whereas imbalances such as anaemia, haemorrhage, and hypoproteinaemia decrease blood viscosity.

The relationship between vessel length and resistance is simple; the longer the vessel, the greater the resistance. In a 'healthy' person the viscosity and length of vessels normally remain unchanged, and thus may be considered as 'constant' variables. In health, changes in the diameter of blood vessels provide the main means of varying peripheral resistance.

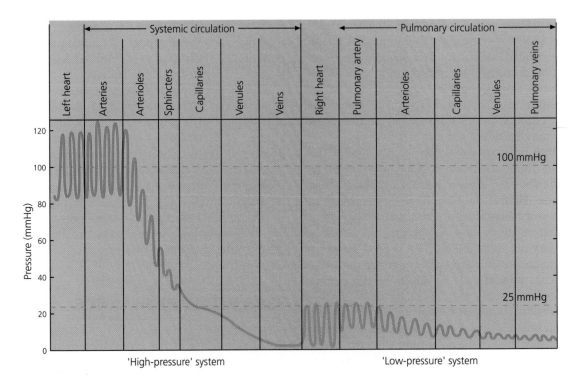

Figure 9.17 Blood pressure changes within the circulatory system. Note the general decline in circulatory pressures within the systemic circuit and the elimination of the pulse pressure oscillations in the arterioles.

The relationship between the diameter of blood vessels and resistance is also simple: the smaller the diameter, the greater the resistance to blood flow. In fact resistance increases to the fourth power of the inverse of the radius, i.e. a halving of the radius increases the resistance 16-fold ($2 \times 2 \times 2 \times 2$).

Normally the peripheral resistance primarily reflects the resistance due to arterioles, in particular their diameter, and is influenced by neural and hormonal mechanisms although tissues have varying degrees of intrinsic control. The vasomotor centre of the brainstem medulla regulates arteriolar diameter via its sympathetic innervation. The normal background level of vasomotor activity sets the vasomotor or sympathetic tone of arterioles, which determines the peripheral resistance under resting conditions (Figure 9.18a). Thus, greater vasomotor sympathetic outflow

increases the resistance due to arteriolar vasoconstriction (Figure 9.18b), and reduction in sympathetic output decreases the peripheral resistance by inducing vasodilation (Figure 9.18c).

Factors affecting vasomotor activity are discussed later in this chapter.

MEASUREMENT OF BLOOD PRESSURE

Arterial pressure is measured using a sphygmomanometer (Figure 9.19). This involves putting an inflatable cuff, usually around the left upper arm, to record blood pressure in the brachial artery (which is taken to be a measure of aortic pressure). A stethoscope is placed over the artery distal to the cuff so that the

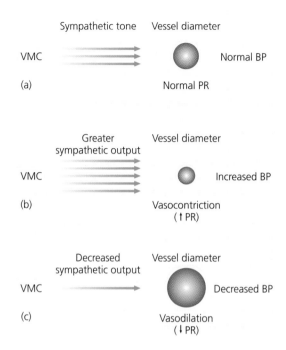

Figure 9.18 Vasomotor centre control of blood pressure via changing the peripheral resistance of arterioles: (a) normal blood pressure (i.e. within homeostatic range); (b) low blood pressure (i.e. below homeostatic range); (c) high blood pressure (i.e. above homeostatic range). VMC, vasomotor centre; PR, peripheral resistance; BP, blood pressure.

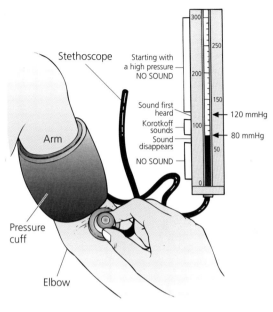

Figure 9.19 Sphygmomanometer measurement of blood pressure.

diastole). The average blood pressure of a young adult male is expressed as 120/80 mmHg. Female values are slightly less.

PULSE AND PULSE PRESSURE

The alternate expansion and elastic recoil of an artery with each left ventricular systole is called the pulse; thus the pulse rate is equivalent to the heart rate. The strongest pulse is in the arteries closest to the heart; it progressively weakens as it passes through the arterial tree, disappearing altogether within the capillary networks. The radial pulse is the most commonly used area to feel and monitor the pulse. Other areas include brachial (arm), carotid (neck – a site frequently used in cardiopulmonary resuscitation) and popliteal (behind the knee) pulses (Figure 9.20). These are all sites where the artery lies superficially, and so can be felt, or palpated.

The pulse pressure comprises the difference between systolic and diastolic pressures, and in

pulse can be heard. The cuff is inflated until the pressure in the cuff reaches 180–200 mmHg, enough completely to compress the brachial artery and stop blood flow. The cuff is then slowly deflated, until the first (Korotkoff) sound is heard through the stethoscope. This sound results from the movement of blood through the no-longer occluded vessel. The mercury column reading at this point corresponds to the systolic blood pressure (i.e. the force at which blood is pumped against the walls during left ventricular contraction). As the cuff pressure falls further, the sound suddenly becomes faint and then disappears as blood movement beyond the previously sealed vessel is no longer impeded. This reading corresponds to the diastolic pressure (i.e. the force of blood in arteries during ventricular

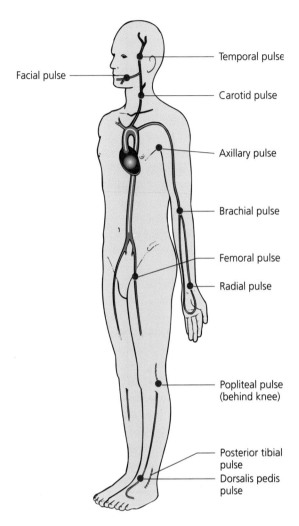

Figure 9.20 Pulse points. Each pulse point is named after the artery with which it is associated.

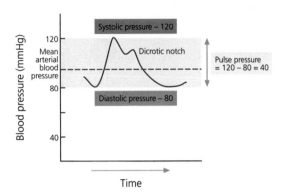

Figure 9.21 Arterial blood pressure: systolic, diastolic, and pulse pressures.

become smaller with increasing distance from the heart. The former decreases because of the friction which blood encounters within blood vessels, the latter because vessels become less elastic. The pressure oscillations disappear in the arterioles (see Figure 9.17), but arteriolar vessels containing precapillary sphincters cause the mean pressure to remain steady at about 25–30mmHg. As blood passes through the capillary beds the pressure falls from 25–30 mmHg at their arterial side to 15–18mmHg at their venous side. The decline is necessary to slow the blood flow so as to aid capillary exchange of plasma constituents with tissue fluid (see later).

VENOUS PRESSURE

Whereas arterial pressure determines the rate of blood flow to tissues, venous pressure influences venous return to the heart, which in turn is an important determinant of the cardiac output. Venous blood pressure is less than one-tenth of arterial pressure. When an individual is standing the venous pressure must overcome gravitational forces so that blood returns and flows within the inferior vena cava. This is made possible with the aid of three previously mentioned factors: valves,

a young adult male this approximates to 40 mmHg (Figure 9.21). The pulse pressure provides information about the condition of blood vessels. Homeostatic imbalances, such as arteriosclerosis (hardening of the vessels) and patent ductus arteriosus (a vessel in the fetus; Chapter 19) record higher pulse pressures.

The mean arterial pressure lies between the systolic and diastolic values (Figure 9.21) and is calculated by adding one-third of the pulse pressure to the diastolic pressure. Both the mean arterial and pulse pressure values muscular pumps produced by muscle contraction in the limbs, and thoracoabdominal pumps, produced by pressure reductions in the thorax and pressure changes in the abdomen, during breathing movements.

In exercise, these factors combine to increase venous return to its maximum so as to enable an increase in cardiac output to a level required for the continuance of the exercise.

THE HOMEOSTATIC CONTROL OF ARTERIAL BLOOD PRESSURE

Although variations in blood viscosity may affect blood pressure, such variations are not normally observed. The three principal factors influencing blood pressure are: the cardiac output, the peripheral resistance, and the blood volume (which alters the cardiac output). (Figure 9.22). The factors are related by the equation:

$$\text{Blood pressure} = \text{Cardiac output} \times \text{Total peripheral resistance}$$

Cardiac output

Cardiac output is the volume of blood ejected into the aorta each minute. Blood pressure varies directly with cardiac output, i.e. an increase in cardiac output increases blood pressure, and vice versa. The reader should recall that:

1 Cardiac output = stroke volume × heart rate, thus changes in either will alter blood pressure.

2 Cardiac output is partly regulated by the cardiac accelerator and inhibitory centres of the brainstem via sympathetic and parasympathetic output respectively.

3 Hormones (such as adrenaline, and thyroxine), ions (such as potassium, sodium, and calcium), physical and emotional factors

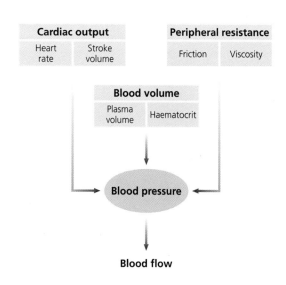

Figure 9.22 A summary of factors that influence blood pressure and blood flow.

(such as depression), temperature, gender, and age all affect the heart rate, its force of contraction (stroke volume), and thus, cardiac output.

Peripheral resistance

As stated earlier, peripheral resistance in a normal healthy individual is the major opposition to blood flow through peripheral vessels and is largely determined by the diameter of the vessels. Peripheral resistance is regulated by the activity of the sympathetic nervous system, which promotes constriction and dilatation of arterioles (Figure 9.18), or by the release of vasoconstrictor hormones.

Blood volume

Blood pressure varies directly with blood volume. The average volume of blood in a human body is 5 litres, and homeostatic imbalances such as haemorrhage may decrease blood pressure by excessively decreasing the blood volume. Conversely, imbalances such as sodium retention (see Chapter 12) induced by aldosteronism (excess of the hormone aldosterone) increase blood pressure by also promoting water retention and hence increasing blood volume. Accompanying the larger volume of blood is a greater stretch on the arterial wall which in turn increases the elastic recoil and this also contributes to the higher blood pressure.

The interrelationships between cardiac output, peripheral resistance, and blood volume determine cardiovascular functioning and their control stabilizes blood pressure to within its homeostatic parameters at rest and also during exercise when these parameters are modified to increase blood pressure to its altered homeostatic set-points. To maintain cellular homeostasis blood pressure must be tightly regulated since pressure changes (especially a decrease) influence the transport of metabolites and 'waste' products of metabolism to and from cells.

Figure 9.23 illustrates a number of short-term and long-term homeostatic regulators of blood pressure. As discussed in Chapter 1, short-term controls act to restore homeostatic equilibria quickly. If they fail, long-term controls must respond, and, if these fail to readdress homeostasis, then illness occurs. Regarding blood pressure controls, these are important in preventing its inappropriate elevation (called hypertension) which can cause mechanical damage to vessels of the heart, brain, and kidneys, or its reduction (called hypotension) which can cause inadequate blood supply or ischaemia and hence necrotic changes to tissues. Short-term controls are neural responses; these adjust cardiac output and peripheral resistance to stabilize blood pressure, and hence tissue blood flow. Various vasoconstrictor hormones support this action but their effects are slower to be initiated. Long-term controls change the blood volume, which alters the cardiac output, and hence blood pressure. These latter regulators are mainly hormonal responses which again highlights the distinction between these two coordination systems. That is, the nervous

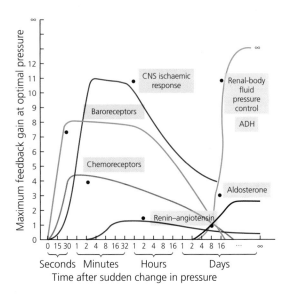

Figure 9.23 Arterial pressure control mechanisms at different times after the onset of an arterial pressure imbalance.

system responds and acts immediately to homeostatic imbalances; the endocrine system is comparatively slower to respond and its course of action is of a longer duration.

Short-term homeostatic control of blood pressure

Neural mechanisms provide the immediate responses to changes in blood pressure and blood gas concentration and prevent an individual from fainting due to an inadequate blood supply to the brain when the individual stands upright very quickly (gravity causes a pooling of blood below the heart on standing which reduces the cardiac output).

Reductions in cardiac output (including those imbalances that decrease blood volume) promote vasoconstriction of blood vessels, except those of the heart and brain, which can be considered a homeostatic adaptive mechanism that maintains blood flow to these vital organs. In these instances, blood pressure is especially controlled by sympathetic activity which is stimulated by afferent information from stretch receptors (baroreceptors) within the circulatory system and/or chemoreceptors of vessels or higher centres in the brain. The latter detect changes in blood gas composition, or blood acidity. Hence these are two classes of reflex in the neural control of blood pressure and blood distribution. These are:

1 The baroreceptor reflex – sensitive to blood pressure changes.

2 The chemoreceptor reflex – sensitive to dissolved gases (oxygen, carbon dioxide and hydrogen ions).

These reflexes are mediated by the brainstem vasomotor centre, and control arteriolar diameter (Figure 9.24a,b).

Baroreceptor reflexes

Baroreceptors are specialized mechanoreceptors which respond to systemic blood pressure changes. Arterial baroreceptors are located mainly in the aortic sinus, carotid sinus, and within the large arteries of the neck and thorax, and monitor blood pressure at the beginning of the systemic circuit. Atrial baroreceptors monitor blood pressure at the end of this circuit. The atrial reflexes differs from the aortic and carotid reflexes in that they monitor stretch within the heart, rather than in blood vessels. For example, an increase in right atrial blood pressure means that blood is arriving faster than it is being pumped out into the aorta; atrial baroreceptors respond by stimulating the cardiac accelerator centre, which increases the cardiac output which in turn removes the potential congestion in the right atrium, thus returning the atrial pressure to normal. In contrast, arterial baroreceptors are high pressure receptors. When there is an increase in systemic blood pressure they have a number of effects. First, they stimulate the cardiac inhibitory centre, and hence vagal nerve activity which depresses the heart rate and so reduces cardiac output. Second, they inhibit the cardiac accelerator centre, and so

reduce sympathetic activity to the heart. This makes the influence of vagal nerve activity even more effective. Finally, they inhibit vasomotor centre activity, causing peripheral vasodilation, which reduces peripheral resistance.

Collectively such responses result in a compensatory decrease in blood pressure (Figure 9.24a).

Conversely, if there is a decrease in blood pressure, then arterial baroreceptors promote the opposite response, by decreasing vagal nerve activity, and promoting sympathetic activity to the heart and blood vessels, causing an increase in cardiac output and peripheral vasoconstriction.

The consequence of such responses is a compensatory increase in blood pressure (Figure 9.24b).

The central role of baroreceptors is to protect the circulation against short-term changes in blood pressure, such as those that may occur with changing posture. Figure 9.23 illustrates their immediacy of response to blood pressure changes, and their ineffectiveness in protecting against sustained blood pressure changes. In patients who have chronic hypertension (i.e. high blood pressure persisting for some years), the baroreceptors seem to be reset to monitor changes at a higher set-point.

Chemoreceptor reflex

Chemoreceptors are located in the aortic arch, carotid sinus (specifically known as the aortic and carotid bodies), large arteries in the neck, and within the central nervous system. They are sensitive to low levels of oxygen (especially those outside the central nervous system) and are even more sensitive to high levels of carbon dioxide and hydrogen ions.

These imbalances are usually a consequence of low blood pressure and inadequate blood flow (Figure 9.24b). In such circumstances chemoreceptors transmit impulses to the cardiovascular centres of the brainstem which in turn reflexly increase blood pressure, and blood flow to the heart, so as to correct the

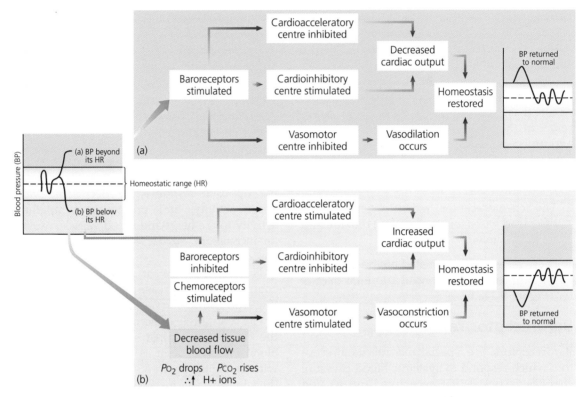

Figure 9.24 Reflexes that assist in the regulation of blood pressure. (a) The baroreceptor reflexes. (b) The chemoreceptor and baroreceptor reflexes.

imbalance(s). The rate and depth of breathing are also increased, which facilitates gas exchange. The chemoreceptors are discussed in more detail in Chapter 11.

Higher centre control

Higher brain centres, such as the cerebral cortex and hypothalamus, although not routinely involved in blood pressure regulation, can modify arterial blood pressure via the medullary centre of the brainstem in response to strong emotions. During the 'fight and flight' response and sexual excitement, for example, the hypothalamus and cerebral cortex stimulate the vasomotor sympathetic reflex, bringing about vasoconstriction and the accompanying increase in arterial pressure. In addition, sympathetic stimulation causes the secretion of adrenaline and noradrenaline from

the adrenal medulla. These hormones mimic and prolong many of the sympathetic responses of Selye's general adaptation syndrome's alarm stage (Chapter 22), including persistent vasoconstriction and the consequential protracted increase in blood pressure.

In times of depression and grief the higher centres decrease the vasomotor sympathetic reflex, and the resultant decrease in blood pressure can cause fainting. The hypothalamus also mediates the redistribution of blood flow and changes in cardiovascular dynamics associated with exercise and changes in body temperature.

Long-term control of blood pressure

Some hormones, such as adrenaline and noradrenaline, act as short-term homeostatic regulators of blood pressure by influencing cardiac function and peripheral resistance. Others, such as angiotensin II, erythropoietin, aldosterone, atrial natriuretic factor and anti-diuretic hormone (ADH) are longer-term regulators which act by influencing blood volume and/or peripheral resistance (Figure 9.25a,b).

Angiotensin II

Angiotensin II, a powerful vasoconstrictor, is produced by activation of a plasma precursor, angiotensinogen, by the enzyme renin (which converts angiotensinogen to angiotensin I) and angiotensin-converting enzyme (ACE which converts angiotensin I to angiotensin II). Renin is secreted from specialized kidney cells which detect a fall in blood pressure, or in response to vasoconstrictor activity to this area. ACE is found in the lung and is activated by the presence of angiotensin I. Angiotensin II also stimulates the secretion of ADH and aldosterone, the latter of which stimulates the renal retention of sodium, and hence, water. In addition, angiotensin stimulates the hypothalamic thirst centre, so that the individual seeks fluid; the high levels of ADH and aldosterone ensure that much of the additional water consumed will be retained, hence elevating blood volume and blood pressure (Figure 9.25a). Renin is not secreted when the blood pressure and blood volume are high.

Erythropoietin

Erythropoietin is secreted by kidney cells in an indirect response to a decrease in blood pressure and in a direct response to a considerable decrease in the oxygen-carrying capacity of blood, as occurs when one ascends to altitude prior to acclimatization. This hormone stimulates erythrocyte production which results in an increased blood pressure and oxygen carrying capacity of blood (Figure 9.25a).

Atrial natriuretic factor

An increase in venous return, as experienced when blood volume is high, causes an overstretching of the atrial wall which stimulates the release of a natriuretic factor; in turn this hormone decreases blood volume and blood pressure by stimulating peripheral vasodilation, increasing sodium and water losses via the kidneys, antagonizing the effects of adrenaline/noradrenaline, ADH, and aldosterone, and decreasing thirst.

As blood volume and pressure are restored there is less stretch and, hence, secretion of this factor – yet another example of negative feedback control.

Antidiuretic hormone (ADH; or vasopressin)

Vasopressin is produced by the hypothalamus and released from the posterior pituitary in response to a low blood pressure (via arterial baroreceptor stimulation) and/or an excessive increase in the osmotic concentration of plasma as a consequence of dehydration (via hypothalamic osmoreceptors). The hormone causes intense vasoconstriction, and also water conservation by the kidneys, which help to reverse changes in blood pressure (Figure 9.25a). A high blood pressure has the opposite effects.

Role of the kidney in the regulation of blood pressure

The kidneys are long-term homeostatic regulators of blood pressure, influencing it via their ability to alter blood volume. For example, when blood volume and blood pressure rise, the kidneys produce more urine, thus decreasing blood volume and causing blood pressure to fall. Conversely, when blood pressure and blood volume are low, the kidneys produce little urine, conserving water and returning it to the circulation, increasing blood volume and blood pressure. These mechanisms of the kidney are responses to the endocrine secretions discussed earlier. The near constancy of blood volume in the adult is an indication of their effectiveness.

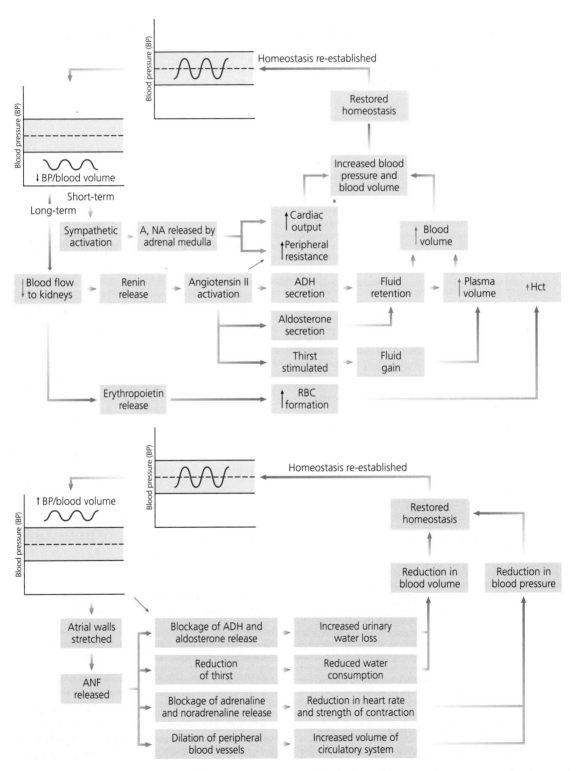

Figure 9.25 The homeostatic regulation of blood pressure (BP) and blood volume. (a) Factors that compensate for decreased blood volume and pressure. (b) Factors that compensate for increased blood volume and pressure. Hct, haematocrit; A, adrenaline; NA, noradrenaline, ANF, atrial natriuretic factor; ADH, antidiuretic hormone; ↑ increased; ↓ decreased.

Role of vascular system in systemic homeostasis

BLOOD FLOW TO TISSUES

Blood flow to tissues must be tightly regulated since it is responsible for:

1 Absorption of nutrients from the gastro-intestinal tract.

2 Gaseous exchange in the lungs.

3 Transport of oxygen, nutrients, hormones, etc., to tissue cells throughout the body.

4 The removal of waste products of metabolism from cells.

5 Processing of blood by the kidneys and other excretory organs.

The flow of blood to specific tissues reflects the metabolic demands of that tissue. At rest, for example, skeletal muscles receive approximately 20% of the total blood volume each minute. During exercise blood is redistributed from other areas (e.g. kidneys and abdominal organs), so that skeletal muscles receive a higher proportion of the (increased) cardiac output to cater for their increased metabolic demands (Figure 9.26).

Velocity of blood flow

The speed at which blood flows varies throughout the systemic/pulmonary circulations and with the specific stages of the cardiac cycle. Obviously, the greatest velocity is recorded in the aorta during ventricular systole. Furthermore, since velocity is inversely related to the cross-sectional area of blood vessels, the flow rate decreases as the aorta branches, being slowest within the capillary beds, and this is essential as the capillaries are the exchange vessels (Figure 9.27a). Flow speeds up again in the venous system as blood collects from the different tissues and is returned to the heart (Figure 9.27b).

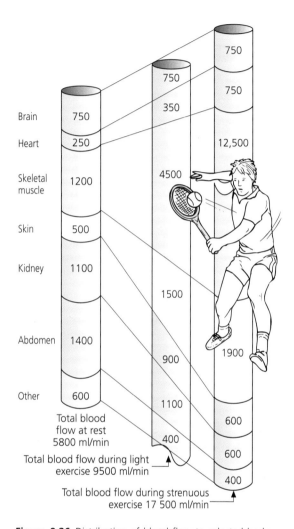

Figure 9.26 Distribution of blood flow to selected body organs at rest, during light exercise and during strenuous exercise.

Tissue autoregulation – local regulation of blood flow

Tissue autoregulation of blood flow is independent of systemic control but is proportional to the tissue's requirements, being regulated by local conditions. Flow is, therefore, increased automatically in response to:

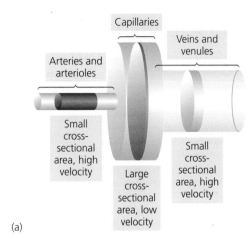

(a)

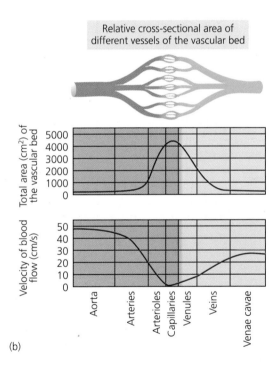

(b)

Figure 9.27 Relationship between cross–sectional area of blood vessels and velocity of blood flow. (a) Relative cross–sectional areas of arteries, capillaries and veins. (b) Relationship between blood flow velocity and total cross–sectional area in various blood vessels of the systemic circulation.

1 Nutrients and oxygen levels falling below their homeostatic range, i.e. when they fail to meet the demands of the tissue.

2 Carbon dioxide levels beyond its homeostatic range. This is the most powerful trigger to autoregulation and could be viewed as resulting from an accumulation of this metabolic product due to inadequate blood flow.

3 The release of metabolically active substances from cells, such as lactic acid, kinins, prostaglandins, potassium and hydrogen ions, which again will occur if blood flow to the tissue was inadequate.

4 The presence of inflammatory chemicals, such as histamine, which promote the protective inflammatory response when the tissue is damaged.

These stimuli cause immediate arteriolar vasodilation and relaxation of precapillary sphincters, thus causing an increased blood flow to the tissues concerned. Autoregulation is considered both as a short-term and long-term regulator of blood flow, which acts to readdress homeostasis in the particular tissues. Cerebral blood flow in particular is regulated by one of the most precise autoregulatory mechanisms in the body. Brain tissue, however, is particularly sensitive to increased carbon dioxide (and the consequential decreased pH), though severely excessive carbon dioxide levels may remove the brain's autoregulatory response, resulting in severe brain damage. Oxygen deficit is a less potent stimulus even though neurons are totally intolerant of ischaemic conditions. Oxygen deficit, however, increases the presence of many of the metabolites noted above and the regulatory mechanisms protect the area from damage by responding to the changing levels of these metabolites.

Blood flow through capillary networks is intermittent due to the contractions and relaxations of the smooth muscle fibres of the arterioles and precapillary sphincters of true capillaries.

CAPILLARY DYNAMICS RELATED TO CELLULAR HOMEOSTASIS

Body fluids are compartmentalized into intracellular and extracellular fluids. The latter is further subdivided into plasma and interstitial (tissue) fluid. Within the extracellular fluid compartment the exchange of fluid between plasma and interstitium is important since it brings nutrients into the proximity of cell membranes and aids the removal of substances secreted by cells ('wastes', hormones, etc.) in the opposite direction. Such exchanges are essential if solutes are to enter and exit intracellular fluid efficiently. In order to prevent excessive loss of fluid from plasma (which would induce hypovolaemia) or an excessive build-up of tissue fluid (called oedema), a similar volume of fluid must be returned to plasma as was extruded from it.

The movement of water and some of its dissolved solutes between plasma and tissue fluid occurs at the capillary level (Figure 9.28). Water is driven out of the plasma largely because the hydrostatic pressure of the arterial end of the capillary is higher than the osmotic (referred to as the oncotic or colloidal) pressure generated by plasma proteins. The hydrostatic pressure decreases along the length of the vessel as water is exuded into the tissue fluid, and eventually is exceeded by the plasma oncotic pressure. Proteins are largely retained within capillaries due to their macromolecular size (though small proteins can be transferred across capillary membranes). Net pressure at the venous end of the capillaries thus favours the return of fluid into the capillary (a small volume of exudate is returned to the circulation via lymph vessels which drain the interstitial spaces). Plasma protein concentration is, therefore, another important factor in the homeostatic maintenance of a normal circulatory blood volume.

EXERCISE: A CHANGE IN CARDIOVASCULAR HOMEOSTATIC SET POINTS

A number of interrelated changes occur during a steady rate or low rate of exercise. For example, the oxygen consumption of exercising skeletal muscles is increased, facilitated by precapillary sphincter relaxation in these tissues as a response to their changing metabolic requirements. Consequently, blood flow increases (Figure 9.26) and blood is returned to the veins at an increased rate. The increased venous return to the heart results from a greater activity in the skeletal muscular 'pumps' which force blood along the peripheral veins. The accompanying increased breathing rate also increases blood flow into the vena cava via the suction pressure created by the thoracoabdominal 'pumps'. A greater venous return to the heart results in an increased cardiac output by mechanisms associated with Starling's and Bainbridge's reflexes, and increased sympathetic activity. As long as the increased cardiac output can supply the increased demand then arterial pressure will be maintained, despite the increase in muscle blood flow. Indeed, the increased cardiac output observed during exercise actually causes an increase in systemic blood pressure as a consequence of an elevated systolic blood pressure; diastolic pressure is little changed.

There are minimal alterations in blood flow distribution to accommodate low levels of exercise, although skeletal and cardiac muscles, together with the skin, exhibit a small increase. The increased skeletal muscular flow is via the release of local factors mentioned earlier which relax precapillary sphincters at these sites. The increased skin blood flow is via hypothalamic–vasomotor centre responses to an increase in body temperature, which causes vasodilation of the skin arterioles and promotes the removal of the excess heat generated by the body. Severe exercise promotes additional physiological adjustments to

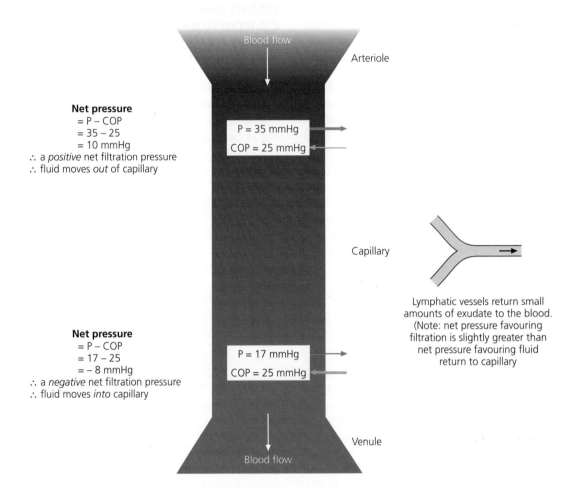

Net pressure
= P − COP
= 35 − 25
= 10 mmHg
∴ a *positive* net filtration pressure
∴ fluid moves *out* of capillary

P = 35 mmHg
COP = 25 mmHg

Blood flow

Arteriole

Capillary

Lymphatic vessels return small
amounts of exudate to the blood.
(Note: net pressure favouring
filtration is slightly greater than
net pressure favouring fluid
return to capillary

Net pressure
= P − COP
= 17 − 25
= − 8 mmHg
∴ a *negative* net filtration pressure
∴ fluid moves *into* capillary

P = 17 mmHg
COP = 25 mmHg

Venule

Blood flow

Figure 9.28 Capillary exchange processes. *P*, hydrostatic pressure within the capillary; π, oncotic pressure due to plasma proteins; ⌁, direction of fluid (+ solutes) flow into/out of capillary; (oa), direction of blood flow through capillary.

accommodate the massive increase in the peripheral distribution of blood to skeletal muscles. In addition to metabolic factors, these include:

1 Sympathetic stimulation of the cardiac accelerator centre, which accounts for a cardiac output increase of up to 20–35 l/min, depending upon the fitness of the individual.

2 Redistribution of blood flow to skeletal muscles via:

(a) a shutdown of blood flow to 'non-essential' organs (e.g. kidneys, gut) by vasomotor sympathetic stimulation to their arterioles;

(b) an increased blood flow to skeletal muscle, heart, and lungs via reduced vasomotor sympathetic activity to their vasculature.

With training, one's cardiovascular fitness is improved by the increased myocardial bulk which develops. This increases the stroke volume, and, hence, cardiac output and the trained individual has a lower heart rate for a given cardiac output when compared with an untrained individual. Sebastian Coe, the famous 1500 metre runner of the 1980s, claimed to have a resting heart rate of just 36 beats/min (compared with the adult average of 72 beats/min). This would still have been sufficient to maintain blood flow to his tissues, due to his large stroke volume. Such a heart rate associated with a non-athletic person, however, is clinically referred to as a brady-cardia, since the accompanying lower stroke volume would be insufficient to deliver blood to the surrounding tissues.

Examples of homeostatic control system failure and principles of correction

Cardiovascular malfunctions may be conveniently classified as cardiac and circulatory homeostatic imbalances. It cannot be overemphasized, however, that neither malfunction exists in isolation without compromising the other's homeostatic function, together with the homeostatic functions of other tissues and organs because of the interdependence of organ system functioning. Consequently a vast array of clinical problems, ranging from the less severe (e.g. temporary ischaemic pain), to the very severe (e.g. cerebrovascular accidents, kidney failure, pulmonary failure), present themselves when cardiovascular function is impaired.

CARDIAC IMBALANCES

Principal cardiac malfunctions arise from:

1 The physical structure of the heart (e.g. congenital septal and valvular defects).

2 The conduction system (e.g. atrioventricular heart block and bradycardia).

The net result of either is a decreased cardiac output and cardiac reserve which consequentially reduces blood flow to the peripheral tissues. Infections also cause cardiac imbalances. For example, endocarditis is a

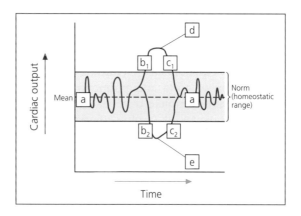

Figure 9.29 Cardiac output – an expression of cardiovascular function.
a, Cardiac output fluctuating within its normal homeostatic parameters.
b_1, Increased cardiac output as occurs: (i) normally when the homeostatic parameters are reset (e.g. exercise); (ii) abnormally, when indicating a homeostatic imbalance, such as right–to–left cardiac shunts (e.g. tetralogy of Fallot, transposition of the great vessels), aortic stenosis (and its associated left ventricular hypertrophy) and tachycardia.
b_2, Decreased cardiac output, as occurs with homeostatic imbalances such as the left–to–right cardiac shunts (atrial septal defects, ventricular septal defects, patent ductus arteriosus), cardiomyopathies, bradycardia, heart failure and incompetent valves.
c_1 and c_2, Correction varies according to the imbalance, i.e. oxygen therapy for the cyanosed patients; drugs or pacemaker to correct conduction imbalances; surgical techniques to correct structural defects.
d, Re–established homeostasis of cardiac output.
e, Homeostatic failure of cardiac output.

localized inflammation of the structures of the endocardium (e.g. valves) and can also promote general imbalances, such as ischaemia and/or infarctions (cardiac muscle death) due to the increased potential for emboli development. A selected few common cardiac imbalances will now be discussed (Figure 9.29).

Congenital heart defects

Most congenital cardiac imbalances result from teratogenic influences during early stages of pregnancy when the heart is developing. Some of these defects are mentioned in Chapter 19; suffice-to-say such defects account for approximately one half of all infant deaths arising from congenital abnormalities. The most frequent are septal defects and a patent ductus arteriosus. Since blood passes from high pressure regions to low pressure regions, cardiac defects involving right-to-left shunts (e.g. teratology of Fallot, transposition of aorta and pulmonary arterial trunk) prevent complete oxygenation of blood and so cause cyanosis (a blue colorization due to low oxygen content of blood). This may be treated initially with oxygen therapy depending upon the severity of the cyanosis, and later with corrective surgical techniques to abolish the shunts and/or vessel abnormalities. Conditions comprising left-to-right shunts (e.g. patent ductus arteriosus, patent foramen ovalis, septal defects) increase pulmonary blood flow and lead to congestive heart failure if uncorrected. Correction involves controlling the consequential pulmonary oedema, providing respiratory support, and restricting fluids. Frusemide, a loop diuretic, may be prescribed if the imbalance does not correct itself, in order to reduce blood volume and cardiac congestion, and again surgical correction may be necessary.

Conduction imbalances

As discussed earlier, the heart rate varies with changing activities. In exercise, an increased heart rate is considered quite normal, since the homeostatic set points are altered to accommodate the increased metabolic demands of the tissues to prevent intracellular homeostatic imbalances. However, if the heart rate is persistently, and markedly, increased or decreased at rest, this usually signals conduction malfunctions – tachycardia and bradycardia respectively. The former is a heart rate beyond its homeostatic parameters (tachy- = fast), whereas the latter is a heart rate below its homeostatic parameters (brady- = slow). Clinically, tachycardia and bradycardia refer to resting heart rates of >100 and <60 beats/min respectively.

Heart failure

The cardiac output is largely determined by the venous return and the normal myocardial pumping activity. If the latter is compromised (despite a satisfactory venous return), it may result in the cardiac output not being able to meet the metabolic demands of the body. In such circumstances the term heart, cardiac, or pump failure is used. Since the heart has two ventricular pumps, it is possible to have left heart failure (as occurs in left-sided myocardial infarction, mitral or aortic valve incompetence, aortic stenosis, systemic hypertension), and right heart failure (as occurs in pulmonary diseases).

In left ventricular failure the output is less than the volume received from the right heart; the left ventricle, therefore, becomes congested with blood, causing imbalances in:

1 The chambers and vessels preceding the left ventricle, i.e. an increased volume, hence pressure, occurs in the left atrium, pulmonary veins, and capillaries. The latter may cause pulmonary oedema which compromises gaseous exchange, and if severe can be life-threatening. A back-up of blood will also cause congestion of the right ventricle.

2 The vessels and tissues after the left ventricle, i.e. the decreased cardiac output reduces tissue perfusion, the severity of which is

directly related to the depressed cardiac output. Renal function may be impaired, causing fluid retention, and so exacerbating the cardiac congestion.

In right heart failure, the right ventricular output is less than the volume returned from the systemic circulation; congestion therefore occurs behind the right ventricle in the systemic venous circulation. Consequently, oedema occurs at various peripheral sites, such as the wrist and ankles. The liver and spleen become distended, thus compromising their functions. When both sides of the heart fail, the term congestive heart failure is used.

Short-term homeostatic control mechanisms compensate in acute heart failure; long-term homeostatic controls compensate in chronic heart failure. Acute failure, as occurs in myocardial infarction, means that the damaged ventricular myocardium cannot pump out its returning blood, the consequence being a decreased cardiac output, heart congestion, and an increased right atrial pressure.

The decreased cardiac output induces a decreased arterial pressure which stimulates the baroreceptor reflex and promotes appropriate vasomotor sympathetic activity. This precipitates an increased myocardial contractility and vessel vasoconstriction, which improves the arterial pressure. Increased venous return further increases right atrial pressure and this increases the ventricular end diastolic volume and thus the force of contraction (Starling's effect). In addition, sympathetic activity redistributes blood flow away from non-essential organs (e.g. guts, kidney, skin) to vital organs (brain and heart).

In chronic heart failure an additional compensatory mechanism occurs. That is, the increased interstitial fluid volume that is observed (oedema) occurs at the expense of plasma volume and so decreases cardiac output further. The renin–angiotensin system is activated by the reduced blood pressure and sympathetic activity along with the secretion of aldosterone and antidiuretic hormone. Such responses provoke the 'compensated heart failure mechanisms', that is, by increasing blood volume, increasing venous return, and increasing the force of contraction (Starling's effect), all of which aids the restoration of the cardiac output. In severe failure these mechanisms can increase blood volume so much that the myocardium is pushed beyond its physiological parameters of contraction, resulting in ventricular congestion, and consequently an enlarged heart. A vicious circle (i.e. a positive feedback) ensues which eventually, if uncorrected, results in death. This is referred to as 'decompensated heart failure'. Correction involves the administration of drugs such as cardiac glycosides (e.g. digitalis) which increase the force of ventricular contraction, thus improving its emptying, thereby increasing cardiac output and improving renal function. In addition, they decrease the heart rate and this extends the diastolic period, thus increasing myocardial oxygen supply (it should be recalled that, unlike other tissues, coronary blood flow is higher during diastole than during systole when myocardial vessels may be crushed by the contraction).

Cardiomyopathies

Cardiomyopathy is a degenerative condition of myocardial cells, whereby the myocardium becomes thin and weak, the ventricles enlarge, and the muscle tone becomes incapable of maintaining an adequate cardiac output; consequently heart failure results. Cardiomyopathies frequently arise secondary to other imbalances, such as chronic alcoholism, coronary arterial disease, pathogenic infections, and multiple sclerosis. They also occur as primary imbalances as there are several inherited forms of the condition. Correction is therefore aimed at removing the underlying primary causal factor (for example, alcohol abstinence). However, this is not always possible, as in the inherited cases, when correction necessitates a heart transplant.

HOMEOSTATIC FAILURES OF THE CIRCULATION (Figure 9.30)

This section focuses on imbalances in which there is:

1 An inability to maintain arterial pressure, e.g. hypertension and hypotension.

2 An insufficient oxygen supply to the myocardium, e.g. coronary arterial disease resulting in coronary ischaemia and myocardial infarction.

3 An inadequate blood flow to the cells, e.g. shock, atherosclerosis, and arteriosclerosis.

Hypertension

Hypertension refers to a circulatory imbalance whereby blood pressure is sustained that is beyond the normal homeostatic parameter for a particular age group, i.e. 20-year-old hypertensives have pressures in excess of 140/90 mmHg; 50-year-olds – 160/90 mmHg; 75-year-olds – 170/105 mmHg. Hypertension may occur when the muscle and elastic components of arterial walls are replaced by fibrous tissue. Consequently, the walls of small and medium arteries become thick, hard, inflexible, and their lumens are narrowed. Large arteries, however, may lose their elasticity and dilate, resulting in an exacerbated pulsating flow. At the bends and branches of the arterial tree there is an increased tendency for blood clotting as platelets and fibrin are deposited. Consequently, the original imbalance of hypertension leads to an increased risk of other homeostatic imbalances, such as thrombosis, ischaemia, and infarction, which compromise the functioning of those organs affected, again reflecting the interdependency of homeostatic functioning. Blood vessels most commonly affected are cerebral, coronary, and renal vessels – thus cerebrovascular accidents, myocardial infarctions and renal diseases are common clinical manifestations of hypertension.

In 10–15% of all cases, hypertension results from other imbalances and so is called secondary hypertension. Causes include:

1 Excessive renin release, as occurs with kidney damage, leading to excessive angiotensin generation, and hence an increase in peripheral resistance.

2 Hypersecretion of aldosterone (Conn's syndrome) and cortisol and hence an excessive blood volume, as occurs with:
   (a) hypothalamic and/or pituitary tumours which causes excessive release of adrenocorticotrophic hormone (ACTH), the stimulant for adrenocortical hormone, e.g. aldosterone and cortisol secretion, and/or,
   (b) adrenal cortical tumour which displays an excessive reaction to ACTH, and/or,
   (c) a failure in the negative feedback mechanisms which control ACTH and adrenal steroid release.

3 Hypersecretion of antidiuretic hormone due to hypothalamic tumours, or a failure in the feedback mechanisms. Excessive release of this hormone exerts its hypertensive effects by increasing peripheral resistance, and by promoting water retention.

Correction involves anti-hypertensive therapy aimed at the primary imbalance, or at compensation for the imbalance, for example:

1 Diuretic drugs which increase urinary sodium and water loss and so reduce blood volume.

2 Beta-blocker drugs (e.g. propranolol) which decrease heart rate, cardiac output, and hence blood pressure.

3 Relaxation techniques which decrease sympathetic activity, reducing cardiac output and promoting a decreased peripheral resistance.

In 85–90% of hypertensive individuals no obvious secondary cause can be determined, since it is almost certainly multifactorial and is likely to be produced by a combination of genetic and environmental factors. This form

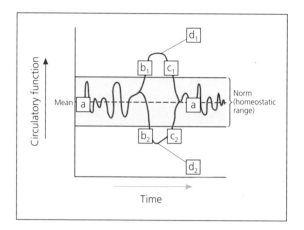

Figure 9.30 Circulation – an expression of cardiovascular function.
a, Circulatory function fluctuating within its homeostatic range.
b_1, Increased circulatory flow as occurs: (i) normally with increased oxygen supply to the myocardium and muscle cells when the homeostatic flow parameters are reset as in exercise; (ii) abnormally, as occurs in hypertension.
b_2, Decreased circulatory flow as occurs in the homeostatic imbalances of: (i) hypotension; (ii) ischaemic disease, myocardial infarctions, cerebrovascular accidents and thrombotic changes in vessels.
c_1, Clinical correction is dependent upon the underlying imbalance, i.e. anti–hypertensive therapy used in hypertension may be via diuretics, β–blockers, or relaxation therapies.
c_2, Clinical correction of the imbalance, (i) i.e. hypotension is treated by anti–hypotensive drugs *or* treating the underlying cause of the imbalance (e.g. hypothyroidism causes hypotension); (ii) glycerol trinitrate, angioplasty, streptokinase therapy in myocardial ischaemia; (iii) peripheral vasodilators in tissue ischaemia.
d, Continued imbalance because of the irreversibility of the underlying cause, e.g. d_1, prolonged hypertension leading to cerebrovascular accident, myocardial infarction, renal failure, etc., or d_2, prolonged hypotension leading to death due to cerebral ischaemia/infarction.

of hypertension is referred to as primary or essential hypertension.

Hypotension

Hypotension refers to a circulatory imbalance whereby there is a sustained systolic blood pressure below 100 mmHg. Acute hypotension is one of the most important indicators of circulatory shock (see below), whereas chronic hypotension may be associated with:

1 Poor nutrition resulting in anaemia and hypoproteinaemia.

2 Addison's disease, i.e. an inadequate secretion of cortisol and aldosterone from the adrenal glands leading to diminished blood volume, and cardiac function.

3 Hypothyroidism, i.e. an inadequate secretion of thyroid hormones leading to a reduced cardiac function.

4 Severe tissue wasting, as occurs in cancer patients, resulting in lowered peripheral resistance and blood pooling.

Hypotension produces an inadequate blood supply to the brain, which may result in unconsciousness. Depending upon the cause, this may be brief (fainting), or prolonged, the extreme of which leads to death. Postural hypotension, which induces a transient loss of consciousness (called syncope), is common in the elderly, who suffer a temporary hypotension and dizziness when they rise suddenly from a lying or sitting position. This arises because of a decreased sensitivity of the baroreceptor reflex as a consequence of ageing.

Correction of hypotension is aimed at removing the underlying cause and with anti-hypotensive drug therapy, including cardiac stimulants or vasoconstrictors.

Shock

Circulatory shock refers to any condition in which blood vessels are inadequately filled, thereby producing a tissue blood flow that is inadequate for cellular homeostatic requirements. The lack of cellular metabolites results in intracellular imbalances, e.g. insufficient oxygen produces hypoxia and promotes anaerobic respiration; the persistent build-up of 'waste' products causes cell death, and organ damage ensues. Shock is classified as hypovolaemic (i.e. due to low blood volume), cardiogenic (i.e. of cardiac origin), vascular (i.e.

of blood vessel origin), neurogenic (i.e. of neural origin), and anaphylactic (i.e. as a consequence of an allergic reaction).

Hypovolaemic shock (hypo- = low, -volaemic = blood volume) is the most common form of this imbalance, causes of which include:

1 Severe acute haemorrhage.

2 Extensive superficial burns (when there is excessive loss of tissue fluid leading to further exudation from the blood plasma).

3 Severe vomiting and diarrhoea (when excessive loss of gut fluid promotes further secretion from the blood plasma).

In hypovolaemia there is:

1 An increased heart rate which acts to improve cardiac output and readdress this homeostatic balance. The resultant rapid 'thready' pulse is an initial sign of this condition (the 'thready' nature of the pulse reflects a diminished pulse pressure).

2 An intense vasoconstriction which acts to re-establish blood volume by forcing blood from blood reservoirs (spleen and liver, etc.) into the circulation to enhance venous return, and by increasing peripheral resistance, both of which stabilize blood pressure. If blood loss continues, blood pressure drops sharply as compensatory mechanisms are exceeded; this is serious and is a late sign of shock.

Figure 9.31 illustrates the homeostatic controls involved in redressing the blood volume after haemorrhage.

Cardiogenic shock (pump failure) results from a sudden reduction in cardiac output, as occurs in acute heart disease, such as myocardial infarction. In vascular shock, blood volume is normal and constant, and inadequate circulation results from a huge drop in peripheral resistance as a consequence of extreme vasodilation, leading to pooling in the large veins. Consequently, a decrease in venous return, cardiac output, and arterial pressure results. The most common causes of this imbalance are loss of vasomotor (neural) tone, and septicaemia as a consequence of a severe Gram-negative bacterial infection, since bacterial toxins are potent vasodilators. Extensive peripheral vasodilation also occurs in anaphylactic shock, a dangerous allergic reaction which is discussed in Chapter 10.

Neurogenic shock may occur as a result of a sudden acute pain and/or severe emotional experience. Both stimulate a parasympathetic (vagal) slowing of the heart rate, thereby reducing the cardiac output and arterial pressure. The venous return may be reduced by venous pooling of blood. These changes decrease cerebral flow which may cause a temporary loss of consciousness (fainting) – a phenomenon known as a vasovagal 'attack'.

Arteriosclerosis

Several types of arteriosclerosis exist, some more dangerous than others. Arteriosclerosis associated with ageing is a progressive degenerate arterial imbalance, whereby the artery walls gradually lose elastic fibres, and hence lose their cushioning effects on pressure oscillations. These vessels become stiff, hard, relatively inelastic, and eventually their lumen is narrowed as they become infiltrated with collagen and calcium. Systolic pressure peaks are therefore much higher in the arteriosclerotic vessels. This exposes their walls to greater stresses and increases the risk of cerebrovascular accidents and myocardial infarctions. The risks are further elevated if one is also hypertensive from additional factors.

Atherosclerosis

Atherosclerosis is a type of arteriosclerosis characterized by patchy change, called atheromatous plaques, within the blood vessel walls (Figure 9.32). Plaques consist of cholesterol compounds, excess smooth muscle, and fibroblastic cells. They grow and spread along the arterial wall, forming a swelling which

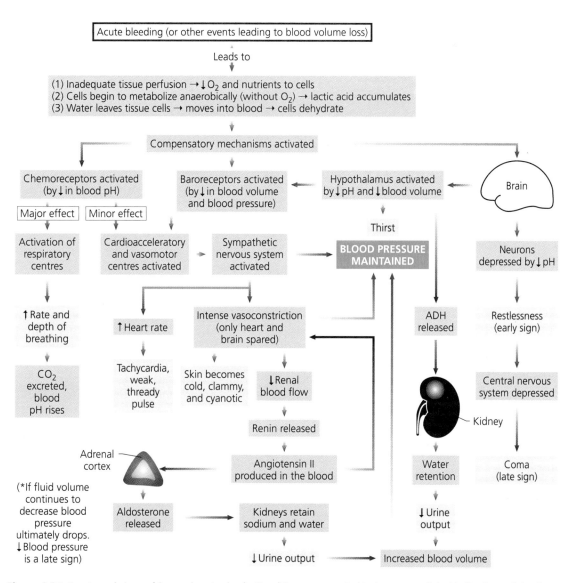

Figure 9.31 Events and signs of hypovolaemic shock. Conditions represented in boxes are clinical indications of shock.

protrudes into the lumen and thus compromising blood flow to the organs affected. The origin of plaques is debatable, although vascular 'fatty streaks', if not absorbed (an homeostatic control process), are thought to be precursors. Streaks are evident in autopsies of children as young as 6 years of age and may be of genetic and/or environmental origin. Arteries most commonly affected are those of

the heart, brain, lower limbs, and small intestine. Atherosclerosis is therefore an obvious cause of coronary artery disease, cerebral vascular accidents, and tissue ischaemia.

Atherosclerosis predisposes one to other imbalances such as:

1 Thrombosis – i.e. when the endothelial lining over the plaque breaks down,

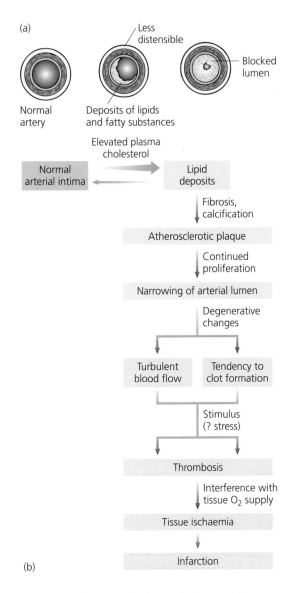

Figure 9.32 (a) Atherosclerotic vessel changes. (b) Mechanism producing atherosclerosis and tissue infarction.

2 Aneurysm formation – i.e. if the arterial wall is weakened by the plaque, a local dilatation of the wall, called an aneurysm, may develop. Rupture of this causes haemorrhaging.

Ischaemic heart disease

Ischaemic heart disease is a homeostatic imbalance which reflects myocardial oxygen insufficiency, arising from a narrowed or occluded coronary artery. The narrowing and the occlusion may be caused by atherosclerotic plaques alone, or by plaques becoming complicated by a thrombotic narrowing leading to angina (cardiac pain), or myocardial infarction if the vessel becomes occluded.

If the atheroma progresses slowly, a collateral arterial supply grows, effectively acting as a homeostatic control to replace the malfunctioned atheromatosed vessel. If, however, a sudden severe narrowing or occlusion occurs, the collateral circulation has insufficient time to develop, consequently a myocardial infarction may occur.

Failure of myocardial homeostasis thus requires clinical intervention to re-establish it. The angina patient, for example, is given vasodilator drugs (e.g. glyceryl trinitrate), or beta-blockers (e.g. propranolol) to increase coronary flow or reduce oxygen requirements by the myocardium. The infarcted patient may require a coronary vessel bypass operation to readdress cardiac integrity, i.e. if a large area of the myocardium is affected and/or major vessels are occluded.

Angina pectoris literally means 'choked chest'. It is a chest pain associated with a temporary decrease in the delivery of blood to the heart muscle. Angina may result from a variety of causes:

1 Increased physical demands on the heart which cannot be met by the coronary circulation;

2 Stress-induced spasms of the coronary arteries;

platelets are activated and stimulate the clotting cascade. The developing thrombus (or emboli) may cause ischaemia and infarction. In fact, 90% of myocardial infarctions in the Western world are due to coronary atherosclerosis (Figure 9.32b).

3 Hypertension (which increases excessively the oxygen demands of the heart);

4 Fever which elevates cardiac activity and hence its oxygen needs;

5 Hyperthyroidism (i.e. excessive release of thyroid hormones), which also increases cardiac activity;

6 Aortic stenosis (a narrowing of the aortic valve);

7 Atherosclerosis.

If the coronary arteries become completely occluded then blood flow to the tissue beyond the occluded site ceases, and the myocardial tissue dies. This is a heart attack (myocardial infarction or coronary). Occlusion may be caused by a thrombus or embolus (i.e. a homeostatic failure of the clotting process) in one of the coronary arteries. The after effects depend partly on the size and location of the infarcted (necrotic) area. In chronic ischaemic heart disease, small infarcts may give rise to myocardial weakness, angina, and heart failure. If the ischaemic heart disease is acute, then one or more large arteries are occluded and the atheroma is usually complicated by thrombosis. Consequently a large infarct results, and death may ensue as a result of acute heart failure, ventricular fibrillation (i.e. a lack of coordination of the cardiac cycle), rupture of the ventricular wall, or pulmonary or cerebral embolism (leading to respiratory or cerebral failure).

Summary

1 The cardiovascular system is the body's transport network and is adapted to maintain intracellular and extracellular homeostasis.

2 The cardiovascular system comprises a double circulation, i.e. there are pulmonary and systemic circuits. The former's role is to oxygenate blood to within its homeostatic parameters. The latter's role is to deliver oxygen, nutrients, etc. to tissue cells throughout the body to maintain their intracellular homeostasis.

3 The heart has two ventricular pumps: the right pump supplies the pulmonary circuit; the left pump supplies the systemic circuit.

4 The heart wall contains three layers (epicardium, myocardium and endocardium), and there are four chambers (paired, upper atria and lower ventricles).

5 Valves ensure unidirectional flow through the heart and venous system.

6 The heart sounds 'lubb-dupp' correspond to the closing of the atrioventricular and semilunar valves respectively during the functional 'cycle' of cardiac contraction. Heart murmurs are evidence of stenosed or incompetent valves.

7 Coronary vessels deliver blood to the myocardium. Their partial or complete occlusion compromises myocardial function and leads to the homeostatic imbalances of angina and/or myocardial infarction.

8 The cardiac cycle describes the sequence of events that occur with each heart beat. The cycle principally consists of diastolic (relaxing and filling) and systolic (contracting and emptying) stages.

9 The cardiac output, a clinically important homeostatic parameter, is calculated by multiplying the heart rate by the stroke volume. Changes in either will change the cardiac output.

10 The heart rate is intrinsically controlled and extrinsically modified by the autonomic nervous system and the endocrine system. It varies according to age, gender, temperature, and level of activity.

11 The stroke volume varies according to changes in the venous return, which alter the stretch within the chambers (Starling's law), to the

period of ventricular filling, and to autonomic neural activity.

12 Most blood vessels share a common macroscale structure, consisting of three tunicae (intima, media, and externa). Their microstructure, however, is adapted for their specific homeostatic function.

13 The path of blood flow is from the heart → arteries (elastic and muscular or distributing vessels) → arterioles (smallest arteries) → capillaries (exchange vessels) → venules (smallest veins) → veins (drainage vessels and blood reservoirs). The latter vessels take blood back to the heart.

14 Blood flow is calculated by dividing the blood pressure differential between arterial and venous vessels by the peripheral resistance provided by the vasculature, particularly arterioles. Blood pressure provides the force necessary to produce blood flow along the vessels.

15 Arterial blood pressure is calculated by multiplying the cardiac output by the total peripheral resistance.

16 Arterial blood pressure is measured by a sphygmomanometer. It is expressed as systolic and diastolic values. Blood pressures increase with age and with homeostatic imbalances, such as arteriosclerosis, hypertension, etc., and decrease in imbalances, such as hypotension, shock, heart failure, etc.

17 Blood pressure is normally maintained within its homeostatic range via a number of short-term and long-term blood pressure homeostatic controls. These can be broadly divided into neural and endocrine mechanisms respectively.

18 Cardiovascular homeostatic parameters are reset in 'normal' homeostatic adaptive states, such as exercise and pregnancy.

19 The medulla oblongata of the brainstem contains the cardiac centres and the vasomotor centres. These centres control cardiovascular function.

20 Homeostatic imbalances of the cardiovascular system can be broadly subdivided into cardiac and circulatory imbalances. Each compromises the function of the other and that of other organ systems due to the interdependency of body systems.

Review Questions

1 Describe how cardiovascular function aids the maintenance of intracellular homeostasis.

2 Which blood vessels are known as:
(a) the distributing vessels;
(b) the precapillary resistance vessels;
(c) the exchange vessels;
(d) the capacitance vessels.

3 List the major differences and similarities between arteries, capillaries, and veins.

4 Describe the route taken by blood as it moves from the right atrium to the kidneys and back to the right atrium.

5 Draw a labelled diagram of the heart to include its conduction system.

6 Compare the intrinsic rhythm of the SA node with that of other components of the heart's conduction system.

7 List the normal ECG waves. What do these components represent?

8 Compare the effects of parasympathetic and sympathetic stimulation on the heart's conduction system. List the factors which influence such activity.

9 Describe what is meant by the 'vagal brake'.

10 List the 'stages' of the cardiac cycle and briefly describe the electrical events that precede each mechanical event.

11 How is cardiac output directly and indirectly determined?

12 What are the contributory factors of the cardiac output?

13 How does the heart rate affect the cardiac output?

14 What is Starling's law of the heart?

15 Explain how an athlete's low resting heart rate does not compromise cardiac function.

16 Explain why the maintenance of arterial blood pressure is so important to intracellular homeostasis.

17 What are the primary determinants of blood pressure?

18 Explain what causes a pulse in an artery and identify the common locations where the pulse point is most easily felt.

19 List and briefly explain the short-term and long-term regulators of blood pressure.

20 How do varicose veins develop? What complications can arise from varicose veins?

21 Explain how circulatory function is altered by:
(a) atherosclerosis;
(b) hypertension;
(c) hypotension;
(d) aneurysms;
(e) haemorrhage.

22 Define 'shock' and list the major types of shock.

23 Distinguish between ischaemia and infarction.

10

The lymphatic and immunity systems

Introduction: relation of the lymphatic system to cellular homeostasis

Introduction: relation of the immune system to cellular homeostasis

Overview of the anatomy and physiology of the lymphatic system

Details of the physiology of the lymphatic and immune systems I: lymph formation

Details of the physiology of the lymphatic and immune systems II: immune responses and defence mechanisms

Examples of homeostatic control system failures and principles of correction

Summary

Review questions

Introduction: relation of the lymphatic system to cellular homeostasis

Blood distributes oxygen and other metabolites to the body cells, and removes their waste products. Cells are bathed in tissue, or interstitial, fluid, which acts as an intermediary fluid between blood and cells. The lymphatic system is an extensive, branched tubular network adapted for the prevention of tissue fluid accumulation. Excess fluid is returned back to the circulation, and so the lymphatic system is important in the homeostatic maintenance of all body fluids. The system also acts as an intermediary between the digestive and circulatory systems following absorption of a meal, whereby it is concerned with the transportation of long chain fatty acids (Chapter 7). In addition, the lymphatic system has immunological defence functions which are concerned with filtering and destroying potential environmental pathogenic hazards. Figure 10.1 summarizes the homeostatic functions of the lymphatic system.

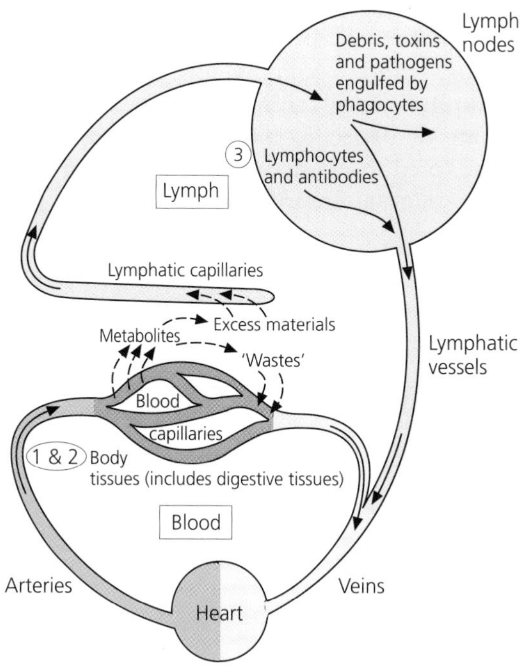

Figure 10.1 A diagram summarizing the homeostatic functions associated with the lymphatic system: 1, regulation of body fluids; 2, fat absorption; 3, defence functions.

Introduction: relation of the immune system to cellular homeostasis

The human body's external and internal defences continually act to maintain cellular homeostasis by combating harmful environmental agents. Frequently, these agents are pathogens, i.e. disease-causing organisms, or pathogenic secretions called toxins. Alternatively, environmental pollutants, such as asbestos or coal dust particles, may also trigger an immune response. Individuals have different resistances and susceptibilities to infections, depending upon the efficiency of the responses.

Resistance is comprised of complementary non-specific and specific defence mechanisms as follows.

NON-SPECIFIC IMMUNITY

Non-specific resistance is the immunity present at birth. These defence mechanisms are the same for everyone and they are divided into external physico-chemical barriers, such as the skin and tears, and internal (bodily) reactions including the phagocytic response, that provides immunological surveillance against pathogenic microbes and their toxins.

SPECIFIC IMMUNITY

Specific resistance is the immunity acquired during life. It develops mostly after birth when an individual becomes exposed to potential environmental hazards. Specific immunity is the lymphocytic response: it involves activating specific lymphocytes (= 'lymph cells') and stimulating them to release their secretions (cytotoxic substances and antibodies) in response to 'foreign' substances entering the body. Fetuses and neonates receive antibodies from their mothers via the placenta and breast milk, respectively. This passive immunity gives resistance for approximately 3 months until the transferred antibodies are eventually destroyed by the liver. A programme of vaccination is therefore required soon after birth which ensures acquisition of active immunity against pathogens which have the potential to produce serious diseases, such as diphtheria, tetanus, and poliomyelitis. This active immunity is long-lasting.

Both non-specific and specific immunities are adapted to maintain the equilibrium of the body's internal environment.

Overview of the anatomy and physiology of the lymphatic system

LYMPHATIC VESSELS AND THE LYMPHATIC CIRCULATION

The lymphatics, or lymphatic capillaries, are thin, blind-ending vessels present in all body tissues, except in the spleen and in those areas not directly serviced by the circulation (such as the cornea of the eye), the central nervous system, and bone marrow. The lymphatics of the skin travel in loose subcutaneous adipose tissue, generally following veins, whereas visceral lymphatics generally follow arteries, forming plexuses around them. Lymph (i.e. tissue fluid inside the lymphatics) is produced at approximately 1.5 ml/min throughout the body. The lymphatics merge, forming larger vessels, the largest of which drain into two large ducts called the right lymphatic duct and the thoracic duct.

These ducts empty their contents into blood within the neck, at the junction of the left subclavian and jugular veins (Figure 10.2). By preventing tissue fluid accumulation this drainage helps to ensure that a constant blood volume and composition is maintained. If, however, the return of lymph is blocked, as in the case of the parasitic worm condition elephantiasis, then tissue fluid accumulates distal to the obstruction resulting in oedema.

RETURN OF LYMPH TO THE CIRCULATION

The flow rate of lymph is very slow compared with that of blood. Two factors control lymph flow rate, and hence its return to blood:

1 Tissue pressure. When tissue fluid pressure (i.e. volume), rises above its homeostatic range, there is a greater formation of lymph which enhances its flow rate.

2 Lymphatic pump. Lymph vessels have valves which promote unidirectional movement towards the neck region, so lymph can be returned to the blood circulation. The movement is encouraged via compression exerted by muscles, and other tissues, surrounding the lymphatic vessels. These muscles and tissues are referred to as the lymphatic pumps. Increased metabolic rates (such as those experienced by exercise) increases the efficiency of lymphatic pumps. This is a homeostatic necessity, since increased metabolic rates are associated with a greater blood flow to the high metabolizing cells, resulting in greater tissue fluid formation. Consequently, a greater lymph formation results, producing a greater flow rate of lymph to maintain blood volume.

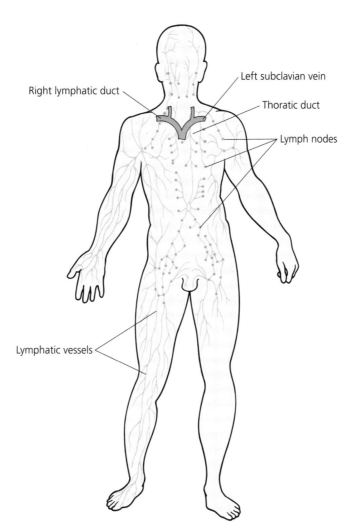

Right lymphatic duct

Left subclavian vein

Thoratic duct

Lymph nodes

Lymphatic vessels

Figure 10.2 Diagram representing the main vessels of the lymphatic system (those of the left limbs are omitted for clarity). Right lymphatic duct drains the right side of the head and neck, and the right arm.

THE LYMPHOIDAL SYSTEM

In addition to fluid and solute of the interstitium, lymph also contains specialized cells which form an important part of the mechanism by which the body defends itself against infection by micro-organisms. The various organs which comprise the lymphoidal system may be classified as primary or secondary (Figure 10.3), and it is in the former organs that lymphocytes (= 'lymph cells') are produced. These organs are the bone marrow, thymus, and fetal liver. As discussed later, the lymphocytes generated in the primary lymph organs migrate to the secondary organs, those being the spleen, lymph nodes and other lymphatic tissue throughout the body.

Lymph nodes

Lymphatic nodes are oval-shaped masses of lymphatic tissue encapsulated by dense connective tissue. The organ consists of:

1 Cortex, containing B lymphocytes aggregated into primary follicles. Following stimulation by antigen (i.e. non-self substances or cells) these develop into a focus of active proliferation (a germinal centre) and are then termed secondary follicles. These follicles are in intimate contact with the antigen-presenting cells.

2 Paracortex, contains T-lymphocytes.

3 Medulla, contains both T- and B-lymphocytes.

The roles of the T- and B-lymphocytes will be described in a later section. Each node has internal extensions of fibrous capsule, called trabeculae, which dip through the outer cortex and inner medullary regions of the node (Figure 10.4). Nodes exist individually and are randomly located, for example the urogenital and respiratory mucous membranes, or as multiple nodular complexes located at specific sites, for example tonsils, Peyer's patches, appendix, spleen, and thymus gland.

Afferent vessels transport lymph into node sinuses (a series of irregular channels), after which it circulates into one or two efferent vessels located at the node's hilum, a 'hillock' shape at the exit. Efferents are wider than afferent vessels, and they contain valves that open away from the nodes, and encourage unidirectional flow.

Nodular filtering action: a homeostatic function

Antigenic substances become entrapped in the lymph nodes as they filter the lymph passing

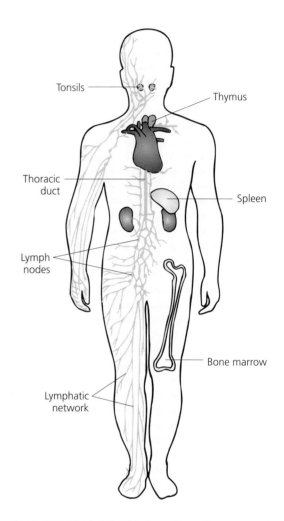

Figure 10.3 The lymphoid system. The various organs of the lymphoid system are classified as *primary* or *secondary*. The primary organs (e.g. bone marrow, thymus, fetal liver) are the sites where lymphocytes are produced. Lymphocytes generated in the primary lymphoid organs migrate to the secondary organs, mainly, the spleen and lymph nodes and various lymphoid tissues throughout the body.

through the lymphatic network during its passage from the periphery to the thoracic ducts. They are destroyed via:

1 phagocytosis by macrophage cells;

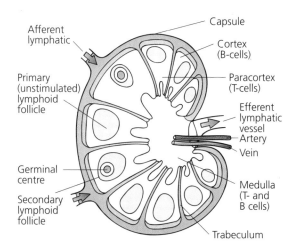

Figure 10.4 Structure of a lymph node. The organ consists of (1) cortex, (2) paracortex, (3) medulla, and (4) connective tissue capsule. Lymphocytes and antigens (if present) enter into the node through the afferent lymphatics. The lymph drains through the node (sinuses) and passes out of the medulla of the node through the efferent lymphatic vessel. The B-cells in the cortex are aggregated into primary follicles; subsequent to stimulation by antigen they develop a focus of active proliferation (germinal centre) and are termed secondary follicles. These follicles are in close contact with antigen-presenting dendritic cells. The paracortex contains T-cells and the medulla contains both T- and B-cells. Each node has its own blood supply.

2 cytotoxic secretions (e.g. interleukin, interferon, etc.) produced by T-lymphocytes;

3 antibodies secreted by B-lymphocytes.

The thymus gland

The thymus is positioned in the upper thorax above and anterior to the heart, between the lungs, and behind the sternum. It extends backwards into the root of the neck (Figure 10.3). The gland's size increases until puberty; it then begins to involute during adolescence and, by middle age, has returned to its size at birth. Despite this reduction in size during adulthood, evidence suggests that the thymus continues to function throughout life. The effectiveness of its lymphocytes in response to antigenic insults declines, however.

Structure of the thymus

The thymus is a bilobed gland encapsulated by fibrous tissue. Each lobe has a peripheral cortex and a central medulla. The former consists of small, medium, and large tightly packed lymphocytes; the latter consists mainly of epithelial cells and diffused scattered lymphocytes. Internal capsular extensions (trabeculae) divide the organ into lobules, which consist of an irregular branching framework of epithelial cells responsible for the production of thymic secretions and lymphocytes.

Homeostatic functions of the thymus

The thymus is primarily responsible for the production and support of T-cells. Such cells originate in the bone marrow where stem cells differentiate into specialized lymphocytes in a process called lymphopoiesis. The majority of these cells enter the thymus, where they develop in the cortex into stem T-lymphocytes. These undergo mitosis, and upon maturation move into the medulla. These mature cells either enter and remain in systemic blood, enter systemic blood and are transported to lymphoidal tissue, or remain in the thymus gland to become the future generations of T-lymphocytes.

Thymic epithelial cells also produce thymosin. This hormone is responsible for the maturation of the thymus and other lymphoidal tissue.

The spleen

The adult spleen is the largest collection of lymphoidal tissue in the body. It is approximately 12 cm in length, 7 cm wide and 2.5 cm thick, and has an average weight of 150 grams. The organ is positioned in the left of the abdomen lying between the fundus of the stomach and diaphragm.

Structure

Anteriorly, the spleen's encapsulated surface is covered with peritoneum. The organ's oval shape is determined by structures which are in close proximity (Figure 10.5a). It contains a number of surface features including:

1 a gastric impression: the organ's soft consistency enables its shape to change according to the stomach's contents;

2 a renal impression;

3 a colonic impression;

4 a smooth and convexed diaphragmatic surface, which conforms to the concaved surface of the adjacent diaphragm.

The organ is divided into an outer red pulp, which contains sinuses filled with blood, and a centrally located white pulp consisting of lymphatic tissue. This latter contains lymphocytes and macrophages (Figure 10.5b). Entering and leaving the spleen hilum are the splenic artery and vein, efferent lymphatics, and a nerve supply.

Blood in the splenic artery flows into the spleen's sinuses. These have distinct pores between lining endothelial cells, allowing blood to come into close association with the splenic pulp cells.

Homeostatic functions of the spleen

The spleen performs the same functions for blood that lymph nodes perform for lymph:

1 Phagocytosis. The spleen is a part of the reticuloendothelial system, and so it is concerned with the breakdown of erythrocytes. Bilirubin, iron, and the protein globin

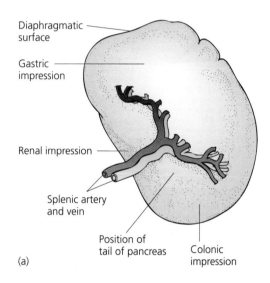

(a)

(a)

(b)

(b)

Figure 10.5 (a) Spleen. Its oval shape is determined by the structures in close proximity to it. (b) Diagram of a section of a spleen.

are released from haemoglobin, and are passed to the liver by splenic and portal veins. Leucocytes, thrombocytes, and antigenic microbes are also phagocytosed in the spleen. This organ has no afferent lymphatic vessels, however, and so is not exposed to infections spread via the lymphatic system.

2 Development of lymphocytes. The spleen produces T- and, in particular, B-lymphocytes.

In addition, the spleen acts as a blood reservoir, releasing blood on demand, for example following severe haemorrhage. This release is controlled by the sympathetic nervous system and is a homeostatic mechanism which helps to maintain the composition of body fluids. During early fetal development the spleen also synthesizes blood cells for the developing circulatory system (Chapter 8).

Details of the physiology of the lymphatic and immune systems I: lymph formation

It was discussed in Chapters 5 and 9 how positive filtration pressures at the arterial side of blood capillaries result in the exudation of fluid from plasma and the formation of tissue fluid. Negative filtration pressures at the venous end of the capillary ensure that tissue fluid is returned to the blood. The return, however, cannot compensate totally for the loss, and thus there is a potential for the accumulation of tissue fluid. In addition, because capillary walls are slightly permeable to protein, there is a slow but steady loss of blood protein to tissue fluid. These proteins cannot be returned to the circulation across capillary walls, since there are insufficient fluid pressures to move them in that direction.

The lymphatics drain the tissue fluid that is in excess of its homeostatic range and so return the proteins to blood. The endothelial cells of lymphatic vessels are not tightly bound, but they overlap and the regions of overlap function as one-way valves. These permit the entry of fluid (and proteins) into the vessels, but prevent their return to the interstitial spaces. Accumulation of tissue fluid causes the tissues to swell, and the increased tissue fluid pressure opens the endothelial valves further, so more fluid can flow into the lymph capillaries. The larger capillaries also contain semilunar valves. These are quite close together, and each causes the vessel to bulge, giving the lymphatic system a beaded appearance (see Figure 10.2). As discussed earlier, these valves aid normal lymphatic flow. On its return journey to blood, lymph flows through one or more lymph nodes. Their homeostatic function is to filter the lymph of potential antigenic material, and then destroy pathogens and their toxins (described in a later section).

The large thoracic duct receives lymph from vessels below the diaphragm, and from the left half of the head, neck, and chest, and empties into the venous system, close to the junction of the left internal jugular and left subclavian veins. The smaller right lymphatic duct ends at a comparable location on the right side. It drains lymph from the right side of the body above the diaphragm (see Figure 10.2).

The lymphatic system is therefore a homeostatic mechanism for the maintenance of body fluid composition and volume. Clinical conditions that inhibit such a return may influence fluid distribution to such an extent that death can occur in less than 24 hours, if the balance is not restored.

Details of the physiology of the lymphatic and immune systems II: immune responses and defence mechanisms

This section is concerned with discussing:

1 how one's external defences are adapted to prevent the entry of environmental hazards into the body;

2 how one's internal defences operate following external defence failure.

3 how immunization, monoclonal antibodies, and transplantation are used for the benefit of the individual;

4 what happens when the immune mechanisms malfunction.

Both external and internal defence mechanisms exhibit non-specific and specific responses. It was mentioned in the introduction how non-specific immunity is the body's natural resistance to disease. Its two roles are to prevent the entry of pathogenic hazards into the body, and to prevent the spread of those hazards which have successfully gained entrance to the body.

EXTERNAL DEFENCE MECHANISMS

The non-specific components of the external defence mechanisms include (Figure 10.6):

1 skin and mucous membranes;

2 digestive secretions;

3 tears;

4 lysozymes;

5 urination and defecation.

Skin and mucous membranes

The skin and mucous membranes are the body's first line of resistance. Both act as physi-

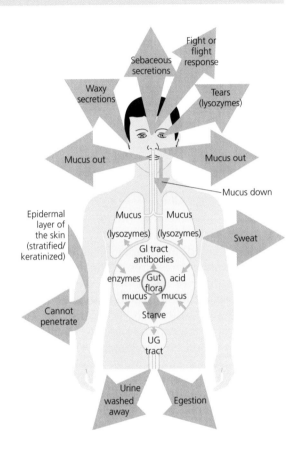

Figure 10.6 The physical and chemical barriers of natural immunity.

cal barriers which prevent pathogenic agents from entering their target tissues. For example, the viruses that cause hepatitis must gain access to liver cells. These organisms, however, must first penetrate external barriers to enter blood, which then transports them to their target sites.

Skin

The intact skin is the most effective external barrier of the body. It provides a watertight barricade protecting the internal organs from infection. The effectiveness only becomes apparent when there is widespread damage to the skin. For example, with serious burns, infection becomes a real danger, and infection prevention and control are major considerations in burn treatments. The skin contains two principal layers, the outer epidermis and inner dermis (Chapter 17). Together they provide both physical and chemical protection.

PHYSICAL FACTORS

The epidermis is a stratified squamous epithelium and some of its cells are keratinized (Chapter 17). These characteristics make this tissue a formidable physical barrier for the entrance of potential pathogenic materials, and the intact healthy epidermis is rarely penetrated by bacteria. When the epidermis and the dermal blood vessels are damaged, however, the individual is potentially exposed to bacterial infection, in particular staphylococcal (a type of bacterium) infections, since their natural habitats include hair follicles and sweat glands. Other pathogens are also common in the environment; for example, it is common for tetanus-causing bacteria to be introduced into the circulation (e.g. in gardening injuries). Since skin wounds are common, tetanus immunization programmes have been developed which prevent the consequence of infection.

CHEMICAL FACTORS

The epidermal surface is moist due to the secretory and excretory products of sweat and sebaceous glands. Sweat and sebum secretions are acidic (pH 5.5) in nature and this pH discourages the growth of alkali-liking microbes whose enzyme systems cannot operate in such conditions. The acid pH, however, encourages growth of microbes whose enzyme systems favour this environment. These organisms must still penetrate the stratified epidermis if they are to cause visceral infections. Sweat and sebum also contain bactericidal chemicals (chemicals that kill bacteria), antibodies, and lysozymes, which contribute to the homeostatic functions of protection and defence. Sebum, for example, inhibits the growth of certain bacteria, such as streptococcal bacteria which cause scarlet fever, and those which are the main cause of sore throats.

Perspiration, therefore, actively removes some microbes from the skin's surface. Changing climatic conditions can, however, alter the skin's resistance to certain infections. For example, hot humid environments, in which sweat evaporation is limited, encourage fungal infections, such as athlete's foot.

Skin derivatives, such as hair and nails, protect the epidermis from mechanical abrasion and consequential damage from hazardous stimuli. Ceruminous secretions (earwax) also acts as an external barrier to microbes.

The skin's interactive role with the body's specific immune responses are discussed later.

Mucous membranes

Mucous membranes line those body cavities which open to the external environment. The principal cavities concerned are the respiratory, digestive, and urogenital tracts. The membrane's goblet cells produce mucus, and this viscous secretion prevents membrane desiccation, and its adhesive properties trap particles, such as microbes, and so prevent their spread. In some areas cilia remove the entrapped materials from the body. For example, respiratory epithelia move mucus to the throat. This stimulates coughing or sneezing reflexes to remove the mucoidal mixture to the external environment (unfortunately this is also a highly effective way of spreading infection). Alternatively, the mixture is swallowed, and gastrointestinal secretions usually destroy any microbes present (see below).

The pH characteristics of mucus, together with the presence of lysozymes and antibodies, contribute to epithelial defence functions, but mucous membranes are less effective than the skin at inhibiting microbial penetration. Infection is therefore more frequent. Common microbial infections of the respiratory, digestive and urogenital mucous membranes include colds, influenza, gastroenteritis and sexually transmitted infections.

Digestive secretions

Saliva

In addition to its digestive properties, saliva has defence functions which include:

1 washing and cleansing the teeth, gums and mouth, thus removing food particles which otherwise would encourage bacterial growth. The consequential formation of acids leads to dental caries, loss of teeth, or gum abscess.

2 discouraging the growth of acid-liking microbes by inactivating their enzyme 'systems' due to its slightly alkaline constitution (pH 7–8).

Gastric juice

Food (and the inevitable presence of microbes) is swallowed and passed to the stomach. In this region, gastric acid (pH 2–3) destroys alkaliliking microbes and all important bacterial toxins. Conversely, the stomach's pH encourages growth of acid-liking microbes which may have bypassed salivary deactivation.

Intestinal juice

The intestinal alkaline fluid (pH 7–8) destroys acid-liking microbes.

Digestive secretions therefore have important external defence properties, by denaturing microbial enzymes, and so promoting microbial death. Gastrointestinal tract infections such as gastroenteritis occur when these defence functions are overwhelmed.

Lachrymal secretions (tears)

Tears are continually being produced and secreted and blinking spreads them over the eye surfaces. Tears only become evident, however, when they are secreted in excess (an homeostatic imbalance). Hypersecretion may be due to the presence of large microbial colonies or irritants on the eye surface, or to emotional behaviours.

Lachrymal secretions, together with its entrapped dust particles and microbes, are directed towards the nasal passageways via the lachrymal ducts. Pathogenic materials are then usually destroyed by respiratory and digestive defences.

Lysozymes

Lysozymes are catalytic enzymes (nucleases, proteases, lipases carbohydrases, etc.) which are capable of 'digesting' potential pathogens. Lysozymes are abundant in tissue fluids, tears, saliva, and nasal secretions. Their effects are widespread.

Urination and defecation

Urine and faecal matter are potential media for the growth of pathogenic organisms. Frequent urination and defecation helps to prevent excessive growth of these colonies.

Memory and stress response

Once the individual has become conditioned to identify potential environmental threats, for example the expected presence of pathogenic microbes or corrosive acids, then one's memory and the stress response is involved in avoiding such potential hazards.

INTERNAL DEFENCE MECHANISMS

External defences are mainly non-specific and non-specific immune responses are also observed internally in the inflammatory and phagocytic responses by particular cells to non-self antigens. Internal defence mechanisms, however, also include the specific immune responses which act against specific antigens.

Non-specific responses: inflammation

Inflammation occurs when cells are damaged by antigenic components. This response has both protective and defensive roles, and acts to restore tissue homeostasis by neutralizing and destroying antigens at the site of injury. Inflammation is an internal defence mechanism representing a coordinated non-specific response to tissue injury. That is, the processes involved are the same in response to any antigenic insult or wound damage. The appearance of the inflamed area, however, depends upon two factors as follows.

Strength of environmental hazard (or stimulus) applied

The weakest stimulus produces a reflex vasoconstriction causing the inflamed area to pale, whereas stronger stimuli produce vasodilation of capillary networks, then arterioles, bringing a flush to the tissue. The strongest stimulus produces a raised 'wheal' around the lesion or wound. Such inflammation is usually associated with redness, pain, heat, and swelling. The injured site may lose its functions, but this depends upon the actual site and the extent of the injury.

Pathogenicity (ability to cause disease)

Microbes with a greater pathogenicity cause a greater degree of inflammation.

Stages of inflammation

Inflammation is a complex process which results from a series of responses. Histamine is released from mast cells, basophils (a type of white blood cell), platelets, and damaged cells at the site of injury. Mast cells also release serotonin and heparin and injured cells also release kinins and prostaglandins. Basophils only release their active substances once antigens interact with their surface antibodies (see later). The collective responses to these chemicals are to increase the permeability of capillaries in the area, increase blood flow to the area, bring more cellular defenders to the injury site, and remove toxic products and dead cells from this region.

The vasodilatory effects of histamine, kinins, and prostaglandins also elevate the local temperature. This may act as a homeostatic defence mechanism, since it is likely to affect the functions of microbial enzymes.

Debris and bacteria are attacked by the phagocytic white blood cells called macrophages and neutrophils which are chemically attracted to the infected area. Circulating neutrophils also attack pathogens or toxins which may have entered the blood. Eosinophils, another type of white blood cell, become involved if the antigenic materials are coated with antibodies of the IgG class (see later).

Clotting factors and 'complement' proteins also enter the area of damage and become activated. The resulting clot acts to isolate the area and prevent the spreading of antigenic material, whilst activation of the complement system, which consists of more than a dozen components, acts as a cascade to damage microbes by stimulating inflammation and by stimulating phagocytic activity.

Antigenic materials, such as foreign protein, micro-organisms, and microbial toxins, which have accumulated and/or been presented to phagocytes at the site of inflammation, also stimulate the body's specific defences.

Non-specific responses: phagocytosis

Microbes which have penetrated external defences must be kept in check by internal resistance mechanisms. Phagocytosis is the body's first line of cellular defence against microbial invasion. The process is sometimes so efficient that microbes are removed as potential sources of infection before the lymphocytes have become aware of their presence.

Two broad classes of phagocytes exist: microphages and macrophages (micro- = small; macro- =large).

Microphages

These phagocytes include the white blood cells called neutrophils and eosinophils. Microphages circulate and police the body by entering injured peripheral tissues. Neutrophils have the greater phagocytosing capacity, since they are more abundant, and more mobile than eosinophils (Chapter 8).

Macrophages

These phagocytes are also white blood cells, but are enlarged monocytes. They are classified as 'wandering' or 'fixed' macrophages. The former migrate to areas of infection, whereas the latter are permanent residents of specific tissues, for example the reticuloendothelial, or kupfer cells, of the liver. The term 'fixed' is misleading, since these cells can be transported to nearby damaged tissue.

Phagocytic giant cells can be produced if several phagocytes accumulate together. This occurs in response to large and highly active antigenic material and increases the capacity of such cells to destroy the material. Phagocytosis is greatly enhanced if the particles are coated, or opsonized, with specific antibodies, and further enhanced by certain components of the complement system (see later).

Phagocytosis as a homeostatic process

Before phagocytosis begins, mobile microphages and macrophages must move through capillary walls (a process called diapedesis) to the vicinity of antigenic material. As a matter

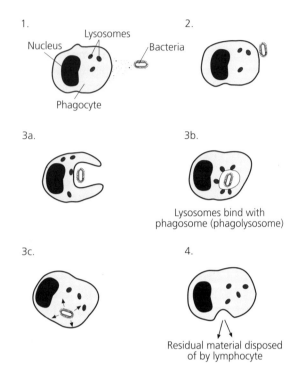

Figure 10.7 Phagocytosis. 1 Chemotaxis. 2 Adhesion. 3 (a) Ingestion; (b) intracellular digestion; (c) intracellular absorption of useful products. 4 Disposal (exocytosis).

of convenience, the process of phagocytosis is divided into four stages (Figure 10.7).

CHEMOTAXIS

Chemicals released from pathogens (e.g. toxins), from lymphocytes (e.g. macrophage-attracting substances), and from damaged tissue and surrounding tissues (e.g. histamines), attract phagocytes to the area in a process called chemotaxis. Some microbial chemicals, however, may repel phagocytes, and these contribute to the microbe's own homeostatic defences!

ADHERENCE

Adherence involves a firm contact being made between the phagocyte's plasma membrane and the antigen. Phagocytes have a number of membrane chemicals, which have sticky properties and aid microbial adherence. Complement or antibody-coated bacteria promote the adherence, and this is referred to as optimization of immune adherence. Adherence sometimes proves to be a difficult process but is facilitated by trapping the microbe against a roughened surface (e.g. blood clot), or a solid surface (e.g. blood vessel). This activity is referred to as non-immune, or surface, phagocytosis.

INGESTION AND INTRACELLULAR DIGESTION

Phagocytes employ cytoplasmic streaming to produce cell membrane projections called pseudopodia (podia = feet) which engulf, or ingest, the material to be phagocytosed. The engulfed antigen becomes surrounded by a membrane-lined vacuole, or phagosome, which becomes cytoplasmically bound and lysosomes (Chapter 2) coalesce with it, forming a larger structure called a phagolysosome or a secondary lysosome. Lysozymes are released into the vesicle, and these enzymes (lipases, proteases, nucleases, etc.) break down complex microbial components into simple molecules. These pass into the cytoplasm of the phagocyte to be utilized in its metabolism. Lactic acid, another component of lysosomes, provides the pH most suitable for lysosomal enzyme activity.

DISPOSAL

Inevitably, some microbial components cannot be degraded, since human genotypes cannot produce all of the enzymes necessary for total microbial destruction. Indigestible or residual material remains vacuolated within the phagocyte until they are ejected from the cell by exocytosis.

Some toxin-producing microbes are not necessarily killed by phagocytosis, but may become killers of the phagocytes themselves through the secretion of their toxins. Others (e.g. tuberculin bacilli) even divide within phagolysosomes and destroy the phagocytes

intracellularly. Yet other micro-organisms (e.g. HIV) remain dormant within phagocytes for long periods before having their effects. Further problems can arise if the phagocytosed antigen cannot be catabolized (e.g. coal dust), thereby causing its intracellular accumulation. These phagocytes then produce an abundance of lysosomes, which fuse with the phagosome in an attempt to destroy the particles. Eventually, phagocytic autolysis (literally 'self-destruction') occurs when lysozymes are released intracellularly.

An increase in cellular respiration accompanies the process of phagocytosis. Consequently, hydrogen peroxide is produced and this chemical is toxic to many bacteria; it therefore contributes to the body's defence operations. Some bacteria counteract this effect by producing an enzyme, catalase, which converts peroxide into water and oxygen. Needless to say, this enzyme production is a useful homeostatic adaptation which gives these bacteria a degree of resistance.

The specific immune response: a homeostatic process

In addition to surviving the above non-specific defences, pathogens must also simultaneously deal with specific (lymphocytic) immune responses if they are to be effective in producing infection or disease. In summary, the non-specific mechanisms have stereotypic actions against all antigenic insults, whereas lymphocytic responses confer specific immunity against particular antigenic insults. Such responses have two closely allied components:

1 A component involved in the production of specific T-lymphocytes, some of which attach themselves to antigenic materials to destroy them. This response is particularly effective against the antigens of fungi, intracellular viruses, parasites, foreign tissue transplants, and cancer cells. This is referred to as cellular, or cell-mediated, immunity,

since it is mainly reliant upon the secretion by these cells of cytotoxic and other substances, which include lysozymes, macrophage-attracting substances, and interferon. The latter is specifically released when the antigen is a virus. It is important in controlling viral infections by preventing their replication whilst inside host cells. Thus, since antibodies cannot enter cells, interferon succeeds where antibodies fail.

2 A component involved in the production and secretion of specific antibodies into the circulation. Antibodies are produced by B-lymphocytes in an attempt to destroy a particular antigen. Thus, if antigen 1 penetrates the external defences, antibody 1 is produced against it, whereas if antigen 2 enters the body, antibody 2 is produced, etc. These cells confer humoral, or antibody-mediated, immunity, which is particularly effective against bacteria and viral antigens.

Prior to considering cell-mediated and antibody-mediated reactions, it is necessary to discuss the origin of the cells involved, and the structure of antigens and antibodies.

LYMPHOCYTE PRODUCTION AND DESTRUCTION: A HOMEOSTATIC PROCESS

Embryologically, T-cells (responsible for cellular immunity), and B-cells (responsible for humoral immunity) are derived from bone marrow lymphocytic stem cells, which themselves have originated from stem cells within the bone marrow (Figure 10.8). The majority of lymphocytic stem cells migrate to the thymus, where they are processed into T-lymphocytes. Processing bestows immunological competence; i.e. cells develop the capacity and ability to differentiate into cells that perform specific immune reactions. Competence is conferred by the thymus shortly after birth, and for a few months post delivery. Removal of the gland prior to processing

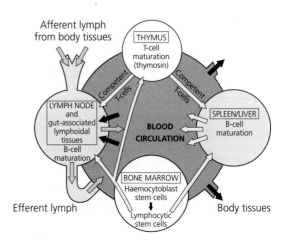

Figure 10.8 Lymphocyte development and circulation. Lymphatic stem cells from the bone marrow which mature in the thymus are called T-cells. Those that migrate to the spleen, liver, and lymph nodes mature into B-cells. T-cells also migrate to the spleen and lymph nodes from the thymus. T- and B-cells circulate in the blood and lymph.

impairs the development of cell-mediated immune responses.

Competent T-cells leave the thymus and become embedded in lymphoidal tissue of the fetal liver, spleen, lymph nodes and the gut-associated lymphoidal tissue (adenoids, tonsils, appendix, etc.). Thymosin, a hormone, and other thymic secretions stimulate further T-cell development.

The remaining lymphatic stem cells are destined to become B-cells. They are processed in the bone marrow, and then migrate to the lymphoidal tissue mentioned above. The presence of both T- and B-cells means that these tissues are now capable of stimulating both cellular and humoral immunities, in response to antigenic insults. Consequently, the thymus gland and bone marrow sites are called the primary lymphoidal organs, whereas the above lymphoidal tissues are called the secondary lymphoidal organs.

'Adult' lymphocyte production, or lymphopoiesis, is maintained in the bone marrow and lymphatic tissue. Lymphocytes have long lifespans compared with most body cells; approximately 80% survive 4 years, and some live for 20 years or more. Cell production must match destruction to maintain the homeostatic functions of the immune system and the ageing process is associated with increased destruction and decreased production rates. It is, therefore, not surprising that the elderly are more susceptible to infections and diseases.

ANTIGENS

Materials which induce specific immune reactions are called antigens; usually they are not normal constituents of the body. Sometimes, however, the distinction between self and non-self fails, and antibodies attack the body's own antigens, in a variety of conditions known as the autoimmune diseases (see later). Antigens consist of a variety of chemicals. They are usually conjugated proteins, such as nucleoproteins, lipoproteins, and glycoproteins, with molecular weights in excess of 10 000. Others are lipids and polysaccharides.

Non-self cells such as bacteria, viruses, fungi, and transplanted cells, are referred to as immunogens. The immune response against immunogens is a reaction to their cellular antigens. Immunogenic antigens may be:

1 plasma membrane receptors (Figure 10.9a);

2 cell surface structures, such as cilia, flagella, etc.;

3 secretions, such as bacterial toxins;

4 non-microbial antigens, such as incompatible blood cells, transplanted tissues and organs, and allergic substances (allergens), such as pollen grain, fur, feathers, wheat, food additives, etc. Allergens cause the production of specialized antibodies in hypersensitive or allergic immune responses (see later).

Non-self materials are classified according to whether they promote immunogenicity and/or reactivity. Immunogenicity is the ability to stimulate the production of specific antibodies,

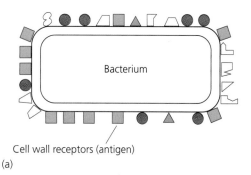

Cell wall receptors (antigen)

(a)

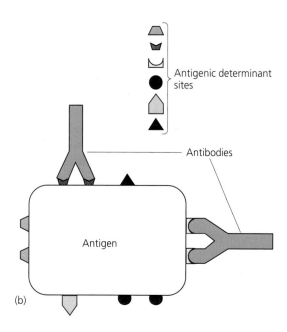

Antigenic determinant sites

Antibodies

Antigen

(b)

Figure 10.9 (a) The immunogen is the bacterium which may have many antigens or antigenic determinants. (b) Relationship of an antigen to antibodies. The majority of antigens contain more than one antigenic determinant site (i.e. they are multivalent). However, the majority of human antibodies are bivalent (i.e. they have two reaction sites that are complementary to the antigenic determinant sites). Each antibody has reaction sites for specific antigenic determinant sites only.

whereas reactivity is the ability to react specifically with relevant antibodies.

Complete antigens possess both important features. Partial antigens (or haptens) do not stimulate antibody production. Thus, such antigens have reactivity, but not immunogenicity. The immune response to haptens depends upon their combination with other antigenic substances.

Antibodies target an antigen's exposed surface, known as the antigenic determinant site (Figure 10.9b). The number of sites is known as the valence. Most antigens are multivalent; for example, the antigen of individual micro-organisms may have thousands of sites. Two sites are needed to induce antibody formation. Partial antigens have only one antigenic site which explains why they do not individually stimulate antibody production. Haptens (which include several antibiotics, e.g. penicillin), however, may become bound to carrier molecules. These larger conjugated compounds have two or more antigenic sites, and have become by definition complete antigens, and are capable of stimulating antibody production.

ANTIBODIES

Antibodies are produced and secreted in response to the presence of antigens (antigenic insults). They are found in all bodily tissues, although their greatest presence is within blood. Antibodies are very large proteins called gammaglobulins, and, since they are a part of the immune response, they are often referred to as immunoglobulins (abbreviated as Igs). Major categories are given Greek letters and include IgG (Ig gamma), IgA (Ig alpha), IgM (Ig mu), IgD (Ig delta), and IgE (Ig epsilon).

Since antibodies are proteins they consist of polypeptide chains. Most consist of two pairs, being comprised of a pair of 'heavy' chains (chains of more than 400 amino acids), and a pair of 'light' chains (consisting of 200 amino acids). The partner of each pair is identical, thus an antibody consists of identical halves, joined by disulphide (sulphur–sulphur) bonds (Figure 10.10). Each half consists of a heavy and a light chain, also held together by disul-

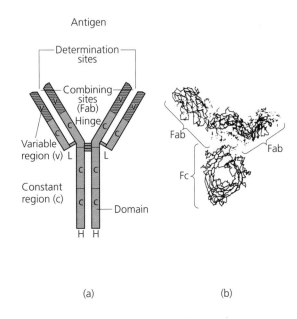

Figure 10.10 The antibody molecule and its combination with antigen. (a) A diagrammatic representation of an antibody molecule. Antibodies consist of four polypeptide chains – two identical light (L) and two identical heavy (H) chains joined by disulphide bonds. The site at which the antibody molecule combines antigen is a relatively small area of the variable region. This combining site is formed by both the light and heavy chains. Flexibility at the hinge region permits the two combining sites to bind with antigens in different configurations. The shape of the combining site is complementary to a particular determination site (DS) on the antigen. Consequently other DSs on the antigen are recognized by different antibodies. (b) The antibody molecule model is based on X-ray crystallography studies.

phide bonds. Within each chain there are two distinct regions:

1 A constant region. This region is identical in the number, type, and sequencing of its constituent amino acids in all antibodies of the same class (i.e. either IgG, IgM, etc.). The constant portion, however, differs between antibody categories, and is thus responsible for distinguishing between the different types of immunoglobulins and their

Table 10.1 The structure and function of antibodies

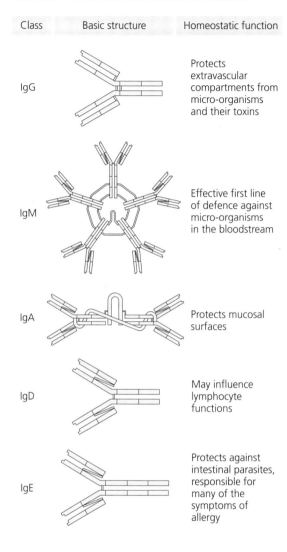

Class	Basic structure	Homeostatic function
IgG		Protects extravascular compartments from micro-organisms and their toxins
IgM		Effective first line of defence against micro-organisms in the bloodstream
IgA		Protects mucosal surfaces
IgD		May influence lymphocyte functions
IgE		Protects against intestinal parasites, responsible for many of the symptoms of allergy

biological functions. Immunologists refer to this as the Fc part of the molecule.

2 The variable region. The variable portion differs for each antibody, allowing antibodies to recognize and specifically attach themselves to particular antigens. The combining site, at which the antibody molecule combines with the antigen, is located in a relatively small area of the variable region and is formed by both the light and heavy chains. Immunologists refer to the arms of the molecule which combine with antigens as the Fab parts.

Binding converts the normal T-shaped antibody molecule into a Y-configuration, and it is this transformation which activates the antibody. Each 'arm' of the Y-configuration contains a combining site and the flexibility at the hinge region permits the two combining sites to bind with the antigens in different configurations. The shape of the combining region will be complementary to the particular determination site on the antigen. Other determination sites on antigens with different structures will be recognized by different antibodies. This 'lock and key' binding of antibody and antigen sites gives immune responses their specificity. Most antibodies have just two combining sites for the attachment of antigens, and are said to be bivalent. IgM and IgA antibodies have a higher valency because they are respectively pentamers and dimers of the basic divalent unit. The structure and homeostatic function of immunoglobulins are summarized in Table 10.1.

The combining sites of the antibodies react with antigens to form macromolecular complexes in a variety of ways which neutralize, agglutinate, precipitate, lyse or opsonize the antigen (Figure 10.11). Others prevent the adhesion necessary for microbes to penetrate the skin and mucous membranes.

Neutralization

Bacterial toxins cause disease by binding to specific cells. Neutralization involves those antibodies, called antitoxin, which include some IgGs that bind to the determination sites of the toxin chemicals, thus neutralizing their toxicity. This interaction may alter the toxin's shape, thus removing its specific binding properties and preventing its interaction with cell membranes, or destroy the antigen by increasing its susceptibility to phagocytosis.

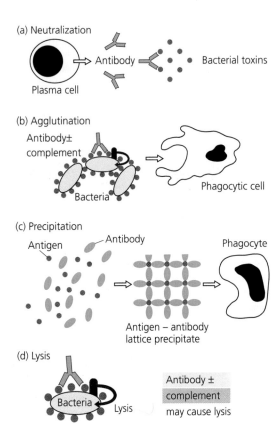

Figure 10.11 Antibody–antigen complexing.

Agglutination

Specialized antibodies called agglutinins which include some IgGs and IgMs, together with complement proteins, cause immunogens coated with non-self antigen to clump together. This is referred to as agglutination, and makes bacteria more susceptible to phagocytosis. The principles of agglutination reactions concerned with blood grouping procedures have already been described in Chapter 8. The modern pregnancy test, based upon agglutination inhibition, is discussed in Chapter 18.

Precipitation

Specialized antibodies called precipitants (including some IgGs and IgMs) react with soluble antigens via many cross-linkages to form an insoluble precipitate, which is more readily phagocytosed.

Lysis

Some IgG and IgM antibodies attach to immunogen surface antigens and directly cause cellular rupture (lysis), hence causing their death. Alternatively, antibody–antigen formation enhances the fixation of complement proteins, which also results in lysis.

Opsonization

Certain microbes, such as bacteria, have specialized structures ('slippery' plasma membranes) which, perhaps, are homeostatic adaptations to prevent phagocytosis. Opsonization is the coating of such microbes with antibodies (opsonins include some IgEs, IgGs and IgMs), and some complement proteins. This roughens their surfaces, enhancing the likelihood of adhesion and subsequent phagocytosis.

Prevention of bacterial adhesion

The IgAs present in mucus, sweat, and digestive secretions coat bacteria, decreasing their capacity for attachment to body surfaces, thus minimizing their penetration of our external defences.

ACTIVATING THE LYMPHOCYTIC RESPONSE: A HOMEOSTATIC PROCESS

Very few antigens appear to bind directly to antigen-reactive T- or B-lymphocytes. Instead some are presented to the lymphocytes on the surface of the macrophages following phagocytosis; these are known as antigen-presenting cells or APCs (Figure 10.12). A much more important group of APCs are the non-phagocytic dendritic cells. These cell types are widely distributed throughout the body, and appear

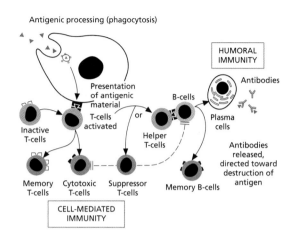

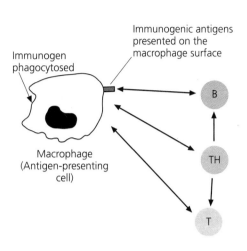

Figure 10.12 Lymphocyte response: B, B-cells; TH, T-helper cells; T, T-cells.

Figure 10.13 Interactions between macrophages, T-cells, and B-cells. Non-phagocytic dendritic cells also present antigenic material to activate the lymphocytic responses.

to trap the antigen, thereby preventing its spread. They then initiate local immune responses. Dendritic cells of the lymph nodes and spleen trap circulating antigens in the lymph and blood and present them to the resident lymphocytes. Similarly, dendritic cells present in non-lymphoidal tissues trap antigen, and then the complex moves towards the lymphoidal tissues. The structure of the spleen and lymph nodes is such that the APCs and lymphocytes are in very close contact. Immunogenic antigens, such as those associated with incompatible blood transfusions, transplanted organs, cancers, or 'self' antigens that have changed, also sensitize T-lymphocytes. A lymph node under antigenic stimulation shows T- and B-cell proliferation, and becomes enlarged in the process.

Upon contact with antigen, macrophages secrete a chemical called interleukin-1, which is a lymphokine (i.e. it increases the activity of lymphocytes) and is responsible for promoting lymphoidal T- and B-cell proliferation. Proliferation itself stimulates further macrophagic activity and hence further proliferation (i.e. positive feedback mechanism). Macro-

phages, dendritic cells, T- and B-lymphocytes thus cooperate with one another to provide immunity against antigenic insults (Figure 10.13).

T-lymphocytes and cell-mediated immunity

There are thousands of different T-cells, but only those specifically programmed to react with the specific antigen present are activated. Sensitized T-lymphocytes divide mitotically, giving rise to clones, that is cells which are identical to one another and to their parent cells (Figure 10.14). The major difference is that the parent cells cannot destroy immunogens. Clones include the following.

Killer (cytotoxic, or null) T-cells

Killer cells become attached to immunogenic antigens. They kill foreign cells by secreting the following cellulotoxic substances:

1 Lymphotoxins. These destroy immunogens directly, by producing 'holes' in their plasma membrane, resulting in lysis.

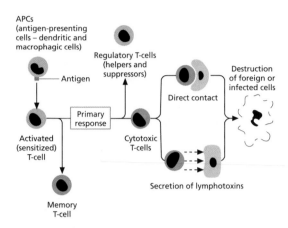

APCs
(antigen-presenting
cells – dendritic and
macrophagic cells)

Regulatory T-cells
(helpers and
suppressors)

Antigen

Destruction
of foreign or
infected cells

Direct contact

Activated
(sensitized)
T-cell

Primary
response

Cytotoxic
T-cells

Memory
T-cell

Secretion of lymphotoxins

Figure 10.14 Cell-mediated immunity. Activated or sensitized T-cells undergo mitosis and differentiate into memory T-cells, regulatory (helper and suppressor) T-cells, and cytotoxic (killer) T-cells.

2 Lymphokines. These powerful proteins give most of the protection provided by killer cells but act in a variety of ways. Lymphokines include:
  (a) transfer factors. These proteins recruit lymphocytes by transforming non-sensitized T-lymphocytes into sensitized T-cells;
  (b) macrophage-chemotaxic factor. This chemical attracts macrophages, and thus intensifies phagocytosis of the antigen;
  (c) macrophage-activating factor. These factors directly increase the phagocytic activity of macrophages;
  (d) migration inhibitory factor. This inhibitory chemical prevents the migration of macrophages, and thus encourages their continued presence at the site of infection;
  (e) mitogenic factor. This protein induces rapid division of uncommitted or non-sensitized T-cells.

3 Interferon. This antiviral agent prevents viral replication in infected cells and enhances killer cell activity, which results in the destruction of the host cells.

4 Lysozymes. The lytic actions of these enzymes have previously been explained.

The stimulation of killer T-cells is known as cell-mediated immunity, since their secretions are toxic to immunogens (non-self cells). Normally, individual immunogens stimulate both cellular and humoral immune responses; however one type usually predominates depending upon the invading immunogen. Some killer T-cell secretions promote non-specific responses and can result in the loss of 'self' tissue in the locality.

Helper T-cells

Helper lymphocytes assist plasma cells (those derived from B-lymphocytes) to secrete antibodies. In addition, helper cells secrete the chemical interleukin-2 (a lymphokine) which amplifies the proliferation of killer cells. Prior to this, however, interleukin-2 must be activated by interleukin-1, secreted from macrophages, thus demonstrating the interdependency of white cell types in controlling the homeostatic functions of defence. In addition to stimulating lymphocyte proliferation, interleukins also:

1 amplify inflammatory and macrophagic responses;

2 elevate body temperature, which interferes with the rate of bacterial cell multiplication;

3 aid scar tissue formation by increasing fibroblast activity during wound healing;

4 promote ACTH secretion, and the subsequent release of the metabolic hormone cortisol;

5 stimulate mast cell production (i.e. cells which secrete histamine and other substances as a part of the response to antigens).

Suppressor T-cells

These lymphocytes restrain killer cell and B-cell activities, and so help to moderate responses. This is important as it limits the effect of cytotoxic secretions on 'self' tissue in the locality.

The interaction between suppressor and helper T-cells, therefore, regulates the immune response. The ratio of these cells can be used to indicate the presence or absence of infection, and the stage of infection. For instance, a 2:1 ratio of helper to suppressor T-cell occurs when there are no signs of infection. Early in the infection cycle, however, a higher ratio of helper cells (and hence killer cells, B-cells, and their antibodies) exists which promote the removal of non-self antigens. Conversely, several weeks onwards, a high suppressor to helper cell ratio (and hence to killer and plasma B-cells and their corresponding antibodies) is observed and the response declines.

Delayed hypersensitivity T-cells

These cells secrete various lymphokines, including migration-inhibitory and macrophage-activating factors, in response to the presence of allergens. Destruction of the allergens at their site of entry means that these cells have key roles in delaying or preventing allergic (hypersensitive) reactions.

Amplifier T-cells

Amplifier lymphocytes somehow exaggerate the activities of helper, suppressor, and B-cell descendants. There are specific amplifier cells for helper cells, and others for suppressor cells, etc.

Memory T-cells

Memory cells retain the ability to recognize previously encountered non-self antigens, so that second and subsequent exposures lead to a rapid 'secondary' immune response (Figures 10.15 and 10.16). Immunity of this kind is thus conferred for a long time, and often for life.

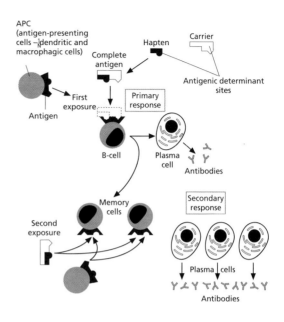

Figure 10.15 Humoral immunity.

Production of memory cells in response to administered antigens forms the basis of vaccination programmes.

Natural killer (NK) lymphocytes

NK cells are similar to killer cells, in the sense that they lyse target cells. The difference is that NK cells directly kill those cells with altered surface membrane antigens without the need to interact with other lymphocytes, or antibodies. Since it is believed that cancerous cells have abnormal surfaces it is possible that secretion of interferon by NK cells plays a prime role in destroying viral infected or damaged cells that might otherwise form tumours. NK cells are considered to be the 'first line of defence' in specific immunity. Cancer patients

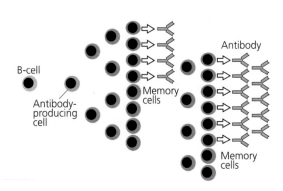

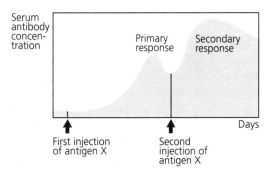

Figure 10.16 The primary and secondary antibody responses and clonal expansion. To demonstrate primary and secondary responses, a test animal is injected with antigen (X) and the serum antibody concentration assayed on successive days. The antigen stimulates B-cell differentiation into memory cells and antibody-producing plasma cells. Antibody concentration reaches a peak, and then declines as the plasma cells die. This is known as the primary response. Signs and symptoms usually appear. A minority of antigen-stimulated B-cells survive as memory cells. When the same antigen is encountered on a subsequent occasion, antibody is produced more rapidly and in a greater quantity as a result of the clonal expansion following the first contact with antigen. This is the secondary response. Signs and symptoms are either very mild or absent.

have a reduced number of NK cells, and interestingly the level of decrease corresponds to the severity of disease.

Specific and non-specific defences are therefore coordinated by physical interactions, and by the release of chemical messengers. In addition to lymphocytic secretions, the monocytes and macrophages also secrete monokines, such as the tissue tumour necrotic factor. This protein is responsible for:

1 slowing down tumour growth processes;

2 killing sensitive tumour cells;

3 stimulating the production of those white blood cells called granulocytes (granulo-cytopoiesis);

4 promoting the activity of phagocytic granulocytes, called eosinophils;

5 increasing T-cell sensitivity to interleukin chemicals.

Skin and T-cell interactions

The skin's epidermal cells have active integrative roles with the body's specific immune responses. For example, when antigens penetrate the keratinized cell layer of the epidermis they bind to cells called Langerhan cells. These cells present the antigenic material to epidermal T-helper cells, activating them. Langerhan cells also interact with epidermal suppressor T-cells, but usually the helper cells predominate, and instigate the destruction of the antigenic substances. If, however, Langerhans cells are destroyed, for example by UV radiation, or are bypassed, then these antigens react directly with suppressor cells, causing their predominance.

Humoral immunity – B-cells and antibody production

The body contains thousands of specialized B-cells which carry (or express), on their surface, antibody molecules which act as receptors for antigens. Each antibody is capable of responding only to a specific antigen. When a B-cell is exposed to an antigen, small B-lymphocytes (influenced by interleukin from activated macrophages) become larger plasma cells.

These produce and secrete into the blood and lymph specific antibody of the same type as that expressed originally on the surface of the parent cell (even though B-cells remain in lymph). The antibodies are thus transported to the site of antigenic invasion.

Within the plasma cell's lifespan (4–5 days to a few weeks), they are capable of producing approximately 2000 antibody molecules per second; their high metabolic rate explains their brief existence. Some B-cells do not possess the genetic capability to differentiate. These remain as memory B-cells, which, together with T-memory cells, are programmed to recognize original antigens on their second and subsequent invasion of the body. They are therefore responsible for stimulating that which is called the secondary immune response.

Primary and secondary immune responses

Plasma cells initiate antibody production in the primary immune response. The speed of this response is determined by the time it takes for antigenic activation of the appropriate B-cell, and for that specific B-cell's multiplication and differentiation. Consequently, there is a gradual sustained rise in circulating antibody concentration, peaking at approximately 1–2 weeks after the initial exposure. Antibody concentration subsequently declines, assuming that the individual is no longer exposed to those antigens. The decline in antibody production parallels the death of the plasma cells, which have a limited lifespan due to their high rate of metabolism. If one recovers from a microbial infection upon first exposure without having to use medication, then it is because the primary immune response has provided sufficient defence to aid recovery. If, however, the primary response has not provided sufficient defence, then an illness 'drags on' and recovery must be facilitated by using medication (such as antibiotics) .

Memory B-cells may also differentiate into plasma cells, and become antibody producing, but only upon the second exposure to the original antigen. Memory cells have long lifespans, with some surviving 20 years or more, and this secondary (anamnestic, or memory) response occurs immediately with antibodies rapidly being secreted in vast amounts. Peak values are higher and occur much more quickly compared with those of the primary immune response. The secondary response is usually so swift that signs or symptoms of the illness do not appear, since the microbe is destroyed quickly and efficiently. The immediate antibody upsurge of the response may have pathological consequences, however, particularly if normal cells are also destroyed by the response, since this could trigger a massive widespread inflammatory response.

The anamnestic response forms the basis of immunization programmes, i.e. the initial immunization sensitizes the body, so that if the immunogen is encountered in the future through infection, or a booster dose of the antigen is administered, then the body experiences the anamnestic response. Booster dosages are required because antibodies and memory cells have a limited metabolic lifespan and therefore the antigen must be given periodically to maintain high antibody titres.

Figure 10.16 highlights the principal differences between primary and secondary immune responses.

There is a lag phase between antigen exposure and antibody production. This largely depends upon the pathogenicity of the organism concerned, the organism's mode of entry, and if it is a primary or secondary immune response.

In summary, immunity is a set of reactions stimulated in response to the invasion of the body by non-self substances or antigens (Figure 10.17). Such a response is said to be:

1 Adaptive, i.e. an antigenic invasion produces a response to the environmental (antigenic) insult.

2 Highly specific for different antigenic insults.

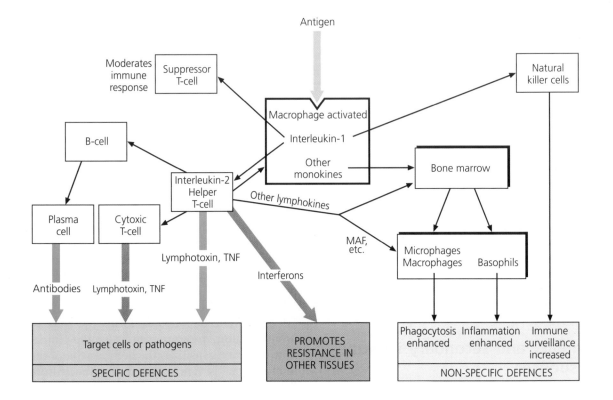

Figure 10.17 A summary of cellular and chemical interactions associated with the immune response.

3 Xenophobic, i.e. the body distinguishes between self and non-self antigenic materials.

4 Anamnestic, i.e. there is a memory component of the immune response, allowing both primary and secondary responses to occur.

Immunological competence

Immunological competence is the ability to produce an immune response to an antigenic insult. Cellular immunity occurs from approximately the third month of gestation, but active humoral immunity appears much later. The fetus, however, receives IgGs from the maternal circulation until delivery, although this is referred to as passive immunity as it is not the response of fetal tissue. In the seventh month of gestatory development, the fetus develops IgA and IgM immunological competence if exposed

to the relevant antigens. The mother also provides IgAs post-natally in breast milk, although this passive immunity is gradually lost. Maternal IgGs decline within the first 2 months following birth, since they have a short biological life, and because there is no anamnestic immune response in the baby. During this period the infant is vulnerable to infection and this necessitates the implementation of vaccination programmes soon after birth. During childhood the antibody titres gradually rise towards adult levels, and the population of memory B- and T-cells progressively increases as one encounters different antigens, until their decline as a consequence of the ageing process (Chapter 19).

Tolerance

Tolerance is the term given when the immune system does not respond to an antigen, as is normally the case with respect to the body's own tissues.

Stress and immunity

Prolonged distress induces homeostatic failure (Chapter 22) and it is generally accepted that distress depresses one's immune responses. Interleukin-1, secreted from macrophages, stimulates the secretion of the hormone ACTH from the pituitary gland and this has a direct action to lower antibody production, and to stimulate the secretion of glucocorticoids from the adrenal glands. These steroidal hormones have anti-inflammatory effects and their long-term secretion inhibits the immune response, lowering one's resistance to disease as a consequence (Figure 10.18). These inhibitory mechanisms are as follows:

1 Depression or cessation of the immune response. Glucocorticoids inhibit mast cell activity and so decrease the availability of histamine, the initiator of inflammation. Capillaries remain impermeable to protein, and this reduces the availability of fibrinogen, complement, and other cellular defences important in the inflammatory response. This inhibition can halt inflammation totally.

2 Inhibition of interleukin production and secretion. This depresses the stimulation of killer cell proliferation and other responses associated with interleukin.

3 Reduced number of phagocytes. This impairs non-specific processes by interfering with phagocytosis, and also impairs the antigenic processing and presentation to lymphocytes.

4 Reduced number of lymphocytes.

Consequently, one becomes more susceptible to diseases ('diseases of adaptation' according to Selye's stress theory, Chapter 22) when one's immune system is depressed by chronic distress. It appears, though, that stress (i.e. eustress), can sometimes enhance immune responses. Eustressful experiences are,

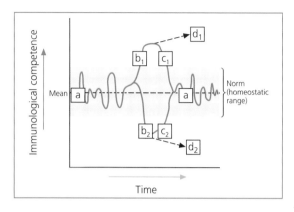

Figure 10.18 Immunological competence: a homeostatic process.
a Normal homeostatic sensitivity and functioning of the immune system's component parts (i.e. cellular/humoral responses).
b_1 Hypersensitive immune response. This can be (1) a temporary hypersensitive response to an overexposure to immunogenic and non-immunogenic antigens, e.g. as occurs in the secondary immune response, so that signs and symptoms are mild or do not appear; (2) a pathological hypersensitive response reflecting a homeostatic imbalance, e.g. as occurs in allergies, tissue rejection following transplantation, and autoimmune diseases.
b_2 Hyposensitive immune response. This can be (1) a temporary response which does *not* necessarily reflect an infection *or* illness, as occurs in acute bouts of distress; (2) a pathological response as occurs with immune deficiency syndromes and chronic bouts of distress.
c_1 and c_2 Normal function restored.
d_1 Terminal autoimmune allergic reaction (shock).
d_2 Terminal immunological deficiency syndromes, e.g. AIDS.

however, time-dependent, and generally short-lived, before they transfer to distress and this could explain why most research has identified the association between stress and loss of immunity.

Immunology and cancer

Cancer cells possess specific surface antigens characteristic of tumours. The immune system usually recognizes these as being non-self, and thus attempts to destroy them; this is called immunological surveillance. Although sensitized macrophages are involved in the response, there is general agreement that cell-mediated responses are especially involved in tumour destruction; sensitized killer cells react with tumour-specific antigens, initiating their lysis. Some cancer cells, however, employ the phenomenon of 'immunological escape'. Explanations accounting for such an escape include:

1 Tumour cells shed their specific antigens, and therefore evade the initial recognition necessary for immunological surveillance.

2 Decreased immune functioning makes people more susceptible to cancer, and this supports the increased incidences of cancer observed with the use of immunosuppressive therapy in transplant patients, in people suffering from chronic distress, and with age.

Monoclonal antibodies

Scientists have been able to fuse individual B-cells with rapidly dividing tumour cells, and the resultant hybridoma cells are plentiful long-term sources of antibodies specific against one antigen; hence the term monoclonal. Such antibodies are of diagnostic importance in allergies, pregnancy, and diseases such as hepatitis and cancer, as the use of highly specific antibodies offers greater sensitivity, speed, and specificity in comparison to conventional diagnostic tests. They are used independently, or in combination with radioactivity or chemotherapy, in the treatment of cancer, and the clinical application of monoclonal antibodies to prevent cancers is exciting, since such antibodies selectively locate and destroy cancer cells, but cause little or no damage to surrounding healthy cells. This treatment, therefore, overcomes some of the major adverse effects of isolated chemotherapy and radiotherapy. The use of monoclonal antibody vaccines may also prove to be useful to counteract tissue and organ transplant rejection, and to treat autoimmune diseases.

ACQUIRED IMMUNITY

An individual can acquire immunity to infectious diseases either naturally or artificially, both of which can be passive or active (Figure 10.19).

Passive natural immunity

Passive natural immunity is acquired before birth with the passage of maternal antibodies across the placenta, or after birth in lactating infants with the passage of antibodies present in breast milk.

The actual antibodies transferred by the mother depends upon her active immunity. Passive immunity is short-lived, since the child's lymphocytes are not activated and the maternally derived antibodies are not replaced as they are metabolized.

Active natural immunity

Active natural immunity involves stimulating the body to produce its own antibodies. It is acquired via:

1 Having the disease, i.e. during an illness B-lymphocytes differentiate into plasma cells

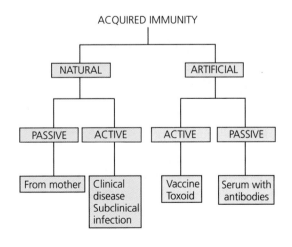

Figure 10.19 Summary of types of immunity.

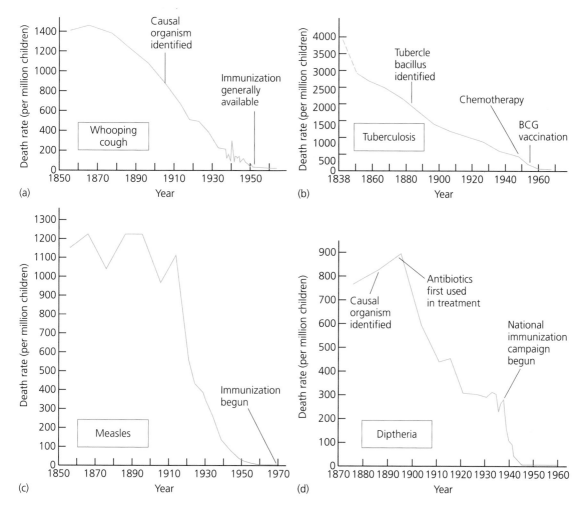

Figure 10.20 Graphs indicating the success of vaccination. (a) Whooping cough: death rates of children under 15, England and Wales. (b) Respiratory tuberculosis: death rates, England and Wales. (c) Measles: death rates of children under 15, England and Wales. (d) Diphtheria: death rates of children under 15, England and Wales.

which produce and secrete immunoglobu-lins in sufficient quantities to overcome the infecting antigenic material. Upon recovery and during convalescence, lymphocytes retain the ability to produce these specific antibodies against the antigens previously encountered, since there is a memory component associated with immunity.

2 Having a subclinical infection. In this situa-tion, the infection is not severe enough to cause clinical manifestation of disease. It

does, however, stimulate B-lymphocyte activity.

Passive artificial immunity

Passive artificial immunity is acquired by giving individuals ready-made antibodies using human or animal sera. Antibodies are obtained from convalescing individuals, or from horses which have been artificially immunized. Use of such anti-serum is administered prophylactically to prevent development of a disease in individuals who have been exposed to the infection, or therapeutically, after the disease has developed.

The antibody-containing serum from other species, however, can manifest itself as a dangerous hyperimmune response in susceptible humans. This has led to the removal of horse serum treatment in patients infected with the tetanus organism, for example.

Active artificial immunity

Active artificial immunity develops in response to the administration of dead, or live but artificially weakened, microbes as vaccines, or of detoxified microbial toxins as toxoids. Vaccines and toxoids retain antigenic properties and therefore stimulate the immune response without causing disease. The first vaccination of this kind was performed by Edward Jenner in 1796, who used the fluid extracted from cowpox blisters to confer immunity against the similar virus of smallpox. Modern immunization programmes have reduced the incidence of many serious diseases, including whooping cough, tuberculosis, measles, diphtheria (see Figure 10.20), cholera, rubella, smallpox, typhoid, and poliomyelitis.

Immunization can confer either lifelong immunity against infections, such as whooping cough and mumps, or short-lived immunity against certain other infections. Tetanus immunization, for example, is effective for just a number of years. Some immunities, however, may last for only a few weeks, before revaccination is necessary.

The apparent loss of immunity to an infective microbe may result from contact with different microbial strains, that are capable of producing the same clinical manifestations. Influenza viruses, for example, have rapid mutation rates and even a slight mutation produces different antigenic properties; hence we are constantly subjected to different bouts of influenza.

Examples of homeostatic control system failures and principles of correction

HOMEOSTATIC IMBALANCES OF THE LYMPHATIC SYSTEM

There are multiple clinical conditions associated with lymphatic homeostatic imbalances. The purpose of this section is to consider two ways in which lymphatic function can be jeopardized. These are (1) the spread of disease, leading to lymphatic infections and/or tumours, and (2) lymphatic obstruction.

Spread of disease

Lymph capillaries drain tissue fluid which may contain pathogens and/or tumour cells and if these are not phagocytosed they may settle and multiply in the first lymph node they encounter, thus producing localized infections or tumours. Alternatively, subsequent to proliferation, they may spread to other lymph nodes, blood, or other parts of the body using the body's transporting systems. Consequently, each new site of infection or (metastatic) tumour, becomes a further source of infection or malignant cells via the same routes, thus producing infections or tumours elsewhere, such as tonsillitis, appendicitis, glandular fever, lymphomas, thymomas, splenomas, etc.

Common lymphatic infections

Infections and tumours, and also the presence of excessive amounts of abnormal material such as bacteria and their toxins, can all cause lymph node and lymph organ enlargement (Figure 10.21). This is reversed when the infection subsides (either naturally or by using clinical intervention, for example, antibiotic therapy), and/or the tumour or abnormal particle is destroyed or moves on. Reinfections, new tumours or reintroduced abnormal particles, however, result in tissue fibrosis and a continued enlargement. Lymphatic organs which become chronically inflamed, and are associated with abscess formation, may require surgical removal to reduce the incidence and severity of subsequent infections.

Splenomegaly (enlargement of the spleen) usually occurs secondary to other conditions, such as circulatory disorders and infections, or cirrhosis of the liver. Hyperactivity of the spleen increases its phagocytic activities and leads to reduced blood cell counts (anaemia, thrombocytopenia, and leucopenia). Surgical removal, called splenectomy, is the only known cure for this condition.

Rupture of the spleen because of its soft consistency is quite common in traumatic injuries, such as broken ribs. Rupture causes severe intraperitoneal haemorrhage and may lead to shock. A splenectomy is performed to prevent the patient bleeding to death. A missing or non-functional spleen causes hyposplenism. This does not pose a serious problem, although such individuals are more prone to microbial infection, and thus special immunization programmes are recommended.

Hypertrophy of the thymus is associated with autoimmune disease of the thyroid, called thyrotoxicosis.

Common tumours

Lymphoidal tumours are classified as Hodgkin's and non-Hodgkin's lymphomas. Hodgkin's, a malignant disease, is initially a homeostatic imbalance of cell division (called

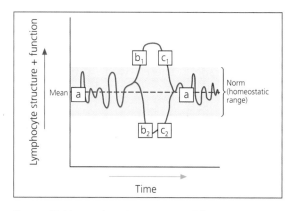

Figure 10.21 Lymphocytic structure and function: a homeostatic process.
a Normal lymphocytic function and structure.
b_1 Hyperplasia of lymphatic tissue and organs. Tumours are examples of permanent failures of hyperplasia: e.g. lymphomas (Hodgkin's and non-Hodgkin's); thymoma (rare, but occurs in myasthenia gravis); splenomas (hypersplenism). Pathogenic infections are examples of temporary hyperplasia: e.g. tonsillitis (bacterial infection); glandular fever (viral infection); splenomegaly (secondary infected site). These are signs when the immune system is attempting to restore homeostasis.
b_2 Homeostatic failures associated with hypoplasia of lymphoidal tissue and organs, e.g. hyposplenism (missing or functionless spleen).
c_1 Clinical correction involves: (1) radiotherapy; (2) chemotherapy; (3) surgical removal (only cure for hypersplenism) or, more commonly, a combination of the above to remove permanent hyperplastic failures. Correction of temporary hyperplastic failures depends upon type of infection, e.g. antibiotic therapy for tonsillitis, rest for glandular fever.
c_2 Correction involves special immunization programmes.

hyperplasia) in superficial lymph glands, which metastasize to other lymphoidal tissues throughout the body.

Although white blood cell counts are elevated, the cells are immature. Specific complications include a deficiency of cell-mediated immunity and thus an increased susceptibility to microbial infections. This disease was formerly always fatal; however, isolated bouts of radiotherapy, or combined radio-chemotherapy, have considerably improved the prospects of securing one's remission for long periods. The effectiveness of treatment depends largely on the stage of disease when the treatment is begun.

Non-Hodgkin's tumours occur in lymphoidal tissue and bone marrow and are classified as follows:

1 Low grade. These well differentiated tumour cells progress slowly, and death occurs usually after a period of years.

2 High grade lymphomas. These poorly differentiated tumour cells progress rapidly and death occurs in weeks or months.

Thymoma (thymus tumours) and splenomas (spleen tumours) are rare. Node and organ enlargement due to tumour growth usually necessitates surgical removal, since complications may arise due to growth interfering with the functions of adjacent structures.

Lymphatic obstruction

Tumours, depending upon their site and growth, can cause obstruction inside lymphatic vessels, or inside nodes. In addition, if external to the lymphatic vessel, they may cause sufficient external pressure to restrict lymph flow. Surgery performed to remove lymph node cancers and to prevent metastasis can also result in lymphatic obstruction.

The accumulation of lymph as a result of the obstruction to lymph flow results in a swelling, called lymphoedema, the extent of which depends upon the size of the obstructed vessel.

Lymphoedema also occurs as a consequence of local inflammation, and the subsequent lymphatic fibrosis which enhances this condition.

COMMON HOMEOSTATIC IMBALANCES OF IMMUNE RESPONSES

Disorders involving abnormal immune system responses can be categorized as being problems arising from either inadequate or excessive sensitivity. The former include the immune deficiency diseases, which result from inadequate humoral and/or cellular immune responses. Such an imbalance may be inherited or acquired. Excessive sensitivity involves homeostatic imbalances arising from the immune mechanisms responding too well, or too often. Such imbalances result in allergies, tissue rejection following transplantation, or autoimmune diseases (Figure 10.18).

Immune deficiency diseases

Individuals who either lack, or have defective, immune system components are said to have immune deficiencies. Some of these are inherited and some, such as AIDS, are acquired via transmissible viruses. Children suffering from DiGeorge's syndrome are born without a thymus, and so are highly susceptible to those infections usually combated by T-cell-dependent immunity. Death may occur unless a healthy thymus graft is transplanted. Other children are born with B-cell deficiencies and so are subjected to infections usually combated primarily by antibodies. These children require repeated injection of serum antibodies from healthy donors.

Acquired immune deficiency syndrome (AIDS)

AIDS develops subsequent to infection by human immunodeficiency virus (HIV). Typically, the initial infection stimulates antibody production; IgMs are produced up to one month following the humoral response, whilst IgGs appear at approximately one month post-infection, and continue to rise throughout the remainder of the year; these antibodies are produced in response to HIV's core proteins. Interestingly, the inappropriately named 'AIDS' test identifies these antibody markers of HIV infection (perhaps it should therefore be referred to as the anti-HIV test, since it is not a test for AIDS, or even the HIV!). Eventually however, HIV depresses the body's immune system, primarily by attacking helper T-cells, and thus inhibiting their central role in immunity. In this way one homeostatic imbalance of T-cell deficiency leads to a failure of other interdependent homeostatic functions, for instance:

1 A reduced antibody production, since helper cells stimulate immunoglobulin secretion by plasma cells.

2 Fewer killer T-cells, since helper cells secrete interleukin-2, which stimulates killer cell proliferation.

In addition, HIV also infects monocytes and macrophages. The viruses mainly remain dormant in these cells, but do decrease their host cells' secretion of interleukin-1, which is needed for the stimulation of interleukin-2 release. Suppressor T-cells are relatively unaffected by HIV.

Overall, HIV infection grossly impairs normal immune functions, and consequently normally harmless microbes can initiate potentially fatal infections; the impairment of the host's defences allows the development of cancer and opportunistic infections of various kinds. The appearance of an opportunistic (or indicator) disease signifies that one has AIDS. The two commonest diseases that kill AIDS patients are *Pneumocystis carinii* pneumonia (PCP) and Kaposi's sarcoma (KS). The former is a rare form of pneumonia, caused by a protozoan, the latter is a rare malignant skin cancer. AIDS patients are also subjected to infections of the central nervous system, which eventually produce neurological imbalances such as AIDS dementia.

To date AIDS appears to be invariably fatal. At present, treatment consists of fighting infections as they occur, of experimenting with antiviral medication, or more recently via the use of immune system stimulants.

The triggers for the conversions of an HIV infection to early symptoms of AIDS (called AIDS related complex, or ARC), and from ARC to AIDS remain a mystery. Each transition has different signs and symptoms due to different homeostatic imbalances. The presence of these imbalances at specific times perhaps may help to explain why HIV infection leads to ARC or AIDS.

Severe combined immunodeficiency (SCID)

SCID is an inherited failure to develop cellular and humoral immunities, either as a consequence of a lack of both T- and B-cells, or because they are inactive. Consequently, even mild infections can be fatal. Bone marrow transplants from a compatible donor, usually a very close (i.e. genetically similar) relative, have been used to colonize the sufferer's lymphatic tissue with functional lymphocytes. Although the immunodeficient child cannot reject the bone marrow tissue, the bone marrow can reject the child since it contains immunologically active lymphocytes which react against the child's tissues.

Hypersensitivity: excessive antibody production

Hypersensitivity occurs either because the body is exposed to an excessive amount of antigen, because the antibody is secreted in too high a quantity, or because the antibody and T-cells are directed against one's own body as in autoimmune diseases. Hypersensitive reactions are of four main types as follows.

Type I (anaphylaxis) reactions

An allergy is a hyperimmune response to an antigen, in this case called an allergen, to which most people have no noticeable response. The symptoms of allergies, such as hay fever and asthma, following exposure to allergens, (i.e. pollen, antibiotics, etc.), are dramatic and occasionally lethal.

Type I reactions occur within a few minutes of being sensitized to an allergen. Some people produce IgEs and these bind to the surface receptors of mast cells and basophils (Figure 10.22). These cells are found in and underneath the mucous membranes in the nose, throat,

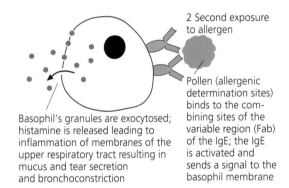

1 Plasma cell encounters allergen for the first time. Antibodies (IgE) are secreted and combine with receptor sites on mast cell

2 Second exposure to allergen

Pollen (allergenic determination sites) binds to the combining sites of the variable region (Fab) of the IgE; the IgE is activated and sends a signal to the basophil membrane

Basophil's granules are exocytosed; histamine is released leading to inflammation of membranes of the upper respiratory tract resulting in mucus and tear secretion and bronchoconstriction

Figure 10.22 Immediate (type I) anaphylactic hypersensitivity as occurs in hay fever.

eyes, and lungs. Binding causes a person to produce an allergic response, since such an interaction causes cells to release the chemical mediators of anaphylaxis (e.g. histamine, serotonin, and prostaglandins). These are responsible for increasing blood capillary permeability, increasing smooth muscle contraction, and increasing secretion of mucus. Consequently, a person may experience oedema, redness, breathing difficulties, and a 'runny' nose, along with other inflammatory responses.

Eosinophil (another white blood cell) counts are elevated during an allergic response, as a homeostatic response, since these cells are thought to exert anti-inflammatory effects by absorbing histamine.

Anaphylactic reactions, such as hay fever and bronchial asthma, may remain localized.

Others are considered systemic; for example, acute anaphylaxis may produce circulatory shock (in this instance called anaphylactic shock) and asphyxia, both of which can be fatal without clinical intervention.

Some sensitized people can become accustomed to allergens, if they are presented with them gradually and in increasing dosages. That is, they become desensitized. Children often grow out of allergies for this reason. Since only some people are allergic, this suggests that the tendency to produce IgEs in response to specific allergens may be genetically determined.

Type II (cytotoxic) reaction

Cytotoxic reactions involve IgG, IgM, or IgA antibodies which bind to antigens on body cells, mainly blood cells. This interaction activates the complement system and these proteins cause:

1 Mast cell secretion of histamine and kinins, which cause a local vasodilation and an increased permeability of capillary walls. They are also responsible for bronchoconstriction, which gives rise to inadequate gaseous exchange by the lung.

2 The chemical attraction of neutrophils (a type of white blood cell) to the site of inflammation, enhancing phagocytosis by activating macrophages. Complement enzymes attached to the antigens, and to antibodies, identify the cells to be phagocytosed.

Affected cells are thus phagocytosed and/or destroyed (Figure 10.23). Incompatible ABO blood transfusions (Chapter 8) promote such a reaction, when agglutinated cells from the donor are lysed by recipient phagocytes.

Drugs, such as methyldopa, may also produce haemolytic anaemias in the susceptible person, because the drug coats erythrocytes and promotes immune attack. Similarly, bacterial endotoxins, such as those released from *Salmonella*, also cause erythrocytic haemolysis. Cytotoxic reactions may also result in the chronic failure of transplanted organs, which

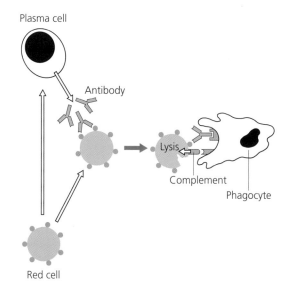

Figure 10.23 A diagram representing the mechanism of cytotoxic hypersensitivity. In this example surface antigens on a red cell stimulate antibody production. When the antibody binds to the red cells three arms of the immune response may be triggered: i.e. (1) Cells containing Fc receptors bind to the red cell via the bound antibody and lyse it. Phagocytes also contain Fc receptors and engulf the cell. (2) Complement is activated by the antibody and red cell antigen complex. (3) Complement lyses the red cell and opsonizes it for attachment by phagocytes with complement receptors.

may become necrotic due to thrombosis of the donated organ. This is caused by an antibody response to the endothelium of the donated organ's blood vessels, causing it to be damaged and resulting in the adherence of platelets and thrombus formation.

Type III (antibody mediated) reactions

Type III reactions cause antibody–antigen complexes to be deposited in various tissues, for example in joints, causing arthritis, in the heart, causing myocarditis, and in renal glomeruli causing glomerulonephritis.

The complement system, if in the presence of IgGs or IgMs, may also be activated.

A localized type III reaction (or Arthus reaction) occurs when antigens are injected; a local vasculitis and inflammatory response occurs, as a result of immunoglobulins forming complexes with the injected antigens. This sometimes occurs in the diabetic who has developed IgG antibodies against some antigenic component of their insulin preparations.

Type IV (cell-mediated) reactions

Cell-mediated (delayed-type) reactions involve T-cells, and are often not apparent for a day or more. They become apparent when allergens bind to tissue cells, causing them to be ingested by macrophages, and the antigens are then presented to the T-cells. Consequently, T-cell proliferation is responsible for the destruction of allergens. An example of a type IV reaction is a positive tuberculosis (Mantoux) skin test.

The symptoms of hypersensitive reactions can develop within minutes of the allergic, or anaphylactic response. It must be understood that hypersensitive reactions are normal homeostatic protective responses which, if in excess (i.e. in severe cases), can result in extensive peripheral vasodilation, producing a fall in blood pressure, and possible circulatory collapse. Localized allergic reactions, such as those created by pollen exposure in hay fever sufferers, produce unpleasant but less severe symptoms.

Adrenaline administration counteracts some of the responses to histamine and antihistamine drugs. Treatment of severe anaphylaxis involves antihistamine and corticosteroid injections, in addition to respiratory and/or circulatory support.

Autoimmune diseases

Self antigens do not normally initiate immune responses. However, self cells are sometimes destroyed by autoimmune responses. This type of reactivity may be important in the normal homeostatic control of body function, for example in wound healing by removing dead tissues and cells. At other times autoimmune responses are less beneficial. When autoimmunity noticeably damages otherwise healthy tissues it causes autoimmune diseases such as:

1 Diabetes mellitus. Autoantibodies may destroy the beta-islets of Langerhans, thus causing the hypoinsulinism associated with juvenile-onset diabetes.

2 Hashimoto's thyroiditis. Anti-thyroid antibodies may impair the activity of the thyroid gland.

3 Myasthenia gravis. Autoantibodies interfere with the function of motor end plates at neuro-muscular synapses, preventing the transmission of nerve impulses to motor muscles. They do so by decreasing the sensitivity of muscle membrane receptors to the transmitter chemical acetylcholine, or alternatively by destroying the neurotransmitter itself. Whichever the case, it is not surprising that these patients have weak muscles that fatigue easily and eventually may become paralysed.

4 Rheumatoid arthritis, or rheumatoid disease. Autoantibodies to certain immunoglobulins result in deposition of complexes within synovial joints, eventually leading to destructive changes. Other tissues such as the lungs and blood vessels may also be affected.

Tissue rejection in transplantation

As discussed in Chapter 8, the antigens on erythrocytes are used to categorize one's blood group status. Antigens of other body cells (called histocompatibility antigens) are used to determine an individual's tissue type. Transplanted tissues and organs thus possess non-self antigenic material, and recipients therefore produce antibodies and an immune response against transplanted antigens which may cause transplant rejection. The possibility of rejection is minimized by tissue typing, and immuno-suppressant therapy.

TISSUE TYPING

Tissue typing involves matching the donor and recipient human lymphocytic antigens (HLA).

Histocompatibility antigens are determined by several hundred genes at the HLA loci on chromosome 6. A great variation of HLAs therefore exists since there are thousands of possible genetic, and thus antigenic, combinations; a complete match is extremely unlikely. The closer the HLA match between donor and recipient, the greater the likelihood of transplant success. Despite international cooperation to match donors with recipients, immune rejection is still the main hazard in transplantation. Tissues with a similar genetic make-up are less likely to be rejected. Thus:

1 autografts (grafts from the person's own body tissues), have no non-self antigens and are obviously not rejected;

2 isografts (grafting from 'identical' genetic make-up, i.e. monozygotic twins) have little risk of rejection;

3 allograft or homograft (grafting between members of the same species, but not genetically identical individuals) have a higher rate of rejection;

4 xenograft or heterograft (using grafts from different species) have a higher rate of rejection.

Immunosuppressant therapy Subsequent to transplantation, patients receive immunosuppressant therapy in an attempt to prevent rejection. These drugs are aimed at T-lymphocytes, since these cells are most active in rejection. Unfortunately, immunosuppressants are non-specific, and suppression of the patient's natural defences to otherwise trivial pathogens may result in disease, which may threaten life. For example:

1 Corticosteroids, used for preventing transplant rejections, in the treatment of severe allergies, and for autoimmune conditions, operate by gradually destroying lymphoidal tissue, which directly depletes T- and B-cells. Their main action, however, is to decrease the activities of phagocytic cells. Thus, they make recipients more susceptible to infections.

2 Cytotoxic drugs, used to inhibit lymphocytic mitosis, also non-specifically inhibit mitosis of other cells, for example, in the bone marrow, gastrointestinal tract, and skin cells. Consequently, they can produce undesirable side-effects, such as thrombocytopenia, anaemia, leucopenia, hair loss, skin disorders, gastrointestinal upsets, etc.

Summary

1 The lymphatic system is closely associated with the cardiovascular system. It transports excess tissue fluid to the blood, helps defend the body against disease-causing microbes, and transports long-chain fatty acids absorbed from the gut into the blood.

2 Lymph is formed in blind-ending tubes which are closely associated with capillary networks. It then flows into lymphatic vessels that drain into the two major thoracic collecting ducts, which return lymph to blood at the junction of the subclavian and jugular veins.

3 Lymph flow is aided via:
   (a) the squeezing actions of surrounding skeletal muscles;
   (b) low pressure in the thorax created by breathing movements;
   (c) the presence of valves.

4 Any condition which interferes with the flow of lymph results in the clinical condition called oedema.

5 Lymph nodes are clinically important as they are the production centres for lymphocytes. They also contain macrophages, and so filter foreign particles present in the lymph.

6 The spleen resembles an enlarged lymph node. It acts as a blood reservoir.

7 The body has a number of external defence mechanisms which provide formidable barriers against antigenic invasions.

8 Inside the body, the antigenic material encounters non-specific defence mechanisms (phagocytic response) and specific defence mechanisms (lymphocytic responses). The phagocytic and lymphatic responses are extremely effective at promoting recovery from infection.

9 The phagocytic response consists of inflammation and phagocytosis.

10 Monocytes give rise to macrophages.

11 The lymphocytic response is comprised of the cellular (T-cell) and the humoral (B-cells) immune responses. T- and B-lymphocytes secrete cytotoxic substances and antibodies respectively in response to 'antigenic insults'.

12 Stem cell lymphocytes originate in the bone marrow.

13 The thymus produces T-lymphocytes, and a hormone thymosin (thymone) which stimulates other lymphoidal tissue to produce T-cells.

14 The bone marrow and other sites of the body produce B-lymphocytes.

15 The memory component of the immune response ensures a quicker and boosted response following subsequent detection of an antigen, resulting in the majority of situations presenting no signs and/or symptoms of a disease should the antigen enter the body once again.

16 Immunization gives protection against a variety of infections.

17 The two principal problems associated with homeostatic failure of the lymphatic system are lymphatic obstructions and the spreading of infections.

18 A knowledge of the location of lymph nodes and the direction of lymph flow is important in predicting the source of infection, and the spread of cancers.

19 The immune system is instrumental in policing the body's tissues in order to ensure the correct functioning of cells.

20 Homeostatic failures of the immune system are principally concerned with hypoactivity and hyperactivity of immune responses.

Review Questions

1 Describe the homeostatic functions of the lymphatic system.

2 Outline the clinical importance of lymph nodes.

3 Describe the relationship between plasma, tissue fluid and lymph.

4 What factors promote the flow of lymph?

5 Why are the spleen, the thymus, and gut-associated lymph nodes considered organs of the lymphatic system?

6 Define immunity.

7 Define an antigen.

8 What is a pathogen?

9 List the external defence mechanisms which act to prevent the entry of environmental hazards ('antigenic insults').

10 Differentiate between the specific and non-specific immune responses.

11 Describe the structure of an antibody.

12 How is the body able to distinguish between self antigens and foreign antigens?

13 Describe the functions of complement in response to bacterial invasion.

14 Distinguish between the specialized and distinctive roles of T- and B-lymphocytes.

15 Differentiate between the primary and secondary immune responses.

16 What is immunization and how does it work?

17 Why are heterograft transplants rejected?

18 What is autoimmunity?

19 Give examples of established autoimmune diseases.

20 Discuss in broad terms the homeostatic failures associated with the immune system.

The respiratory system

11

Introduction: relation of the respiratory system to cellular homeostasis

Overview of the anatomy and physiology of the respiratory system

Details of the physiology of the respiratory system

Role of the respiratory system in homeostasis

Examples of homeostatic control system failures and principles of correction

Summary

Review questions

Introduction: relation of the respiratory system to cellular homeostasis

Chapter 3 described how the energy requirements of cellular metabolism are provided mainly by the catabolism of glucose and also of fatty acids and amino acids. Efficient energy production requires the presence of oxygen, i.e. it is produced aerobically.

Oxygen requirements of tissues vary according to their metabolic activity. Thus, cardiac muscle uses about 10 ml of oxygen per 100 g of tissue per minute when we are at rest, whereas skin uses only 0.3 ml per 100 g per minute. The influence of metabolism on oxygen consumption is strikingly illustrated by skeletal muscle tissue in which oxygen utilization may increase 15-fold during exercise.

Tissue oxygen requirements are met by four main processes:

1 Oxygen exchange between the air (or more precisely lung) and blood.

2 Oxygen carriage by the blood.

3 Adequate perfusion of tissues with blood.

4 Oxygen exchange between blood and cells.

Tissues are provided with blood by the cardiovascular system and the control of tissue perfusion is described in Chapter 9. The present chapter will describe the other three processes.

Although an adequate oxygen supply is essential for normal cellular function, it is also the case that metabolic 'wastes' must be removed in order to prevent a disturbance of intracellular homeostasis. Under normal circumstances the production of energy by oxidizing (i.e. using oxygen) glucose yields carbon dioxide and water, i.e.

$$\begin{array}{cc} C_6H_{12}O_6 & 6O_2 \\ 1 \text{ Molecule} \quad + & 6 \text{ Molecules} \\ \text{of glucose} & \text{of oxygen} \end{array}$$

$$\downarrow$$

$$\begin{array}{cccc} 6CO_2 & + & 6H_2O & + & \text{ENERGY} \\ 6 \text{ Molecules} & & 6 \text{ Molecules} & & (\text{ATP} + \text{heat}) \\ \text{of carbon} & & \text{of water} \\ \text{dioxide} \end{array}$$

Carbon dioxide will combine with water to form carbonic acid and so must be excreted to prevent an accumulation of harmful hydrogen ions in body fluids. Virtually all of the carbon dioxide produced by metabolism is ultimately excreted to the air via the lungs, and this chapter will also describe those processes involved. Excess water produced by metabolism is excreted by various routes (See Chapter 12).

Overview of the anatomy and physiology of the respiratory system

The term 'respiration' is widely used to describe those processes occurring in the lung (= external respiration) and also those biochemical reactions involved in energy production within cells (= internal respiration). This chapter is particularly concerned with external respiration, and the carriage of gases by blood, and this section introduces the anatomy and physiology of the lung and airways.

The oxygen required by cells must come from the air around us, and that air also provides a suitable medium for the excretion of carbon dioxide. Our lungs, therefore, are basically organs which provide a large surface area, and as thin a barrier as possible, for adequate gas exchange to occur between blood and environment.

At rest an adult breathes in about 500 ml of air with each breath and has a breathing rate of about 10–12 breaths/minute i.e. about 5–6 litres of air are breathed in (and out) each minute. The cells of the body at rest use some 250 ml of oxygen per minute, and produce some 200 ml of carbon dioxide. During exercise, however, oxygen requirements may be as high as 3.5–4 l/min and the volume of air breathed is increased to perhaps 80–100

l/minute. Lung function, therefore, must be controlled according to metabolic needs. In fact, control of lung function ensures that the gas composition of arterial blood is held almost constant and this facilitates normal cell and tissue function; it is a homeostatic mechanism.

Chapter 3 described how the production of energy from glucose produces the same amount of carbon dioxide as the oxygen consumed and it might, therefore, seem odd that the production of carbon dioxide by the body is normally less than the volume of oxygen consumed. This occurs mainly because a proportion of our energy production comes from the metabolism of fats (which produce less carbon dioxide per volume of oxygen used). The volume of carbon dioxide produced divided by the volume of oxygen used gives a parameter called the respiratory quotient. Thus,

$$\frac{\text{Volume of } CO_2 \text{ produced}}{\text{Volume of } O_2 \text{ consumed}} = \frac{200 \text{ ml/min}}{250 \text{ ml/min}} = 0.8$$

The respiratory quotient is a useful index as to which metabolic fuel predominates – for

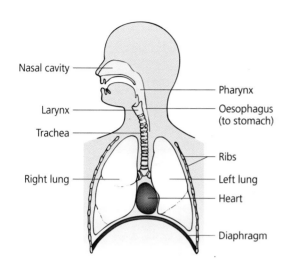

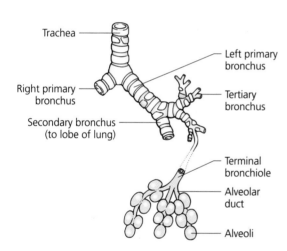

Figure 11.1 (a) Position of the lungs within the thoracic cavity, and (b) the respiratory 'tree'.

carbohydrate alone the value is 1 whereas for fats it is 0.7. The above value of 0.8 reflects a mixed metabolism of fats and carbohydrate.

Lungs are paired organs lying within the thoracic cavity. The left lung has two lobes whilst the right has three – the left lung is smaller than the right because of space occupied by the heart (see Figure 11.1a). The lungs and chest wall are lined with serous membranes called the visceral pleural membrane and

parietal pleural membrane respectively. The narrow space between these two membranes forms the fluid-filled pleural cavity and it is the pressure changes generated within this cavity by movements of the chest that promote air movement into the lungs during breathing. The pleural cavity is therefore an integral component of the breathing mechanism.

The lungs and heart are totally separated from the abdomen by a sheet of skeletal muscle – the diaphragm – which is dome-shaped prior to lung expansion but flattens during breathing in (Figure 11.2).

THE RESPIRATORY 'TREE'

The macrostructure of the lung may be likened to that of a tree, in which the continuously dividing airways represent the branches. The general anatomy of the lung and its airways is shown in Figure 11.1b.

The nasal cavity is a large cavity lined with a ciliated glandular epithelium. The area is well supported with blood. The epithelium is effective at warming (via heat from blood), filtering (by cilia), and moistening (via mucus) the air on breathing in. Projections, called conchae, increase its surface area. These processes continue within the cavities at the back of the mouth, the pharynx. The opening to the latter is called the glottis and is closed off during swallowing by a small flap called the epiglottis. The larynx consists of cartilage and ligaments and forms the 'Adam's apple'. Elastic fibres and muscle within the larynx form the vocal cords.

From the larynx the inspired air enters the trachea which is a tube of fibrous and muscular tissue some 12 cm in length and 2.5 cm in diameter and lined with ciliated mucosal epithelium. The trachea is strengthened by 16–20 C-shaped rings of cartilage which prevent it from collapsing. The absence of cartilage posteriorly prevents friction rub with the oesophagus during swallowing. The trachea bifurcates into the left and right primary bronchi (singular, bronchus). The

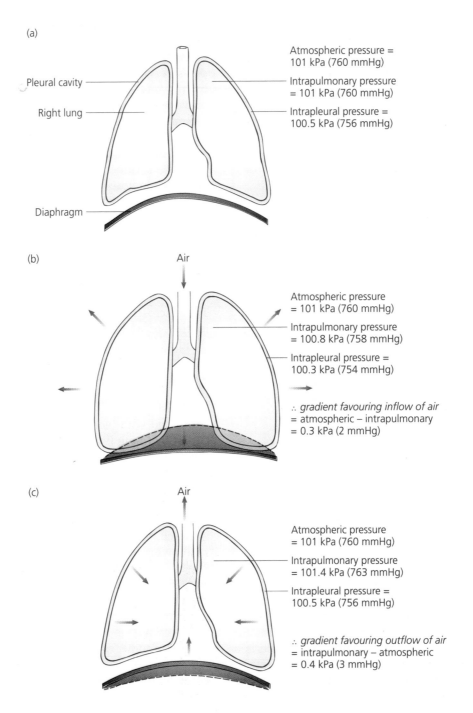

Figure 11.2 Pressure gradients during inspiration and expiration. (a) At end of normal expiration. (b) During inspiration. (c) During forced expiration.

right branch is larger and more vertical than the left so any particles still remaining in the air tend to be lodged in the right lung. The primary bronchi are generally similar in structure to the trachea, but are of smaller diameter. One primary bronchus goes to each lung where it divides into smaller secondary and tertiary bronchi. Each secondary bronchus supplies a lobe of a lung. Cartilaginous structures become less well defined in these smaller bronchi, which later divide into numerous even smaller branches called bronchioles. Although less than 1 mm in diameter, these divide further and thus continue the extensive network of branches of the 'tree'.

Bronchioles do not contain cartilage but consist of smooth muscle, and ultimately terminate in alveolar ducts which open into minute clusters of cup-shaped or globular sacs called alveoli (singular, alveolus). Each alveolus is of the order of 0.3 mm in diameter. Alveoli are richly supplied with blood capillaries and the barrier formed by the capillary endothelial cells and the alveolar epithelial cells forms the surface across which gas exchange occurs between the lung and blood.

Being globular and extremely numerous (approximately 300 million in total) alveoli provide a huge surface area for gas exchange between the alveoli and the blood. It has been estimated that the surface area of a pair of lungs is approximately 70 m².

Since only the alveoli provide the gas exchange surfaces, it follows that much of the airways do not participate in this exchange. The nasal cavity, pharynx, trachea, bronchi, and bronchioles therefore comprise a 'dead space' for gas exchange. These airways will be filled with air during inspiration, and with alveolar gases following expiration. The dead space has an important role in the homeostatic regulation of blood gas concentrations (see next section).

The airways are lined with cells which have important roles in moistening the inspired air, which prevents dehydration of the alveoli, and in trapping particulate matter in the air. Thus, the airways contain goblet cells (see Chapter 2) which secrete mucus, whilst other cells possess masses of cilia which waft the mucus and trapped particles in the direction of the throat where they are swallowed.

GENERAL PRINCIPLES OF LUNG FUNCTION

Analysis of the gases in alveoli after inspiration shows that they have become enriched in oxygen and depleted of carbon dioxide. This is not surprising since inspired air is comprised of approximately 21% oxygen and only 0.03% (effectively 0) carbon dioxide. The remaining 79% is mainly nitrogen. The changes in lung gas composition during inspiration, however, are relatively slight mainly because the airways and alveoli will still contain 'old' alveolar gas at the end of expiration (note that the alveoli do not completely deflate). On breathing in, the inspired air will therefore mix with a relatively large volume of lung gas and so the dilutional effect that the air has on lung gases will not be pronounced.

The changes in gas composition in alveoli during inspiration, though not pronounced, are sufficient to generate the necessary pressure gradients to promote oxygen diffusion into the blood and carbon dioxide from the blood. Being gases, the diffusion of oxygen and carbon dioxide across membranes will only occur if a pressure gradient is available to drive the movement.

Finally, if a major role of the lung is to provide adequate oxygen for tissue function elsewhere in the body, then the process would be self-defeating if the lungs themselves were to utilize much of the oxygen taken in during inspiration simply to sustain the respiratory movements required to inflate or 'deflate' the lungs. In fact the energy requirements of the lung are relatively small – during a normal resting inspiration/expiration cycle the lungs consume less than 1% of the total uptake of oxygen. The low energy requirements are facilitated by the anatomy of the lung, described in more detail in the next section.

Details of the physiology of the respiratory system

INSPIRATION AND EXPIRATION

Inspiration requires inflation of the lungs, expiration requires deflation. Although this appears a simple process, inflation or deflation can only occur if the appropriate air pressure gradients are generated which will move gases in and out of the lungs (see Figure 11.2).

Inspiration

According to Boyle's law, if the volume of a container is increased the pressure of gas within the container will decrease. Thus, lung inflation is caused by the contraction of external intercostal (inter- = between; -costal = rib) muscles which raise the rib cage upwards and outwards, and also of the muscular diaphragm which, by flattening the 'dome' of this muscle sheet, distends the thoracic cavity (see Figure 11.2). When we are at rest, contraction of the diaphragm alone may be all that is required to provide adequate ventilation of the lungs; this is called diaphragmatic breathing. Both mechanisms are necessary during physical activity and with severe respiratory effort accessory muscles such as the sternocleidomastoid muscle of the neck region are also utilized (Figure 11.3). The extra muscle contraction will increase the energy expended simply to maintain the appropriate level of breathing but this still represents only about 3% of the total oxygen consumption.

Expansion of the thoracic cavity lowers the pressure within the lung. To be precise, expansion of the thoracic cavity lowers the pressure within the fluid-filled pleural cavity which in turn 'pulls' the lung outwards (remember that the lungs are not directly attached to the chest wall), thus lowering pressure within the airways. It can be seen from Figure 11.2 that the subatmospheric pressure generated is only very slight, producing a gradient between the alveoli and the air of only 2 mmHg, yet this is adequate to draw some 500 ml of air into the lungs. Inflation at such low pressure gradients suggests that the resistance to air flow within the lung must be very low. This is in fact the case and results from the way the airways divide. Thus, although the airways decrease in diameter as they divide, the large increase in the number of branches actually increases the total cross-sectional area. Consequently, it is the nasal cavities and the pharynx which normally provide the main site of airway resistance, especially if there is inflammation and excess mucus because we have a cold! A low airway resistance is physiologically important because if it was high the energy expended in muscle contraction to generate the large pressure gradients necessary to inflate the lungs would be excessive and cause fatigue.

Expiration

In contrast to the active process of inspiration, expiration at rest is passive. The terminal bronchioles and alveoli contain elastin fibres (Figure 11.4) which stretch as the lung inflates during inspiration. The ease with which the lung can be inflated is measured as the compliance which is calculated as:

$$\text{Compliance} = \frac{\text{change in volume}}{\text{change in pressure}}$$

Thus, if the lung could be inflated without causing a large change in pressure (clearly beneficial in view of the small gradients normally required – see above) this would indicate a highly compliant or elastic lung. The naturally high compliance of lungs means that, should inspiration stop and the inspiratory

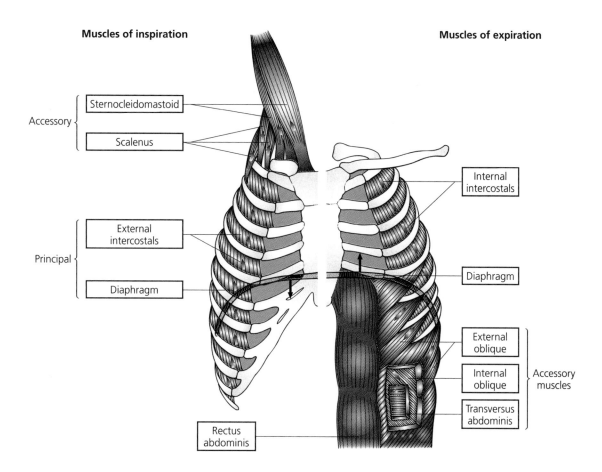

Figure 11.3 Muscles of inspiration and expiration.

muscles relax, the lungs will simply recoil like a piece of stretched elastic and so expel the gases. This passive nature of expiration helps to keep oxygen usage during breathing to a minimum. It can only be effective, though, because the resistance to air flow is extremely low since again only a small pressure gradient is developed (Figure 11.2). The importance of airway resistance is illustrated graphically in Figure 11.5.

Expiratory effort can be increased if necessary by contracting the internal intercostal muscles, which lower the rib cage and move it inwards, and by contracting accessory muscles such as the rectus abdominis muscle of the abdomen (Figure 11.3). Such processes are important if breathing rate and depth are to be increased, as in exercise. A forced expiration also provides a useful means of clinically monitoring airway resistance since, for a given resistance, a predicted rate of gas flow should be attainable in health. The expiratory rate is measured using a peak flow meter, i.e.

$$\text{Rate} = \frac{\text{volume expired}}{\text{time taken}}$$

Finally, there is a potential danger that the walls of the alveoli will touch and adhere to each other after expiration. Alveolar membranes must be kept moist to avoid dehydration, and contact between wet surfaces produces powerful adhesion because of the phenomenon of surface tension (try lifting a sheet of glass off a wet kitchen top!). Respiratory movements are inadequate to overcome such adhesion forces and so the collapse of alveoli must be prevented. Alveoli do not, in fact, totally deflate following expiration. In addition they are also coated with a detergent-like chemical, a phospholipid called surfactant, which is secreted by cuboidal epithelial cells of the alveoli (see Figure 11.4) and which acts to lower the surface tension within the alveoli. Surfactant is not produced in quantity by the lungs until about the 24th week of fetal development and this is a major factor in the survival of very premature babies.

PULMONARY AND ALVEOLAR VENTILATION, AND DEAD SPACE

From Figure 11.1 it is clear that a volume of lung gas will remain within the major airways after breathing out. This gas will re-enter the alveoli during the next inspiration, closely followed by the fresh air. At the end of inspiration a portion of the inspired air will then fill the major airways. Since these parts of the respiratory tree do not exchange gases with the blood, they form a 'dead space'. The importance of the dead space is that it forms a component of the functional residual capacity (see later) after expiration and also that, on breathing in, only a proportion of the inspired air will actually reach the alveoli. Both aspects prevent large fluctuations in the composition of gas in the alveoli and, therefore, of the blood, and so are an aid to homeostasis. Thus, for an inspired volume of 500 ml, approximately 150 ml will fill the dead space and only 350 ml will enter the alveoli.

Dead space can be envisaged as being the volume of gas contained in non-exchanging parts of the lung (= anatomical dead space) or,

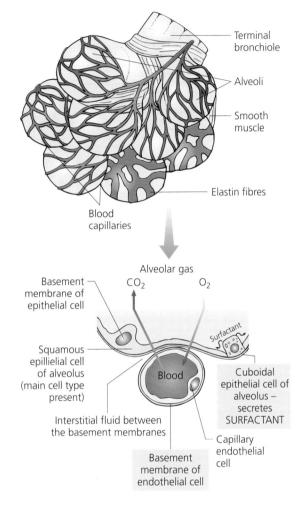

Figure 11.4 Alveoli and the alveolar-capillary membranes.

alternatively, as being that volume of inspired air which does not take part in gas exchange (= physiological dead space). The main difference between these definitions is that the first makes the assumption that all alveoli take part in normal gas exchange with the blood. This is usually the case and the anatomical and physiological dead spaces are more or less equal. A pathological disturbance of alveolar function may interfere with gaseous exchange, however, and the alveoli affected will thence become part of the dead space, i.e. the physiological dead space will then exceed the anatomical dead space.

The volume of air breathed in per minute is called the pulmonary ventilation, or respiratory minute volume. Because of the dead space it cannot be assumed that the pulmonary ventilation gives a measure of the ventilation of the alveoli (= alveolar ventilation). This is illustrated by the following example:

Volume inspired   = 500 ml
per breath
Breaths per minute   = 10
Dead space   = 150 ml

Respiratory   = volume/breath ×
minute volume   breaths/minute
                        = 500 ml × 10
                        = 5.0 l/min

Alveolar ventilation   = (inspired vol −
                            dead space) ×
                            breaths/min
                        = (500 − 150) × 10
                        = 350 ml × 10
                        = 3.5 l/min

If the volume inspired is doubled (to 1000 ml), but the breathing rate is halved (to 5 breaths per minute):

Respiratory minute   = 1000 ml × 5
volume   = 5.0 l/min

i.e. unchanged, but,
alveolar ventilation   = (1000 − 150) × 5
                        = 850 ml × 5
                        = 4.25 l/min

i.e. increased.

In this example the increased volume inspired per breath has a pronounced effect on the rate of alveolar ventilation and this is one of the major responses observed in exercise, in which alveolar ventilation must be substantially increased in order to increase the rate of gas exchange. Breathing rate is also increased during exercise, of course, which increases alveolar ventilation still further.

The airways, therefore, must exhibit a range of functional changes according to need and

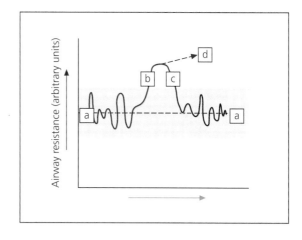

Figure 11.5 Airway resistance homeostasis.
a Normal airway resistance. Alveolar ventilation appropriate with minimum effort.
b Increased airway resistance due to, e.g. constriction of bronchioles (as in asthma), resulting in poor alveolar ventilation and increased respiratory effort.
c Intervention to reduce bronchoconstriction by reducing anxiety and/or drug administration, leading to restoration of adequate alveolar ventilation.
d Failure of intervention to correct increased airway resistance leading to further deterioration of alveolar ventilation and gas exchange.

these changes can be assessed using spirometric function tests. These tests can also provide an aid to the diagnosis of disordered lung function.

PULMONARY AIR VOLUMES AND CAPACITIES: SPIROMETRY

The volume of air inspired per breath at rest is called the tidal volume and averages about 500 ml. We can consciously (or unconsciously during exercise), increase the volume breathed in and also deflate the lung further than is observed at rest, and so it is clear that the lungs are not fully inflated after normal inspiration nor are they fully deflated after expiration; i.e. there are inspiratory and expiratory reserve volumes (see Figure 11.6). In addition it is also clear that the lung contains a volume of gas

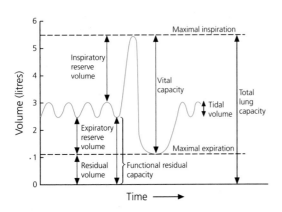

Figure 11.6 Spirometer recording (spirogram) of principal lung volumes and capacities. Note that the zero line cannot be ascertained directly.

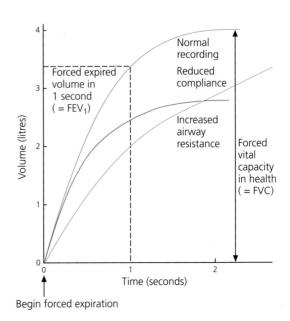

Figure 11.7 'Vitallograph' traces of vital capacity measurement to illustrate the use of FEV_1 as a diagnostic tool. Note that FVC varies between individuals, expecially in the diseased state. Values stated are examples for this illustration.

even after maximal expiration has occurred as deflation of the alveoli is incomplete and some gas fills the dead space; there is a residual volume (of about 1.5 litres). The expiratory reserve plus the residual volume represents a volume of gas into which inspired air will normally mix and is called the functional residual capacity (about 2.5 litres in volume) and this is approximately equal to half the maximum or total lung capacity. In other words the normal resting operation of the lung occurs with the lung being always about half inflated.

If we maximally inflate the lungs and then breathe out maximally, the volume of gas expired from the lungs represents the maximum volume of gas which can be possibly expelled from the lung in a single breath and this is called the vital capacity (about 4–4.5 litres in volume in men, slightly less in women). If we add the vital capacity to the residual volume then this also gives the total lung capacity (about 5.5–6 litres in volume). Note that a capacity consists of two or more distinct volumes.

Lung volumes and capacities are measured using a machine called a spirometer. There are various kinds of spirometer, some of which are portable and may simply measure, for

example, the vital capacity (using a 'Vitallograph' – see Figure 11.7). Measurement of the forced vital capacity, that is, the maximal expired volume from a full lung, expired as fast as possible, is a useful clinical assessment of airway resistance. Thus, in health, more than 80% of the vital capacity should be expelled in the first second. This is called the forced expiratory volume in 1 second or FEV_1. With increased airway resistance this proportion falls according to the severity of the condition (Figure 11.7).

The residual volume cannot be measured directly, but an indirect method may be used by determining the effect of the residual gases to dilute an inert marker gas such as helium after inspiration. The degree of dilution can then be used to calculate the residual volume.

Although the various lung capacities and volumes provide an indication of the relationships between various airway components and lung function, ultimately there must be gas exchange across the respiratory surface and this is considered in the next section.

PARTIAL PRESSURES AND THE EXCHANGE OF GASES BETWEEN ALVEOLI AND BLOOD

Oxygen and carbon dioxide exchange between the alveoli and blood is a simple process of diffusion, the rate of which is determined by the pressure gradient which exists across the alveolar–capillary membranes, and by the nature of the 'barrier' produced by the membranes. Anatomically the membranes consist of squamous epithelial cells of the alveoli and the endothelial cells of the pulmonary capillaries (Figure 11.4). The barrier is exceedingly thin (only about 0.4 μm) and so blood cells are brought into close proximity to the lung gases. The gases, however, still have to traverse across the intracellular fluids of the cells which form the membranes, and across the interstitial fluid between them. Much of the resistance to gas diffusion is therefore caused by fluids, and so the solubility of oxygen and carbon dioxide in water is another consideration in the exchange process.

The discussion prior to this point has only considered the total pressure of gases within the lung and in the air. In order to understand the exchange of individual gases within the mixture found in the lung it is important that the concept of partial pressures is understood, since it is these individual pressures that form the gradients which promote gas diffusion.

As the name implies, partial pressures are the pressures generated by individual gases within a gas mixture. According to Dalton's law each gas in a mixture of gases exerts its own pressure. Thus the total pressure of a gas mixture will be the sum of the individual partial pressures. For example 21% of air is comprised of oxygen. If the total air pressure is, say, 101 kPa (760 mmHg) the partial pressure of oxygen will be $21 \times 101/100$, that is, about 21 kPa (160 mmHg). When applied to gas exchange in the lungs, partial pressures produce the driving force for the movement of individual gases and, provided that sufficient time is available, there will eventually be an equilibration between the partial pressure of a gas dissolved within the alveoli and that of the same gas within the blood (see Figure 11.8). Note that gases dissolved in a fluid also exert a pressure and, according to Henry's law, the quantity of gas dissolved will be proportional to the partial pressure of the gas and its solubility in the liquid (assuming temperature is constant). Under normal circumstances venous blood passing through the lung will equilibrate with alveolar gas in about 0.2 seconds. In fact it usually takes red blood cells about 0.7 seconds to pass through pulmonary capillaries when the body is at rest so there is a considerable 'reserve'.

Analysis of alveolar gases after inspiration shows that the partial pressure of oxygen averages 13.3 kPa (100 mmHg). This is lower than air because alveolar gas contains a higher proportion of carbon dioxide and is saturated with water vapour (which will also exert a partial pressure). The partial pressure of carbon dioxide within the alveoli averages 5.3 kPa (40 mmHg) after inspiration – remember that the lungs contain a large volume of gas after expiration has finished so that, although air is virtually carbon dioxide-free, inspiration will not reduce the alveolar carbon dioxide composition to zero. The average partial pressures of alveolar gases, pulmonary arterial blood, pulmonary venous blood and air are compared in Tables 11.1 and 11.2.

The presence of a relatively high partial pressure for oxygen in alveolar gases is important because oxygen is poorly soluble in water and its diffusion will be facilitated by the high pressure. Diffusion from alveoli into blood is also facilitated by the presence of a large exchange surface area, and by an extensive capillary network around alveoli which slows the rate of blood flow and therefore provides

(a) Gas pressures in solution

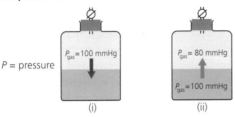

P = pressure

(i)   (ii)

(b) Partial pressures

Let the total pressure of a gas = 150 mmHg. If 66.6% of the gas is oxygen, then the (partial) pressure due to oxygen (Po_2) will be $150 \times 66.6/100 = 100$ mmHg. If 33.4% of the gas is carbon dioxide, then the (partial) pressure due to carbon dioxide (Pco_2) will be $150 \times 33.4/100 = 50$ mmHg

In solutions,

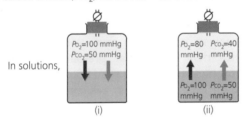

(i)   (ii)

(c) Representative values for lung/blood gas exchange after inspiration

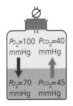

Figure 11.8 Partial pressures of gases. (a) Gas pressures in solution: (i) gas diffuses into solution until pressures in the solution and above the solution equilibrate; (ii) reducing the gas pressure above the solution now favours diffusion of the gas out of the solution until the pressures equilibrate again. (b) Partial pressures: (i) as in (a(i)), oxygen and carbon dioxide will enter the solution until the pressures above and in the solution equilibrate; (ii) if the pressures of oxygen and carbon dioxide above the solution are now reduced, both gases will tend to diffuse out of the solution, until pressures equilibrate again. (c) Representative values for lung/blood gas exchange after inspiration. The partial pressure gradient for oxygen favours diffusion of the gas into the solution ($\equiv$ blood), whilst the gradient for carbon dioxide favours diffusion out of the solution into the gases above it ($\equiv$ lung), i.e. gas exchange in the lung is promoted by the respective partial pressure gradients for oxygen and carbon dioxide.

more time for the exchange to occur. In contrast, the solubility of carbon dioxide is much higher than that of oxygen and adequate diffusion of the gas from the blood into the alveoli takes place with much lower partial pressure gradients.

From Table 11.1 it can be seen that the partial pressures of oxygen and carbon dioxide dissolved in blood leaving the lung (= pulmonary venous or systemic arterial blood) is the same as that of the alveolar gases after inspiration. In other words equilibration between the blood and alveolar gas occurs. It must be stressed, however, that the values shown for alveolar gases are averages. In fact the gas composition in alveoli, and hence in blood leaving these alveoli, varies between regions of the lung and regional disturbances in the ventilation or blood perfusion of the lung are amongst the most common causes of low blood oxygen content (= hypoxaemia; hypo- = less than normal; -aemia = of the blood).

VENTILATION/PERFUSION RATIO

At rest we breathe in (and out) some 5 litres of air per minute. The rate of blood flow through

Table 11.1 Representative partial pressures of gases in air (dry), inspired air (water saturated), alveolar gas, and expired gas (= alveolar gas + dead space air)

	Air (dry) kPa (mmHg)	Inspired air (wet) kPa (mmHg)	Alveolar gas kPa (mmHg)	Expired gas kPa (mmHg)
Oxygen	21.2 (159.8)	19.9 (149.6)	13.3 (100)	15.6 (117)
Carbon dioxide	0.03 (0.2)	0.03 (0.2)	5.3 (40)	3.8 (29)
Nitrogen	79.8 (600)	77.5 (583)	76.2 (573)	75.4 (567)
Water vapour	0 (0)	6.3 (47)	6.3 (47)	6.3 (47)
TOTAL	100.9 (760)	100.9 (760)	100.9 (760)	100.9 (760)

Atmospheric pressure is taken to be 100.9 kPa (760 mmHg). Note how the saturation of inspired air with water vapour changes the values for other gases – the sum of the pressures must remain the same.

the lungs is about 5–6 l/min at rest and so the ratio of ventilation/perfusion averages, between 0.8 and 1.0. This near matching of gas and blood movements within the lung ensures optimal oxygenation of haemoglobin, and adequate removal of carbon dioxide. The ventilation/perfusion ratio, therefore, is an important aspect of respiratory, and tissue, homeostasis. The ventilation/perfusion ratio (sometimes written as V/Q) varies between regions of the lung, however, and the value of 0.8 represents a mean. Alveoli at the base of the lung are better perfused and better ventilated than those at the apex. This is because:

1 Alveoli at the base are more deflated during expiration than ones at the apex and therefore expand more easily on the next inspiration.

2 Blood flow to the base of the lung is enhanced by gravity (note the anatomical position of the lung relative to the heart in Figure 11.1). Gravity also reduces the perfusion of alveoli at the apex (in the upright position) since blood pressure in the pulmonary arteries is only of the order of 25/8 mmHg and this will barely maintain blood flow to the lung apex.

Table 11.2 Representative partial pressures and gas composition of blood entering the lungs (mixed venous blood) and blood leaving the lungs (pulmonary venous blood)

	P_{O_2} kPa (mmHg)	P_{CO_2} kPa (mmHg)	Vol O_2 ml/100 ml blood	Vol CO_2 ml/100 ml blood
Mixed venous blood	5.3 (40)	6.0 (45)	14	52
Pulmonary venous blood (systemic arterial blood)	13.3 (100)	5.3 (40)	19.7	48
CHANGE	+8.0 (+60)	−0.7 (−5)	+5.7	−4.0

Net changes as blood passes through the lungs are shown.
Note that the changes in oxygen and carbon dioxide content of blood as it passes through the lungs are produced by disproportionate changes in their partial pressures.

Table 11.3 Regional variation in the rates of ventilation and blood perfusion in the lungs

	Ventilation (l/min)	Perfusion (l/min)	V/Q	P_{O_2} kPa (mmHg)	P_{CO_2} kPa (mmHg)
Zone*					
Apex	0.24	0.07	3.3	17.5 (132)	3.7 (28)
Base	0.82	1.29	0.63	11.8 (89)	5.6 (42)
Whole Lungs	5	6	0.83	13.3 (100)	5.3 (40)

Ventilation/perfusion ratios (V/Q) are shown as are the regional partial pressures of oxygen and carbon dioxide. Average values for the lungs as a whole are shown for comparison.
*Note that zonal values between apex and base are not included, but will contribute to values for whole lungs.

Despite being better ventilated and perfused at the base of the lung, in relative terms the alveoli there are better perfused than they are ventilated, whilst alveoli at the apex are better ventilated than they are perfused. The ventilation/perfusion ratio actually increases vertically through the lung and has an effect on the gas composition of blood leaving these areas, as shown in Table 11.3.

Thus, regional variations in the ventilation/perfusion ratio within the lung will result in blood of differing gas composition leaving those areas. Subsequent mixing of blood produces the final composition found in pulmonary venous (i.e. systemic arterial) blood. The significance of ventilation/perfusion matching is that areas of the lung may pathologically exhibit diminished ventilation or perfusion and the resultant mismatch will then alter the final composition of pulmonary venous blood. Ventilation/perfusion mismatches are amongst the commonest causes of lung-induced oxygen deficiency in the tissues (= hypoxia).

A limited correction of mismatch is possible physiologically. Thus localized hypoxaemia (low blood oxygen content) as a consequence of reduced ventilation of an area of the lung (resulting in a very low ventilation/perfusion ratio) causes vasoconstriction and so directs blood to areas of high ventilation/perfusion ratio. The overall ventilation/perfusion ratio will therefore be homeostatically maintained near to normal. Such a response is limited, however, and will not be effective if large areas of the lung are affected.

GAS CARRIAGE BY BLOOD

The carriage of gases by the blood is facilitated by the red pigment, haemoglobin, present in red blood cells.

Structure of haemoglobin

Haemoglobin begins to be synthesized in the early stages of differentiation of the red blood cell, when the cell is still nucleated. A molecule of haemoglobin consists of four molecules of a globulin protein called globin, and four molecules of a pigment called haem (Figure 11.9). The globin components account for more than 95% of the total protein within the cell. Like all proteins globin consists of a chain of amino acids. The globin molecules within a haemoglobin molecule are not identical,

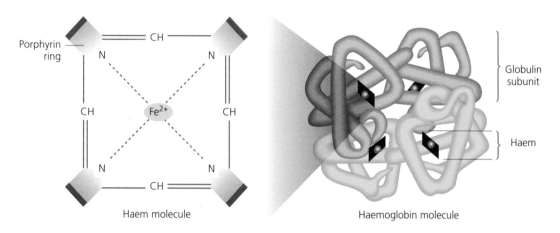

Figure 11.9 A molecule of haemoglobin, showing 4 molecules of globin and 4 molecules of haem. The haem molecule consists of a porphyrin ring surrounding an iron ion (as Fe^{2+}).

however, because of slight differences in their amino acid composition.

Four types of globin are known and they are given Greek letters to distinguish them. Each haemoglobin molecule has only two types present. Most haemoglobin of adults (abbreviated as HbA) contains two molecules of alpha globin and two of betaglobin. In some (HbA_2) the beta globin is replaced by delta globin, although functionally this type of haemoglobin is similar to HbA. In contrast, some two-thirds of the haemoglobin of the fetus has two alpha and two gamma globins in its molecule and this difference from the adult type has a significant effect on the relationship between haemoglobin and oxygen. The fetal type is an important adaptation to uterine life, and is discussed in a later section.

Haem molecules are complex structures and are an example of a group of organic chemicals called porphyrins. Porphyrins are usually associated with a metal ion and each haem molecule has an iron ion at its core. A haemoglobin molecule, therefore, contains four ions of iron, each of which can combine reversibly with an oxygen molecule.

The globin part of the haemoglobin molecule can combine reversibly with carbon dioxide or hydrogen ions, and has an important role in the transportation of carbon dioxide by blood, and in the regulation of the acid–base status of blood.

There are 200–300 million molecules of haemoglobin in each mature red blood cell, and this means that each 100 ml of blood contains approximately 13–15 g of haemoglobin. This amount, together with the properties of the pigment, ensure that the blood can transport adequate amounts of respiratory gases. This is particularly so for oxygen as this gas is poorly soluble in blood plasma; carbon dioxide can also be carried dissolved in plasma, and also as bicarbonate ions produced by its chemical reaction with water. Haemoglobin deficiency, therefore, has greater implications for oxygen carriage than for the transportation of carbon dioxide.

Carriage of oxygen

Oxygen is mainly carried in association with haemoglobin. Thus:

$$\text{Hb} + \text{O}_2 \rightleftharpoons \text{HbO}_2$$
$$\text{Haemoglobin} + \text{Oxygen} \rightleftharpoons \text{Oxyhaemoglobin}$$

When fully saturated with oxygen, haemoglobin (at a normal concentration of 15

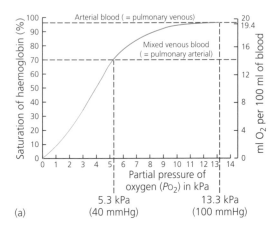

(a)

5.3 kPa
(40 mmHg)

13.3 kPa
(100 mmHg)

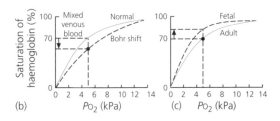

Figure 11.10 Oxygen carriage by haemoglobin. (a) At pH = 7.4, PCO_2 = 5.3 kPa, temperature = 37 °C. (b) Shifted curves due to increased acidity, temperature, and PCO_2 (Bohr shift) aids unloading. (c) Shifted curve for fetal haemoglobin aids loading.

g per 100 ml of blood) will carry about 19 ml of oxygen per 100 ml of blood. Only another 0.3 ml of the gas per 100 ml of blood will be transported dissolved in the plasma, i.e. almost 99% of oxygen carried by oxygenated (arterial) blood is transported as oxyhaemoglobin. Functionally, the pigment must bind reversibly with oxygen otherwise the gas will not be released in the tissues. The local partial pressure of oxygen is the determining factor.

Where the partial pressure of oxygen is relatively high, as occurs in the lung, haemoglobin rapidly picks up oxygen to form oxyhaemoglobin, and blood leaves the lungs with its haemoglobin virtually saturated with

oxygen. Indeed the affinity is such that even blood perfusing those areas of the lung with a low ventilation/perfusion ratio, where the partial pressure of oxygen is less than the average 13.3 kPa (100 mmHg), is still almost saturated with oxygen. This accounts for the 'plateau' phase of the oxygen–haemoglobin dissociation curve (Figure 11.10a). Within the tissues, the low partial pressure of oxygen causes the gas to dissociate from haemoglobin.

Deoxygenation of blood in the tissues causes the blood to become considerably darker in colour than arterial blood, yet venous blood usually still contains considerable amounts of oxygen. Thus, the haemoglobin of 'mixed' venous blood is still some 70% saturated with oxygen and the blood will contain about 14 ml of oxygen per 100 ml. One important feature of the association between oxygen and haemoglobin is that, should the partial pressure of oxygen be decreased locally, for example in exercising skeletal muscle, oxygen is unloaded very rapidly from the pigment as indicated by the steep slope of the dissociation curve (Figure 11.10a). Oxygen loading is therefore facilitated in the lungs, unloading in the tissues. The relationship between oxygen and haemoglobin is therefore vital for cellular homeostasis.

Factors influencing the relationship between oxygen and haemoglobin

Another feature of the properties of haemoglobin is that its relationship with oxygen can be shifted. Thus, under conditions found locally in highly active tissues (viz. an increased partial pressure of carbon dioxide, increased acidity, and increased temperature) the position of the dissociation curve shifts to the right, referred to as the Bohr shift (Figure 11.10b). Although this does not affect oxygen loading in the lung, it means that for a given (low) partial pressure of oxygen more of the gas is off-loaded from the haemoglobin. The enhanced release of oxygen helps to maintain the increased metabolism.

Fetal haemoglobin, which differs slightly from that of the adult, has a dissociation curve toward the left of that of adult haemoglobin (Figure 11.10c). This means that the pigment will have a greater saturation with oxygen for a given partial pressure. Although this may seem detrimental in terms of unloading oxygen within the fetal tissues, in fact it is an important aid in the loading of oxygen across the placenta from maternal blood which has already lost some of its oxygen.

These examples illustrate how the position of the dissociation curve in relation to partial pressures of oxygen has important physiological implications. One further example of note is the adaptation observed at high altitude, when the individual is exposed chronically to an atmosphere with a low partial pressure of oxygen. Under these circumstances the release of oxygen from haemoglobin is enhanced by elevation in red blood cells of the substance 2,3-diphosphoglycerate (2,3DPG). This combines reversibly with haemoglobin and causes it to release its oxygen by shifting the dissociation curve to the right. This adaptive measure helps to maintain an adequate oxygenation of tissues, even under conditions of low atmospheric partial pressure of oxygen, and so performs an important homeostatic function.

Carbon dioxide

In contrast to oxygen, carbon dioxide is a highly soluble gas and so a specific pigment to carry this gas in blood is unnecessary. Haemoglobin has a role in carbon dioxide transport, however, and about 23% of the carbon dioxide produced by respiring cells is carried by the pigment (after it has given up its oxygen) in the form of carbaminohaemoglobin (Figure 11.11a). Most (70%) carbon dioxide carried by blood, however, is found combined with water to form bicarbonate ions. Only 7% is carried simply as dissolved gas, but this component is important because it is dissolved gas which produces the partial pressure and therefore determines the amount of carbon

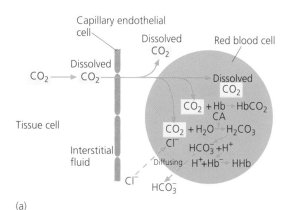

(a)

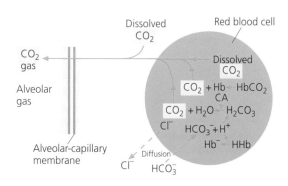

(b)

Figure 11.11 Carbon dioxide carriage: loading and unloading. (a) Loading in tissues. Note that the amount of CO_2 dissolved determines formation of carbaminohaemoglobin ($HbCO_2$) and also bicarbonate ions (in presence of carbonic anhydrase (CA) enzyme). Note also the importance of deoxygenated haemoglobin (Hb). (b) Unloading in lungs. Note that, as dissolved CO_2 diffuses into the alveolus, the gas is released from carbaminohaemoglobin and from bicarbonate. Also note that actions of carbonic anhydrase (CA) now favour formation of CO_2 and H_2O (see 'Effects of substrate availability', Chapter 3).

dioxide combined with haemoglobin and with water. Partial pressure gradients also determine the direction of gas movement across cell membranes.

The formation of bicarbonate ions from carbon dioxide is promoted within red blood cells by the enzyme carbonic anhydrase. Carbonic acid is initially formed and weakly dissociates into bicarbonate and hydrogen ions (see Chapter 5), thus raising their concentrations within the red blood cell. Since this rise in 'substrate' availability will promote the reformation of carbonic acid (through its influence on enzyme actions – see Chapter 3), and so promote its dissociation back into carbon dioxide, it is essential that the ion concentrations are reduced. This is achieved in two ways.

First hydrogen ions are buffered by combination with deoxygenated haemoglobin:

$$
\begin{array}{ccc}
H^+ & Hb & HHb \\
\text{Hydrogen} + \text{Haemoglobin} \rightarrow & \text{'Reduced'} \\
\text{ion} & & \text{haemoglobin}
\end{array}
$$

Secondly, the elevated concentration of bicarbonate ions favours their diffusion into the plasma. As the ions are lost from red blood cells the further dissociation of carbonic acid is promoted and so even more acid will be formed from carbon dioxide (thus promoting further uptake from tissues), i.e.

$$
\begin{array}{ccc}
CO_2 & + & H_2O \\
\text{Carbon dioxide} & & \text{Water} \\
\text{(from tissues)} & &
\end{array}
$$

$$\updownarrow$$

$$
\begin{array}{c}
H_2CO_3 \\
\text{Carbonic acid} \\
\text{(in RBCs/plasma)}
\end{array}
$$

$$\updownarrow$$

$$
\begin{array}{ccc}
HCO_3^- & + & H^+ \\
\text{Bicarbonate ions} & & \text{Hydrogen ions} \\
\text{(buffered by Hb)} & & \text{(diffuse into plasma)}
\end{array}
$$

The disturbance in the electrical balance of plasma produced by the diffusion of bicarbonate ions out of red blood cells is corrected by the influx of other negatively charged ions, in fact chloride ions, into the blood cells (called the chloride shift). The buffering of hydrogen ions and the efflux of most of the bicarbonate ions (i.e. of base) prevents an acid–base disturbance within red blood cells and the electrical

balance between the intracellular fluid and the plasma is maintained.

When blood reaches the lung the processes are reversed. Thus:

1 Carbon dioxide dissolved in plasma and within blood cells will diffuse across the alveolar-capillary membranes reducing its partial pressure in blood and raising it in the alveoli.

2 As the partial pressure in blood decreases, carbon dioxide will be released from carbaminohaemoglobin.

3 As carbon dioxide is removed from blood, the dissociation of carbonic acid to carbon dioxide and water will be promoted. This in turn will favour the formation of more carbonic acid from bicarbonate and hydrogen ions, i.e.

$$
\begin{array}{ccc}
HCO_3^- & & H^+ \\
\text{Diffuses into} & + & \text{Released} \\
\text{red cells} & & \text{from Hb}
\end{array}
$$

$$\updownarrow$$

$$
\begin{array}{c}
H_2CO_3 \\
\text{Carbonic acid}
\end{array}
$$

$$\updownarrow$$

$$
\begin{array}{c}
CO_2 + H_2O \\
\text{Diffuses} \\
\text{into alveoli}
\end{array}
$$

The whole process is facilitated by the enzyme carbonic anhydrase and ensures that carbon dioxide is excreted.

4 As bicarbonate ions diffuse in, chloride ions move out of the red cells back into the plasma so that electrical balance is maintained.

Thus, carbon dioxide carriage by blood is very different from that of oxygen. At physiological values there is no sigmoid-shaped relationship between the partial pressure of carbon dioxide and the volume of gas being carried which would be analogous to that of the oxygen–haemoglobin dissociation curve.

Rather, the relationship is virtually linear and a slight change in partial pressure induces a pronounced change in the amount of carbon dioxide carried.

GAS EXCHANGE BETWEEN BLOOD AND TISSUES

As with the exchange of gases between lung and blood, that between blood and tissues (or rather intracellular fluid) requires the presence of favourable pressure gradients (see Figure 11.12). The partial pressure of oxygen within cells is relatively low, on average about 5.3 kPa (40 mmHg), since cells utilize oxygen in metabolic processes This is considerably lower than that of the arterial blood perfusing the tissues (13.3 kPa or 100 mmHg) so a substantial gradient exists for oxygen transfer. As in the lung, equilibration between the two compartments occurs and venous (deoxygenated) blood leaving the tissues will also have a partial pressure of oxygen which averages 5.3 kPa, although the actual value will vary from tissue to tissue according to metabolic activity.

Cells continually produce carbon dioxide through metabolism and its partial pressure in intracellular fluid will be higher than that of arterial blood – 6.0 kPa (45 mmHg) on average and 5.3 kPa (40 mmHg) respectively. Again equilibration will occur so venous blood will have an average partial pressure of carbon dioxide of 6.0 kPa. Again note the small pressure gradients required to transfer adequate amounts of this soluble gas. Such a small gradient, though, leaves little scope for adaptation to an increased partial pressure of carbon dioxide in arterial blood arising perhaps as a consequence of poor cardiac or lung function; the carbon dioxide content of intracellular fluid will rise as a consequence. This in turn will generate more carbonic acid (i.e. hydrogen ions) and disturb cell homeostasis. This problem is normally avoided by the homeostatic regulation of the partial pressure of carbon dioxide in arterial blood.

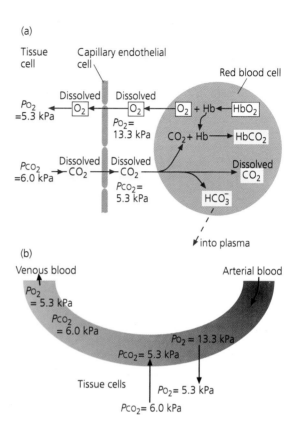

Figure 11.12 Gas exchange between blood and tissues.
(a) Summary of gas exchange. Partial pressure values are averages based on arterial and mixed venous blood.
(b) Equilibration of blood and tissue gases.
Note the large diffusional pressure gradient for O_2 but only a small gradient for CO_2, reflecting differences in solubility of the two gases.

NEURAL CONTROL OF THE RESPIRATORY SYSTEM

The partial pressures of oxygen and carbon dioxide in systemic arterial blood are usually determined by lung function. Breathing movements are largely involuntary, although they can be changed consciously. They are controlled by the rhythmical discharge of nerve impulses from the respiratory centres of the brainstem and pass down the spinal cord. Some impulses are relayed via nerves arising

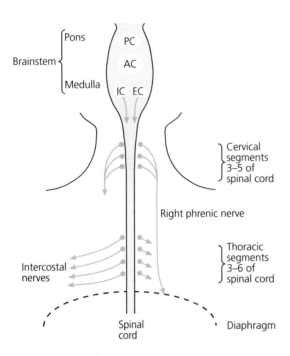

Figure 11.13 Respiratory centres and innervation of the thoracic muscles: PC, pneumotaxic centre; AC, apneustic centre; IC, inspiratory centre; EC, expiratory centre.

in the 3rd–5th cervical segments of the cord (see Chapter 13) and these nerves form the left and right phrenic nerves which innervate the diaphragm (Figure 11.13). Other impulses are relayed to nerves exiting from the 3rd–6th thoracic segments of the cord and these form the intercostal nerves which innervate the internal and external intercostal muscles. Further spinal nerves innervate the accessory muscles of inspiration and expiration.

Three major respiratory centres of the brainstem have been identified (Figure 11.13) and breathing movements result from an integration of nervous activity from these centres.

1 Inspiratory/expiratory centres of the medulla area. Impulses to the inspiratory and expiratory muscles originate from these centres. The final neural output, however, is controlled by the apneustic and pneumotaxic centres.

2 Apneustic centre of the medulla area. This centre excites the inspiratory centre and so inspiration would be continuously stimulated if its activities were not inhibited at appropriate moments in the respiratory cycle. Inhibitory impulses originate from the pneumotaxic centre (see below) and also from afferent inputs from stretch receptors present in the lung, intercostal muscles and diaphragm (which pass to the brainstem via the vagus nerve). The role of stretch receptors is illustrated by the Hering–Breuer reflex, in which overinflation of the lungs causes a cessation of activity in the nerve cells that stimulate the contraction of inspiratory muscles. During forced expiration, impulses from the apneustic centre also directly stimulate the expiratory centre, which in turn stimulates contraction of internal intercostal muscles and the accessory muscles of expiration.

3 Pneumotaxic centre of the pons area. Impulses from this centre inhibit the apneustic centre and so promote expiration.

Although stretch receptors in the thorax help to regulate breathing movements, lung function can clearly be modified by a variety of factors.

FACTORS THAT MODULATE RESPIRATORY RHYTHM

The respiratory centres of the brainstem receive neural inputs from a variety of sources including chemoreceptors, thoracic stretch receptors and higher brain centres, perhaps, but not necessarily, stimulated by sensory information from around the body (Figure 11.14).

Chemoreceptors

An essential role of the lung is to maintain homeostatically the gas composition of arterial

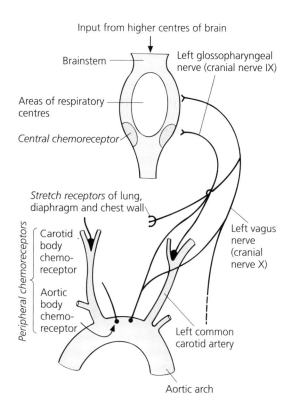

Input from higher centres of brain

Brainstem

Left glossopharyngeal nerve (cranial nerve IX)

Areas of respiratory centres

Central chemoreceptor

Stretch receptors of lung, diaphragm and chest wall

Left vagus nerve (cranial nerve X)

Peripheral chemoreceptors

Carotid body chemo- receptor

Aortic body chemo- receptor

Left common carotid artery

Aortic arch

Figure 11.14 Sensory (afferent) input into respiratory centres of brainstem.

blood, which is continuously monitored by chemoreceptors that respond to changes in either oxygen or carbon dioxide (and acidity) content.

The oxyhaemoglobin curve shows, however, that a change in the partial pressure of oxygen from the normal 13.3 kPa (100 mmHg) to about 10.5 kPa (80 mmHg) has little effect on the volume of oxygen carried by blood. This lower partial pressure normally still represents an adequate pressure gradient to drive the diffusion of oxygen into cells. For carbon dioxide, however, a similar proportionate increase in its partial pressure from 5.3 kPa to 6.4 kPa would represent an increase in carbon dioxide content from 44 to 52 ml/100 ml of blood, and a subsequent increase in the acidity of body fluids. It

is therefore not surprising that even small changes in the partial pressure of carbon dioxide provide a stimulus to change lung function, whilst only a relatively substantial decrease in that of oxygen will promote a noticeable response.

The respiratory chemoreceptors are found centrally and peripherally.

Central chemoreceptors

These receptors do not actually monitor blood gases. They monitor the acidity of the cerebrospinal fluid (Chapter 5) which is separated from the circulatory system by the 'blood–brain barrier'; this is actually a secretory epithelium (e.g. the choroid plexus, see Chapter 13). The epithelium is impervious to hydrogen ions in the blood but is freely permeable to carbon dioxide. Thus if the partial pressure of carbon dioxide is elevated in arterial blood the gas will diffuse into the cerebrospinal fluid, form carbonic acid, and so increase the acidity.

Central chemoreceptors are associated with the medulla area of the brainstem (Figure 11.14) and are therefore ideally placed to modify the outputs from the respiratory centres.

By their nature central chemoreceptors do not monitor oxygen concentrations. Also, being outside the circulatory system, their responses to an elevated blood carbon dioxide content will be relatively slow. They appear to be involved in modulating the basal respiratory rhythm and are especially important in adaptations to prolonged exposure to low oxygen environments (for example at high altitude – see below).

Peripheral chemoreceptors

These chemoreceptors are found in the walls of the aortic arch and at the bifurcation of each of the common carotid arteries in the neck (an area called the carotid body). Changes in the partial pressure of carbon dioxide (and the acidity) of arterial blood stimulates these receptors and impulses are relayed to the brainstem (Figure 11.14).

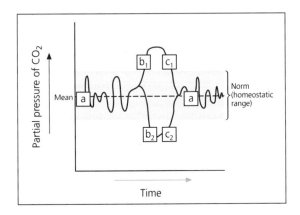

Figure 11.15 Homeostatic regulation of the partial pressure of carbon dioxide in arterial blood.
Note, this does not take into account special circumstances in which a change in CO_2 is a deliberate homeostatic response, e.g. altitude acclimatization or acid–base regulation.
a Homeostatic range for the partial pressure of CO_2, i.e. excretion = production.
b_1 Elevated partial pressure of CO_2 due to excretion < production.
b_2 Decreased partial pressure of CO_2 due to excretion > production.
c_1 Restoration of value to homeostatic range by increased excretion (lung function stimulated by chemoreceptor activation).
c_2 Restoration of value to homeostatic range by decreased excretion (lung function diminished).
Note that, at rest, production rates of CO_2 are not homeostatically altered.
d Maintained elevation in partial pressure of CO_2 due to excretion << production as a consequence of inadequate alveolar ventilation (due to lung disease or respiratory centre depression) or of venous blood being shunted away from lungs. Causes excessive acidity of body fluids.
e Excessive decrease in partial pressure of CO_2 due to excretion >> production as a consequence of lung disease or hyperventilation due to pain or anxiety. Causes excessive alkalinity of body fluids.

Peripheral chemoreceptors respond rapidly to changes in the partial pressure of carbon dioxide in arterial blood and will quickly adjust breathing movements. They also respond to a modest decrease in the oxygen content of arterial blood but small reductions in the partial pressure of oxygen have little effect. It would be incorrect, however, to assume that changes in blood oxygen have only a weak involvement in the regulation of lung function. If small degrees of hypoxaemia are accompanied by an increased partial pressure of carbon dioxide, the respiratory response to the elevated carbon dioxide is potentiated as the chemoreceptors become sensitized.

The role of chemoreceptors in the homeostatic regulation of the partial pressure of carbon dioxide is illustrated in Figure 11.15.

Inputs from other receptors

Numerous receptors influence respiratory movements when stimulated – some only acutely. These are muscle/joint proprioreceptors stimulated in exercise, chemoreceptors of the nasal mucosa, larynx, and trachea stimulated by airborne irritants, touch receptors of the pharynx stimulated by the presence of food, and pain receptors.

All produce reflex changes in respiratory movements. Exercise-induced changes are discussed below, but other stimuli may promote:

1 Sneezing – a short inspiration followed by a forced expiration with the glottis open.

2 Swallowing – inhibits breathing movements.

3 Coughing – short inspiration followed by a series of forced expirations against a closed glottis. Sudden opening of the glottis releases the high pressure developed in airways and carries away the irritants.

4 Hiccoughing – spasmodic contractions of the diaphragm with the glottis closed.

Psychic and emotional factors

The respiratory centres of the brainstem also receive impulses from higher centres of the brain. We can therefore alter breathing movements voluntarily, control expiration in singing or speech, inspire deeply with spasmodic expirations in weeping and laughing, prolong expiration in sighing, inspire deeply in yawning and produce rapid movements in fear and excitement. The functions of many of these responses are not understood.

RESPIRATORY ADAPTATIONS TO EXERCISE AND ALTITUDE

Exercise

Oxygen consumption and carbon dioxide production in heavy exercise may be of the order of 4 l/min (the maximal oxygen consumption rate is called the V_{O_2}max) compared with 250 ml/min and 200 ml/min respectively at rest. Increased oxygen demands during exercise, and increased carbon dioxide excretion, are met by increasing the alveolar ventilation rate through increased breath volume and breathing rate. In this way as much as 100 litres or more of air may be inspired per minute (compared with about 6 litres at rest).

An increased breath volume is made possible because the inspiratory and expiratory reserve volumes are utilized. This increased ventilation results from a modification of outputs from the respiratory centres and must also include an overriding of afferent impulses from stretch receptors within the thorax so that greater inflation can be achieved.

Efficient ventilation during exercise is also facilitated by a reduction in airway resistance. Earlier in this chapter it was described how airway resistance is low, and that the nasal cavity and pharynx provide the greatest site of resistance. Mouth breathing is utilized in exercise and this bypasses the nasal cavity. The smooth muscle of the bronchioles is also relaxed to dilate the terminal airways, and this is induced by the actions of the sympathetic nervous system (and adrenaline), which is stimulated during physical activity.

As a result of respiratory changes the average gas composition of arterial blood does not alter during exercise and this helps to maintain cellular homeostasis, although venous composition will change as tissues use more oxygen and produce more carbon dioxide. What promotes the increased ventilation is still unclear, but the response must result from a stimulation of receptors somewhere in the body. Possible afferent pathways include nerve impulses from muscle or joint receptors, from chemoreceptors within the pulmonary circulation and from potassium-sensitive receptors, since potassium ions are released from exercising muscle cells and their concentration in blood rises sharply during exercise.

Altitude

The atmospheric pressure falls on ascending from sea level, which means that the partial pressure of oxygen also decreases. This in turn will lower the partial pressure of oxygen in alveolar gas and hence in arterial blood and tissues (i.e. hypoxia will result). Note though that arterial carbon dioxide content will be unaffected since even at sea level its partial pressure in air is negligible. Thus, any increased ventilation promoted by the hypoxia (detected by peripheral chemoreceptors) will be quickly reversed as the elevated ventilation removes too much carbon dioxide (chemoreceptors are particularly sensitive to changes in carbon dioxide).

With adaptation, however, the hypoxia begins to exert a dominant influence on respiration and the body begins to tolerate the consequential decrease in carbon dioxide content. Adaptation occurs because the buffering capacity of the cerebrospinal fluid (which bathes the central chemoreceptors) is altered. As a result a change in carbon dioxide content does not alter the fluid's pH (see Chapter 5 for a discussion of buffers) and so the receptors are not stimulated. This means that the hypoxic stimulation of the peripheral chemoreceptors can now be expressed as an increased lung ventilation.

Other adaptations to altitude include an elevation in the 2,3DPG content of red blood cells, which facilitates the unloading of oxygen in the tissues, and an increased red blood cell count (hypoxia stimulates the release of erythropoietin). The additional red cells make more haemoglobin available to carry oxygen. Total lung capacity may also be increased.

Role of the respiratory system in homeostasis

All cells require oxygen and must excrete carbon dioxide; the respiratory system therefore plays an essential role in all tissue functions. Adequate gas exchange requires an integration of respiratory and cardiovascular functions, coordinated by the nervous system, and an appropriate blood gas composition. Disturbance of normal oxygen uptake will therefore produce widespread changes in organ function, with those having either a high metabolic rate or a poor capacity to resort to anaerobic metabolism being the first affected.

Thus neural coordination and heart function will quickly be affected, and these in turn will exacerbate the hypoxia of other tissues.

Inadequate carbon dioxide excretion will promote an acidosis due to the accumulation of carbonic acid in body fluids. Hydrogen ions are highly reactive and one of their major adverse effects is to disrupt the structure and actions of enzymes. Widespread changes in cellular homeostasis will result, causing a depression of systemic functions, leading to further homeostatic disturbance.

Examples of homeostatic control system failures and principles of correction

Disturbances of blood gas composition promote inadequate oxygenation of tissues (hypoxia) and/or deficient or excessive carbon dioxide concentrations (called hypocapnia and hypercapnia respectively). Tissue hypoxia may be due to inadequate perfusion with blood (and is called stagnant hypoxia), to low haemoglobin content of blood (called anaemic hypoxia), or to inadequate uptake of oxygen by the lungs (called hypoxic hypoxia). Hypercapnia results in excessive generation of carbonic acid and so promotes acidosis, whereas hypocapnia induces an alkalosis. Hypercapnia is frequently, but not always, associated with hypoxia, particularly stagnant and hypoxic hypoxia.

The homeostatic regulation of the circulatory system, and of blood haemoglobin content, are described in other chapters. This section is particularly concerned with primary disorders of lung function.

HYPOVENTILATION AND HYPERVENTILATION

Alveolar ventilation is normally adjusted to match the respiratory needs of the body. Underventilation (hypoventilation), resulting for example from brainstem depression, a primary lung disorder, spinal cord damage between the level of entry and exit of respiratory nerves and the brainstem, damage to the respiratory peripheral nerves or the respiratory muscles themselves, or to excess pleural fluid (pleural effusion) causes increased alveolar partial pressure of carbon dioxide but a decreased partial pressure of oxygen. Similarly, overventilation (hyperventilation) resulting, for example, from extreme anxiety states, reduces the partial pressure of carbon dioxide but raises that of oxygen. Systemic arterial gas pressures will also exhibit these changes, although hyperventilation will hardly increase the amount of oxygen carried by blood since haemoglobin is normally saturated anyway. Treatment depends upon the underlying cause. A primary lung disorder may necessitate the use of oxygen-enriched mixtures, or even artificial ventilation, to alter the composition of alveolar gases. Keeping the subject upright also helps to ensure that diaphragmatic movements are not impaired by abdominal viscera.

OBSTRUCTIVE AIRWAY DISEASE

Asthma and bronchitis are common examples of disorders in which airway inflammation, excessive airway secretions, or bronchoconstriction, increases airway resistance. The additional resistance is overcome by increasing the inspiratory effort. Expiration at rest is passive in health and the elevated resistance necessitates the use of muscular contraction to generate sufficient intrathoracic pressure to force gases out of the lung. Obstructive airway disease, therefore, increases the energy required simply to maintain breathing movements.

In chronic airway disease, the severity of the increased resistance prevents adequate expiration, leading to an increased functional residual capacity and, consequently, a decreased inspiratory reserve. Oxygen content of alveolar gas declines, whilst that of carbon dioxide increases, and similar changes are observed in the blood. There is a reduced capacity to increase the breath volume during physical exertion, with the result that the individual fatigues easily.

Conditions may become so severe that areas of tissue become necrotic. Thus, in emphysema, airways may collapse during expiration, exacerbating the problem. Loss of functioning alveoli increases the physiological dead space.

Reversal of the cause of obstruction, for example by using bronchodilator or anti-inflammatory drugs, may alleviate acute problems. Severe disorders may necessitate ventilation using gases enriched with oxygen. With chronic disease, however, care must be taken not to remove carbon dioxide too rapidly from blood as these individuals exhibit adaptation to the hypercapnia induced by their condition. The elevated carbon dioxide content of blood becomes a new 'set-point' about which breathing movements are regulated. Thus, returning the blood gas composition to 'normal' will be interpreted as hypocapnia. Correction of hypoxia, and the induction of hypocapnia, will therefore remove the patient's stimuli to breathe.

RESTRICTIVE LUNG DISORDERS

Restrictive disorders, such as asbestosis and silicosis, prevent the normal inflation of the lung and so are primarily disorders of inspiration. Reduction of lung elasticity as a consequence of lung fibrosis ('scarring') causes a reduction in compliance and a decreased vital capacity. Inadequate ventilation of alveoli disturbs the alveolar gas composition, resulting in oxygen deficiency and carbon dioxide excess.

VENTILATION/PERFUSION INEQUALITIES: SHUNTS

Shunts may result from an anatomical defect, such as a heart septal defect, which causes some venous blood to bypass the lungs, or by poor ventilation/perfusion matching by the lungs, which produces a similar effect. The main problem is that hypoxaemia is induced with consequences for tissues. The greater the shunt effect the more severe the consequences. Treatment depends upon the causes but ventilation/perfusion mismatch may necessitate the use of artificial ventilation, including positive pressure ventilation, in an attempt to improve lung function.

ADULT RESPIRATORY DISTRESS SYNDROME

This is a condition in which gas exchange in the lungs is impaired because of the presence of exudate (pulmonary oedema) in the alveoli, thus increasing the thickness of the diffusion barrier. Hypoxia results. The precise cause of this condition is still unclear but it is frequently observed after a severe trauma. Artificial ventilation will be required to raise the alveolar partial pressure of oxygen and so increase the gradient for diffusion to occur. The best means to remove the accumulated fluid is debatable. Colloid infusions may be used to increase the oncotic pressure of plasma, thus withdrawing fluid from the lungs by osmosis, but may increase blood viscosity and impair blood flow through the lungs.

Infant respiratory distress syndrome is characterized by a deficiency of surfactant, leading to alveolar collapse.

PNEUMONIA

This arises as a consequence of viral or bacterial infection of the alveoli. Inflammation of alveolar cells occurs, and fluid exudate accumulates. Both interfere with the alveolar-capillary membranes and impair gas exchange. Treatment is largely aimed at reducing the inflammation and curing the infection.

Summary

1 The carriage of oxygen (O_2) and carbon dioxide (CO_2) to and from tissues, and the exchange of these gases with air, is vital for life.

2 When a person is at rest, 5–6 litres of air are taken into, and breathed out of the lungs each minute. Physical exercise may increase this to 80–100 l/min by increasing the depth of each breath and the rate of breathing. Such changes in lung ventilation ensure that the gas composition of systemic arterial blood remains almost constant.

3 The amount of energy required to maintain breathing movements is minimized by low airway resistance and a high compliance (elasticity).

4 The 'vital capacity' represents the maximum volume of gas which can be taken into the lungs, and expired from them, in a single breath. The vital capacity is used clinically to assess airway resistance and compliance.

5 Gas exchange occurs across the lung alveoli; the rest of the airway comprises a 'dead space'. This, together with the volume of gas left in the lungs after expiration, constitutes the 'functional residual capacity' or FRC. Inspired air mixes with the FRC gas and produces a slight enrichment of the O_2 content and a slight depletion of the CO_2 content.

6 Gases diffuse down pressure gradients. The air in the lung consists of a mixture of gases and the partial pressure exerted by each gas is physiologically more significant than the total pressure of the whole mixture. Lung ventilation ensures that the partial pressure gradients are conducive to the diffusion of oxygen into blood, and of carbon dioxide out of blood.

7 Alveolar gas composition and blood perfusion varies throughout the lungs and the partial pressures of gases in systemic arterial blood represent the mean of those in the alveoli after inspiration.

8 Oxygen is poorly soluble in water and is carried in the blood combined with the pigment haemoglobin. The O_2 is released from the pigment in tissues, where the partial pressure of O_2 is reduced by utilization of the gas. The release is facilitated by conditions associated with high rates of metabolism, such as high temperature and low pH, and this is called the Bohr shift.

9 Carbon dioxide is a soluble gas and is carried from tissues dissolved in blood, or in combination with water to form bicarbonate ions. Some is combined with haemoglobin. The lower partial pressure of CO_2 found in the lungs promotes the conversion of bicarbonate to CO_2, the release of CO_2 from haemoglobin, and diffusion of the gas out of the blood.

10 Lung ventilation is controlled by neural activity from centres within the brainstem. The centres are modulated by neural inputs from various areas, in particular from chemoreceptors in the arterial system and in the brainstem. These especially monitor pH and so provide a means of evaluating the CO_2 content of blood and cerebrospinal fluid, since the gas forms carbonic acid in water. Other inputs originate from stretch receptors in the lung, from higher brain centres and from joint receptors.

11 Some homeostatic set-points are altered during exercise, and following ascent to high altitude, and promote the respiratory changes observed.

12 Disorders of lung function most frequently result from increases in airway resistance, loss of lung compliance, ventilation/perfusion equalities, alveolar inflammation, and pulmonary oedema.

Review Questions

1 Distinguish between the different types of respiration.

2 How is gaseous exchange accomplished:
(a) at the alveoli–pulmonary capillary interface?
(b) at the systemic capillary–tissue fluid–cellular interfaces?

3 Discuss how speech and coughing relate to breathing.

4 What is the relation between alveolar pressure and atmospheric pressure during inspiration?

5 What is the relation between alveolar pressure and atmospheric pressure at end-expiration?

6 Define:
(a) tidal volume, (b) vital capacity, (c) inspiratory reserve volume, (d) residual volume.

7 Which of the lung volumes given below can be measured using a simple spirometer?
(a) Tidal volume.
(b) Vital capacity.
(c) Inspiratory reserve volume.
(d) Residual volume.

8 What are the average volumes in mls of the tidal volume, vital capacity, inspiratory reserve volume and expiratory reserve volume?

9 Which of the following conditions in the red cell shifts the O_2 dissociation curve to the right?
(a) Rise in P_{CO_2}.
(b) Reduction in temperature.
(c) Reduction in pH.

10 What happens to oxygen–haemoglobin formation when CO_2 is given off by the blood in the lungs?

11 What is the ratio of hydrogen carbonate to carbonic acid if the arterial blood is to be maintained at pH 7.4?

12 What is meant by the ventilation/perfusion ratio?

13 What causes:
(a) a high ventilation/perfusion ratio?
(b) a low ventilation/perfusion ratio?

14 List the factors which influence the transport of O_2 from the atmosphere to the tissue cells.

15 What are the respiratory adaptations to:
(a) hypoxia, (b) hypercapnia, (c) hypocapnia, (d) exercise.

16 Which of the following factors is the most important control of ventilation?
(a) pH. (b) P_{CO_2}. (c) P_{O_2}.

17 In what circumstances is O_2 therapy used?

18 How does smoking affect lung function?

19 What happens to airway resistance in the following conditions?
(a) Bronchoconstriction.
(b) Airway obstruction.
(c) Increased lung volume.
(d) Emphysema.
(e) Pneumothorax.

20 Distinguish between obstructive and restrictive lung diseases.

The kidneys: Excretion and body fluid homeostasis

Introduction: relation of excretion to cellular homeostasis, and routes of excretion

Overview of the anatomy and physiology of the kidneys

Details of kidney physiology and body fluid homeostasis

Role of excretion in homeostasis

Examples of homeostatic control system failures and principles of correction

Summary

Review questions

Introduction: relation of excretion to cellular homeostasis, and routes of excretion

Chapter 5 described how the biochemical reactions which constitute cell metabolism, largely take place mainly in the aqueous environment provided by the intracellular and extracellular fluids. The composition of these fluids must be homeostatically maintained appropriate to cell function. In the broadest sense this means:

1 ensuring the availability of metabolic substrates;

2 removal of metabolic 'waste' products;

3 maintenance of an appropriate water content, hence cell volume;

4 maintenance of appropriate electrolyte concentrations;

5 maintenance of appropriate metabolic enzyme availability.

The provision of metabolic substrates requires the functional integration of the major physiological homeostatic systems and their roles are considered in other chapters. This chapter is concerned with describing how metabolic products ('wastes') and substances absorbed from the gut in excess of the body's utilization and storage capacities are removed from the body.

EXCRETION, DEFECATION, AND SECRETION

Excretion may be defined as the processes by which substances are eliminated from the body in urine, faeces, sweat, and expired gases. All contain substances that have been derived from body fluids. Even faeces contain various substances, such as bile salts and bile pigments, which have been added during the formation of 'stools' in the bowel. The formation of faecal stools, and the process of faecal elimination, called defecation, are described in detail in Chapter 7. Some faecal material, that is indigestible components such as fibre, does not come into contact with intracellular metabolism and this distinguishes them from excretory materials.

Secretion is the extrusion of substances and/or water across cell membranes into extracellular fluid. This may involve the fusion of intracellular vesicles with the membrane followed by the release of the vesicular contents, as in the secretion of hormones, enzymes, or neurotransmitters. Alternatively, it may involve the transport of substances using membrane carrier processes, for example into forming urine within the kidney, the forming of sweat within sweat glands, or the forming of faecal stools in the lumen of the bowel, and these may ultimately be excreted from the body. Secretion, therefore, may play an integral role in the determination of the final composition of excreted material.

Excretory losses may be homeostatically controlled, or they may be 'obligatory'. An example of the latter is the continued production of urine even when we are dehydrated. In addition, water will always be lost via sweat, especially if we are hot, and as water vapour in respiratory expiration. Another example of 'obligatory' loss is the presence of electrolytes in urine, sweat, and faeces which, though of variable composition, will always contain salts. Obligatory losses only contribute to homeostasis under normal conditions. When there is already a homeostatic imbalance involving a depletion of body fluids, such as dehydration or hypovolaemia (low blood volume), such losses are detrimental.

WHY EXCRETE?

Metabolism produces a variety of substances which cannot be utilized (i.e. used in their principal form by the body, or stored or transferred into other components of the body) and which, if allowed to accumulate, will eventually disturb cell processes. Two major 'waste' products are carbon dioxide (from carbohydrate metabolism) and urea (from protein metabolism). Both are lipid-soluble and so their passage from cells is not hindered by the cell membrane. They are also highly soluble in water and will readily dissolve in body fluids. Their exit from cells is by diffusion but this will only be efficient if their concentrations in extracellular fluids, primarily in tissue fluid, are kept correspondingly low. Creatinine is another 'waste' substance that is produced in significant quantities. It is a product of creatine (an energy source) metabolism in muscle and must be transported across the cell membrane since it is not lipid-soluble. The rate at which it leaves muscle cells will still be influenced, however, by its extracellular concentration.

The term 'waste' might also be used to describe substances produced by cells which, although functionally important, must be removed once their action is complete. Hormones, for example, must be removed from body fluids, or at least be inactivated, to stop their activities as required. Inactivation is carried out in the liver and the products are usually excreted.

In addition to products of metabolism, our body fluids are also continually influenced by substances absorbed from our diet. Many of these are in excess of body requirement and some may not be utilized at all. For example, ingested carbohydrates and lipids that are in excess of needs are placed into stores; little is normally excreted. In contrast, other dietary

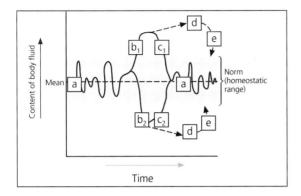

Figure 12.1 General homeostatic schema in relation to excretory needs.

a Fluctuations of solute concentrations in body fluid within the 'normal' range.

b_1 Increase in solute concentration due to dietary intake and/or metabolic production in excess of excretion rate.

b_2 Decrease in solute concentration due to excretion being in excess of dietary intake/metabolic production.

c_1 and c_2 Restoration of solute concentration to within homeostatic range by appropriate changes in intake/metabolic production and/or excretory rate.

d Failure of homeostatic controls leading to persistently disturbed body fluid composition.

e Clinical intervention to change excretion rate, intake, and/or metabolic production.

constituents such as water-soluble vitamins, minerals, and water cannot be stored to any degree and therefore any excess must be removed from the body.

Thus the solutes dissolved in our body fluids are continually being added to via metabolism or via dietary uptake. The maintenance of body fluid composition necessary for intracellular

homeostasis, therefore, is dependent upon excretion of the excesses, and requires the rate of excretion of each substance to be equal to the rate at which it is added to the body fluids (see Figure 12.1). In other words, excretion rates must be homeostatically regulated.

ROUTES OF EXCRETION

It has already been noted that there are various routes for excreting substances. In summary the substances excreted by each route are:

1 The gut (faeces): bile salts, bile pigments, small amounts of electrolytes, and water.

2 The kidneys (urine): metabolic byproducts (e.g. urea, creatinine), electrolytes, and water.

3 The lungs (expired gases): carbon dioxide, and water vapour.

4 The skin (sweat): electrolytes, water, and some metabolic byproducts (e.g. urea).

The functions of the gut, lungs, and skin are covered elsewhere in this book. The aim of this chapter is to examine in detail the role of the kidneys in maintaining body fluid homeostasis. It has already been noted that excretion must be appropriate to bodily needs and further discussion must therefore also include how kidney function is itself regulated so that fluid homeostasis is maintained.

Overview of the anatomy and physiology of the kidneys

The kidneys are paired organs situated in the superior and posterior aspects of the abdomen wall, lying outside the peritoneum on either side of the vertebral column and embedded in adipose tissue. Each weighs approximately

140 g and may be described as being bean-shaped (though some beans are kidney-shaped!) The right kidney lies a little lower than the left as a consequence of displacement by the liver (Figure 12.2a).

autonomic nerves and a ureter (Figure 12.2b). The latter transports urine to the urinary bladder for storage prior to urination, or micturition.

The function of efferent renal nerves has been debated for years. Certainly neural activity can cause intense vasoconstriction following extensive haemorrhage as part of the homeostatic response to restore systemic arterial blood pressure, or during heavy exercise when blood is redirected toward exercising muscles. Nerve activity can also be recorded under less traumatic circumstances, however, and has been shown to influence the urinary excretion of sodium, although transplanted kidneys, which are denervated, do not exhibit a deficiency in sodium handling, presumably because of compensatory mechanisms.

Afferent renal nerves may provide sensory information which enables the function of each kidney to be matched.

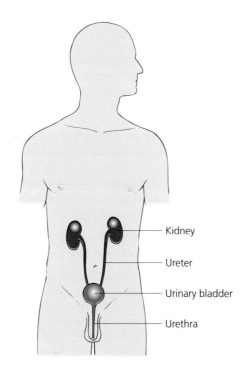

(a)

(b)

Figure 12.2 The urinary system. (a) Components of the urinary system. (b) Renal vessels and nerves.

Each kidney receives blood via a direct branch of the abdominal aorta, called a renal artery, and is supplied with efferent (motor) branches of the autonomic (mainly sympathetic) nervous system. Leaving each kidney is a renal vein, which drains directly into the inferior vena cava, afferent (sensory)

COMPOSITION OF URINE

Urine is characteristically yellow/amber in colour because of the presence of pigments, called urochromes, derived largely from the metabolism of bile (Chapter 7). The colour varies with diet (e.g. the reddish colour after eating beetroot) and also the urine concentration (from a deep yellow to almost colourless). Fresh urine is normally clear but may be cloudy due to the presence of mucin secreted from the linings of the urinary tract.

Urine also has a characteristic odour but on standing develops an unpleasant smell of ammonia as urea within it undergoes bacterial decomposition.

As might be expected, urine is a complex solution of various ions and organic solutes. 'Typical' urine composition is shown in Table 12.1 and for reference is compared with that of the body fluid from which it is formed, the blood plasma. Such values for urine must be considered only as a guide, since urine volume

Table 12.1 Comparison of solute concentrations in plasma, urine, and the glomerular filtrate

	Plasma (mmol/l)	Urine* (mmol/l)	Glomerular filtrate (mmol/l)
Sodium	140	200	140
Potassium	4	50	4
Calcium	1.3†	5	1.3
Chloride	105	150	113
Bicarbonate	25	2	27
Glucose	4	Trace	4
Urea	4	250	4
	(g/l)	(g/l)	(g/l)
Protein	70	Trace	0.2

*These are only representative values. Concentrations vary according to conditions. See text for details.
†Represents ionized calcium, not total (approximately 50% of calcium in plasma is bound to proteins).

and concentration vary considerably according to our state of hydration, and also because the concentrations of many solutes may change independently. The comparison is useful, because it illustrates how the concentrations of many electrolytes are enriched in urine, as also are those of nitrogenous waste. The latter account for a considerably greater proportion of the total solute concentration in urine than in plasma, and this emphasizes the importance of urine as a route to excrete these substances.

Urine should contain only trace amounts of blood cells, perhaps 100 red cells per ml of urine, compared with 500 million per ml of blood. An increase in the numbers present is indicative of structural damage to the kidney. Similarly, urine is normally virtually protein- and glucose-free, compared with concentrations of 70 g/litre and 5 mmol/l in blood plasma, respectively, and an increase would again indicate underlying disease.

Bearing in mind that urine is initially formed from blood plasma, there is clearly considerable modification of its composition during its formation. In order to understand how this can occur, and what influences such changes, it is important that the reader understands the anatomy of the kidney and how kidneys function. Prior to reading the next sections, it would be advantageous for the reader to consult Chapter 2 regarding the processes which govern the movement of solutes and water across epithelia and cell membranes.

Filtration

Urine is initially formed as an ultrafiltrate of blood plasma within the outer, or cortical, layer of the kidney (Figure 12.3a), that is to say a fluid is formed which will contain water and solute molecules other than those which are large, such as proteins (though smaller proteins may gain access). Blood cells are retained within the circulatory system. The composition of the filtrate will therefore be in many ways similar to that of plasma (see Table 12.1) but very different from that of the final urine.

The filtrate is produced across microscopic filters, some 100–150 μm in diameter, called glomeruli (glomerulus, singular; Figure 12.4a), of which there are over a million in each kidney. Each glomerulus is basically a tuft of blood capillaries which provides a large surface area available for filtration; the total area for both kidneys is of the order of 2 m² (about the size of a large bath tub). The filtrate is produced into individual cup-like receptacles called Bowman's capsules, each of which forms the terminus of a kidney tubule (renal tubule or nephron). The tubule extends into the kidney mass. A single glomerulus and its Bowman's capsule is sometimes referred to as a Malpighian corpuscle. The filter itself consists of two layers of cells: the endothelial cells of the blood capillaries and the epithelial cells of Bowman's capsule, and their basement membranes. The capillary endothelium is penetrated by pores, as also is the Bowman's capsule epithelium. It is these pores, together with the matrix of the basement membranes, which allow the passage of smaller solute molecules (such as electrolytes, glucose) but prevent the passage of large molecules and blood cells.

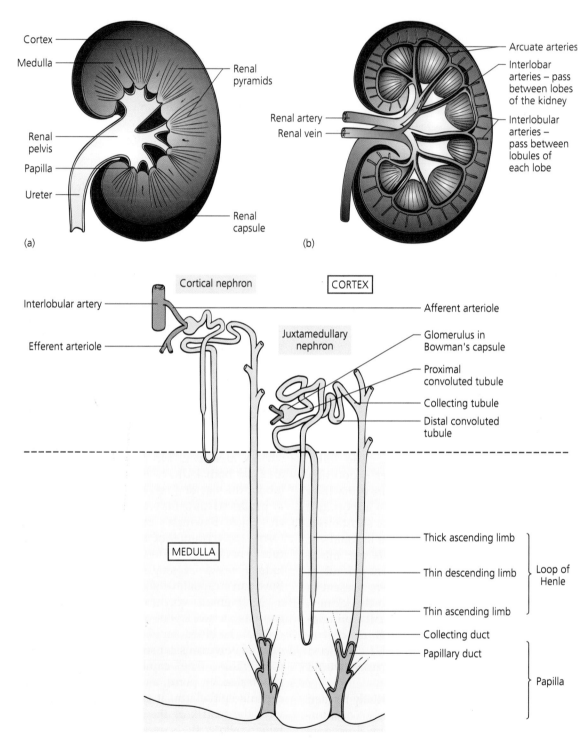

Figure 12.3 (a) General anatomy of the kidney. (b) Vasculature of the kidney. (c) Anatomical segmentation of the renal tubule. Note the two types of nephron – one with a short loop which does not extend into the medulla (cortical nephrons) and one with very long loops which extend deep into the medulla (juxtamedullary nephrons).

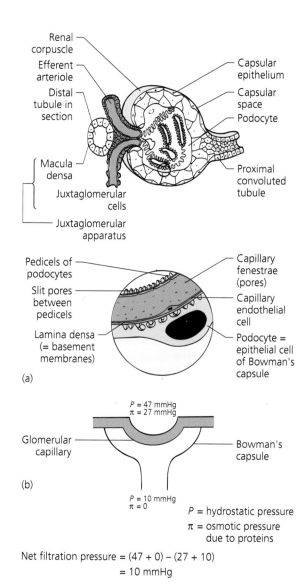

Figure 12.4 The renal glomerulus: (a) structure; (b) forces promoting filtration.

Net filtration pressure = (47 + 0) − (27 + 10)
= 10 mmHg

P = hydrostatic pressure
π = osmotic pressure due to proteins

P = 47 mmHg
π = 27 mmHg

P = 10 mmHg
π = 0

Reabsorption and secretion

Modification of the glomerular filtrate occurs as a result of transport processes present within the cell membranes of renal tubular cells.

Reabsorption is a term used to describe the movement of solutes and water out of the lumen of the tubule and back into the circulatory system. This is distinct from 'absorption', as applied to the gut, in which the uptake of substances into the blood plasma occurs for the first time. In the kidney the fluid in the tubule has already been produced from plasma. Both processes are homeostatic control mechanisms which help to regulate the solute and water composition of the extracellular and intracellular fluids.

Secretion was defined earlier in this chapter. In the kidney the term is usually used to indicate the addition of substances into the tubule fluid from cells lining the tubules. These secretions are constituents of the final urine.

The concentrations of urinary constituents are determined by how much is filtered, reabsorbed and/or secreted by the tubules. Some substances, such as creatinine, are exclusively filtered but are not reabsorbed or secreted to any degree, and so their excretion in urine is determined by how efficiently the kidneys are filtering. This is clinically useful because creatinine excretion can be used to determine the rate of glomerular filtration (see 'clearance methodology' later).

On the other hand, potassium ions filtered by the kidney are almost entirely reabsorbed by early parts of the renal tubule, and the potassium which appears in urine has largely been secreted into later tubule segments. The rate of secretion is appropriate to the body's needs to excrete the ion and can be so efficient that more potassium can be excreted in urine than could possibly be the case if filtration alone was relied upon. Similarly, some of the organic acid byproducts of metabolism are secreted into early tubule segments and this contributes to their efficient excretion.

Many other solutes in the filtrate, such as sodium ions, are not secreted to any degree by the tubules. Rather their excretion is finally determined by how much has been reabsorbed from the filtrate as it passes along the tubule. For many solutes this rate of reabsorption is also adjustable according to needs.

STRUCTURAL AND FUNCTIONAL ASPECTS OF THE RENAL TUBULE OR NEPHRON

The renal tubule can be subdivided into segments of different anatomical arrangement and functions. These are (1) the glomerulus/ Bowman's capsule, (2) the proximal tubule, (3) the loop of Henle, (4) the distal tubule, and (5) the collecting ducts (see Figure 12.3c).

Glomerulus/Bowman's capsule

The structure of the glomerular filter was described earlier. The rate at which fluid is passed across the glomeruli into the Bowman's capsule is called the glomerular filtration rate, abbreviated as GFR. For both kidneys the total GFR is about 125 ml/min in young adults, which is equivalent to about 180 l/day. This is a considerable volume and requires the presence of a force sufficient to drive the process. This is provided by the pressure gradient which exists across the filter, largely due to the hydrostatic pressure of blood in the capillaries.

The driving, or filtration pressure, in the capillaries is, to a certain extent, counteracted by the colloidal osmotic pressure generated by plasma proteins, most of which are not filtered from plasma. This is the same situation as occurs in other capillary beds. However, the hydrostatic ¨pressure in those capillaries declines along the vessel until it is exceeded by the colloidal osmotic pressure, with the result that most of the fluid exuded out of the capillary in the early stages is now drawn back into it again (see Chapter 5). This reversal of fluid movement is not observed in the kidney because the hydrostatic pressure is maintained at a much higher value than in capillaries elsewhere. The higher pressure is achieved by the presence of an efferent arteriole as blood exits the glomerulus, in addition to the conventional arteriole as blood enters (the afferent arteriole). The resistance to flow provided by

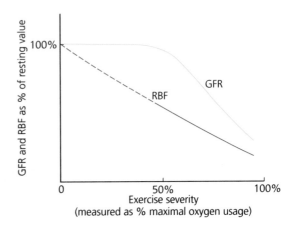

Figure 12.5 Comparison of changes in glomerular filtration rate (GFR) and renal blood flow (RBF) during exercise. Note the maintenance of a 'normal' GFR during exercise up to about 50% of maximal oxygen uptake.

the narrowed efferent arteriole prevents a pressure drop in the glomerulus. The constrictor activities of, for example, sympathetic nerves on the efferent arteriole also helps to maintain the glomerular capillary pressure, and hence the filtration function of the kidney, during moderate exercise when blood flow to the kidney is reduced (Figure 12.5).

The maintenance of a high rate of filtration requires a high degree of blood flow to the kidney. Together the two kidneys receive 1200 ml of blood per minute and this represents about 20% of the entire cardiac output (remember that the kidneys comprise only about 0.4% of body weight). Of this blood, some 700 ml will be plasma, the remaining volume being occupied by blood cells. Thus the kidneys filter out 125/700, or approximately 20%, of the plasma flowing through them. This is called the filtration fraction.

The rate at which glomerular filtrate is formed under normal circumstances is thought to be kept virtually constant under the precise control exerted by the kidney itself; it is autoregulated (auto- = self). Homeostatic maintenance of the glomerular filtration rate requires regulatory responses to be made to any change in the rate. The precise mechanism

Table 12.2 Illustration of the renal responses necessary to maintain sodium and water balance should the glomerular filtration rate (GFR) change

GFR	Urine volume	Volume reabsorbed	Na+ filtered	Na+ excreted	Na+ reabsorbed	Creatinine filtered (= creatinine excreted)
(ml/min)	(ml/min)	(ml/min)	(mmol/min)	(mmol/min)	(mmol/min)	(mmol/min)
Normal						
125	1	124	17.5	0.15	17.35	12.5
Elevated						
160	1	159	22.4	0.15	22.25	16.0
Difference from normal		+35			+4.9	+3.5
Decreased						
90	1	89	12.6	0.15	12.45	9.0
Difference from normal		−35			−4.9	−3.5

Note the elevated GFR means an increased energy cost if the kidneys are to retain additional water and sodium in order to maintain water/sodium homeostasis.
Note the decreased GFR may seem to represent an energy saving as less water/sodium needs to be reabsorbed. There are consequences, though, for substances dependent upon filtration for their excretion, e.g. creatinine.
The need for homeostatic control of the GFR is evident.

responsible is still debatable and may involve detecting a change in capillary hydrostatic pressure, a change in the rate of renal blood flow, or a change in the composition and volume of tubule fluid as a consequence of a changed rate of fluid flow within the tubules. The importance of keeping the filtration rate near constant is illustrated in Table 12.2.

Proximal convoluted tubule

The filtrate produced by the glomerulus enters the renal tubule from the Bowman's capsule, the first segment of which is called the proximal tubule. The major modification of the filtrate composition and volume begins in this segment. The term 'proximal' describes its position, being close to the centralized structure, in this case the Bowman's capsule.

Most of the proximal tubule is convoluted and so this section is called the proximal convoluted segment or pars convoluta. The convolutions increase its length and, therefore, the surface area available for reabsorption and secretion. The convoluted section is found in the cortical region of the kidney (see Figure 12.3), and continues as a straight section, called the pars recta, which takes the tubule toward the medulla region. The surface area of the proximal tubule is further increased by the presence of finger-like microvilli on the inner or luminal surface of the tubule cells. The simple columnar epithelium of the proximal tubule also has other features related to its function. In particular, it is 'leaky' to water and is rich in cell transport mechanisms which, together with the large surface area, help to increase its capacity to reabsorb fluids and solute from the filtrate. Some 80% of the filtrate is reabsorbed by the time the filtrate has reached the end of the proximal tubule.

Some solutes, such as glucose, amino acids, and small proteins, are almost completely reabsorbed by the proximal tubule. As a result the final urine is virtually free of these solutes and this is important if these valuable nutrients are not to be wasted. Other solutes, such as organic acids produced by metabolism, are secreted into the tubule fluid by the tubule cells. In general the reabsorption of solutes and water occur in the same proportion and so the osmotic pressure of the fluid in the proximal tubule remains much the same as that of plasma.

In contrast the final excreted urine can be very dilute (with an osmotic pressure less than that of plasma) or very concentrated (with an osmotic pressure far in excess of that of plasma). The dilution and concentrating processes occur in tubule segments beyond the proximal tubule.

Loop of Henle

Fluid enters the loop of Henle from the proximal tubule (see Figure 12.3). The loop is a hairpin-like structure which carries the remnants of the filtrate into the medullary region of the kidney via its descending limb and thence back out into the cortex again via its ascending limb. In fact the loops penetrate the medullary region to varying degrees; about 15% of tubules have loops which extend deep into the medulla (juxtamedullary nephrons), whilst most of the remainder do not penetrate it at all (cortical nephrons). In contrast, none of the tubule loops of the aquatic beaver (which does not have problems of dehydration) penetrates the medulla, whereas those of desert rodents are all very long indeed. This variation between species gives a clue to the importance of the loop of Henle in water conservation and its function will be considered in detail later. Two important features need to be highlighted at this point, however:

1 Fluid passing down the descending limb of the loop becomes more concentrated as water is reabsorbed (by osmosis) from the tubule and solutes (mainly sodium chloride) diffuse into it.

2 Fluid leaving the ascending limb of the loop always has an osmotic pressure less than that of plasma as electrolyte (mainly sodium chloride) reabsorption has occurred without the simultaneous reabsorption of water. This limb is frequently called the 'diluting segment' and the importance of active transport in this section in determining the final urine output is illustrated by the effectiveness of 'loop' diuretic drugs (diuretic = promote urination) which inhibit the transport mechanism.

Distal nephron

Fluid leaving the ascending limb of the loop of Henle enters into another convoluted section of tubule which used to be called the distal 'convoluted' tubule. Although the name persists it is now considered doubtful that the segment forms a distinct anatomical part of the tubule. Rather it seems to form a transition between the cells and processes of the ascending limb of the loop and the collecting system of tubules.

The collecting tubules form part of a collection system in which a number of individual tubules join together before emptying into common collecting ducts. The convoluted section of tubule and the collecting tubules are collectively called the distal nephron.

By the time fluid leaves the loop of Henle only some 15% of the filtrate volume remains; 85% has been reabsorbed along the proximal tubule and loop of Henle. More significantly, the reabsorption of sodium chloride by the ascending limb of the loop of Henle has resulted in dilution of the fluid and so its osmotic pressure is considerably less than that of the plasma and hence the fluid leaving the proximal tubule. The dilution process continues along the distal nephron as solutes (again mainly sodium chloride) are reabsorbed. Some water may follow by osmosis but this is a section of tubule which has a variable water permeability and may be almost impermeable.

Fluid entering the distal nephron is virtually potassium-free; almost all of the potassium filtered from plasma by the glomerulus is reabsorbed by earlier segments. Potassium ions are then added to the tubule fluid by secretion from the cells of the distal tubule, loosely in exchange for sodium ions. Hydrogen ions too are usually secreted and this is the main site of urinary acidification. As was explained earlier, secretion means that, if necessary, the urine can contain more of a solute than would be the case if filtration and reabsorption were the only processes available, and so represents an efficient excretory mechanism.

Collecting duct

The collecting duct descends back into the renal medulla (see Figure 12.3c). Solute and water reabsorption continues in this segment but the water permeability is variable. Thus, solute reabsorption can if necessary occur at a rate which, if water permeability is low, will result in further dilution of the tubule fluid. Alternatively, water reabsorption in excess of solutes can be promoted and this will concentrate the tubule fluid. The collecting duct, therefore, has an important role in the determination of the final osmotic pressure of the urine.

The collecting ducts eventually drain into the renal pelvis. From here the urine is transported to the bladder by peristaltic contractions of the ureter, assisted by gravity.

SUMMARY OF RENAL TUBULE FUNCTION

The renal tubule is anatomically and functionally divided into five parts:

1 Glomerulus/Bowman's capsule. The glomerulus produces a filtrate of plasma into a Bowman's capsule, a distended blind terminus to the tubule.

2 Proximal tubule. This is the site of reabsorption of 80%+ of the filtrate volume and solutes. Some solutes such as glucose are almost completely reabsorbed. Fluid osmotic pressure remains similar to that of plasma.

3 Loop of Henle. This is the site of fluid dilution (ascending limb). There is some reabsorption of water from the descending limb of the loop.

4 Distal nephron. This is the site of continued solute (especially sodium) reabsorption, but also of potassium and hydrogen ion secretion. There is variable water reabsorption.

5 Collecting duct. This is the site of continued solute reabsorption; water reabsorption is variable. It is responsible, with the collecting tubules of the distal nephron and with the loop of Henle, for generating a hypertonic urine, i.e. urine which has an osmotic pressure greater than that of plasma.

It is clear that segments beyond the proximal tubule are largely responsible for the final modification of urine volume and composition. Thus, dilute urine may be produced at a rate of about 16 ml/min (1 l/hour) and very concentrated urine at a rate of 0.3 ml/min (20 ml/hour). On average, urine is produced at about 1 ml/min (60 ml/hour) and has an osmotic pressure about twice that of plasma.

The two kidneys filter at a rate of 125 ml/min, so a urine production rate of 1 ml/min represents a reabsorption of more than 99% of the filtrate. This is extremely expensive in terms of energy usage since water reabsorption by osmosis is mainly linked to the active reabsorption of solutes. In fact, the kidneys account for about 10% of the body's resting oxygen consumption. However, there are important advantages of such a high rate of filtration. These are:

1 Without a high rate of filtration the excretion of substances that are not transported by renal tubule cells (e.g. creatinine) would be low since little would be filtered from the plasma (see Table 12.2). Looked at in another way, novel substances produced by

metabolism, or ingested in the diet, would not be excreted efficiently unless transport processes to secrete them into tubule fluid were present, and this might not be the case.

2 A high rate of filtration allows a high degree of flexibility in the regulation of solute excretion, particularly of sodium, and of water. This is illustrated by the reduction in the concentrating ability of failing kidneys as inadequate sodium chloride filtration reduces the effectiveness of salt transport in the loop of Henle.

THE URINARY BLADDER AND MICTURITION

Urine formed by the renal tubules passes down to the urinary bladder via muscular ureters, partly assisted by gravity. These are basically tubes of about 25 cm long and 0.5 cm in diameter which undergo peristaltic contractions to move the urine away from the renal hilum.

The bladder is a hollow organ, largely comprised of smooth muscle, which lies within the pelvic girdle but behind the symphysis pubis (Figure 12.6). In the female it lies anterior to the uterus and vagina, and in the male is situated anterior to the rectum. The bladder is outside the peritoneal cavity and extends upwards as it inflates, between the peritoneum and the external body wall.

The bladder wall has three layers: an outer or serous layer (which is an extension of the peritoneum), a middle layer of smooth muscle, and an inner transitional epithelial layer. The muscle layer is itself divided into three layers: outer and inner layers of longitudinal muscle fibres and a middle layer of circular muscle. This arrangement means that contraction causes the bladder to reduce in length and diameter, thus emptying it effectively.

Most of the inner surface of the bladder is extremely folded. This, and the transitional type of epithelium, allows considerable distension of the bladder as it fills. Upon emptying, the bladder returns to its folded appearance.

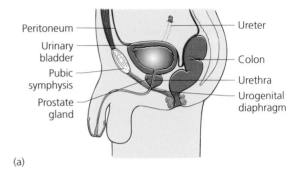

(a)

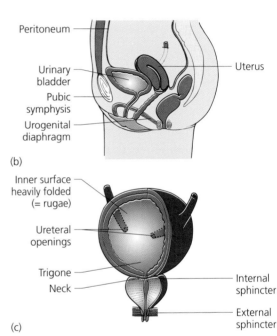

(b)

(c)

Figure 12.6 General anatomy of the urinary bladder: (a) male; (b) female; (c) detail.

The base of the bladder has a smooth triangular-shaped area, called the trigone, formed between the points of entry of the ureters and the exit of the urethra, or tube to the exterior.

Where the urethra leaves the bladder, the circular involuntary muscle layer is arranged so as to produce a functional sphincter – the internal sphincter (Figure 12.6c). A second sphincter, the external sphincter, is formed from striated (voluntary) muscle of the pelvic floor.

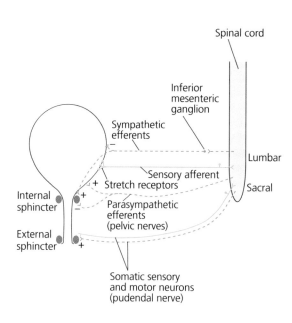

Figure 12.7 Neural control of the urinary bladder: +, contraction when efferent nerves stimulated; −, relaxed when efferent nerves stimulated.
Note that for the bladder to *fill*, parasympathetic efferent activity must decrease and sympathetic activity increase. For the bladder to *empty*, parasympathetic efferent activity must increase and sympathetic activity decrease.

The pressure within the bladder rises during filling but, when there is about 200 ml of urine present, the muscle layers relax (though the internal sphincter remains closed) and so the pressure does not rise even as filling continues. Eventually a point is reached (when the bladder contains about 400 ml of urine) when

addition of further urine causes a marked rise in pressure. In fact the sensation of a 'full bladder' is perceived prior to this point but the sensation becomes more intense. Bladder emptying, or micturition, can be suppressed at this stage but must occur once the bladder holds about 600–700 ml of urine.

Visceral afferent (sensory) nerve fibres provide information on the degree of bladder distension, or more precisely of the tension of the bladder wall, and of pain. These fibres enter into the spinal cord in the lower (11th and 12th) lumbar segments (Figure 12.7). Sensory activity causes an increase in parasympathetic motor (efferent) nerve fibre activity in those fibres supplying the bladder muscle. The main body of the bladder contracts, and the internal sphincter reflexly dilates. At this point relaxation of the external sphincter will allow micturition to occur. Control of this sphincter, however, is voluntary (but only to a degree) and can even be closed once micturition is in progress.

Control of the internal sphincter arises through the activity of sympathetic motor nerve fibres. Sensory information regarding the tension of the bladder wall is relayed up the spinal cord to the sensory cortex of the brain. Final output to the sphincter's sympathetic fibres is generated from areas within the brainstem. The fibres themselves originate from the lower lumbar segments of the spinal cord and when stimulated close the sphincter. This means that spinal injury will usually result in loss of both involuntary and voluntary bladder control. Delayed maturation of the brainstem areas involved also means that control is not established until about 1.5–2 years of age.

Details of kidney physiology and body fluid homeostasis

Kidney function can be looked upon as 'clearing' the plasma, and other body fluids, of various solutes and water. This section describes the concept of 'clearance', and explains how renal function is regulated so that body fluid homeostasis is maintained.

RENAL CLEARANCE AND ITS USE TO MEASURE THE GLOMERULAR FILTRATION RATE

The renal clearance of a substance is defined as being the volume of plasma which contains the amount of that substance excreted per unit time. The greater the clearance rate, the faster the substance is removed from the circulatory system. The clearance of a substance is calculated using the equation:

Clearance of substance S =

$$\frac{\text{urine conc. of } S \times \text{urine (in ml/min) volume/min}}{\text{plasma conc. of } S}$$

Clearance values can be determined for any substance found in urine. For example, the methodology is valuable in determining how efficiently a drug is removed from plasma after it has been administered. Dosages of a drug are calculated according to how long it remains at effective concentrations in blood. Thus, if its clearance rates are low, and liver metabolism of the drug is also low, then the drug remains effective for a long period of time and so lower or more infrequent doses are required.

Any clinical assessment of kidney function would be limited without knowledge of how well the kidneys were filtering. Clearance methodology also provides a technique to measure the rate of filtration by determining the clearance of a substance which is freely filtered by the kidneys, but which is neither reabsorbed nor secreted by the nephron. The excretion of such a substance is therefore determined by how efficiently it is filtered from the plasma. As mentioned earlier, creatinine is one such substance and its use to measure glomerular filtration rate is illustrated as follows.

The amount of creatinine excreted per minute in the urine is calculated as:

$$\text{Urine conc.} \atop \text{of creatinine} \quad \times \quad \text{urine volume/minute} \qquad \text{(eq.1)}$$

(abbreviated as $[\text{creat.}]_{\text{urine}} \times \dot{V}$)

The concentration of creatinine in a urine sample is easily measured, and the minute volume readily calculated from noting the time interval between emptying the bladder and dividing the total urine volume by the time in minutes.

The amount of creatinine filtered during that time is given by the equation:

$$\text{Plasma conc.} \atop \text{of creatinine} \quad \times \quad \text{glomerular filtration} \atop \text{rate/minute} \qquad \text{(eq.2)}$$

(abbreviated as $[\text{creat.}]_{\text{plasma}} \times \text{GFR}$)

Since all of the creatinine filtered is excreted it follows that equations 1 and 2 must be equal:

Creatinine filtered = Creatinine excreted

i.e.

$$[\text{creat.}]_{\text{plasma}} \times \text{GFR} = [\text{creat.}]_{\text{urine}} \times \dot{V}$$

i.e.

$$\text{GFR} = \frac{[\text{creat.}]_{\text{urine}} \times \dot{V}}{[\text{creat.}]_{\text{plasma}}}$$

If V is in ml/min then the calculated GFR will also be in ml/min.

This is a form of the general clearance equation given above, and, strictly speaking, measures the clearance rate of creatinine. As

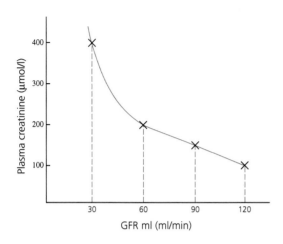

Figure 12.8 Influence of reductions in glomerular filtration rate (GFR; creatinine clearance) on plasma creatinine concentration. Graph assumes that metabolic production of creatinine remains constant. Note the reciprocal relationship: halving the GFR doubles the plasma creatinine concentration.

we have seen, though, the properties of creatinine mean that its clearance value is equal to the glomerular filtration rate. Thus, the rate of glomerular filtration can be calculated using a simple blood sample and a timed urine collection. For the method to work, however, the concentration of creatinine in plasma must remain constant during the entire urine collection period.

Various other substances are used clinically to monitor the glomerular filtration rate. Unlike creatinine, they are not normally found in body fluids and so have to be administered. The polysaccharide inulin is one such substance but must be infused to keep its plasma concentration constant. A timed urine collection also has to be made. To speed up a patient's progress through the clinic a substance such as ethylene ditetraacetic acid (EDTA) may be used. Radioactive isotopes of EDTA are used for ease of analysis and the EDTA is injected, rather than infused. The GFR is then calculated from the rate at which the concentration of EDTA in plasma declines

during a period of an hour or so (i.e. how rapidly it is being 'cleared'). A similar principle applies to the use of plasma creatinine concentration to monitor the rate of decline of GFR in patients who have chronic renal failure. Addition of creatinine to plasma from muscle normally occurs at a fairly constant rate, and so any increase in the plasma concentration reflects a decrease in its clearance (i.e. a decline in GFR; see Figure 12.8).

THE HOMEOSTATIC CONTROL OF BODY FLUID COMPOSITION AND VOLUME

For many organic constituents, such as creatinine and urea, their excretion is predominantly determined by how much is filtered from the plasma. The rate at which the kidneys filter, however, is normally maintained fairly constant, which would suggest that their concentrations in body fluids could fluctuate depending upon how much is produced by tissues. In practice this is generally not the case as any increases in their plasma concentration will result in more being filtered, since the amount filtered is determined by the kidneys' filtration rate in ml/min and the concentration of the substance in plasma. The concentrations of these substances in extracellular fluid do not change dramatically unless their production is markedly increased. The process is limited, however, and regulation is not as precise as for those substances which are reabsorbed or secreted to varying degrees by the renal tubules. Changes in plasma creatinine and urea concentrations are amongst the first consequences of kidney failure.

The remainder of this section looks at how kidney function is altered in response to homeostatic disturbances in (1) water balance, (2) sodium balance, (3) potassium balance, (4) calcium balance and (5) acid–base status. The importance of regulating these factors, and the kinds of receptor necessary to detect changes have already been described in Chapter 5.

Regulation of water balance (regulation of body fluid osmotic pressure or osmolarity)

It was noted in Chapter 5 that the osmotic movement of water across cell membrances ensures that the osmotic pressure of intracellular and extracellular fluids remains in equilibrium. To maintain a constant cell volume and intracellular composition homeostatically it is therefore essential that changes in the osmotic pressure of extracellular fluid are detected, so as rapidly to promote a change in renal water excretion.

The regulation of water balance is not simply a question of increasing or decreasing urine volume. A urine excreted with the same osmotic pressure as plasma will reduce the water content of the plasma but will not affect its osmotic pressure. The effects of overhydration, when plasma is diluted and so its osmotic pressure is decreased, will be more rapidly corrected by the excretion of a large volume of dilute urine (i.e. by excreting water more efficiently than solutes), whilst the effects of dehydration, when plasma osmotic pressure is elevated, will be better corrected by excretion of a small volume of highly concentrated urine (i.e. by excreting solutes more efficiently than water).

The role of the loop of Henle, distal nephron, and collecting ducts in the process of urinary concentration and dilution was noted previously. To understand how changes occur, the function of these tubule segments needs to be considered in more detail.

Urinary concentration and dilution

As illustrated in Figure 12.9, it is in the ascending limb of the loop of Henle that dilution of the tubule fluid begins. This occurs because the electrolytes, especially the more abundant sodium and chloride ions, are extracted (by active transport of chloride ions and positive movement of sodium ions) out of the fluid but

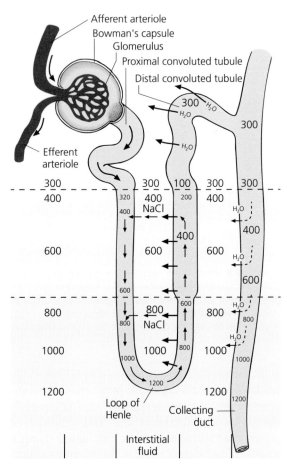

Figure 12.9 The loop of Henle countercurrent multiplier mechanism in the production of a concentrated (i.e. hypertonic to plasma) urine. The reabsorption of water by the distal nephron is facultative and depends on the presence of ADH. The fluid dilution seen as fluid leaves the loop of Henle will continue if ADH is absent so that the urine will have a high volume but low concentration, i.e. the process becomes one of urine dilution.

Note that numbers refer to sodium concentration (sodium chloride is the main solute involved) in the tubule fluid and in the interstitial fluid outside the tubule.

Arrows indicate the movement of sodium (in the loop of Henle) and water (in the distal convoluted tubule and collecting duct).

the osmotic movement of water with these salts is prevented by the tubule being virtually impermeable to water.

Figure 12.9 also shows that fluid concentration actually increases in the descending limb of the loop. This segment is very water-permeable. As the electrolytes (mainly sodium and chloride) transported out of the ascending limb accumulate in the interstitial fluid bathing these parts of the tubule, water is passively absorbed from the descending limb by osmosis. Some of the solutes also diffuse into the tubule from the interstitium. These actions have three functions:

1 As water is absorbed from the descending limb, and solute is added to it, the resultant concentration of electrolytes in the tubule fluid stimulates the reabsorption process in the ascending limb, i.e. the loop acts as a countercurrent system which enhances its effect – hence it is called a countercurrent multiplier.

2 The stimulation of electrolyte reabsorption from the ascending limb results in their further accumulation in the interstitial fluid, and so the osmotic pressure of this fluid within the renal medulla increases. This is important because it enhances the processes described in the descending limb, and provides a large osmotic concentration to drive water reabsorption, if necessary, from the collecting tubules/ducts.

3 They therefore contribute to the water-reabsorptive function of the kidney.

The action of the ascending limb ensures that fluid leaving the loop of Henle is more dilute than plasma. If this dilution process continues then the final urine will also be less concentrated than plasma. Osmotic pressure is measured in terms of osmolarity (in mosmol/l, see Appendix A) and whereas that of plasma is about 285 mosmol/l, that of urine may be as low as 50 mosmol/l, indicating a considerable dilution effect.

The dilution of tubule fluid can only continue if the collecting tubules and collecting ducts have a low permeability to water, otherwise water will be absorbed by osmosis and the effect will be lost. Remember that the collecting duct passes through the renal medulla which has a very high osmotic

pressure as a consequence of electrolyte reabsorption by the ascending limb of the loop of Henle. Should the collecting tubules and ducts become permeable to water then it can be envisaged that water will pass out of the tubule by osmosis until the osmotic pressure of the tubule fluid equilibrates with that of the interstitial fluid (Figure 12.9). The urine will then have a low volume but a high concentration (up to about 1400 mosmol/l – about five times that of plasma).

The absorbed water is returned to the circulatory system via small capillaries, called the vasa recta. These are arranged in hairpin 'loops' within the medulla, and lie parallel to the loop of Henle and collecting ducts. Since the generation of a very concentrated tissue fluid within the renal medulla is vital for the urinary concentrating mechanism, it is important that blood flowing through these capillaries does not remove the solutes. The rate of blood flow through the vasa recta is relatively slow and solutes diffuse into the blood as it descends into the medulla. On ascending again the blood passes through areas of the medulla which have a gradually decreasing tissue fluid concentration (the nature of the loop of Henle activities generates this concentration gradient, being most concentrated in the deepest areas around the tip of the loops). Because the blood flows slowly there is ample time for much of the solute accumulated by the blood to diffuse back out again into the tissue fluid. In this way the solute concentration gradient within the medulla is conserved.

One additional component to the urinary concentrating mechanism is the role of urea. Urea is a product of amino acid metabolism, and it has been known for many years that people on a low protein intake have a reduced urinary concentrating ability.

Urea is freely filtered from the plasma and a proportion of the filtered urea is reabsorbed by the tubule. Cell membranes are permeable to urea and, as its concentration rises in the tubule fluid as a consequence of water reabsorption, urea passively diffuses out of the tubule. This effect is only partially effective, and urea excretion rates are usually quite high. In producing a concentrated urine, water reabsorption out of the collecting ducts causes a considerable increase in the concentration of urea in the tubule fluid. Another change to the collecting ducts that is observed in these circumstances is an increase in their permeability to urea, particularly in the terminal part of the tubule. Diffusion of urea out of the tubule fluid is therefore enhanced, which adds to the solute content of the interstitial fluid. This promotes further osmotic movement of water and increases the concentrating capacity of the kidney.

Water homeostasis

The switch from producing a high volume, dilute urine to a low volume, concentrated one is produced by antidiuretic hormone (ADH; anti- = against; diuretic = promote urination). Central to the determination of urine concentration and volume, then, is the degree to which ADH is released from the posterior pituitary gland. This depends upon the osmotic pressure of the plasma and how much it has deviated from its homeostatic set-point of about 285 mosmol/l.

Any change in plasma osmotic pressure outside its homeostatic range is detected by specialized nerve cells, called osmoreceptors, within the hypothalamus. These are found associated with aggregates of nerve cells called the preoptic nuclei and the paraventricular nuclei. Nerve cells of the preoptic nuclei synthesize antidiuretic hormone (their terminals lie in the posterior pituitary) and it is this hormone which increases the permeability of the distal tubules and collecting ducts to water. Nerve cells from the paraventricular nuclei may also produce the hormone but in addition are important in modulating our perception of thirst.

The process is illustrated by the response to dehydration. As shown in Figure 12.10, a rise in body fluid osmotic pressure as a consequence of dehydration promotes a release of ADH and a feeling of thirst. Often under-

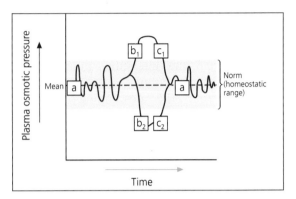

Figure 12.10 Water homeostasis: a schema for the regulation of water balance (via the regulation of body fluid osmotic pressure).
a Osmotic pressure of fluids within normal range.
b_1 Increased plasma osmotic pressure due to dehydration (i.e. water excretion > intake). This is sensed by hypothalamic osmoreceptors.
b_2 Decreased plasma osmotic pressure due to overhydration (i.e. water intake > excretion). This reduces activity of hypothalamic osmoreceptors.
c_1 Restoration of osmotic pressure to normal by increased renal water reabsorption, mediated by release of ADH from posterior pituitary (hypertonic urine produced). Water may also be drunk due to stimulation of thirst.
c_2 Restoration of osmotic pressure to normal by decreased renal water reabsorption as a consequence of decreased ADH release (hypotonic urine produced).

played, thirst is a major part of the mechanism by which body fluid osmotic pressure is normalized, provided that drinking water is available. Water ingestion and a reduction in renal water excretion (producing a concentrated urine) act together to return the body fluid osmotic pressure to normal.

Overhydration promotes the opposite response and inhibits the release of ADH. Thus, the collecting ducts remain hardly permeable to water and a copious, dilute urine is produced.

The responses to changes in water balance are rapid. Drinking a litre of water promotes a measurable increase in urine production within about 15 minutes and the whole litre will be excreted within 1.5–2 hours. The response is aided by the osmoreceptors being highly sensitive to changes in osmotic pressure, with associated rapid changes in

ADH release. Provided that water is available to drink, the mechanism ensures that our water balance is maintained within the limits of ±2% of the homeostatic set-point.

Sodium homeostasis and the regulation of extracellular fluid volume

Table 12.1 shows that, apart from its protein content, blood plasma is basically a solution of sodium chloride with other electrolytes and various organic substances added. This means that sodium and chloride ions are the main contributors to the mineral (or crystalloid) osmotic pressure of plasma.

Sodium chloride in our diet is almost entirely absorbed by the small intestine and distributes throughout the extracellular fluid; it is prevented from accumulating in cells by the membrane Na^+/K^+ exchange pump. Any change in sodium and chloride concentration of the extracellular fluid will be detected as a change in the osmotic pressure of plasma and will be quickly corrected by promoting a change in water balance by the mechanism described in the previous section. Water will also be absorbed from the gut with the electrolytes.

A change in the sodium and chloride content of extracellular fluid will at most, therefore, only transiently alter the fluid's sodium and chloride concentration, but there will be a change in the fluid volume as a consequence of a change in water balance. Note that, although the change in volume represents a change in water balance, this is quite different from the situation described in the previous section which was not associated with a concomitant change in sodium balance. Thus, if the kidneys respond to the increased extracellular fluid volume by increasing water excretion, this will simply cause the concentration of sodium chloride (and the osmotic pressure) of the extracellular fluid to increase and this will then promote water conservation again. Clearly excess sodium and water must be excreted together.

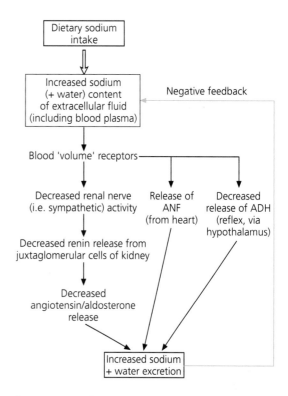

Figure 12.11 Endocrine responses to an elevated blood volume, resulting in increased sodium and water excretion.

Changes in sodium balance are detected by monitoring the extracellular fluid volume. More precisely, the blood component of that fluid compartment is monitored by receptors associated with the circulatory system. The location of these receptors is still debatable, though some have recently been identified in the atria of the heart.

An increased blood volume promotes the urinary excretion of sodium (and water) and the response appears to be effected by hormones (Figure 12.11). Two hormones that have been implicated in the response are aldosterone (a steroid from the adrenal cortex) and atrial natriuretic factor (ANF, a peptide from the cardiac atria; natriuretic = sodium-excreting). It has been known for many years that aldosterone promotes the reabsorption of sodium by the distal nephron. An expansion of blood volume causes a decreased release of

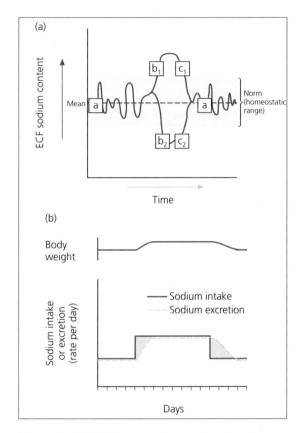

Figure 12.12 (a) The homeostatic regulation of sodium balance.
a Homeostatic range for sodium content (and volume) of extracellular fluid (ECF).
b_1 Increased ECF sodium content resulting from dietary intake being in excess of excretion rate.
b_2 Decreased ECF sodium content resulting from excretion rate being in excess of dietary intake.
c_1 and c_2 Restoration of ECF sodium content (and volume) to homeostatic norm by appropriate changes in sodium intake and sodium (+ water) excretion.
(b) The delayed homeostatic response to changes in sodium intake. The delay in producing a new balance state can be seen to increase body fluid sodium content (shaded area) and volume, as evidenced by the change in body weight.

Both hormones have other actions (see below and Chapter 15) and neither can be said to be solely sodium-regulating. In addition, the decrease in sympathetic nervous activity which occurs when blood volume is expanded (necessary to prevent an increased arterial blood pressure – see Chapter 9) also reduces renal sodium reabsorption and there may debatably be a role for an increased glomerular filtration rate. The control of sodium balance is therefore multifactorial.

The presence of a 'natriuretic hormone' which promotes sodium excretion when blood volume increases has been speculated upon for many years. This 'hormone' remains to be identified, although a body of evidence supports its existence. It does not appear to be the same as ANF, which was discovered during the 1980s. The regulation of sodium balance is complex and incompletely understood.

Sodium homeostasis is outlined in Figure 12.12a. This graph does not, however, show how slow the renal responses are to blood volume changes. Figure 12.12b illustrates what happens when someone is placed on a higher dietary sodium intake. The renal excretion of sodium increases gradually over a period of days during which time sodium will have accumulated (with water) in the extracellular fluid. Thus, a change in sodium balance does not produce complete correction – individuals on a high sodium intake will have a higher extracellular fluid volume (and possibly blood volume) than those on a low sodium intake. This is the basis of the Health Promotion recommendation that we moderate our salt intake.

Potassium regulation

It is described in Chapters 5 and 13 how the concentration gradient of potassium ions across cell membranes is a major determinant of the resting electrical potential of the membrane. The electrical potential is important for a number of reasons, but from a clinical

aldosterone and this is mediated by changes in the activity of the sympathetic nervous system and of the intermediary hormone, angiotensin (see Chapter 9). ANF appears to act by inhibiting sodium reabsorption by the collecting tubules and ducts.

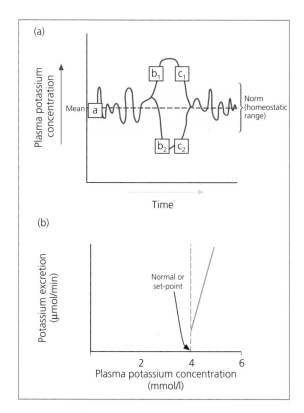

Figure 12.13 Potassium balance.
(a) The sensitivity of renal responses (and hence the narrowness of the homeostatic range) to changes in plasma potassium concentration is shown.
(b) The regulation of plasma potassium concentration.
a Fluctuations in plasma potassium concentration within the homeostatic range.
b_1 Elevated potassium concentration when dietary intake is in excess of excretion. This stimulates the release of aldosterone.
b_2 Reduced potassium concentration when excretion is in excess of dietary intake. This inhibits aldosterone release.
c_1 Restoration of 'normal' values due to increased potassium excretion (via the actions of aldosterone on the kidney).
c_2 Restoration of 'normal' values due to decreased potassium excretion.

important that this low concentration is maintained. In particular, short-term fluctuations must be avoided since the limited compensatory adjustment of intracellular concentration that can occur takes time. It is not surprising that the potassium concentration of blood plasma is closely monitored (by receptors in the adrenal glands). Changes promote a rapid renal response, as can be seen in Figure 12.13a. The increased potassium excretion observed when plasma potassium concentration is increased is primarily due to the release of aldosterone from the adrenal gland. This hormone was mentioned earlier in relation to sodium balance. It acts by stimulating sodium reabsorption by the distal nephron, but in doing so promotes the secretion of potassium ions into the tubule fluid. Unlike sodium, the regulation of potassium balance appears to involve just this hormone. Disorders of the adrenal cortex can have severe effects on the ability to maintain potassium homeostasis.

The homeostatic regulation of potassium is outlined in Figure 12.13b.

Calcium regulation

Calcium ions have a number of functions, including being a trigger for muscle contraction. Calcium ions in extracellular fluid also determine the 'threshold' electrical potential at which nerve and muscle cell membranes are stimulated (Chapter 13). About 50% of the calcium found in blood plasma is reversibly bound to plasma proteins and this component will not be physiologically active. The concentration (about 1.25 mmol/l) of the 50% which are free must be closely regulated. Their concentration can change rapidly if the proportion bound to proteins is altered. This is particularly dependent upon the acid–base status of the plasma, the regulation of which is covered in the next section.

Unlike sodium, potassium, and chloride ions, which are almost entirely absorbed from our foods and are not stored by the body, calcium stores (as bone) are very large and

view it is essential that the potential is maintained as fluctuations can have dramatic effects on the sensitivity of nerve and muscle cell membranes to stimulation.

Potassium concentration in extracellular fluid is normally of the order of only 4 mmol/l (compared with 140 mmol/l for sodium). It is

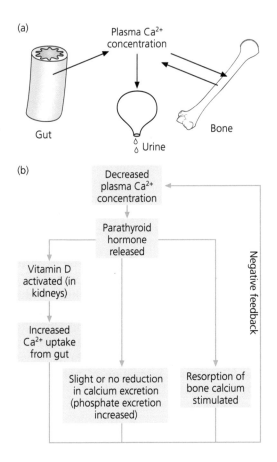

Figure 12.14 Calcium homeostasis.
(a) Unabsorbed calcium in the gut and also bone calcium provide a 'reservoir' which can be drawn upon if required. Note that plasma calcium concentration takes priority over bone calcium content.
(b) Illustration of the role of parathyroid hormone.
Note increased Ca^{2+} concentration decreases parathyroid hormone release and stimulates calcitonin release. Responses are therefore reversed.

only some 50% of our dietary calcium may be absorbed. Calcium in bone is constantly being deposited and resorbed into the extracellular fluid and the concentration of calcium in that fluid must be seen to be a balance between the addition from gut and bone, and the loss into bone and in urine (Figure 12.14a). The handling of this ion is therefore very different from that of the ions mentioned previously.

The movement of calcium in and out of bone is controlled by the hormones calcitonin and parathyroid hormone respectively. Parathyroid hormone is released when plasma calcium ion concentration decreases. The hormone promotes bone resorption but this also releases phosphate ions, and these are excreted through the actions of the hormone to inhibit phosphate reabsorption by the proximal tubule of the kidney, thus helping to maintain phosphate homeostasis.

The conversion (in the kidneys and liver) of inactive vitamin D to the active form also requires the presence of parathyroid hormone. This vitamin promotes the uptake of calcium from the gut and is widely regarded as a hormone rather than a vitamin. The release of parathyroid hormone stimulated by a decreased plasma calcium ion concentration will therefore promote the activation of vitamin D and so increase the uptake of calcium from food in the gut.

Changes in renal calcium excretion have only a small role in the regulation of plasma calcium ion concentration. The role is, nevertheless, important in the overall scheme.

Calcitonin is released when plasma calcium ion concentration is increased above normal. It promotes calcium uptake into bone, and also opposes the actions of parathyroid hormone. Together the two hormones maintain a constancy of the plasma concentration (Figure 12.14b).

Acid–base regulation

The need to regulate body fluid pH (e.g. hydrogen ion concentration) was highlighted in Chapter 5. The sensitivity of cell processes to changes in pH means that any changes in hydrogen ion concentration must be quickly corrected. This is basically achieved by the excretion of carbon dioxide (since this is a major source of acid in body fluids) via the lungs, and by the excretion of hydrogen ions via the kidneys, although this changes relatively slowly. The metabolic production of acid occurs throughout the body, however, and the need to regulate acidity at tissue level prior to the excretion of excess hydrogen ions is provided by chemical 'buffers' (Chapter 5). Buffers are present in intracellular and extracellular fluids but, as with the ions discussed above, it is important that extracellular acidity is monitored and regulated as this will help maintain intracellular pH. Thus, the physiology of acid–base regulation is primarily that of the regulation of the carbon dioxide content, the hydrogen ion concentration and the buffer (particularly bicarbonate) concentration of the blood.

The process is illustrated by the response to an elevated acid load, perhaps generated metabolically. As plasma hydrogen ion concentration rises this stimulates the peripheral chemoreceptors and lung ventilation is increased; more carbon dioxide is exhaled than usual and this reduces the acid load from this source. Should the elevated acidity still persist then hydrogen ion secretion by the renal distal tubule will be promoted, causing an increased acidity of the urine (urine pH is normally about 6–7 but has a range of 4.5–8). Hydrogen ion secretion in the proximal tubule will also be enhanced but this process only promotes bicarbonate reabsorption and does not increase urine acidity; bicarbonate ions in the filtrate are reabsorbed in the proximal tubule by a process which involves combining them with hydrogen ions secreted by tubule cells to produce carbon dioxide and water, which are easily reabsorbed. Bicarbonate ions are then reformed by reversing the reaction in the tubule cells. The released hydrogen ions are resecreted. The additional reabsorbed bicarbonate resulting from this process will maintain the buffering capacity of plasma; in chronic circumstances it may even be increased.

The regulatory process is such that moment-to-moment changes in metabolic rate produce

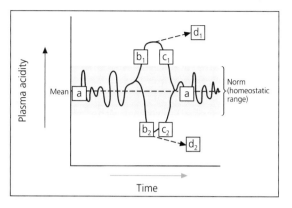

Figure 12.15 Outline of the regulation of plasma acidity. a Fluctuations in plasma pH within the homeostatic range. b_1 Elevated acidity due to production of hydrogen ions (from CO_2 and/or amino acids) in excess of excretion rates (via lung and kidney respectively). b_2 Reduced acidity due to excretion of CO_2 and/or hydrogen ions in excess of hydrogen ion production (from metabolism). c_1 Restoration of normal plasma pH by increased lung ventilation (to remove excess CO_2) and via increased excretion of hydrogen ions in urine. c_2 Restoration of normal plasma pH by decreased lung ventilation (to cause CO_2 retention) or by decreased excretion of hydrogen ions in urine (note urine may become alkaline as base excretion exceeds that of acid). d_1 Persistent elevation of plasma acidity due to *either* chronic CO_2 retention, increased amino acid metabolism, *or* excessive loss of base (e.g. in chronic diarrhoea). d_2 Persistent reduction of plasma acidity due to *either* excessively high lung ventilation, excessive buffer chemical, *or* excessive loss of acid (e.g. in vomiting).

at most only slight, perhaps undetectable, changes in the partial pressure of carbon dioxide of blood and in the plasma concentration of bicarbonate. The acidity changes become more pronounced if there is an excessive change in acid production, for example during exercise when lactic acid from muscle cells adds to the acid 'load'.

Acid–base homeostasis is summarized in Figure 12.15.

Role of excretion in homeostasis

Urine contains a diverse range of substances and the excretion of 'waste' products and excesses is essential for the homeostatic maintenance of all systems in the body. This is clearly illustrated by considering the clinical aspects of chronic renal failure when excretion is diminished and inadequate.

Chronic renal failure is sometimes referred to as 'uraemia' because of the accumulation of urea and other nitrogenous wastes that occurs in the blood and tissues. Such retention (though it is unclear which substances are the main factors) promotes disturbances of cell function which generally lead to further imbalances in intracellular chemistry. Cardiovascular, haematological, gastrointestinal, neurological, skeletal, hormonal, respiratory, skin, and reproductive functions are all disturbed.

Loss of renal function also results in a failure to maintain water and electrolyte homeostasis. Sodium and water retention lead to an elevated extracellular fluid volume, producing oedema and, possibly, hypertension. A metabolic acidosis occurs as hydrogen ion excretion is diminished. Phosphate excretion is reduced, resulting in the release of calcium from bone (the product of plasma calcium $\times$ phosphate concentrations must be kept constant if calcium deposition is to be avoided) and results in bone disorders. Plasma potassium concentration may be elevated. Lethargy and nausea are common symptoms and episodes of diarrhoea and vomiting may exacerbate the ion disturbances.

The kidneys' endocrine function is also compromised, leading to hypertension (renin is released, promoting the generation of the vasoconstrictor angiotensin II; Chapter 9), anaemia (as erythropoietin secretion is diminished; Chapter 8), and further calcium disturbance (as vitamin D_3 is not activated).

Renal failure produces gross disturbances of body fluid composition. Various other conditions, particularly those involving the endocrine system, disturb the excretion of individual solutes but the effects again may be widespread.

Examples of homeostatic control system failures and principles of correction

Disturbances of solute or water homeostasis arise because of poor intake (i.e. malnutrition), excessive metabolic production, or excessive/deficient renal excretion. The latter may arise because of a genetic defect, renal infection, an effect of poisons or drugs, or may be secondary to endocrine disturbances. Some of the most frequent disturbances induced are those of water, sodium, potassium, calcium, and hydrogen ion homeostasis, the conse- quences of which have been outlined in this and previous chapters (Chapter 5). Retention of nitrogenous products of metabolism has already been mentioned in relation to renal failure. Gout results from an excess of uric acid, a product of the catabolism of nucleic acids that is excreted in the urine. Gout may be caused when a persistent and excessively high production of uric acid overwhelms the capacity to excrete it, leading to its retention in blood (hyperuricaemia). Being poorly soluble in water, uric acid crystals are deposited in tissues, especially joints. Gout, therefore, may occur as a consequence of renal failure, or of overproduction.

Inadequate renal function has various causes. The most common ones which arise from a primary disorder of renal function are: (1) renal infection, (2) renal obstruction, (3) renal failure, and, (4) bladder infection.

RENAL INFECTION

Glomerulonephritis

Glomerulonephritis is an inflammation of the glomeruli commonly caused by allergic responses to toxins, by drug abuse, and by 'heavy' metal poisoning. There may also be a genetic component in some individuals. There are many kinds of glomerulonephritis according to which cell type is affected. Symptoms include excessive urinary loss of blood cells and plasma proteins, called haematuria and proteinuria respectively, as a consequence of increased glomerular permeability.

Interstitial nephritis

Interstitial nephritis is damage to the interstitium of the renal cortex and is caused by infection and certain drugs.

Pyelonephritis

Pyelonephritis is a bacterial infection of renal tubules, interstitium (primarily in the medulla), and the renal pelvis, which causes inflammation.

All three above-mentioned conditions are normally acute but can lead to the loss of renal tissue and scarring. Acute renal failure (see below) may ensue and may even progress to chronic renal failure.

RENAL OBSTRUCTION

Calculi (kidney stones)

Calculi normally consist of calcium and uric acid, i.e. substances with a low solubility. Deposition occurs when their concentrations in urine are abnormally high, particularly if urine pH is also appropriate. Blockage of the ureter, kidney pelvis, or tubules results in urine retention, kidney distension and considerable pain. Stones may be removed by surgery, or may be disintegrated using ultrasound.

Hydronephrosis

Hydronephrosis is the accumulation of urine within the renal pelvis because of ureteral obstruction, urethral obstruction, the presence of calculi, or by tumours. The renal pelvis dilates and hypertrophies and the elevated pressure may even cause ischaemia and resultant tissue atrophy. Treatment is aimed at removing the blockage and correcting the underlying disorder.

RENAL FAILURE

Chronic renal failure is a slow progressive decline in glomerular filtration rate and hence in kidney function, perhaps as a consequence of prolonged renal infection but also as a consequence of ageing. The disturbances produced are described in an earlier section. The condition is irreversible and treatment ultimately involves dialysis and/or renal transplantation.

Acute renal failure is a short-term loss of glomerular function due to tubular necrosis (caused by toxins or some drugs), acute glomerulonephritis or pyelonephritis, acute ureteral obstruction, obstruction of the renal artery or vein, or due to prolonged arterial hypotension. Many of the symptoms are similar to those of chronic renal failure. Urine production is normally inadequate for only a week or two at most, and recovery is characterized by a diuretic phase followed by a gradual return to normal function. Full recovery may take several months, however, and for some may not occur at all. The condition is poorly understood and treatment is mainly aimed at controlling body fluid composition until recovery occurs.

BLADDER INFECTION

Cystitis is an infection of the urinary bladder which may cause painful micturition. A major concern is that the infection may 'back-track' up the ureters and cause pyelonephritis.

Summary

1 Metabolism, and our diets, provide excesses of substances which, if retained in the body, will eventually disturb cellular and systemic functions. The main route for their excretion is via the urine.

2 Urine is initially formed as a filtrate of blood plasma and at this point contains all the solutes found in plasma, other than large proteins. The composition and volume of the filtrate is modified as it passes along the renal tubules, by solute reabsorption and by secretion of solutes by the tubular cells.

3 The bulk (normally 99%+) of the filtrate is reabsorbed, primarily by the proximal tubule. Separate renal handling of solute and water reabsorption by the loop of Henle, distal nephron, and collecting ducts means that the final urine can be more dilute or more concentrated than plasma, with consequential effects on plasma osmotic pressure. The process is largely controlled by antidiuretic hormone.

4 The urinary excretion of many metabolic products, such as urea, is primarily determined by the kidney filtration rate. That of electrolytes and glucose is determined by how much is reabsorbed from the filtrate or how much is secreted into it.

5 Virtually all of the glucose and amino acids filtered by the kidneys is reabsorbed and the urine is characteristically free of them.

6 Electrolyte excretion is mainly controlled by hormones.

7 Homeostatic control of solute excretion is essential because of the pronounced effects that retention or excessive loss have on systemic functions.

Review Questions

1 Differentiate between excretion, secretion, and defecation.

2 List the functions of the kidneys.

3 What is the basic structural and functional unit of the kidney?

4 Explain:
  (a) why the overall diameters of the efferent and afferent arterioles are different.
  (b) how this difference enables the afferent arteriole to control the volume of blood filtered in a given time.

5 Describe the morphological features of juxtamedullary and cortical nephrons.

6 Describe the structure of the filtration barrier in the nephron and discuss the forces which bring about glomerular filtration.

7 How are urea and urine formed?

8 Discuss the regional specialization of the nephron with respect to ultrafiltration reabsorption and secretion.

9 Calculate:
  (a) the renal clearance of a substance X, given that the concentration of substance X is 0.2 mg/ml, but it is excreted at a rate of 0.2 mg/min.
  (b) how long it takes 1 litre of plasma to be cleared of substance X.

10 What is the role of ADH in water balance?

11 What is the function of the bladder?

12 Give an account of acid–base balance in man and discuss its control.

13 Discuss the statement that 'the kidney is the ultimate regulator of homeostasis'.

14 Outline the process of micturition.

15 How is blood pressure involved in kidney function? Name the enzyme which increases blood pressure in the Malpighian bodies.

Coordination I: The nervous system

Introduction: relation of nerves to cellular homeostasis

Overview of neural anatomy and physiology

Details of neural physiology: the electrochemical impulse

Overview of functional anatomy of the brain

Overview of functional anatomy of the spinal cord

Overview of the functional anatomy of the autonomic nervous system

Role of the nervous system in homeostasis

Examples of homeostatic control system failures and principles of correction

Summary

Review questions

Introduction: relation of nerves to cellular homeostasis

It was emphasized in Chapter 1 that the processes of physiological homeostasis include recognition that a parameter has changed, and an initiation of an appropriate corrective response (i.e. a negative feedback). The change is detected by specialized receptor cells, many of which are either modified nerve cells or are cells associated with nerve cells (Chapter 14). Coordination of the homeostatic response to change is mediated by hormones (Chapter 15) and/or nerve cells, both of which promote a change in the functioning of their particular target cells and tissues.

Nerve cells, or neurons, thus play a central role in many homeostatic mechanisms. Since these mechanisms act to ensure that the intracellular environment is optimal for a cell's particular function, the importance of nerve cells in regulating cell and tissue function throughout the body is self-evident.

Many homeostatic functions are self-regulating in that the detection of a change in a physiological parameter invokes an involuntary response, frequently without any conscious awareness. In contrast, we have considerable voluntary control over the nerves and skeletal muscles of posture and movement, although there are involuntary aspects to their control also, for example in the reflex withdrawal of a limb in response to pain. Changes in skeletal muscle tone may be a response to a localized stimulus or may act to enable us to perform some kind of physical activity; both contribute to body homeostasis as a whole and therefore to cellular homeostasis.

The neural network is extensive and complex. Even more complex are the brain and spinal cord as these are responsible for interpreting the sensory data and producing the appropriate neural output. The different elements which constitute the anatomy of the nervous system, and its physiology, will therefore be considered as separate subsections, in an attempt to simplify a complicated topic.

Overview of neural anatomy and physiology

WHAT IS A NERVE?

Nerves form an extensive network of conducting pathways which spread throughout the body and provide a means of rapid communication between parts of the body.

A cross-section through a nerve shows that it consists of a tough outer connective tissue covering of collagen, called the epineurium (epi- = outer), and inner bundles of sectioned neurons (Figure 13.1). Bundles of neurons are separated from each other by more connective tissue, called the perineurium (peri- = surround), and by blood vessels. The latter send out fine capillary branches which enter the neuronal bundles to supply the cells with nutrients. Each neuron is surrounded by a further, more delicate, connective tissue layer, called the endoneurium (endo- = inner).

Nerves, then, are conduits for collections of nerve cells, or more precisely the long processes, or fibres, of these peripheral nerve cells, bundled together rather like wires in an electrical cable. The diameter of the nerve is determined by how many nerve fibres are present, and so changes along its length as nerve fibres enter or exit the nerve to supply tissues.

Within the bundles of nerve cells are other cells called Schwann cells, and these play an essential role in producing an insulative layer

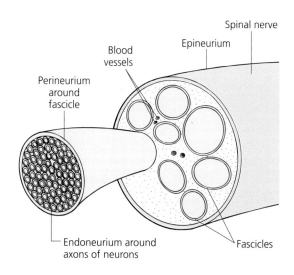

Figure 13.1 Section through a peripheral nerve.

of a substance called myelin around many nerve cells. The importance of this insulation is discussed later in relation to its influence on the conduction of nerve impulses.

ORGANIZATION OF THE NERVOUS SYSTEM

The nervous system may be broadly divided into two anatomical components: the peripheral

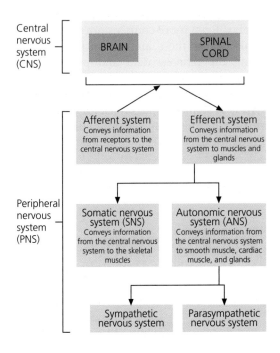

Figure 13.2 General layout of the nervous system.

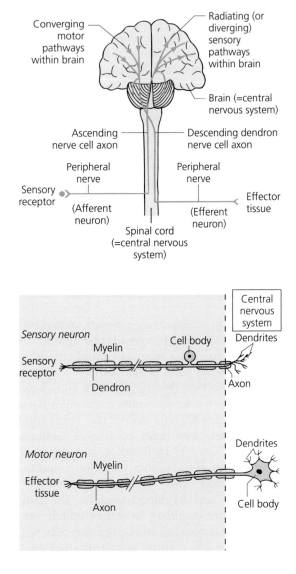

Figure 13.3 Sensory and motor pathways, and neurons, within the nervous system.
Note that a peripheral nerve contains both sensory and motor (efferent) neurons, i.e. they are 'mixed' nerves.

nervous system of nerves which conduct impulses to and from tissues, and the central nervous system in which processing of information occurs.

Components of the peripheral nervous system

Spinal and cranial nerves

The peripheral system can be subdivided according to functional aspects and the tissues served (Figure 13.2). Thus, autonomic nerves mediate those changes in tissue functions which are generally involuntary, and so coordinate the function of most organs (viscera) in the body. Somatic nerves include those nerves which determine the contraction of voluntary muscles, and in particular mediate the control of posture and movement.

Although autonomic nerves are those which primarily alter the function of visceral organs, the roles of the autonomic and somatic branches sometimes overlap in that control. For example, breathing involves contraction and relaxation of the diaphragm and intercostal muscles and this is mediated by somatic nerves (in this case the phrenic nerves), but it is autonomic nerves that influence airway resistance. Similarly the contraction or relaxation of the urinary bladder is an autonomic function, but bladder emptying also requires voluntary relaxation of the external sphincter muscles of the pelvic floor, unless bladder distension is excessive in which case relaxation becomes involuntary!

In certain cases, autonomic function may even be voluntarily overridden. For example, the ability to empty an unfilled urinary bladder voluntarily is achieved by the exercising of voluntary control of those autonomic nerves involved. Similarly, stress relaxation techniques also demonstrate limited conscious control of the resting heart rate, which is a parameter under the involuntary control of the autonomic nervous system.

Nerves of the autonomic and somatic branches each contain neurons which transmit electrical impulses from sensory receptors (see Chapter 14) to the central nervous system, and those which carry impulses from the central nervous system to the tissues (Figure 13.3). These are called afferent and efferent neurons, respectively, and form afferent and efferent nerve 'pathways'. Those efferent nerve cells which cause tissue activities to change are frequently referred to as 'motor' neurons. Afferent neurons of the somatic and autonomic nervous systems are called sensory neurons, because the information they convey originates at sensory receptors, and visceral afferents, because they originate in the viscera, respectively.

Most peripheral nerves enter or exit the central nervous system via the spinal cord, at which point they are generally called spinal nerves, of which there are 31 pairs (Figure 13.4). Thus each spinal nerve contains afferent and efferent neurons of the autonomic and somatic nervous systems and it is only at some distance from the cord that the two systems can be distinguished. Spinal nerves enter/exit the spinal cord between the vertebrae (Figure 13.4) and so may be some distance from the brain. Clearly the spinal cord must contain neural pathways of both the somatic and autonomic systems, and these will conduct the neural activity to and from appropriate parts of the brain.

The remaining peripheral nerves are notable because they do not pass via the spinal cord. Most of these innervate tissues of the head and neck and connect directly with the brain. Collectively they are called the cranial nerves of which there are 12 pairs (see Figure 13.26 and Table 13.4). Not all only innervate tissues of the head, however. For example, the vagus is an extremely long nerve which passes through the thorax and abdomen, and innervates the organs of these areas.

The cranial nerves may contain afferent neurons, mainly originating from the eyes, ears, nose, mouth, facial tissues, and arteries of the neck or efferent neurons, which supply various muscles, salivary glands, etc., or both. For some of these nerves the efferent neurons are solely autonomic or somatic. For example, movement of the eyeballs requires stimulation of the ocular muscles of the orbit of the eye via the oculomotor nerve (a somatic function), whilst basal control of the heart involves the vagus nerve (an autonomic function). Some cranial nerves, however, contain neurons of both systems. For example, the glossopharyngeal nerve mediates contraction of the muscles of the pharynx for swallowing (a somatic function) and also saliva production from certain salivary glands (an autonomic function).

Neuronal structure

Conduction across distances between tissues is facilitated by the neurons being long, perhaps as long as 1–2 m (as in the transmission of certain information from the toe to the brain). It is these elongated neuronal cells that are observed if a nerve is sectioned. In contrast, processing of neural information within the central nervous system usually involves cells which are small and which interact with neighbouring cells close by. All neurons contain cell organelles such as a nucleus and mitochondria, but these are largely localized to the cell body

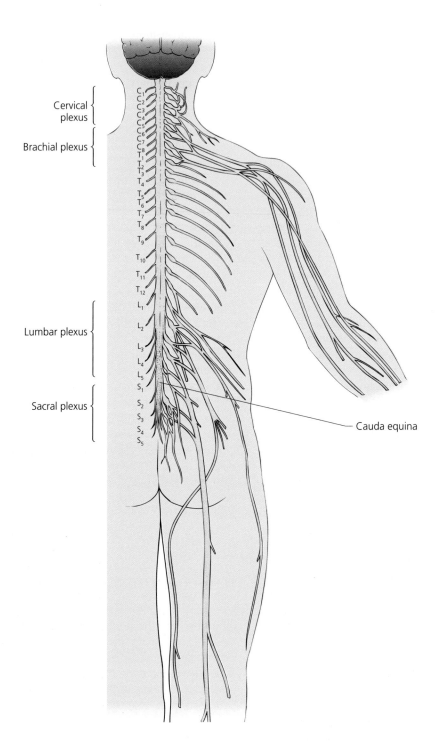

Figure 13.4 General organization of spinal nerves, and the somatic nervous system (plexus = aggregation of nerves or neurons). C, cervical; T, thoracic; L, lumbar; S, sacral. Numbers refer to vertebrae within the respective parts of the vertebral column/spinal cord.

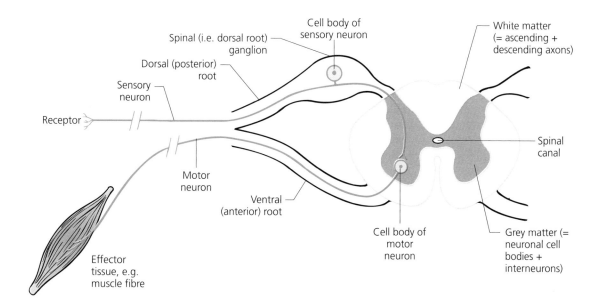

Figure 13.5 Spinal nerve roots and the general appearance of the spinal cord.

(sometimes referred to as the soma) and most of what constitutes the neuron is an elongated process called a nerve fibre. A fibre is anatomically subdivided into the section, called a dendron, between the receptor and cell body, and the axon, that section between the cell body and connections with other nerve cells or efferents. This is illustrated in Figure 13.3.

The cell body of efferent cells is located at the end of the axon either within the spinal cord itself, or (especially within the autonomic system) in neural structures called ganglia (singular ganglion), present within the thorax and abdomen, sometimes at some distance from the spinal cord. For afferent neurons the cell body is found as an 'off-shoot' from the axon, and for most peripheral nerves this is usually close to where the nerve cells enter the spinal cord (Figure 13.5). A distension of the nerve at this point is produced by the large numbers of cell bodies present, as large numbers of afferent neurons are present in a nerve, and this is called a spinal ganglion. Another name is dorsal root ganglion, because afferent cells enter the posterior or dorsal aspect of the cord.

One feature frequently observed in neurons is that their cell bodies and dendron/axon terminals may have extremely fine branching processes called dendrites (dendron = Greek for 'tree'). These are essential because they enable neurons to interact with other cells in the vicinity. The dendrites may come into close proximity with dendrites from other neurons, or with the cell body of other neurons (especially of efferent neurons and brain cells) or with non-nervous tissue (such as skeletal muscle, smooth muscle of the viscera or glandular tissue). Actual physical contact between cells is not usually present, though the 'gap' may only be of the order of 20 nm (20 millionths of a millimetre) wide. The whole structure of the dendritic endings and the 'gap' is called a synapse and plays a central role in whether or not nerve impulses are transmitted from one cell to another. Synaptic function is described in a later section.

Nerve nomenclature

Nerves are frequently named according to where they originated or which tissue they supply. For example, those somatic nerves called the pelvic nerves contain afferent and efferent neurons which pass to/from the pelvic region, while the optic nerve is purely sensory and originates in the eye.

Unfortunately the nomenclature is not always so obvious. The names of many nerves derive from Latin or Greek and may refer to features other than sources or targets. For example, the name of the cranial nerve called the vagus is Latin for 'wandering' and refers to the extent to which this nerve traverses the thorax and abdomen of the body. Branches from the vagus innervate a variety of organs, and the nerve contains both afferent and efferent neurons, and so naming the nerve according to source or target is not feasible.

Nerve nomenclature is therefore complex and is more relevant to students of anatomy than to the intentions of this book. Accordingly nerves will only be named in this chapter when appropriate. Others may be mentioned elsewhere in the book where relevant.

Components of the central nervous system

The neurons of the brain and spinal cord have much the same general anatomy as peripheral neurons in that they consist of a cell body with a dendron, an axon, and dendritic processes. Dendrites permit interactions to occur between a cell and others within the vicinity, whilst dendrons and axons provide a conductive route which enables neurons to interact with those in other parts of the brain, cord and/or muscles or glands. Estimates of the number of cells each brain cell interacts with suggest that a single neuron may be directly associated with tens of thousands of others! The brain contains some 100 000 million neurons, and the potential 'circuitry' is therefore enormous.

Non-neural cells are also evident within the central nervous system. These are called neuroglial cells and estimates suggest that they outnumber neurons by as much as 10:1. They can be subdivided according to their position and function, as outlined in Table 13.1. From

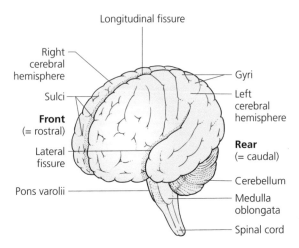

Figure 13.6 External features of the brain (meningeal membranes removed).

Table 13.1, it should also be noted that the Schwann cells mentioned earlier in relation to the contents of a peripheral nerve are also neuroglial cells.

Neural organization of the spinal cord

The organization of neurons within the cord is described in detail in a later section. In general, though, the neurons can be considered under three categories:

1 ascending neurons which pass up the cord to the brain, and so form afferent pathways,

2 descending neurons which pass down the cord from the brain, and so form efferent pathways, and

3 interneurons which are nerve cells that provide connections between various ascending and descending neurons.

Axons of ascending and descending neurons pass along the periphery of the cord, and in cross-section the insulative layer of myelin on many of these neurons makes these areas appear white in colour; hence this is the white matter of the spinal cord. The cell bodies of these neurons, however, are found more

Table 13.1 Neuroglial cells (i.e. non-neuronal cells) of the nervous system

Type	Description	Homeostatic function
Central nervous system		
Astrocytes (astro- = star; -cyte = cell)	Star-shaped cells with numerous processes. Protoplasmic astrocytes are found in the grey matter of the CNS; fibrous astrocytes are found in the white matter of the CNS	Twine around nerve cells to form supporting network in brain and spinal cord; attach neurons to their blood vessels
Oligodendrocytes (oligo- = few; dendro- = tree)	Resemble astrocytes in some ways; processes are fewer and shorter	Give support by forming semi-rigid connective tissue rows between neurons in brain and spinal cord; produce a myelin sheath around neurons of the CNS
Microglia micro- = small; -glia = glue)	Small cells with few processes; derived from monocytes; normally stationary, but may migrate to site of injury; also called brain macrophages	Engulf and destroy microbes and cellular debris; may migrate to area of injured nervous tissue and function as small macrophages
Ependyma (= upper garment)	Epithelial cells arranged in a single layer and ranging in shape from squamous to columnar; many are ciliated	Form a continuous epithelial lining for the ventricles of the brain (spaces that form and circulate cerebrospinal fluid) and the central canal of the spinal cord
Peripheral nervous system		
Neurolemmocyte (Schwann cell)	Flattened cells located along the nerve fibres. Cells encircle the axon many times to form a series of concentric rings. Inner layers contain myelin	Produce insulative sheath of myelin around nerve fibres. Myelin enhances the conduction velocity of 'impulses' along the axon

centrally in the cord and the absence of myelin around the cell bodies makes this area appear darker (hence grey matter).

Neural organization of the brain

Superficially the brain can be observed to consist of a number of structures (Figure 13.6).

Much of the external features of the brain is dominated by the highly convoluted cerebrum. The ridges of the convolutions are called gyri (gyrus, singular) whilst the indentations between the ridges are called sulci (sulcus, singular). The convolutions increase the surface area of the cerebrum (to about 0.2 m²) and this is important because the outer layer of

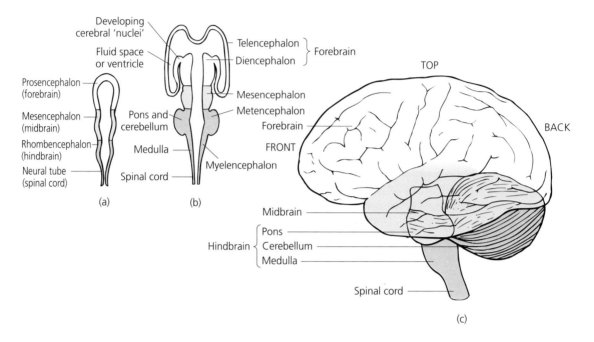

Figure 13.7 An outline of brain development.

the cerebrum, called the cerebral cortex, consists of neurons involved in the processing of information, and so its increased surface area means that more processing tissue can be contained within the skull.

The cortex appears grey as a consequence of the numbers of neuronal cell bodies in these areas. Below the surface, the brain generally appears white because of the presence of myelinated axons. This arrangement of white and grey matter is the reverse of that observed in the spinal cord and reflects the need to conduct activity, via nerve fibres, through the brain mass to the processing areas. Set within the white matter, however, are discrete clusters of nerve cell bodies, which appear as grey matter, and these also provide processing areas. Such clusters are called nuclei (note the distinction between brain nuclei and the nuclei of cells). Axons from such cells connect a nucleus with other nuclei, or perhaps with the cerebral cortex.

The positions of structures within the brain are determined during embryonic develop-ment. The developing brain is first distin-guishable as three enlargements called the forebrain (or prosencephalon), the midbrain (or mesencephalon) and the hindbrain (or rhombencephalon).The forebrain later subdi-vides into two further structures: the telen-cephalon (or end-brain) and diencephalon (or between-brain). Similarly the hindbrain subdi-vides into the metencephalon (after-brain) and myelencephalon (spinal brain).

Such nomenclature is confusing but serves to illustrate how the main brain structures are derived. Thus, in Figure 13.7 it can be seen that the forebrain gives rise to the cerebrum with its underlying nuclei, whilst the hindbrain gives rise to other structures visible as external features: the cerebellum, pons varolii and medulla oblongata. The midbrain consists of nuclei lying above the pons, and tracts of nerve axons conducting information into and out from higher structures. Collectively the midbrain, and the pons and medulla of the hindbrain, are referred to as the brainstem.

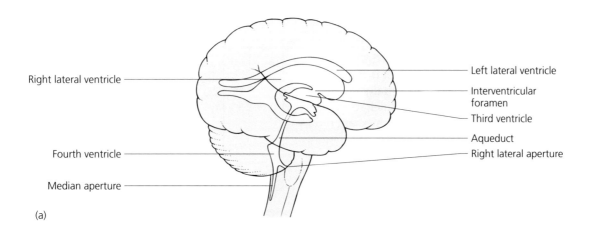

(a)

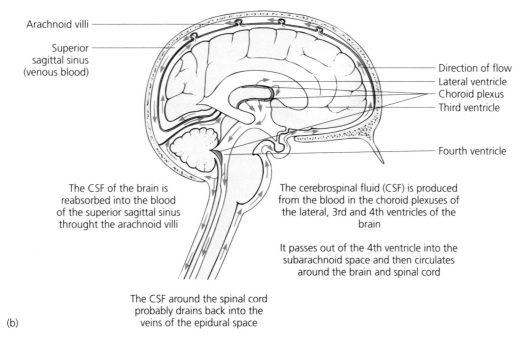

The CSF of the brain is reabsorbed into the blood of the superior sagittal sinus throught the arachnoid villi

The cerebrospinal fluid (CSF) is produced from the blood in the choroid plexuses of the lateral, 3rd and 4th ventricles of the brain

It passes out of the 4th ventricle into the subarachnoid space and then circulates around the brain and spinal cord

The CSF around the spinal cord probably drains back into the veins of the epidural space

(b)

Figure 13.8 The cerebral ventricles, and circulation of the cerebrospinal fluid (CSF). (a) Position of the cerebral ventricles. (b) Circulation of CSF. The choroid plexus is the endothelial tissue which secretes CSF.

Cerebrospinal fluid

The brain and spinal cord do not consist entirely of tissue; fluid spaces are evident. By their nature, neurons are particularly susceptible to changes in their intracellular/extracellular environment and the central nervous system is to a large extent physically isolated from the blood, though the brain is, of course, dependent upon the circulation of blood for its nutrients.

This protects the neurons from the short-term, moment-to-moment fluctuations observed in plasma composition.

Cells of the brain and spinal cord are bathed in cerebrospinal fluid (CSF) which is formed by secretion from the blood by certain epithelial cells, called the choroid plexus, which form villi-like projections from the lining of the main fluid spaces, or ventricles, within the brain (Figure 13.8). Although part of the extracellular fluids of the body, the nature of CSF formation by secretion means that it is physically separate from the other fluids, and its composition and volume are kept under tight homeostatic control.

There are four main ventricles (Figure 13.8a). Three (two large lateral ventricles, and the third ventricle) lie deep within the forebrain, whilst the fourth is in the hindbrain. Most CSF is secreted into the lateral ventricles, which connect with the third ventricle via the interventricular foramina. The third ventricle is connected to the fourth ventricle by the cerebral aqueduct of the midbrain.

The CSF flows from the ventricles into the subarachnoid space (see 'meninges' later) and thence around the brain. Some passes into the subarachnoid space of the spinal cord. Fluid flow is promoted by the action of cilia, although head and vertebral movements help. The fluid is eventually reabsorbed back into the blood plasma via projections of the arachnoid meningeal membrane. Clearly the rate of reabsorption must balance the rate of secretion, if CSF volume is to be maintained. This homeostatic process is illustrated diagrammatically in Figure 13.9. The means of regulation of the process is unclear.

The CSF provides the brain with a protected environment, provides a hydraulic suspension of the brain matter, and also prevents mechanical damage to blood vessels and the membranous linings of the brain by preventing friction with the skull.

The secretory epithelia form a 'blood–brain barrier' as only lipid-soluble substances, or those with transport facilities within the epithelial cell membranes, can cross into the CSF. This barrier is clinically important as drugs must be

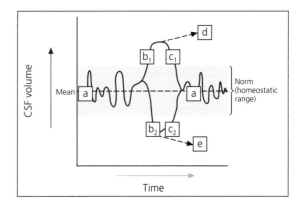

Figure 13.9 Cerebrospinal fluid volume homeostasis.
a The CSF volume, fluctuating within a 'normal' range compatible with normal neuronal function.
b_1 Excessive CSF when rate of production exceeds rate of reabsorption across the arachnoid villi.
b_2 Deficient CSF when rate of production is less than the rate of reabsorption.
c_1, c_2 Restoration of CSF volume by restoring the balance between CSF secretion and reabsorption.
d Persistently elevated CSF volume as a consequence of 'blocked' CSF circulation due to anatomical abnormality or, for example, the presence of a haematoma. e Persistently depleted CSF volume as a consequence of dehydration or the excessive presence of an osmotic agent (e.g. glucose) in blood plasma.

capable of crossing it if brain function is to be affected. General anaesthetics are lipid-soluble and are not influenced by the barrier.

Cerebral and spinal blood flow

The brain is supplied by four arteries (Figure 13.10a). Two arteries originate from the common carotid arteries, each of which divides into an internal and external branch. The external carotid arteries supply the pharynx, larynx, and face with blood, whilst the internal carotids pass deeper and penetrate the base of the skull and supply the brain. The other two arteries supplying the brain are called the vertebral arteries. These ascend the vertebral column, passing through the lateral or transverse foramina of the bones and penetrate the skull via the foramen magnum, through which the spinal cord passes.

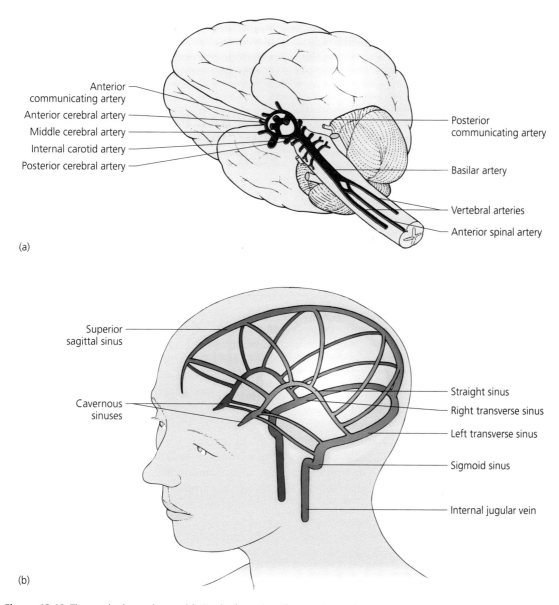

Figure 13.10 The cerebral vasculature. (a) Cerebral arteries. The anterior and posterior communicating arteries join the three pairs of cerebral arteries to form the circle of Willis around the base of the brain. (b) Venous drainage.

On entering the skull, each internal carotid artery divides to form an anterior and a middle cerebral artery, and these supply blood to the anterior half to two thirds of the brain, including cortical and subcortical structures. The vertebral arteries combine to form a single basilar artery. This runs along the ventral aspect of the brain and sends branches into the brainstem and cerebellum. It eventually divides to form a pair of posterior cerebral arteries which supply structures at the rear of the cerebrum.

Although the carotids and vertebral arteries would appear to be responsible for supplying blood to different parts of the brain, the internal carotids and the basilar artery are interconnected at the base of the brain. Communicating arteries branch from the sites of origin of the anterior cerebral and posterior cerebral arteries to form the circle of Willis, which encircles the stalk of the pituitary gland (Figure 13.10). Blood can, therefore, pass from the carotid arteries to the posterior cerebral arteries, or from the basilar artery to the anterior and middle cerebral arteries. In view of its high metabolic activity, and the sensitivity of brain cells to disturbances in their immediate environment, having four arteries supplying the brain and an anastomosis which connects anterior and posterior vessels are adaptations which help to prevent blood flow to the brain being compromised.

Small veins drain the brain and empty into dural sinuses, that is blood spaces within the membrane called the dura mater (a meningeal membrane – see later). The largest of these is called the superior sagittal sinus (Figure 13.10b) which lies within the fold of membrane, the falx cerebri, which runs longitudinally within the cleft between the two cerebral hemispheres. Most venous blood eventually drains into a pair of transverse sinuses, which run forward along the base of the cranium and empty into the internal jugular veins. Venous blood from other parts of the head and neck drain into the external jugular veins.

The spinal cord also has a complex arterial blood supply. Anterior and posterior spinal arteries descend the surface of the cord, and are derived from the vertebral arteries and from cerebellar arteries (branches of the basilar artery which supply the cerebellum). Branches penetrate into the neural matter of the cord. In addition, this blood is joined by arterial blood supplied by small vessels which branch from intercostal, cervical and lumbar arteries and penetrate the cord via spaces between the vertebrae.

GENERAL PHYSIOLOGICAL PRINCIPLES OF NEURAL FUNCTION

The organization of the nervous system reflects its general function: a system of conducting pathways which transmit activity from sensory receptors to processing centres, from which activity is conducted to effector tissues (in other words a homeostatic system). Using appropriate equipment the activity of neurons can be detected as electrical impulses, and the physiology of the nervous system involves mechanisms which enable neurons to change their electrical properties to generate an 'impulse', and to conduct the impulse to other areas.

Neurons must therefore also have properties which ensure that impulses are conducted in the appropriate direction, and are transmitted from one cell to another across the synapse. Synaptic function includes the release of chemicals which interact with the next cell in the pathway, and so are referred to as neurotransmitters. Thus, nerve conduction is a process involving both electrical and chemical events.

The processing of information by the central nervous system is essentially one of an integration of neural pathways, and involves various parts of the brain. Such integration is necessary for all the diverse properties associated with brain function, ranging from the somatic control of posture (Chapter 16), to the autonomic regulation of blood pressure (Chapter 9), to cognitive functions such as memory.

Details of neural physiology: the electrochemical impulse

ELECTRICAL EVENTS

The resting membrane potential

In Chapters 2 and 5 it was emphasized how the phospholipid cell membrane has selective permeability properties: though permeable to some molecules, especially small, uncharged molecules such as urea and carbon dioxide, the permeability to others may be very low indeed, especially electrically charged substances such as ions, or large molecules such as proteins. These properties are important in the maintenance of a different ionic composition of intra- and extracellular fluids (Chapter 5). Thus, sodium has the highest concentration in the extracellular fluids (about 10-fold higher than inside cells), whilst that of potassium is about 30-fold more concentrated within the cells. Likewise, the main anion outside cells is chloride (about 10 times more concentrated than in intracellular fluid), whilst proteins, amino acids, and phosphates are the main negatively charged ions inside cells.

The net effect of this distribution of ions, and hence of electrical charge, is complex and relates to the permeability of the membrane to individual ions, and to its capacity to transport them actively (Figure 13.11). In practice there is a 'leak', albeit slow, of positive charge (i.e. of positive ions) from the cell, mainly as a consequence of the movement of potassium (K^+) ions. Although this leak of charge is largely compensated for (by the sodium/potassium exchange pump of the cell membrane), it is sufficient so that at any given time there is a residual positive charge on the external surface of the membrane. In other words the membrane is polarized, and the situation is usually expressed as the inside of the membrane being negatively charged with

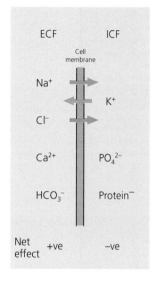

Figure 13.11 Major ionic components of extracellular (ECF) and intracellular (ICF) fluids, and net passive fluxes across the cell membrane. Larger ions such as Ca^{2+}, PO_4^{2-}, HCO_3^-, and protein$^-$ exhibit little passive flux.

respect to the outside (in relative terms the loss of positive charge must mean that there is excess negative charge inside the cell).

The polarity of the cell membrane is therefore rather like that of a battery, and placement of microscopic electrodes across the cell membrane will detect a voltage. The value is minute, however, being of the order of 70 millivolts (usually written as –70mV; i.e. negative inside with respect to outside the cell). The actual value varies slightly between cells but an electrical potential will always be present. This is called the resting membrane potential of the cell and its value particularly depends upon the relative permeability of the cell membrane, especially to sodium and potassium ions.

Nerve and muscle cells are excitable cells as their cell membranes have the capacity to alter their ionic permeability in response to a stimulus. Their membranes contain specific ion 'channels', which are basically proteins through which ions may diffuse. In order to control that diffusion, however, molecular structures must provide 'gating' mechanisms. By regulating the opening or closing of these 'gates' the membrane can determine which ions are free to diffuse across it, and therefore alter the membrane potential.

The voltage measured may move toward electrical neutrality (i.e. by making the inside of the cell less negative, a process called depolarization) or toward an even greater value (i.e. by making the inside of the cell more negative, a process called hyperpolarization), depending upon which ions are free to move across the membrane.

The electrical impulse generated when a nerve cell is stimulated is referred to as an action potential. The generation of an action potential is, in some ways, a disturbance of cell membrane homeostasis. The membrane disturbance is only transient but represents a good example of a changed homeostatic set-point appropriate to body function.

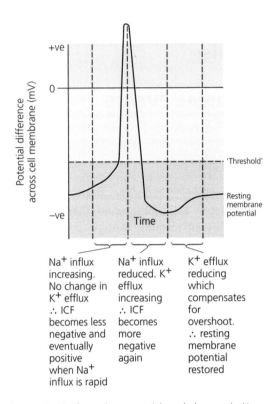

Figure 13.12 The action potential, and changes in Na+ and K+ fluxes across the cell membrane.

The action potential

Nerve cells are stimulated either by activity at a sensory receptor or at a synapse with another neuron (artificially the same effect can be produced by application of a small electric current; hence the devastating effects of electrocution). However produced, stimulation of the neuron causes the membrane to depolarize as sodium channels begin to open and sodium ions (i.e. positive charge) begin to diffuse into the cell, promoted by the concentration gradient and by the net negative charge present within the cell. The value of the membrane potential will therefore begin to move towards electrical neutrality (Figure 13.12).

At a certain value, called the membrane threshold, the sodium channels open fully and sodium ions move rapidly into the cell (Figure 13.12). The movement is so rapid that the

membrane potential actually assumes a positive value (about +30mV, positive inside the cell with respect to outside) because of the influx of positive charge. This part of the action potential can be considered a positive feedback mechanism in which the slight potential change prior to threshold promotes further change, leading to the full response.

Once depolarized to this extent, the cell membrane cannot be restimulated; the membrane must be restored at or close to its original resting membrane potential if the neuron is to be capable of restimulation. Repolarization is achieved by the opening of potassium channels (Figure 13.12) which allow the diffusion of potassium ions (i.e. positive charge) out of the cell down their concentration and electrical gradients. The net loss of positive charge is, in fact, transiently excessive and the

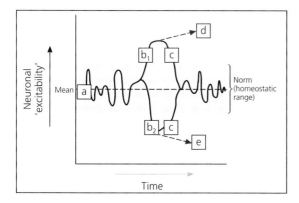

Figure 13.13 Membrane excitability as a homeostatic process.
a Fluctuating membrane excitability within resting range.
b_1 Increased excitability because difference between 'resting' potential and threshold potential is decreased due *either* to a decreased 'resting' potential (as in hyperkalaemia) *or* to a reduced 'threshold' potential (e.g. in hypocalcaemia).
b_2 Decreased excitability because difference between 'resting' potential and threshold potential is increased, due *either* to an increased 'resting' potential (as in hypokalaemia) *or* to an elevated threshold potential (as in hypercalcaemia).
c Restoration of membrane potential to within the normal 'resting' range by physiological restoration of electrolyte imbalances.
d Persistent hyperexcitability due to persistent electrolyte imbalance (e.g. adrenal dysfunction, or respiratory alkalosis).
e Persistent hypoexcitability due to persistent electrolyte imbalance (e.g. in excessive use of potassium-wasting diuretic drugs, or in parathyroid-hormone-secreting tumours).

value of the membrane potential goes beyond its resting value (to about −90mV; inside the cell negative to the outside). This hyperpolarization is actually advantageous as it makes the membrane more difficult to stimulate (i.e. refractory) since a greater depolarization will be required to reach threshold. This means that, once the nerve impulse has moved along a stage in the nerve fibre, retrograde stimulation is unlikely to occur and so the impulse becomes unidirectional. Hyperpolarization also has a role in inhibitory synapses, which are described below.

The whole action potential from depolarization to full repolarization takes place in a

millisecond or so. This extremely rapid response ensures that the impulse can be conducted rapidly, and also that the membrane is quickly available for restimulation.

One further important feature of the action potential is that the membrane becomes fully permeable to sodium ions once the threshold potential has been attained; the response is all or nothing. Graded responses are not possible and the level of activity within a neural pathway is therefore determined by how many action potentials are generated, and conducted, per second.

The ease at which the cell can be stimulated is a measure of its excitability, and depends upon how close the membrane potential is to the threshold potential. Excitability is another example of homeostatic principle in action: the effects of altering parameters which influence either the membrane potential or the threshold potential are illustrated diagrammatically in Figure 13.13. Although there is a need to control excitability, there are situations when it is a physiological advantage to allow the set-point to change. Thus the presence of adrenaline during exercise, or in the stress response, seems to increase excitability (which improves reflex action), and the sinoatrial node of the heart undergoes faster cyclical depolarizations (that generate the heart beat).

Conduction properties of neurons

The generation of an action potential by a nerve cell is only one part of nerve cell function: the electrical activity must be conducted to appropriate tissues. The basic process in propagating a nerve impulse is the destabilization by an action potential of sodium channels in adjacent parts of cell membrane. The resultant depolarization of adjacent cell membrane reaches the threshold potential and another action potential is generated (Figure 13.14a). In this way an action potential is regenerated along successive parts of the membrane, i.e. along the axon or

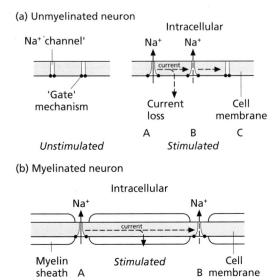

(a) Unmyelinated neuron

(b) Myelinated neuron

Figure 13.14 Sodium channels, membrane currents, and conduction velocities in (a) unmyelinated and (b) myelinated neurons.

In each case 'gates' are fully open at A and so the membrane is fully permeable to Na+ and an action potential is generated. At B, Na+ channels are beginning to open in response to current generated at A so that the membrane potential begins to approach threshold. At C (in part a), the 'gates' are still closed but will subsequently respond to current generated at B.

Note the current decrement in the unmyelinated axon. The presence of myelin (in part b) reduces the decrement so that greater distances between Na+ channels are possible.

dendrite of the cell. How the nature of the action potential ensures unidirectional movement of the impulse was described in the previous section.

The ease of conduction of electric current generated by an action potential will be related to the electrical resistance of the cell membrane, and large diameter axons have a lower resistance than small diameter ones. Large diameter nerve fibres therefore conduct electric current more rapidly (and are also easier to stimulate). The rate at which an axon conducts impulses is called its conduction velocity and for axons without an insulative layer of myelin ranges from 2 to 30 m/s, depending upon axon diameter. Changes in

temperature will also influence conduction velocities, but body temperature is usually homeostatically maintained and so is not a physiological factor. The principle, however, is often used in surgery, and in the treatment of sport injuries using 'freeze' sprays.

In general, only the smallest diameter axons are unmyelinated. The presence of insulative myelin on axons of other neurons conveys important advantages, not least because conduction velocities can be achieved which would otherwise require fibres of extremely large diameter if they were to be unmyelinated and this would make accommodation of large numbers of fibres impossible within the limited space of a nerve.

Myelin is secreted by certain neuroglial cells (Schwann cells in the peripheral nervous system, and oligodendrocytes in the central nervous system). The process of myelination results in the enveloping of the nerve axon by concentric layers of this insulative phospholipid. Myelin reduces the loss of current, generated by an action potential, from the membrane into the surrounding interstitial fluid. The current generated will still decrement, however, largely because of the resistive properties of the cell membrane, noted above.

Clearly there must be gaps within the myelin sheath at which the axonal membrane can be depolarized again to regenerate the current. Such gaps are called the nodes of Ranvier and current (i.e. impulses) can be envisaged as 'jumping' from node to node (note that ion channels will be concentrated only at the nodes – Figure 13.14b). This process is called saltatory conduction in contrast to the continual conduction observed in unmyelinated neurons. For a given fibre diameter conduction velocities will be considerably faster in a myelinated neuron and may reach values of 120 m/s (432 km/h). There is still an influence of axon diameter, however, as this will be a determinant as to the required distance between nodes, and therefore the number of times an action potential has to be generated along the axon.

A range of conduction velocities can be observed within the nervous system and one of

Table 13.2 Nerve fibre classification

Class	Conduction velocity (m/s)	Myelination	Nerve fibre diameter (µm)
A			
Alpha α	50–120	Myelinated	8–20
Beta β	30–70	Myelinated	5–12
Gamma γ	10–50	Myelinated	2–8
Delta δ	3–30	Myelinated	1–5
C	0.5–2	Unmyelinated	<1

Note C fibres normally comprise almost half the nerve fibres in a peripheral nerve, and all the post-ganglionic neurons of the autonomic system.
Note an additional sensory nerve fibre classification is sometimes used in which class I and II fibres correspond to Aα, β and γ fibres, Class III correspond to Aδ fibres and class IV correspond to C fibres.

the main classifications of fibre type relates to conduction velocities and the presence or absence of myelin (see Table 13.2).

CHEMICAL EVENTS

Synaptic conduction

At some point within a neural pathway the activity generated by action potentials in a nerve cell must be transmitted to another cell: either another neuron, a muscle cell, or a glandular cell. If there was physical contact between cells then this would present little difficulty, and the impulse would be conducted as before. Such connections seem to be present in some parts of the brain, and between cells of cardiac muscle (which must also conduct electrical activity). Direct connections do not promote unidirectionality of the conduction of impulses, however, nor do they permit any kind of modulation, and most junctions between neurons, and between neurons and muscle or glandular cells, do not involve physical contact. Such junctions are called synapses.

A synapse is shown diagrammatically in Figure 13.15 from which it can be seen that a small fluid-filled space exists between the neurons. This is called the synaptic cleft and, although microscopically small (of the order of 20 nm across), it represents a significant barrier to the direct conduction of the neural impulse. The neuron that is conducting an impulse terminates at the synapse as a distended bulb-like structure called a synaptic end-bulb (sometimes referred to as a bouton; = terminal button). When reference is made to synaptic function, this neuron is called the presynaptic neuron. The synaptic junction is made with either the next neuron in the pathway, which is referred to as a post-synaptic neuron, or with the (post-synaptic) membrane of a gland or muscle cell.

Microscopically it can be seen that the terminal end-bulb contains thousands of membrane-enclosed sacs, called the synaptic vesicles. Each sac contains a small amount of a chemical which is synthesized in the cell body of the neuron and transported to the end-bulb via the cytoplasm (called axoplasm in nerve cells). When an action potential arrives at an end-bulb of a presynaptic neuron, an influx of calcium ions from the bathing interstitial fluid is promoted and this causes a few of the vesicles to move to the membrane of the end-bulb (called the presynaptic membrane) and to release their contents into the synaptic cleft (Figure 13.15). Molecules of the chemical then diffuse across the cleft and interact with receptor molecules on the surface of the membrane of the post-synaptic cell (i.e. the post-synaptic membrane). This interaction between chemical and receptor induces changes in the ionic permeability of the post-synaptic membrane, and hence in its membrane potential, and collectively these chemicals are therefore called neurotransmitters.

Having interacted with post-synaptic receptors, the neurotransmitter is removed from them by the actions of enzymes, and this leaves the receptors free to interact with further chemical should it be released from the presynaptic membrane. Excess neurotransmitter

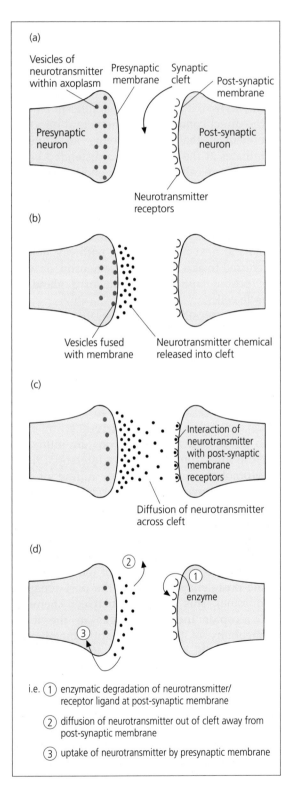

(a)

Vesicles of neurotransmitter within axoplasm

Presynaptic membrane

Synaptic cleft

Post-synaptic membrane

Presynaptic neuron

Post-synaptic neuron

Neurotransmitter receptors

(b)

Vesicles fused with membrane

Neurotransmitter chemical released into cleft

(c)

Interaction of neurotransmitter with post-synaptic membrane receptors

Diffusion of neurotransmitter across cleft

(d)

② ①

enzyme

③

i.e. ① enzymatic degradation of neurotransmitter/ receptor ligand at post-synaptic membrane

② diffusion of neurotransmitter out of cleft away from post-synaptic membrane

③ uptake of neurotransmitter by presynaptic membrane

Figure 13.15 The synapse and modes of activation. (a) 'Resting' synapse. (b) Arrival of action potentials at presynaptic membrane. (c) Activation of post-synaptic membrane. (d) Restoration of synapse to 'resting' state.

within the cleft either diffuses out of the synapse into the interstitial fluid, or is actively transported back into the presynaptic neuron.

A variety of neurotransmitters have been identified (Table 13.3). Whilst some of these cause excitation (i.e. depolarization) of the post-synaptic membrane, others cause inhibition (i.e. hyperpolarization). It is also clear that a given presynaptic neuron can only produce one type of transmitter substance and this determines the nomenclature used to describe a neuron. For example, adrenergic neurons release or respond to noradrenaline at their synapses, and cholinergic synapses involve acetylcholine. Synaptic excitation or inhibition provides the basis for neural processing (described below) and the requirement of the presynaptic release of neurotransmitter also ensures unidirectionality of neural pathways.

Excitatory neurotransmitters

Generally the release of an excitatory neurotransmitter from a single presynaptic end-bulb does not produce an action potential in the post-synaptic neuron. It does cause slight change in the resting membrane potential, however, as sodium channels begin to open, and so brings the membrane potential close to that of threshold. This slight depolarization is called an excitatory post-synaptic potential (or EPSP). Although not triggering an action potential itself, the EPSP makes the membrane more easily stimulated so that, should further neurotransmitter release occur, then the individual EPSPs that are generated may summate to reach threshold and trigger an action potential. This action potential will be propagated along the post-synaptic cell as described earlier.

In practice, EPSPs last for only a few milliseconds and so summation will only occur

Table 13.3 Examples of neurotransmitters and neuropeptides

Substance	Homeostatic actions
Neurotransmitters	
Acetylcholine (ACh)	Released by some neuromuscular and neuroglandular synapses, and at neuronal synapses in the central nervous system. ACh acts mainly as an excitatory neurotransmitter but also has inhibitory functions
Serotonin (5-HT)	Concentrated in certain neurons in the brainstem. Acts as an excitatory neurotransmitter. May induce sleep. Also involved in sensory perception, temperature regulation, and control of mood
Noradrenaline (NA)	Released at some neuromuscular and neuroglandular synapses. Also in neural synapses of the brainstem: mainly excitatory. May be involved in arousal, dreaming, and regulation of mood
Gamma-aminobutyric acid (GABA)	Concentrated in the thalamus, hypothalamus, and occipital lobes of cerebrum; mainly inhibitory
Dopamine (DA)	Inhibitory in substantia nigra of midbrain; involved in emotional responses and subconscious movements of skeletal muscles
Neuropeptides	
Substance P	Excitatory in pain pathways within central nervous system (Chapter 21)
Enkephalins	Inhibitory in pain pathways within the thalamus and spinal cord
Endorphins	Inhibitory as above. May have a role in memory and learning ⎫ (Chapter 21)
Dynorphin	Inhibitory as above. 50 times more powerful than beta-endorphin ⎭

if several adjacent end-bulbs are activated more or less simultaneously (called spatial summation), or if the same synapse is activated a few times in quick succession by the arrival of a train of impulses (called temporal summation).

Inhibitory neurotransmitters

The release of an inhibitory neurotransmitter from a single end-bulb causes a slight hyperpolarization of the post-synaptic membrane as potassium channels and/or chloride channels partly open (which will promote an efflux of positive charge out of the cell, or an influx of negative charge respectively; both therefore increase the negativity of the inside of the cell with respect to the outside). The slight hyperpolarization is called an inhibitory post-synaptic potential (or IPSP) and this can summate with other IPSPs to enhance the hyperpolarization of the membrane. By causing the membrane potential to move further away from the threshold value, IPSPs make the membrane less responsive to excitatory potentials.

Synaptic integration

Neurons, especially those within the central nervous system, may synapse with more than one other neuron. Thus, a cell body of a brain cell may be influenced by synapses from several thousand others, and some of these synapses will be excitatory, others inhibitory. Whether or not the post-synaptic membrane is stimulated depends upon the balance between the summated excitatory and inhibitory synapses that are active at that particular time. Thus a powerful input from inhibitory synapses might prevent the summation of EPSPs and so prevent the depolarization of the post-synaptic membrane from attaining the threshold potential (Figure 13.16).

Inhibitory synapses generally act in one of the following ways (see also Figure 13.17):

1 by preventing depolarization of the end-bulb of an excitatory presynaptic neuron, effectively preventing the release of the excitatory neurotransmitter. This is called presynaptic inhibition;

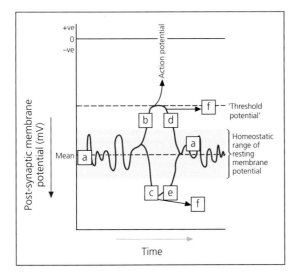

Figure 13.16 Synaptic integration as a homeostatic process.
a 'Resting' membrane potential determined by balance of excitatory and inhibitory inputs.
b Summated excitatory (i.e. depolarizing) potentials in excess of inhibitory potentials, moving membrane potential toward threshold, thus increasing excitability.
c Summated inhibitory (i.e. hyperpolarizing) potentials in excess of excitatory potentials, moving membrane potential away from threshold, thus reducing excitability.
d Restoration of membrane potential to within 'resting' range by *either* decreased excitatory synaptic activity *or* increased inhibitory synaptic activity, i.e. balance of excitatory vs. inhibitory inputs restored.
e Restoration of membrane potential to within 'resting' range by *either* decreased inhibitory synaptic activity *or* increased excitatory synaptic activity, i.e. excitatory vs. inhibitory inputs balanced.
f Persistently increased or decreased membrane excitability by maintenance of imbalance between excitatory and inhibitory inputs.

(a)

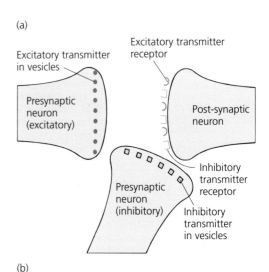

(b)

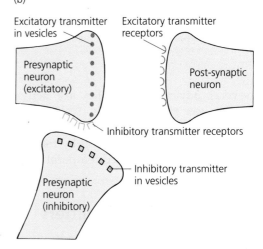

(c)

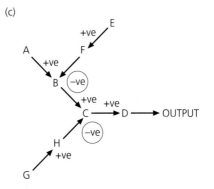

Figure 13.17 Post-synaptic and presynaptic inhibition of synapses, and their role in integrative responses.
(a) Post-synaptic inhibition: interaction between inhibitory neurotransmitters with post-synaptic membranes.
(b) Presynaptic inhibition: interaction between inhibitory neurotransmitter and presynaptic membrane of excitatory neuron. (c) Integration (A–G are neurons). Activity from D is dependent upon presence or absence of inhibitory influences from F and H, and also the integrity of the excitatory neurons throughout the pathway.

2 by prevention of the actions of the neuro-transmitter from the end-bulb of an excitatory neuron. This is an effect on the post-synaptic membrane and is therefore called post-synaptic inhibition.

The importance of synaptic integration is that neural pathways can be modulated by other pathways (Figure 13.17c). In other words, the synapse can be envisaged as being a 'switch' within a neural circuit, which may be 'open' (i.e. excited) or 'closed' (i.e. inhibited). The 'opening' and 'closing' of neural circuits forms the basis of neural processing in the central nervous system, and severe disorders can result if excitatory or inhibitory pathways are abnormally activated (see later section).

Overview of the functional anatomy of the brain

It was mentioned earlier that the brain develops embryologically as three main anatomical structures: the forebrain, the midbrain, and the hindbrain. The cranial nerves and meningeal membranes are the other prominent structures associated with the brain. The functions of parts of the brain are obviously very complex, and much is still not understood. The intention of this section, therefore, is only to provide an overview of brain anatomy and function. From the functional viewpoint, the control of a particular aspect of physiology may involve an integration of activity from various parts of the brain. Accordingly, a summary of some of the integrative aspects of brain function is also provided.

FOREBRAIN

The forebrain consists of perhaps the most obvious external feature of the brain – the highly convoluted cerebrum (or telencephalon) – but also some deeper structures which together comprise the diencephalon.

The cerebrum

The cerebrum is divided into two hemispheres, connected by a large bundle of (mainly) myelinated axons called the corpus callosum (Figure 13.18b). This allows communication between

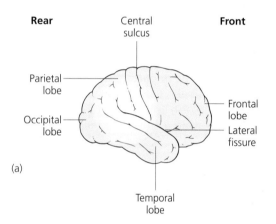

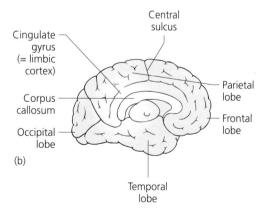

Figure 13.18 Cerebral hemispheres of the forebrain.
(a) External features: lateral view.
(b) The inner surface of the left hemisphere, with the right hemisphere removed.

the two hemispheres and links geographically similar positions of the left and right hemispheres. It is the corpus callosum that is sectioned in a split-brain operation. Each hemisphere consists of outer, or cortical, areas (cortex = 'bark'), and subcortical structures including a number of cerebral 'nuclei' which may interact with each other, with other parts of the hemispheres, or with midbrain and hindbrain structures.

Cortex

The cortex is comprised of 'grey' matter and represents major processing areas. The hemispheres have various functions but some generalizations regarding perceptual functioning can be made. The left hemisphere seems to be more effective at analysing information presented to it in changing sequences and is considered to be important in logic and mathematical analysis ('scientific' functions). The right hemisphere appears more effective in the analysis of shape, form and space ('artistic' functions).

Curiously, the cortex of the right hemisphere also controls the contraction of muscles on the left side of the body, and vice versa. Although both hemispheres must be used together, the occurrence of right or left handedness is taken to imply left or right hemispheric dominance respectively and various studies have suggested that left handedness gives a propensity to artistic abilities.

The surfaces of the hemispheres are divided into four lobes named after the bones of the skull which overlie them, called the frontal lobe, temporal lobe, parietal lobe and occipital lobe (Figure 13.18a). The frontal lobe is separated from the parietal lobe by a large involution called the central sulcus whilst the temporal lobe is delineated by an indentation called the lateral fissure.

FRONTAL LOBES

The frontal lobes are involved in the planning, execution, and evaluation of actions. The cortex includes an area called the motor associ-

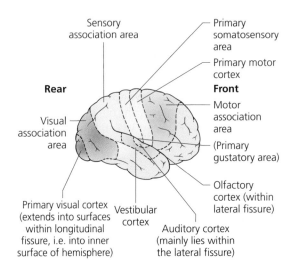

Figure 13.19 Cerebral cortex: general functional anatomy.

ation area (Figure 13.19) in which information concerning planned actions is collated and passed to the primary motor cortex area just forward of the central sulcus. This area determines most of the final efferent output to the muscles. Functions also include the control of facial and neck muscles, and so the frontal lobe is also involved in the control of voluntary eye movements, and speech (this latter especially involves the frontal lobe of the left hemisphere).

PARIETAL LOBES

The parietal lobes are particularly involved in sensory reception and perception. Just behind the central sulcus, directly behind the motor cortex, is an area called the primary somatosensory cortex (Figure 13.19) which receives information from the somatosenses, that is the 'body' senses of touch, pressure, temperature, and pain. Information from this area passes to various parts of the brain including the sensory association area of the parietal lobes. This is a large area which extends into the occipital and temporal lobes (and so receives input from those lobes also), and is involved in the perception of a stimulus, the integration of various stimuli, and also in memory.

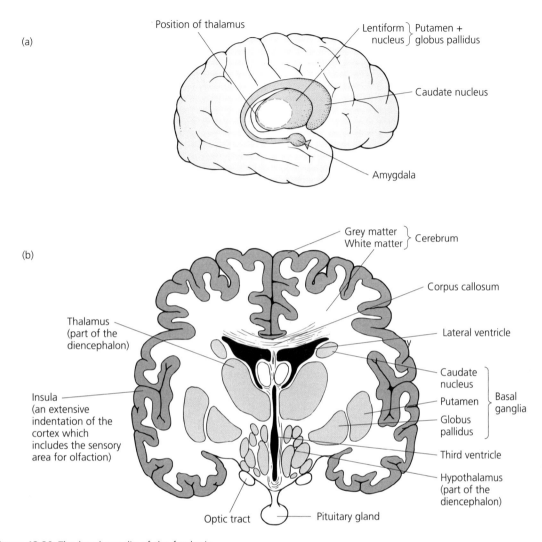

Figure 13.20 The basal ganglia of the forebrain.
(a) Sagittal section to show positions of the main nuclei. (b) Cross-section to show the main nuclei and their position relative to other cerebral structures.

OCCIPITAL LOBES

The occipital lobe consists mainly of the visual cortex (Figure 13.19) and so receives most of its input from the eyes. The primary visual cortex lies within the surfaces of the longitudinal fissure between the two hemispheres.

TEMPORAL LOBES

The temporal lobe has already been mentioned as consisting of part of the sensory association area. It also receives sensory information from the ears and consists mainly of the auditory cortex (Figure 13.19).

Cerebral nuclei

Below the cortex there is substantial white matter, indicative of myelinated axons which convey information through the brain from one area to another. This subcortical region

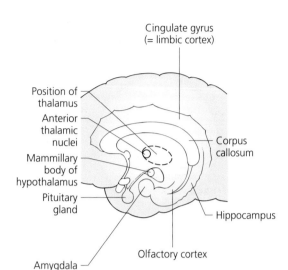

Figure 13.21 Relative positions of major components of the limbic system.

also contains nuclei of grey matter which collectively comprise processing areas called the basal ganglia and the limbic system.

The basal ganglia are a collection of inter-connected structures within both hemispheres which are involved in the control of movement and so interact with the motor cortex. They are illustrated in Figure 13.20, and are described in more detail in Chapter 16.

The limbic system, shown in Figure 13.21, is another collection of interconnected structures surrounding the centre of the forebrain. Two of the most prominent structures are called the hippocampus (named because of its passing resemblance to the shape of a sea-horse) and the amygdala (= 'almond'). Some of the cerebral cortex is also part of the limbic system, especially that along the edge (limbus = 'border') of the cerebral hemispheres, within the fissure between them, which is often referred to as the limbic cortex. Much of the area is readily distinguishable from the rest of the cortex, and is called the cingulate gyrus. The limbic system has various functions, including roles in memory, behaviour, and emotions.

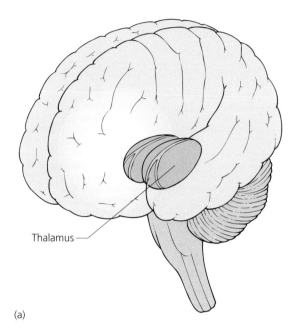

(a)

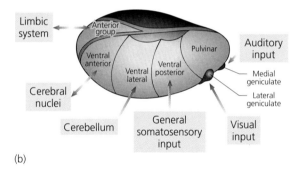

(b)

Figure 13.22 The diencephalon of the forebrain, I: the thalamus. (a) General position of the thalamic nuclei. (b) Thalamic nuclei and their main connections.

Diencephalon

The diencephalon consists of structures deep within the forebrain which separate the cerebrum from the midbrain. There are two major components: the thalamus and the hypothalamus (Figure 13.20b).

Thalamus

The thalamus is a large, bilobed structure, which acts as a relay centre for neural input

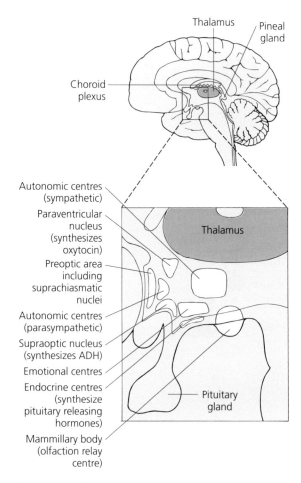

Figure 13.23 The diencephalon of the forebrain, II: the hypothalamus. The functional roles of the major hypothalamic nuclei are shown.

(mainly sensory information) to the cerebral cortex. The thalamus itself is a heterogeneous structure and can be divided into several functional 'nuclei' (Figure 13.22). Axons from these nuclei pass to specific areas of cortex. For example, the lateral (i.e. at the sides of the thalamus) geniculate nuclei receive input from the eyes and relay it to the visual cortex, and the medial (i.e. at the middle of the thalamus) geniculate nuclei receive input from the cochlea of the ear and relay it to the auditory cortex. Not all thalamic nuclei receive sensory information directly, however. For example, the ventral (i.e. at the bottom of the thalamus)

geniculate nuclei receive input from another part of the brain (the cerebellum, see later) and relay it to the motor cortex.

Hypothalamus

The hypothalamus (hypo- = below) is a relatively small structure lying at the base of the brain (Figures 13.20b and 13.23). It is a complex structure, containing several nuclei of cells, and tracts of axons. The nuclei control the autonomic nervous system and, via the pituitary gland, the release of several major hormones. The hypothalamus, therefore, provides an important link between the brain and the functioning of other physiological systems and its role in this respect is described in the relevant chapters. In addition, the hypothalamus is also involved in behaviour organization.

MIDBRAIN

The midbrain (or mesencephalon) lies deep within the brain and consists of two major component parts called the tectum and the tegmentum (Figures 13.24). The midbrain also contains the cerebral aqueduct, the centrally placed channel that connects the third and fourth fluid-filled ventricles of the brain.

Tectum

The tectum (= 'roof') forms the dorsal, or posterior, part of the midbrain. It consists of a number of structures, the main ones being the superior (i.e. upper) and inferior (i.e. lower) colliculi. These appear as four bumps on the brainstem (Figure 13.24a). The superior colliculi receive sensory input from the eyes, via the thalamus, and are involved in the control of eye movement, whilst the inferior colliculi receive input from the ears.

Tegmentum

The tegmentum (= 'covering') lies anterior to the tectum and is a complex structure containing

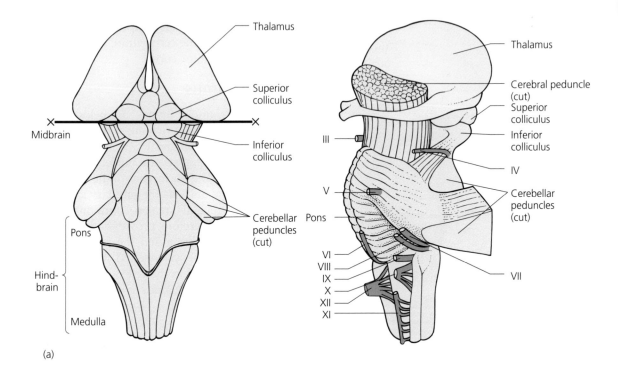

(a)

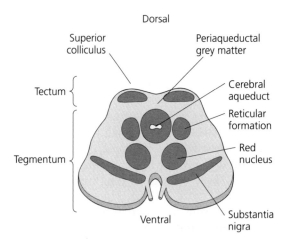

Figure 13.24 (a) Major external features of the brainstem. (b) Section through the midbrain at X–X in (a).

many nuclei. These include some of those involved in the control of movement: the substantia nigra (= 'black substance'; these neurons contain melanin) connects with certain basal ganglia of the forebrain, and the red nucleus projects to the spinal cord and is part of the pathways which convey information out of the brain to the muscles.

The tegmentum also contains part of the reticular (= 'net') formation which is a diffuse area extending into the hindbrain (see below). It receives sensory information from the body and relays it to the cerebral cortex or the thalamus. It is more than just a relay station, however, and has been found to have a role in the sleep/wake cycle and in movement control. Some axons project to the spinal cord and so are efferent pathways from the brain.

HINDBRAIN

The structures of the hindbrain (or rhombo-encephalon) are visible as external features. There are three main components; the cerebellum, pons varolii, and medulla oblongata (Figure 13.25a).

Cerebellum

The cerebellum (= 'little brain') is a large structure behind and below the rest of the brain. In general structure it resembles that of the cerebrum: it has a cortex of grey matter which connects with a set of subcortical structures called the cerebellar nuclei. The cerebellum receives inputs from the eyes, vestibular apparatus of the ears and from somatosensory receptors around the body. Information is then relayed to other areas involved in the control of movement, particularly the cerebral cortex. In addition the cerebellum receives information from the motor cortex regarding the efferent output to muscles.

The activities of the cerebellum provide a 'fine tuning' of movement. The cerebellum, therefore, is important in the coordination of movement for standing and walking, in the production of smooth movement, and in the production of fine movements such as are involved in writing, playing sport, etc.

Pons varolii

The pons (= 'bridge') is visible externally as a large bulge on the brainstem (Figures 13.24a,

13.25a). Some of its composite structures, such as the reticular formation, are continuous with those of the midbrain and medulla, and the tegmentum mentioned above forms the upper part of the pons. There are numerous small nuclei of cells within the pons: many are the nuclei of various cranial nerves whilst others are part of the pathways by which sensory information coming in from the spinal cord passes to appropriate parts of the brain, or form part of the pathways by which efferent activity from motor areas of the brain converge before forming the large efferent tracts called the pyramids (Figure 13.25b).

Converging sensory fibres from the spinal cord form the lemnisci (lemniscus, singular), which traverse the medulla and pons and pass to the thalamus of the forebrain. Another large tract of fibres worth mentioning here are those which form the cerebellar peduncles (Figure 13.24a). These carry sensory information arriving in the pons (via the spinal cord and cranial nerves) to the cerebellum, and also relay information coming out of the cerebellum to the brainstem and cerebral cortex.

Medulla oblongata

The medulla is the section of brainstem which links the brain with the spinal cord. Anteriorly two large tracts of axons pass through the medulla carrying efferent activity to the muscles. These are the pyramids, which are first visible in the pons, and it is in the medulla that the tract from the left side of the brain crosses over (or decussates) to the opposite side of the spinal cord, and so mediates contraction of muscles on the right side of the body, and vice versa (Figure 13.25b). Other large tracts, called the gracile and cuneate fasciculi (there are two of each), are noticeable on the posterior aspect of the medulla. These tracts carry sensory input into the brainstem from the spinal cord.

Internally the medulla is comprised of axonal tracts passing through the brainstem, with associated nuclei, and nuclei of some

(a) External features and position of the cardiovascular centres and respiratory centres

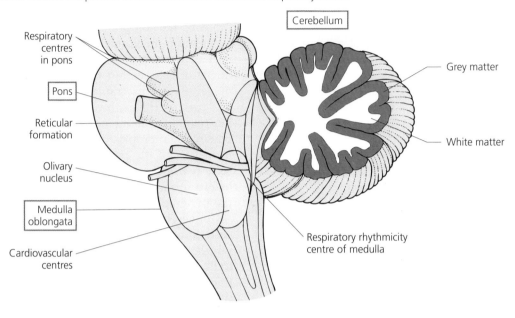

Respiratory centres in pons

Cerebellum

Grey matter

Pons

Reticular formation

White matter

Olivary nucleus

Medulla oblongata

Respiratory rhythmicity centre of medulla

Cardiovascular centres

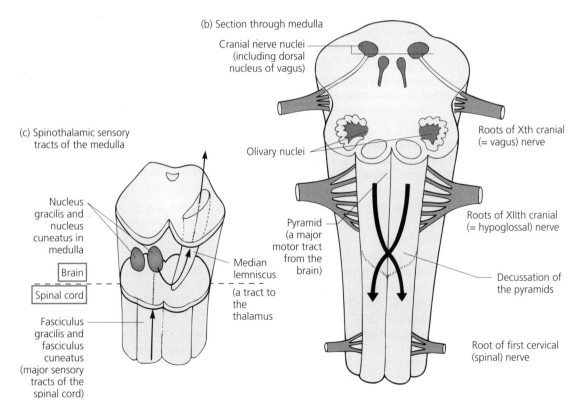

(b) Section through medulla

Cranial nerve nuclei (including dorsal nucleus of vagus)

(c) Spinothalamic sensory tracts of the medulla

Olivary nuclei

Roots of Xth cranial (= vagus) nerve

Nucleus gracilis and nucleus cuneatus in medulla

Pyramid (a major motor tract from the brain)

Roots of XIIth cranial (= hypoglossal) nerve

Brain

Median lemniscus (a tract to the thalamus

Spinal cord

Decussation of the pyramids

Fasciculus gracilis and fasciculus cuneatus (major sensory tracts of the spinal cord)

Root of first cervical (spinal) nerve

Figure 13.25 The hindbrain. (a) External features, and position of the cardiovascular centres and respiratory centres. (b) Section through the medulla, anterior aspect. (c) Spinothalamic sensory tracts of the medulla, posterior aspect.

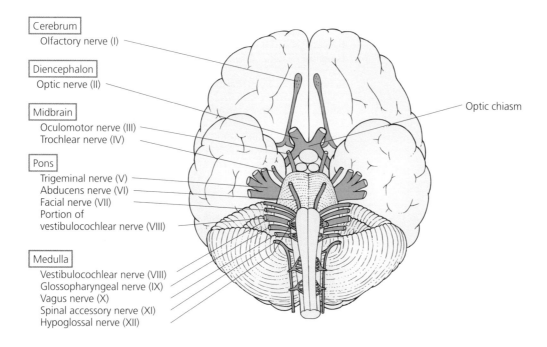

Figure 13.26 The cranial nerves.

cranial nerves. For example, the gracile and cuneate fasciculi terminate at the gracile and cuneate nuclei respectively, from which axons project, as the median lemniscus, toward the thalamus (Figure 13.25c).

The presence of certain cranial nerve nuclei within the medulla also means that this part of the brainstem is particularly involved with coordinating some of the activities of the autonomic nervous system. Diffuse areas of neurons, and various nuclei, comprise the respiratory 'inspiratory' and 'expiratory' centres and the cardiovascular 'accelerator' and 'depressor' areas (Figure 13.25a). Output from the respiratory centres, and hence the regulation of breathing rhythm, is normally controlled by input from an 'apneustic' centre within the pons (see Chapter 11).

In addition to receiving afferent information from autonomic neurons, the medullary areas involved in promoting respiratory and cardio-vascular responses also receive inputs from areas of the hypothalamus (which also receives

input from the limbic system) and these are responsible for the mediation of psychological influences on autonomic responses.

Two oval-shaped protrusions are noticeable on the anterior surface of the medulla (Figure 13.25a,b). These are the olivary bodies, inside which are found the inferior olivary nuclei. These sac-like structures, together with accessory nuclei, act as relay centres for transmission of activity from various parts of the brain and spinal cord to the cerebellum.

CRANIAL NERVES

The cranial nerves are actually part of the peripheral nervous system but are usually considered separately from the spinal nerves because they connect directly with the brain, rather than via spinal pathways. There are 12 pairs of cranial nerves: 10 pairs connect with the brainstem, 2 pairs (olfactory and optic

Table 13.4 Functions of the cranial nerves

Cranial nerve	Branch	Homeostatic Function	Tissues innervated
Olfactory (I)	–	Sensory	From olfactory epithelium of the nose
Optic (II)	–	Sensory	From retinal cells of the eye
Oculomotor (III)	–	Motor	To the rectus muscles (inferior, superior, medial) and inferior oblique muscle that move the eyes. Also to the upper lip area
Trochlear (IV)	–	Motor	To the superior oblique muscle of the eye
Trigeminal (V)	Ophthalmic	Sensory	From areas around the orbits of the eyes, the nasal cavity, the forehead, upper eyelids, and eyebrows
	Maxillary	Sensory	From the lower eyelids, upper lip, upper gums and teeth, the mucous lining of the palate, and the skin of the face
	Mandibular	Mixed	*Sensory* from the skin of the jaw, the lower gums and teeth, and the lower lip. *Motor* to the muscles of mastication, and to the floor of the mouth.
Abducens (VI)	–	Motor	To the rectus muscles (lateral) that move the eyes
Facial (VII)	–	Mixed	*Sensory* from taste receptors (anterior two-thirds of tongue). *Motor* to muscles of facial expression. Includes visceral efferents (autonomic nervous system) to the submandibular and sublingual salivary glands, and tear glands
Vestibulocochlear (VIII)	Vestibular	Sensory	From the vestibular apparatus (balance organs) of inner ear
	Cochlear	Sensory	From hearing receptors of the cochlea of inner ear
Glossopharyngeal (IX)	–	Mixed	*Sensory* from the pharynx, tonsils, and posterior third of tongue. Includes visceral afferents (autonomic nervous system) from carotid arteries and aortic arch. *Motor* to pharynx (i.e. swallowing movements). Also visceral efferents (autonomic nervous system) to parotid salivary glands
Vagus (X)	–	Mixed	*Sensory* from the pharynx, larynx, and oesophagus. Also visceral afferents (autonomic nervous system) from the thorax and abdomen. *Motor* to the larynx, pharynx, and soft palate (swallowing movements). Also visceral efferents (autonomic nervous system) to viscera of the thorax and abdomen
Accessory (XI)	Cranial	Motor	To the pharynx, larynx, and soft palate (swallowing movements)
	Spinal	Motor	To the sternocleidomastoid and trapezius muscles of the neck
Hypoglossal (XII)	–	Motor	To the musculature of the tongue

nerves) connect with forebrain structures (Figure 13.26 and Table 13.4). These are only the initial connections, however. Afferent information carried by the nerves is destined for various parts of the brain, whilst convergence of activity from different areas of the brain produces the information carried by efferent nerve fibres.

The cranial nerves are named according to appearance or function, but there is also a conventional method of numbering them (Figure 13.26 and Table 13.4). Each cranial nerve attaches to the brain at a point close to the 'nucleus' in which its neurons synapse with central nervous system neurons. One cranial nerve nucleus of note within the medulla is the dorsal nucleus of the vagus (the vagus is the Xth cranial nerve) which is the source of parasympathetic nerve cells that supply the thoracic and abdominal viscera (Figure 13.25b). The vagus is a 'mixed' nerve as it contains both sensory afferent and motor efferent nerve axons. Other cranial nerves may be 'mixed' or only sensory or motor nerves (Figure 13.26, Table 13.4).

MENINGEAL MEMBRANES

The brain and spinal cord are lined with three membranes, collectively called the meninges. The outermost layer is called the dura mater, the innermost layer is called the pia mater. Between them is found the arachnoid mater (Figures 13.27).

The dura mater is comprised mainly of collagen and forms a thick, tough protective/supportive layer. The layer around the brain has two components: an inner meningeal layer which is continuous between the brain and spinal cord, and an outer layer which is really the periosteal lining of the bones of the cranial cavity. Intracranial venous sinuses, which eventually return the cranial circulation to the jugular veins, may be found between the layers. The meningeal layer also provides a sheath around the cranial nerves until they exit the skull, and also forms inwardly folding

(a) Around the brain

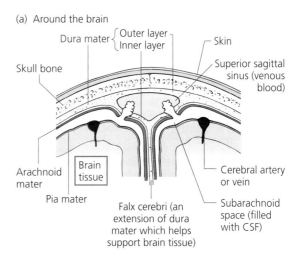

Note: Arachnoid and pia mater are connected by a network of bridging strands (called trabeculae) which help to maintain the patency of the subarachnoid space

(b) Around the spinal chord

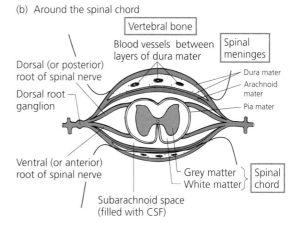

Figure 13.27 The meninges. (a) Around the brain. Note arachnoid and pia maters are 'connected' by a meshwork of bridging strands called trabeculae which help to maintain the patency of the subarachnoid space. (b) Around the spinal cord.

septa which project into the major indentations or sulci of the brain and so help to support it.

The arachnoid mater is a delicate membrane of loose connective tissue. A narrow subdural space separates it from the overlying dura mater, and a much larger space, the subarachnoid space, separates it from the underlying pia mater. This latter space contains cerebrospinal fluid (CSF) and, in certain places, the arachnoid mater penetrates the dura mater to project into the superior sagittal (blood) sinus. These projections are the arachnoid villi and provide the surface for reabsorption of the CSF into the venous circulation. Enlargements of the subarachnoid space in certain parts of the brain, and at the base of the spinal cord, are used clinically to obtain samples of CSF.

The pia mater covers the actual surface of the brain and spinal cord, and also forms a sheath around cranial nerves and spinal nerve roots as they traverse the subarachnoid space. The mater resembles the arachnoid in structure, but is additionally rich in blood vessels which supply the underlying neural tissue. The pia mater also lines the cerebral ventricles and forms the choroid plexus through which the CSF is secreted.

OVERVIEW OF CEREBRAL FUNCTIONAL INTEGRATION

The brain has an extensive role in the control of tissue and organ functions within the body, via the autonomic nervous system, the hypothalamopituitary hormone axis and the mediation of skeletal muscle contraction. These functions are dealt with later in this chapter and elsewhere (Chapters 15 and 16), and this section will only concentrate on some of the brain's cognitive functions. The aim is to present, albeit simplistically, a summary of such functions, the intention being to emphasize the necessity of integrating the activity from various areas of the brain. Much of the physiology of cognitive function is still unknown, and in some instances insight has only been gained in recent years. What constitutes 'consciousness', however, remains an enigma: no physiological basis has been ascertained as yet!

Sleep

The electrical activity of the cortex undergoes four distinct phases during sleep, as shown in

Table 13.5 Electroencephalogram (EEG) patterns and stages of sleep

(a) EEG waveforms

Waves	Frequency (cycles/s)	State of consciousness
Alpha α	8–23	Awake but quiet
Beta β	14–25	Awake, but tense (note: waves are asynchronous during normal increase in mental activity)
Theta θ	4–7	Emotional stress
Delta δ	<3.5	Deep sleep, or anaesthesia (slow wave)

(b) Sleep stages

Sleep stage	Observed EEG
1	Low voltage wave interrupted periodically by bursts of α-waves
2/3	Progressive decline to 2–3 cycles/s, i.e. δ-waves
4 (REM)	Bursts of desynchronized β-waves similar to those in wakefulness. Lasts for 5–30 minutes, recurring approximately every 90 minutes

REM, rapid eye movement sleep, or paradoxical sleep.

Table 13.5. The 'deep' sleep of stage 3 is characterized by the occurrence of synchronized patterns of activity with a slow frequency, and so is called 'slow-wave' sleep. The fourth stage, however, is characterized by alternation between slow waves and patterns of activity reminiscent of more shallow sleep, or even consciousness. Such patterns produce changes in heart and breathing rates, rapid eye movements are observed (and so this is called rapid eye movement, or REM, sleep), and, generally, there is a pronounced muscular paralysis. Dreaming occurs in this stage and it seems to relate to bursts of electrical activity passing from the pons (of the brainstem) to the visual cortex of the occipital lobe. Evidence suggests that sleep (especially stages 3 and 4) is a period during which information is sifted and its emotional impact assessed. Memory is updated accordingly.

Arousal is associated with increased activity in areas of the reticular formation within the upper pons and midbrain regions (Figures 13.24b, 13.25a). The pathways utilize noradrenaline as an excitatory neurotransmitter (which is mimicked by amphetamine abuse) and the activity radiates to the thalamus, hypothalamus, cerebral cortex and other parts of the hindbrain (Figure 13.28). Sleep arises when activity from the reticular formation is inhibited, and this is a site of action of many general anaesthetics and sedative drugs.

Slow-wave sleep seems to involve an inhibitory action of nuclei within the medulla, particularly those called the raphe nuclei, via neurons which utilize the inhibitory transmitter serotonin. REM sleep, which includes a degree of cortical excitation, seems to involve noradrenergic neurons from the reticular formation, and also excitatory cholinergic neurons from various other nuclei within the pons. The latter are probably inhibited during slow-wave sleep but the inhibition is modulated during REM sleep. The pontine nuclei also seem to be responsible for the inhibition of spinal cord motor neurons (causing paralysis) during REM sleep (note that acetylcholine is excitatory, therefore the neurons must synapse with other inhibitory ones for this effect).

Sleep and wakefulness is determined, therefore, by the balance of activities within these various brainstem nuclei. Although these nuclei can be said to induce sleep or wakefulness, what regulates sleep is less clear. The presence of sleep-inducing substances, released into the cerebrospinal fluid, has been implicated but their role remains debatable.

Sleep and wakening is an important biological (i.e. circadian) rhythm which appears to be associated with the suprachiasmatic nuclei of the hypothalamus (a site of putative biological 'clocks'). Neurons from this area pass to the brainstem and cortex.

Memory

Memory is considered to have two components: short- and long-term. Short-term

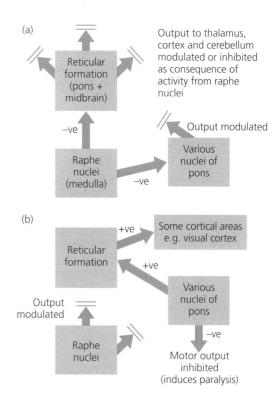

Figure 13.28 Interactions between structures of the brainstem during (a) slow-wave sleep and (b) rapid eye movement (REM) sleep.

memory has a duration of several seconds or a few minutes at most, and has limited volume. Such memories can be converted into long-term ones by consolidation of the information.

Learning can be perceptual (visual), stimulus-response conditioning (an association between two stimuli) or relational (an association between two events). Perceptual learning utilizes the visual association area of the temporal lobe of the cortex, whilst conditional learning involves the amygdala nuclei of the limbic system, which seems to act as a mediator between sensory inputs and behavioural responses. The amygdala, however, has a complex circuitry and receives inputs from various parts of the brain, whilst neurons pass from it to the autonomic nuclei of the brainstem, and to the hypothalamus. Some areas of the cerebellum also appear to be involved in conditional learning.

Relational learning involves the hippocampus (of the limbic system) which consolidates short-term memories. Various nuclei of the thalamus are also involved in the process, and also in the recall of information from long-term stores. Memory also involves the area of cerebral cortex called the limbic cortex.

Short-term memory seems to be associated with the persistent excitability of neurons within the cortex. Such changes seem to reverberate within neuronal circuits, the oscillation of activity remaining for perhaps several minutes before declining. Long-term memory is not associated with persistent neural activity, however. Experimental evidence suggests that the numbers of synaptic connections are increased, and that individual synapses are sensitized or primed so that they are more likely to be stimulated should similar sensory information arrive at a later date.

Acetylcholine is an important excitatory neurotransmitter of memory circuits within the hippocampus and the limbic cortex. Dopamine is also involved (probably as an inhibitory transmitter) in areas of the limbic cortex, whilst endogenous inhibitory or excitatory opiates are important in the amygdala. The complexity of memory is such, however, that various other neurotransmitters have also been implicated, and this is evidence of complex, multiple neuronal circuits.

Speech and language

Areas of the left hemisphere dominate in the comprehension of language and in the production of speech. This seems to be most appropriate considering the general 'analytical' properties of that hemisphere. The right hemisphere includes cortical areas involved in the understanding of the meaning of words, and also applies emotional overtones to the voice.

Comprehension of speech begins within the auditory pathways, particularly in Wernicke's area of the auditory cortex in the superior aspect of the left temporal lobe (Figure 13.29). In contrast, speech is synthesized in a cortical

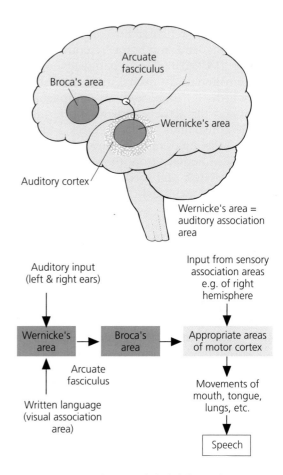

Figure 13.29 Speech areas of the left hemisphere.

area of the left frontal lobe, called Broca's area. This area lies adjacent to the motor cortex responsible for producing movement of the tongue, lips and larynx in the enunciation of speech. It is thought that Wernicke's area in some way contains memories of the features of auditory sounds, turning them into words, whilst Broca's area contains memories of the motor output required to verbalize words. Neurons from Wernicke's area project to Broca's area via a tract of nerve fibres called the arcuate fasciculus.

The 'meaning' of words is stored within parts of the sensory association cortex, and the motivation to speak is supplied by areas of the motor cortex.

Emotional behaviours

'Behaviours' are diverse functions of the brain, but some generalizations can be made regarding the role of the limbic system. Thus, the amygdala nuclei convey a behavioural awareness and ensure that patterns of response are appropriate to an individual's situation. Different areas of the hippocampus are involved in different emotions, such as rage and passivity, and the limbic cortex appears to provide the association required between activity passing to and from various areas of cerebral cortex and the rest of the limbic system.

Aggressive behaviours especially involve medial (offensive behaviour) and dorsal (defensive behaviour) areas of the hypothalamus. Both project to the midbrain for expression. The amygdala is also involved and neurons pass from here to the hypothalamus and midbrain. Interestingly, the amygdala responds to the presence of sex steroids, suggesting a role in sexual aggression.

Sexual behaviour involves various areas. The area of the basal forebrain lying anterior to the chiasma of the optic nerves determines copulatory behaviour and territorial aggression in males, and maternal behaviour in females. The ventromedial nuclei of the hypothalamus determine copulatory behaviour in females. Sexual behaviours are modulated by areas of the limbic cortex.

Overview of the functional anatomy of the spinal cord

The main functions of the spinal cord are to transmit motor activity from the brain to target tissues within the body, and to carry sensory activity from around the body to the brain. The cord, therefore, increases in diameter on ascending the vertebral column as more fibres are incorporated into it. The spinal cord is protected by the vertebrae, passing through the spinal foramen of each bone, and is covered by the three meningeal layers noted earlier.

In fact, the cord is not as long as the vertebral column. On reaching the level of the 2nd lumbar vertebra the cord divides into a mass of neural structures which are the roots of various nerves that enter or exit the cord below this point. The structure is reminiscent of a horse's tail and so is called the cauda equina (see Figure 13.4).

Nerve roots leave the cord and cauda equina at intervals. At each vertebral joint there is a pair of posterior (or dorsal) and anterior (or ventral) nerve roots (see Figure 13.5). The dorsal and ventral roots fuse after leaving the cord within spaces between the vertebrae, called the vertebral foramen, thus forming the spinal nerves of which there are 31 pairs (8 pairs arise from the cervical, 12 from the thoracic, 5 from the lumbar, 5 from the sacral and 1 from the coccygeal vertebrae).

It was noted earlier in this chapter that each spinal nerve consists of sensory (afferent) and motor (efferent) neurons, and it is the sensory neurons which form the dorsal nerve root, whilst the motor neurons form the ventral root. The cell bodies of afferent neurons are found in the same area of the dorsal root and produce the distension called a dorsal root ganglion. The cell bodies of motor neurons lie within the cord itself so there is no comparable ganglionic structure in the ventral root.

STRUCTURE OF THE SPINAL CORD: WHITE MATTER

It was noted earlier that the periphery of the spinal cord appears white in section as a consequence of the presence of myelin, though unmyelinated fibres and glial cells will also be present. The white matter, therefore, consists of

(a) White matter

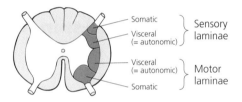

| Descending tracts | | Ascending tracts |

Lateral corticospinal tract (cerebral cortex → cord)

Fasciculus gracilis ⎫ Posterior or
Fasciculus cuneatus ⎬ dorsal columns

Rubrospinal tract (red nucleus of midbrain → cord)

Posterior spinocerebellar tract (cord → cerebellum)

Lateral spinothalamic tract (cord → thalamus)

Reticulospinal tract (reticular formation → cord)

Anterior spinocerebellar tract (cord → cerebellum)

Vestibulospinal tract (vestibular nucleus → cord)

Tectospinal tract (tectum of mid-brain → cord)

Anterior corticospinal tract (cerebral cortex → cord)

Anterior spinothalamic tract (cord → thalamus)

(b) Grey matter

Somatic ⎫
Visceral (= autonomic) ⎬ Sensory laminae

Visceral (= autonomic) ⎫
Somatic ⎬ Motor laminae

Note: Various laminae are present within each group, e.g. substantia gelatinosa within sensory groups

Figure 13.30 Structural organization of the white and grey matter of the spinal cord. (a) White matter. (b) Grey matter.

neuronal fibres which descend or ascend the cord, and is highly organized with neurons forming 'columns' within the cord periphery called dorsal, lateral, or ventral columns according to location. Within the columns, neurons passing to or from similar parts of the brain are arranged into 'tracts' (Figure 13.30a). The dorsal columns are comprised of ascending neuronal tracts which transmit sensory information to the brain. The other columns consist of tracts of ascending (sensory) and descending (motor) neurons.

Ascending tracts

The dorsal columns consist of axons of sensory relay neurons which, on entering the cord, turn to ascend it. They terminate by synapsing with nerve cells within the medulla of the hindbrain, from which neurons cross over to the opposite side before ascending further. Functionally these neurons carry sensory information from mechanoreceptors, particularly cutaneous ones (see Chapter 14). Note that the anatomical arrangement means that the neurons conveying information from such receptors within the foot to the brain must be approximately 1.5 metres in length! (but microscopically thin of course).

Ascending tracts of the lateral and ventral columns consist of neurons which convey information from temperature and pain receptors, as well as pressure receptors of the skin and proprioreceptors of the muscles and joints (see Chapter 14). The neurons synapse with others where they enter the cord; these are sometimes referred to as second-order neurons, the first-order neurons being the afferent neuron from the receptor. Some second-order neurons ascend on the same side as the afferent neuron enters the cord, others cross over to the opposite side before ascending the cord. The destination in the brain of these tracts is considered further in Chapter 14.

Descending tracts

There are a number of descending tracts within the lateral and ventral columns (Figure 13.30a). They are named according to where they originate within the brain, but each tract consists of motor neurons which will eventually synapse with other efferent neurons that pass to skeletal muscles or glandular tissue. Their names and functions are considered further in Chapter 16, where control of muscle function is described.

STRUCTURE OF THE SPINAL CORD: GREY MATTER

The central portion of the cord in section appears as a somewhat H-shaped area (Figure 13.30b). This is the grey matter of the cord, though in life it is actually pink due to blood vessels. It consists of neuronal cell bodies, axons, and glial cells.

Sensory neurons entering the cord via the dorsal root of a spinal nerve enter the grey matter (which at this point is called the dorsal horn) where they either turn to enter the ascending white columns, or relay with small interneurons (association, or relay neurons) which may be entirely confined within the grey matter or project to other parts of grey or white matter. These cells, therefore, provide communication channels, and sites of possible integration, in the cord. Other parts of the grey matter are comprised of the cell bodies of motor neurons, the axons of which project out of the ventral root of a spinal nerve via the ventral or anterior horn. The cell bodies of these cells will relay with descending neurons from the brain, or with interneurons within the grey matter.

Neurons of the lateral areas of the grey matter are particularly involved with the autonomic branch of the peripheral nervous system (see below).

Cells within the grey matter therefore form a laminar arrangement, not columnar as in white matter. In other words there is once again a high degree of neural organization (Figure 13.30b). The types of cell present, and communication, reflect the three main functions of the grey matter, which are: initial processing of incoming sensory information, final processing of outgoing motor activity, and an integrative role modulating motor output in direct response to sensory input without involving the brain (i.e. reflex responses).

Most sensory input into the cord undergoes little or no processing and is relayed intact to the brain. An important exception is that of pain which can undergo considerable modulation, probably within those laminae which comprise the substantia gelatinosa. This modulation is discussed further in Chapter 21.

Spinal canal

The spinal canal lies at the centre of the cord

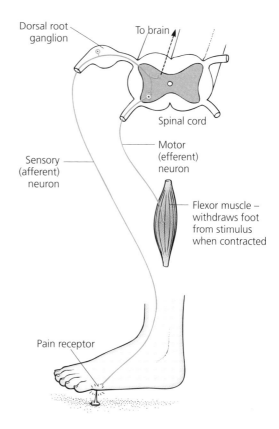

Figure 13.31 A simple monosynaptic reflex arc in response to a painful stimulus.

Note that the brain is *not* involved in the initial response, although information regarding the stimulus and the change in position of the limb will be transmitted to it. The full response will be more complicated than that shown as other postural muscles will be reflexly contracted or relaxed to maintain balance (see Chapter 16).

and extends into the medulla of the hindbrain where it communicates with the fourth ventricle, or fluid space, of the brain. The canal is filled with cerebrospinal fluid, which circulates down the cord and back to the brain by the action of the ciliated epithelium that lines the canal.

OVERVIEW OF THE FUNCTIONS OF THE SPINAL CORD

The spinal cord clearly acts as a conduit for the rapid conduction of information between peripheral nerves and the brain. It is more than an organized 'carriageway', however, and is capable of a limited degree of neural integration. In particular it is involved in the reflex coordination of movement and autonomic function.

Reflexes

Reflexes are responses which do not involve extensive integration of activity by the brain prior to their initiation. The main advantage of having reflex neural pathways is that responses to sensory stimulation can occur much more rapidly than they would if processing by the brain was involved. The process is illustrated by the limb withdrawal reflex in response to pain (Figure 13.31).

Limb withdrawal requires contraction of the flexor muscles which, when stimulated, will move the limb away from the stimulus. For example, standing on a tack stimulates pain receptors at the puncture site, and the afferent activity passes to the spinal cord. Here the afferent neuron synapses directly within the anterior horn of grey matter with the appropriate motor neuron which, when activated, causes the appropriate flexor muscle to contract (Figure 13.31). This is a simple example of a monosynaptic reflex arc, i.e. the whole neural pathway has only one synapse, thus only two neurons, one sensory and one motor are involved. Other reflexes may utilize more synapses, but each synapse introduces a slight delay in the response time.

The role of the reflex in homeostasis is evident in this example, since failure to withdraw the limb could potentially result in more damage to the tissues of the foot. Many reflexes are involved in responses to changes in limb or body position and are considered further in Chapter 16. Other reflexes act via the autonomic nervous system. For example, a reduction in arterial blood pressure is detected by arterial baroreceptors and induces a reflex response which enhances cardiac function and induces selective constriction of arterioles (Chapter 9), thus restoring the blood pressure to normal. In this instance the reflex pathway is via the brainstem, but the same principle applies.

Overview of the functional anatomy of the autonomic nervous system

ANATOMICAL ORGANIZATION OF THE AUTONOMIC NERVOUS SYSTEM

Like the somatic nervous system (described earlier and in Chapter 16), the autonomic nervous system is comprised of both central and peripheral elements. As its name implies, the autonomic system is especially involved in the involuntary control of organ function, although a degree of voluntary control of some organs is possible. The nerves of this system will be comprised of both afferent (sensory) and efferent (motor) nerve cells. In terms of the actions of efferent cells, however, some will stimulate the target tissue, whilst others inhibit it. In this way tissue function can be enhanced

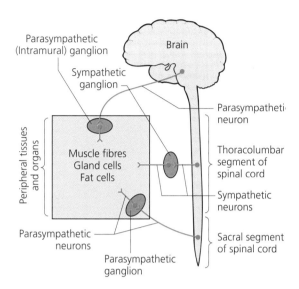

Figure 13.32 General organization of the autonomic nervous system.

or reduced (e.g. increased/decreased heart rates, increased/decreased gut motility), by autonomic nerves which have opposing actions on the tissues and organs they supply.

Accordingly the autonomic nervous system can be subdivided into two sub-branches, called the sympathetic and parasympathetic systems (Figure 13.32), which usually act together in various homeostatic control processes (Figure 13.33). In some instances sympathetic nerves act to stimulate a tissue, and parasympathetic nerves inhibit it, whilst in other instances the reverse is true. For clarity, it is convenient to consider the organization of the two subdivisions separately. It should be noted, however, that autonomic nerves are not comprised entirely of efferent fibres. Visceral and afferent fibres conduct activity from the tissues to the central nervous system and enable aspects of tissue function to be monitored.

Parasympathetic system

The layout of the peripheral nerves of this system is relatively straightforward, and basically consists of the vagus nerve (cranial

nerve X), neurons of various other cranial nerves, and nerves which originate from the sacral (i.e. lower back) region of the spinal cord (Figure 13.33). This is why this is sometimes termed the craniosacral system.

As mentioned earlier, the vagus nerve passes from the brainstem, down through the thorax and abdomen, sending branches to various viscera as it goes along. The parasympathetic functions of the vagus and other cranial nerves are summarized in Table 13.4. Note that few blood vessels are influenced by the parasympathetic system. The sacral nerves help to control lower abdominal functions such as micturition and defecation.

The general layout of the parasympathetic system is, in fact, slightly more complicated than this because the nerves synapse with shorter efferent nerves before interacting with the target tissue. The aggregated cell bodies of the latter nerves form the parasympathetic, or intramural, ganglia (Figure 13.32) and these are usually found very close to the tissues which the efferent cells innervate. The nerve cell axons leading from the cord to the ganglia are therefore usually referred to as preganglionic fibres, whilst the shorter ones are postganglionic.

The parasympathetic nerve cells (afferent and efferent) have connections within the brain (for the sacral nerves there must be neurons within the cord which provide the connections). Various nuclei are involved which have projections to and from sensory areas of the cortex, the thalamus and hypothalamus, and other nuclei of the brainstem.

Sympathetic system

The anatomy of the sympathetic system appears more complex than that of the parasympathetic system. This is because the nerves leave the spinal cord (via the spinal nerve roots) at regular intervals between the 6th cervical and 2nd lumbar vertebrae, hence the term cervicolumbar system. The sympathetic nerves soon dissociate from the spinal

PARASYMPATHETIC

SYMPATHETIC

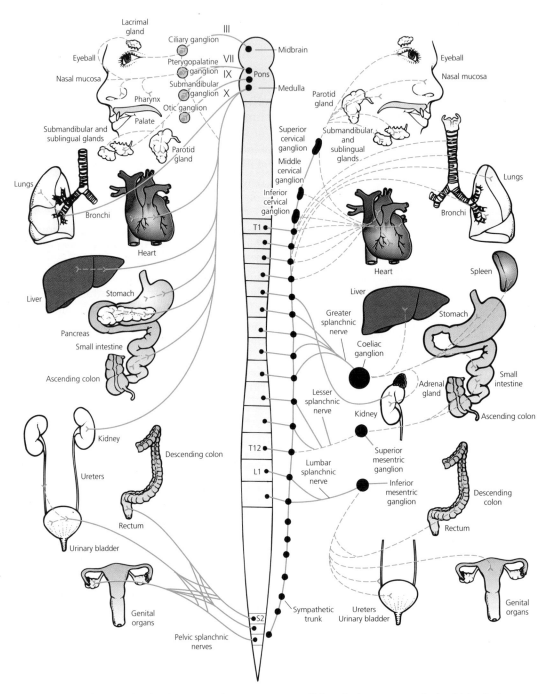

Figure 13.33 Visceral innervation by the autonomic nervous system. Although the parasympathetic division is shown only on the left side of the figure and the sympathetic division only on the right side, keep in mind that each division is actually on both sides of the body. Solid lines: preganglionic neurons; dotted lines: postganglionic neurons.

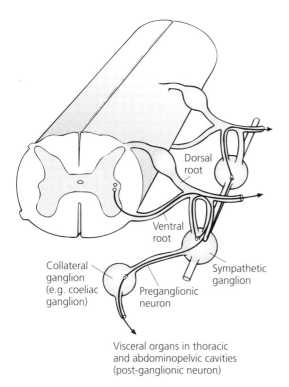

Figure 13.34 Efferent neurons of the sympathetic nervous system.
Note the 'relay' function of the sympathetic ganglia.

nerves, however, and short nerves (containing preganglionic efferent fibres) run to the sympathetic ganglia, which form a chain alongside the vertebral column (Figures 13.33 and 13.34). The post-ganglionic efferent fibres extend from synapses within the ganglia to the target tissues. Slight modifications of this layout are found, however. For example, the coeliac ganglion lies some distance from the cord (Figure 13.33). This ganglion synapses with a number of sympathetic nerves from the cord, and is commonly called the solar plexus.

The sympathetic nervous system clearly involves nerve cells which ascend or descend the spinal cord and will also include various nuclei within the brain. As with the parasympathetic system, connections within the hypothalamus and brainstem are particularly important in sympathetic functions.

SUMMARY OF THE PHYSIOLOGY OF THE AUTONOMIC NERVOUS SYSTEM

The details of the functions of the sympathetic and parasympathetic branches are outlined in Table 13.6 and this section intends only to provide an overview of the integrated functioning of the two branches. The autonomic nervous system is an essential component of homeostatic regulation. As described in Chapter 1, the mechanisms of homeostasis require efferent signalling to change the function of effector tissues, and nerves are vital components of that signalling. The fact that autonomic nerves innervate the viscera means that they play an important role in the control of the internal environment.

The roles of autonomic nerves in regulating the functions of specific systems is highlighted in relevant chapters. The question as to whether it is the sympathetic or parasympathetic nerves which excite the tissue is very much related to the situation under which they are activated. For example, exercise has a marked stimulatory effect on the sympathetic nervous system, and this is responsible for promoting responses which facilitate physical activity. Thus, changes in sympathetic nerve activity:

1 promote cardiac output by increasing the heart rate and force of contraction,

2 induce an initial vasodilatation of muscles (although metabolic factors then become more important in this respect),

3 help to maintain arterial blood pressure, despite pronounced muscle vasodilatation, by inducing vasoconstriction in various other tissues,

4 enhance peripheral vision by inducing dilatation of the pupil, and

5 promote heat loss by stimulating sweat secretion.

Table 13.6 Comparison of sympathetic and parasympathetic nervous system functions

Structure	Sympathetic innervation	Parasympathetic innervation
Eye	Dilates pupil, accommodation for distance vision	Constricts pupil, accommodation for near vision
Salivary glands	Concentrated secretion stimulated	Watery secretion stimulated
Sweat glands	Increased secretion	Not innervated
Cardiovascular system		
Blood vessels		
To skin	Vasoconstriction	
To skeletal muscles	Vasodilatation	
To digestive viscera	Vasoconstriction	
Heart		
Rate and force of contraction	Increases	Decreases rate
Blood pressure	Increases	Decreases†
Adrenal gland	Medulla secretes adrenaline + noradrenaline	Not innervated
Respiratory system		
Diameter of airways	Increases	Decreases
Respiratory rate	Increases	Decreases
Digestive system		
Sphincter muscles	Contract	Relax
General level of activity	Decreases	Increases
Secretory glands	Inhibited	Stimulated
Urinary system		
Kidneys	Decreases urine production	Not innervated
Bladder	Relaxes muscle of bladder, contracts internal sphincter	Contracts bladder muscle, relaxes internal sphincter
Male reproductive system	Increases glandular secretion; ejaculation	Erection

†Indirect effect as consequence of actions on heart rate.

Other actions include promoting glycogenolysis (to provide glucose) and enhanced somatic nerve excitability. These are all excitatory influences.

In contrast, gut motility and secretory activity are inhibited (which is appropriate in view of the concurrent vasoconstriction in the gut) and bronchodilatation occurs (which facilitates lung ventilation). The net effect of the responses of various systems is to maintain cellular homeostasis within the active muscle.

The parasympathetic nervous system tends to be activated in response to emotional experiences, although stress and anxiety are strong stimuli for sympathetic activity. For example, contemplating food induces gastric acid secretion and increases gut motility, and relaxation (which also reduces sympathetic activity) causes heart rate to decrease. Emotional shock promotes bronchoconstriction and may even inhibit the heart to the extent that blood pressure falls and fainting occurs as a consequence of cerebral ischaemia. Sexual stimulation induces penile or clittoral vasodilatation, the main examples of a direct effect of the parasympathetic nervous system on blood vessels.

The opposing actions of the sympathetic and parasympathetic systems on the same parameters of tissue function (e.g. heart rate) raises the question as to how this is achieved at the tissue level. The answer lies in the type of neurotransmitter substance released at the nerve ending, and the responses to that transmitter.

Neurotransmitters of the autonomic system

The significance of excitatory and inhibitory transmitters was explained in an earlier section. In the autonomic system each transmitter can have either excitatory or inhibitory effects on tissues, depending upon the tissue. The principle of each nerve cell being capable of producing only one particular transmitter is still applicable, however.

The nerve endings of post-ganglionic, efferent fibres of the sympathetic nervous system release noradrenaline which interacts with receptors on the post-synaptic membrane (the hormone adrenaline, released when sympathetic nerves to the adrenal gland are stimulated, may also act on these receptors, Figure 13.35). Whether a stimulatory or inhibitory response ensues is mainly determined by the type of receptor present on cells of the target tissue. Thus, receptor subtypes, classified as alpha- and beta-receptors, will be present in appropriate tissues. Further alpha- and beta-subtypes are also found, which modulate the actions still further. In addition, some sympathetic nerve fibres release chemicals related to noradrenaline, called dopamine and serotonin (5-hydroxytryptamine; 5-HT) which interact with their own receptors.

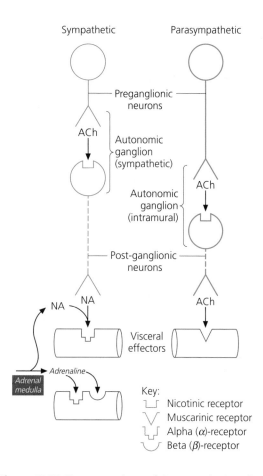

Figure 13.35 Neurotransmitters of the sympathetic and parasympathetic branches of the autonomic nervous system: NA, noradrenaline; ACh, acetylcholine.

Post-ganglionic nerve fibres of parasympathetic nerves release acetylcholine, and receptor subtypes, called muscarinic or nicotinic receptors, also exist for this substance. Just to confuse matters, acetylcholine is also the neurotransmitter released by preganglionic sympathetic nerve fibres (Figure 13.35). This mediates synaptic activity of the ganglia, however, and not the actual interaction with the target tissues.

Role of the nervous system in homeostasis

It should be apparent from this and other chapters that nerves play a vital role in the control mechanisms which regulate the functioning of other tissues and organs. Nerves and hormones provide the efferent (and sometimes afferent) pathways which promote a change in tissue function. Without that influence, physiological systems would be incapable of responding to changes in parameters which have arisen during normal day-to-day activities.

On the one hand, somatic nerves control posture and movement, and are therefore central to one's ability to interact with other individuals, to find and ingest food, and to carry out general physical activities. In contrast, autonomic nerves have a direct influence on our internal environments by affecting how tissues and organs function. Both somatic

and autonomic systems in themselves are dependent upon a broad range of sensory facilities (see Chapter 14) and neural integration for the full expression of their activities.

Although central to systemic functions, it is important to note that nerve cells, as with other cells of the body, must be supplied with nutrients and so are themselves dependent upon a controlled intracellular and extracellular environment in order to function. Frequently nerve cell activities are the first to suffer noticeably when internal environments change. Again, therefore, we see the interaction between systemic functions that is necessary for physical and mental health. It is only through this complex interdependency of systems that the 'characteristics of life' can be maintained.

Examples of homeostatic control system failures and principles of correction

Disorders of the nervous system are widespread and varied. It is the intention of this section to consider simply the major ways in which neural function can be compromised. The consequences of disordered neural function depend upon whether the disturbance influences sensory or motor functions, including somatic muscular control, cognitive functions of the brain, or visceral control (via autonomic functions or errors in hormone secretion).

The pathophysiology of disordered neural function can be categorized as resulting in either an inappropriately increased, or decreased, activity within neural pathways (illustrated in Figure 13.36). Common causes of disturbance are (1) a physical loss of neurons,

(2) cerebrovascular accident, (3) a disturbance in the generation of action potentials of existing neurons, (4) a deterioration in the conduction velocity by which activity passes along neuronal axons, (5) a disorder of synaptic transmission, or (6) a disturbance in the balance between excitatory and inhibitory inputs into neural pathways within the central nervous system.

Infections may also affect various processes. For example, meningitis is an inflammation of the meningeal membranes induced by an infectious agent. Apart from localized effects of the inflammation on adjacent brain/spinal tissue, raised intracranial pressure may occur which will have generalized cerebral effects.

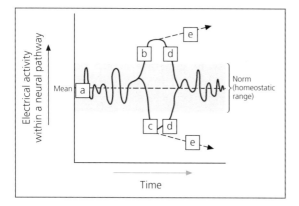

Figure 13.36 Electrical activity within a neural pathway expressed as a homeostatic process.
a Fluctuating activity conducive with 'normal' functioning of neural tissue.
b Increased pathway activity due to increased body temperature (i.e. increased metabolic rate) or to excessive excitatory synapse activity relative to inhibitory synapse activity.
c Decreased pathway activity due to loss of neurons within the pathway, loss of myelin from neurons, interference with membrane ion channels (i.e. by ionic imbalance, decreased temperature or drugs) or to excessive inhibitory synapse activity relative to excitatory synapse activity.
d Correction of changes by restoration of normal body temperature, by drugs, by restoration of normal ion balance or by restoration of inhibitory/excitatory synapse balance.
e Continued disordered activity because of irreversibility of underlying cause, e.g. neuronal loss, myelin loss, excessive inhibitory or excitatory neurotransmitters.

Loss of neurons

The loss of neurons, for whatever reason, will obviously prevent transmission of neural activity along the usual routes. Neurons may be damaged by various means including:

1   direct physical trauma resulting from head injury, or crush effects of a tumour or (in the spinal cord) prolapsed intervertebral discs;

2   indirect physical trauma as in cerebral ischaemia, for example as a consequence of cerebral haemorrhage, and raised intracerebral pressure, due to excess cerebrovascular fluid, as in hydrocephalus and meningitis, or presence of a haematoma;

3   toxin damage, for example the effects of ions of 'heavy' metals on brain development.

Some disorders in which (CNS) neurons degenerate are of unknown aetiology, although autoimmune responses or inherited causes have been implicated (e.g. motor neuron disease; Alzheimer's disease).

Whereas peripheral damage may perhaps induce localized loss of limb function, central damage causes a variety of disorders which can be extensive and devastating. These include cognitive disorders (e.g. cerebral palsy; Alzheimer's disease), motor disorders (e.g. cerebral palsy, epilepsy, motor neuron disease), autonomic disorders (e.g. respiratory dysrhythmias) and endocrine disorders (e.g. pituitary hyposecretion)

Correction may be aimed at removing the underlying cause, such as relieving raised intracranial pressure, or treating an infection. Drug treatments may be used to suppress any inflammation, and tumours may be surgically removed, although additional damage may be incurred in the process. Generally, though, the correction of trauma is limited, and care is directed at alleviating symptoms and providing support. Thus, endocrine deficiencies can be corrected using hormone replacement therapies, but this does not reverse an underlying neural deficit.

In certain circumstances, non-progressive brain damage can be improved, though not reversed, by reinforcement of behavioural or social patterns (e.g. 'conductive therapy' in children with cerebral palsy). This probably promotes the development of new neural synapses within the affected areas. The growth of lateral branches from peripheral nerve axons can also improve some peripheral disorders such as certain neuromuscular conditions (by re-innervating muscle fibres).

Neuronal growth is also effective at restoring limb functions following surgical replacement of severed limbs. There is currently considerable research effort into the possible clinical uses of endogenous chemicals, called nerve growth factors, which promote nerve development.

Cerebrovascular accidents (CVAs)

Cerebrovascular accidents may also cause loss of neurons, or cause an increase in fluid pressure on underlying nerve cells. A CVA, or stroke, occurs when a portion of the brain is deprived of blood, and hence oxygen and glucose. Cerebral thrombosis caused by clot formation at the site of an atherosclerotic plaque, cerebral embolism caused by drifting clots, fatty masses or air bubbles, and cerebral haemorrhages are all common causes of CVA.

Symptoms of CVA depend upon which part of the brain is damaged, and therefore which cerebral artery is affected. Thus, CVAs involving the anterior cerebral artery particularly affect the motor and sensory cortex. Symptoms of a CVA involving the middle cerebral artery will have similar effects but may also include speech and auditory defects. Damage in the posterior cerebral artery will affect the visual cortex, and also the limbic system. Loss of blood supply via the basilar artery may partly be compensated for by blood passing through the circle of Willis. Nevertheless, damage to the cerebellum and brainstem can be severe. Loss of brainstem functions will also affect autonomic control. Initial symptoms of a stroke can be exaggerated by swelling of surrounding tissues, and neural function may improve with time.

Blockages to cerebral arteries can be temporary, and symptoms are short-lived. These are called transient ischaemic episodes and can precede more serious attacks.

Anticoagulant therapy can help to reduce the likelihood of further clotting and so prevent exacerbation of the problem. Surgical intervention may also be necessary to relieve raised intracranial pressure or to improve circulation. Preventive surgery is also possible in some cases. The reduction of risk factors, such as high blood pressure (hypertension), is an important part of Health Promotion strategies.

Disturbance in the generation of action potentials

The capacity to generate action potentials is central to nerve cell functioning, and depends upon a number of factors:

1 The distribution of electrolytes across the cell membrane. The influence of changes in ion concentrations in intra- and extracellular fluids was discussed in Chapter 5: the main ionic influences on neural function are the effects of altering potassium and calcium concentrations within the extracellular fluid. Such disturbances frequently arise as a consequence of disorders of fluid homeostasis induced by endocrine defect, renal failure, or dietary deficiency.

The effect of potassium changes is to alter the resting membrane potential, either depolarizing it toward threshold (in hyperkalaemia) or hyperpolarizing it away from threshold (in hypokalaemia). Calcium ion disturbances influence the 'gating' mechanisms and therefore alter the threshold at which an action potential is generated. Thus hypocalcaemia induces a lowering of the threshold (membrane more excitable) and hypercalcaemia raises it.

2 The presence of ion 'channels' within the membrane. Nerve cells will ordinarily possess such channels. In myelinated axons, however, the channels are concentrated at the nodes of Ranvier. Should the insulative layer of myelin be lost, then current decrement from the membrane may be so extensive that subsequent nodes are not stimulated. This is one of the problems associated with multiple sclerosis.

3 The capacity to open and close the ion channels at appropriate times. Provided that membrane potentials, and the threshold potential, are normal then this should not be a problem. Some drugs, however, interfere with the 'gating' mechanisms. These include local and general anaesthetics.

Temperature is another influence. Physiologically, body temperature will be controlled within tight limits, but hypothermia is a common occurrence, particularly in the elderly, and this will reduce neural function throughout the body.

Deterioration in conduction velocity of existing neurons

A slowing of conduction velocity does not simply mean that response times are delayed. Although reflex responses to stimuli will be depressed if those spinal neurons involved are affected, a slowing of conduction velocity within the brain will also have severe effects on integrated neural circuitry since the output from neurons is determined by the summated excitatory and inhibitory post-synaptic potentials. Summation will be affected if neurons within a circuit are not conducting normally. A common cause of a reduced conduction velocity is when the myelin sheath of axons deteriorates (e.g. in multiple sclerosis).

Hypothermia also reduces conduction velocity via its slowing effect on the generation of action potentials.

Peripherally, inflammatory demyelinating disease (such as the cause of Guillain–Barré syndrome) will also slow conduction. Motor dysfunction causes muscle weakness. Interestingly, sensory activity may actually be enhanced in Guillain–Barré syndrome, presumably as a consequence of altered receptor sensitivity, with the patient experiencing heightened cutaneous sensation of pain, temperature, and touch.

Multiple sclerosis is still poorly understood. Corrective treatment is not yet possible and care is generally aimed at facilitating maximal possible function. The rate of deterioration seems to be slowed by the use of anti-inflammatory drugs which slow the development of sclerotic (scar) tissue in the demyelinated areas. In Guillain–Barré syndrome the care is directed at supporting the patient, with life support if necessary, until recovery occurs. Extensive rehabilitation is usually necessary.

Disorders of synaptic transmission

Synaptic function involves the synthesis and secretion of neurotransmitters, its interaction with receptors on the post-synaptic membrane, removal of excess transmitter chemical, and degradation of the chemical/receptor ligand so that the receptor is free to interact with more chemical when released. Errors can occur at all stages of the process. Myasthenia gravis is a condition in which muscle weakness occurs because of a defect at the neuromuscular synapse, probable causes are a deficiency of available post-synaptic receptors to the neurotransmitter acetylcholine or an excess of acetylcholinesterase. Parkinson's disease and Huntington's chorea are disorders characterized (at least in early stages) by disorders of movement control, and are primarily caused by a deficiency in the release of the neurotransmitters dopamine and gamma-aminobutyric acid (GABA) respectively from certain neurons of the brain.

Correction is aimed at restoring the missing transmitter, for example by administering levodopa, a precursor to dopamine, to Parkinsonian patients, or by prolonging the actions of the transmitter that is released, as in the administration of acetylcholinesterase inhibitors to myasthenia gravis patients.

Imbalance between inhibitory and excitatory neurotransmitters

This overlaps with central nervous system disorders from the previous category. Since the output from neurons within processing areas of the brain is determined by the net effects of excitatory and inhibitory inputs to the neuron, a disturbance in one or other can have drastic effects on brain function. Thus, the movement disorders of Parkinson's disease at least partially result from the lack of the inhibitory transmitter dopamine, leading to excessive expression of excitatory pathways. Similarly, clinical depression seems to be associated with a deficiency of the excitatory transmitter noradrenaline in certain parts of the brain, leading to excessive expression of inhibitory pathways.

Correction is aimed at restoring the balance. This generally means replacing the deficient transmitter. Thus, levodopa (a precursor to dopamine) may be administered to Parkinsonian patients, whilst tricyclic antidepressants, which prevent re-uptake of noradrenaline from the synaptic cleft and therefore prolong its activation of post-synaptic receptors, may be administered in clinical depression.

The role of the synapse in neural circuitry, and in nerve–muscle and nerve–gland interactions is clinically very useful. Various drugs are available which (1) influence neurotransmitter synthesis, (2) influence neurotransmitter release, (3) alter its breakdown from receptors, or re-uptake into the presynaptic cell, (4) act on post-synaptic receptors themselves to stimulate the post-synaptic membrane (these are called agonistic drugs), or (5) interact with post-synaptic receptors without stimulating the post-synaptic membrane, but prevent neurotransmitter from acting on them (these are called antagonistic drugs).

Summary

1 Nerves, or more precisely nerve cells (neurons), provide the means of rapid communication necessary for the short-term regulation of many homeostatic processes, including the control of body posture and movement.

2 The nervous system has two anatomical divisions: the peripheral nervous system which conducts neural activity to and from tissues, and the central nervous system which analyses information before promoting a response.

3 The peripheral system is subdivided into that branch which controls skeletal muscle in the regulation of body posture and movement (called the somatic system), and that which is involved in the regulation of visceral functions (called the autonomic system). In general we can exert considerable conscious control over the former, but the latter is primarily under involuntary control.

4 The central nervous system consists of the brain and spinal cord.

5 Peripheral nerves enter/exit the spinal cord between the vertebrae. Sensory neurons enter the dorsal (or posterior) aspect of the cord, whilst effector (or motor) neurons exit via the ventral (or anterior) aspect.

6 The cord has a precise organization, consisting of tracts of nerve cell fibres which ascend or descend the cord within the 'white' matter, and layers of cells which integrate activity or act as relays within central 'grey' areas. Integrative functions of the cord include the production of reflexes.

7 The brain develops embryologically as three distinct components which increase in complexity during development. The forebrain consists of the cerebral hemispheres (with cortical and subcortical processing areas) and the deeper structures called the thalamus and hypothalamus. The midbrain contains many brain 'nuclei' and fibre tracts, and forms the area between the forebrain and the hindbrain. The latter consists of structures at the top of the spinal cord, including the cerebellum, which have integrative functions particularly in relation to the control of movement and the control of the autonomic system. Collectively some of these structures, with the midbrain, form the brainstem.

8 Nerve cell activity is generated by the movement of electrical charge across the cell membrane, as an action potential. The membrane can be stabilized, however (i.e. the action potential inhibited), by the antagonistic movement of other ions which prevent the action potential being generated. This forms the basis of neural integration, a switching mechanism within the nervous system, and takes place at junctions called synapses between nerve cells.

9 Synaptic function involves the release of neurotransmitters which modulate ionic movements across the membrane of the next cell in the pathway. Some chemicals are excitatory, others inhibitory. Within the central nervous system the ionic environment surrounding the cells is tightly controlled (to enable membrane events to be regulated) by regulating the composition of the bathing fluid, the cerebrospinal fluid.

10 Many cognitive functions of the brain have now been attributed to various brain structures, and involve a variety of neurotransmitters. The balance between excitatory and inhibitory pathways is essential for 'normal' functions.

11 The autonomic nervous system also operates via neurotransmitters and numerous receptor subtypes to these chemicals have been identified and enable the system to exert complex control of visceral functioning. The system is subdivided into the sympathetic and parasympathetic branches which, in general, exert opposing actions on tissues in response to visceral afferent input.

12 Failure of nerve cells to generate action potentials at appropriate times, to conduct the activity along axons, or to integrate synaptic function in an appropriate way, forms the basis of many neural disorders. Complete physical loss of nerve cells will also, of course, disrupt nerve pathways.

Review Questions

1 List the general functions of the nervous system.

2 What is meant by the following:
(a) nerve, (b) neuron, (c) mixed nerve.

3 Explain how neurons are classified according to their structure and function.

4 What are neuroglia cells?

5 Draw a labelled diagram of a synapse.

6 Describe the components involved in a nerve pathway.

7 Describe a reflex arc.

8 Discuss the sequence of events that occur during the generation and conduction of an electrochemical impulse along myelinated neurons, using the following terms: stimulus; receptor; myelin sheath; threshold; 'sodium/potassium pump'; sodium; potassium; action potential; nodes of Ranvier; dendrites, synaptic knob; post-synaptic membrane, synapse; presynaptic membranes; excitatory post-synaptic potential, depolarization, repolarization and polarization.

9 Describe the structure of the meninges.

10 Describe the circulation of cerebrospinal fluid.

11 Describe the structure of the spinal cord.

12 Differentiate between ascending and descending tracts.

13 Describe the structure of the cerebrum.

14 Where are the primary motor and sensory regions located?

15 Name the components of the diencephalon. What are their functions?

16 Where are the basal ganglia and what are their functions?

17 Name the receptors which provide information to the cerebellum.

18 Distinguish between:
(a) Peripheral and central nervous systems.
(b) Somatic and autonomic nervous systems.
(c) Spinal and cranial nerves.
(d) Nerve tracts and plexuses.
(e) Parasympathetic and sympathetic nervous systems.

19 Describe the blood supply to the brain.

20 Name three neuronal disorders and three brain disorders, briefly describing each homeostatic failure.

Coordination II: The senses

14

Introduction: relation of the senses to cellular homeostasis

Overview of the anatomy and physiology of the senses

Details of the anatomy and physiology of the 'special senses'

Role of sensory receptors in homeostasis

Examples of homeostatic control system failures and principles of correction

Summary

Review questions

Introduction: relation of the senses to cellular homeostasis

A 'sense' is a faculty by which the body receives information regarding its internal and external environments. 'Sense' does not necessarily equate with 'sensation' or 'perception', however, as these terms refer to our capacity to be consciously aware of a change in some aspect of our environment. A conscious awareness of a stimulus is frequently not essential; being continually aware of what is happening to body fluid composition, blood pressure or body temperature would not be practical, except when changes are extreme. On the other hand, pain must be perceived to provide us with the information that tissues have been damaged or are threatened.

The sensing of changes to the parameters of our internal environment is central to the whole concept of homeostasis. This normally requires the presence of specialized receptor cells which are sensitive to specific changes within that environment. For example, a rise in the osmotic pressure of plasma is detected by osmotically sensitive receptors within the hypothalamus and corrective responses ensue. In this example the detected change would be indicative of an alteration in body fluid osmotic pressure throughout the body and so the receptors need only be located in an appropriate position. Sensing touch at the finger tips, however, conveys no information of what is happening, for example, to our feet! Touch receptors must therefore be distributed about the body.

The specific type of stimulus detected by a receptor is called its modality, for example touch, pressure, temperature. The properties of receptors are such that many are able to detect individual modalities, such as osmotic pressure; and their responses only relate to the intensity of stimulation. Some receptors are polymodal and can detect different types of stimuli. Thus vision involves the detection of light intensity (brightness) and wavelength (colour), hearing involves the detection of sound intensity (loudness) and frequency (tone), whilst both smell and taste involve the detection of chemical intensity (concentration) and type. The complexity of these 'special' senses is such that the receptors are organized into sense organs – the eye, ear, nose, and tongue. Pain, too, is polymodal and some texts include this as a 'special' sense, although there are no pain sense 'organs' as such. In recognition of the subjectivity of pain, and its particular relevance to health care professions, this 'sense' has been placed into a separate chapter and only brief mention of it will be made in this one.

Most receptors provide information that a change in, or to, the body has already occurred. Those of vision, hearing, and smell, however, all provide additional information on circumstances which may be operative some distance from the body, and so provide a 'predictive' element. A 'predictive' facility enables us to take corrective or avoidance measures if necessary and so either prevent a disturbance in homeostasis or at least minimize it. Similarly, taste allows us to reject a substance which we perceive might be injurious to the body, and pain provides us with a warning that further tissue damage will ensue unless circumstances change.

Receptors are found throughout the body, ranging in structure from complex cells such as those of the retina of the eye, to 'simple' surface molecules on, for example, the post-synaptic membrane of nerve cell junctions or on endocrine cells. All can potentially produce responses to stimulation, i.e. they all detect a change in their immediate environment. The functions of neural and neuromuscular synapses, and of endocrine cells, have been described in other chapters. This chapter is intended to supplement the chapters on neural coordination and will therefore concentrate on those receptor cells which promote activity in sensory nerve cells.

Overview of the anatomy and physiology of the senses

GENERAL PRINCIPLES OF RECEPTOR FUNCTION

Receptors are transducers: they convert energy present within the stimulus (for example, heat, light, energy) into electrical energy by altering the electrical properties of the receptor cell membrane. Electrically charged particles (electrolytes) are abundant within the body fluids and differences in the distribution of electrolytes between the intracellular and extracellular fluids are produced by the specific properties of cell membranes. Receptor cells, and other excitable cells such as nerve and muscle cells, have the capacity to change the ionic permeabilities of their membranes, leading to the movement of certain ions (usually sodium, potassium) into or out of the cell. These ion movements are responsible for the electrical change observed when receptor cells are stimulated and, if 'threshold' is met or superseded, trigger events within the cell which may, for example, promote the release of a neuroendocrine hormone, such as oxytocin from the posterior pituitary gland, or generate action potentials in sensory nerve cells.

Transduction, therefore, requires the generation of small changes in the resting membrane (electrical) potential and such changes are called generator potentials. Generally, the electrical change in a receptor membrane increases with stimulus strength until a 'threshold' is reached when either action potentials are produced or neurohormone release is instigated, depending upon the type of cell. Threshold levels for a specific stimulus determines the receptor sensitivity and are a factor in the efficiency of homeostatic control. Thus receptors will have a low threshold in the homeostatic regulation of parameters with narrow homeostatic ranges.

Receptors may be discrete cells or nerve endings, or the nerve endings may be extensively branched. The latter type extends over the area innervated by its branches and this is called its receptor field. Some receptor fields are large, others small: the smaller the field the greater our ability to 'place' the stimulus. Thus the points of a pair of compasses applied to the finger tips can be discerned as two distinct points even when they are only about 1.5 mm apart, because the finger tips have a high receptor density with small, overlapping receptor fields. Overlap of adjacent receptor fields means that the stimulus is detected by more than one receptor and the information can then be compared. On the back, however, the two points are only separately discerned when some 35–40 mm apart as the receptor fields are large and do not overlap (Figure 14.1).

Receptors of many senses exhibit a decreasing sensitivity in response to continued stimulation, even though the stimulus is still present. Touch is a typical example: life would be unpleasant if we were to be constantly aware of contact with our clothes, or with chairs, or with the ground, or with spectacles, etc. In these instances, once the stimulus has been received, and perhaps acted upon, it becomes more important to detect a new change rather than to remain aware of the old one. Thus these types of receptors adapt to the

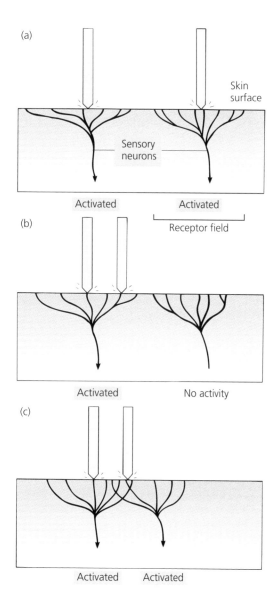

Figure 14.1 Two-point discrimination. In (a) the two points are in contact with the receptor fields of two neurons and so will be discriminated as two contact points. In (b) the points are too close together to be discriminated as separate points of contact. (c) Overlapping receptor fields facilitates the discrimination of two points, even when the points of contact are close together.

stimulus and can respond again if the stimulus changes.

Receptors may be slow-adapting (i.e. tonic) or rapid-adapting (i.e. phasic). The former tend

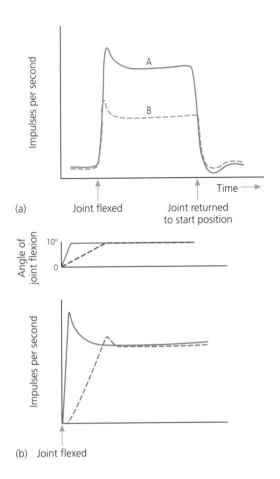

flexed but also how rapidly it was flexed (i.e. its velocity) and even if that velocity changed (Figure 14.2).

Action potentials induced in sensory nerve fibres associated with receptors will usually be conducted to the central nervous system where many will ultimately arrive at the appropriate sensory area of the cerebral cortex. Some will pass to other parts of the brain, such as the hypothalamus or brainstem. Only those which arrive at the sensory cortex can be consciously perceived but even here perception does not always occur.

OVERVIEW OF THE TYPES OF RECEPTOR IN THE BODY

Receptors are usually classified according to either (1) the stimulus they detect, or (2) the environment they monitor.

Classification by stimulus

Mechanoreceptors are usually nerve endings and are sensitive to mechanical deformation. They include receptors of touch, pressure, vibration, and stretch.

Thermoreceptors respond to fluctuations in temperature whilst chemoreceptors are sensitive to changes in the concentration of chemicals within the body fluids.

Nociceptors are responsive to noxious stimuli, and are sensitive to either pronounced mechanical deformation, extreme temperature change, or to chemicals perhaps released from neighbouring cells (i.e. they are types of mechanoreceptor, thermoreceptor or chemoreceptor).

Photoreceptors are sensitive to light. Details of these receptor types and how they are stimulated are provided in the next section.

Classification by environment

The classification of receptors by the environment they monitor places them under the

Figure 14.2 Static and dynamic aspects of joint receptors. (a) Impulse frequency from a joint receptor when the joint is flexed to two different positions (A, B). Note that the receptor activity is maintained and impulse frequency relates to the joint position. (b) Impulse frequency from a joint receptor when the joint is flexed to 14° at two different rates.
Note that the rate of change in receptor activity relates to the rate of change of joint position.

to be those receptors which provide information regarding steady states of the body, such as blood composition and body position. Rapidly adapting receptors are important if states are continuously changing and they convey moment-to-moment information regarding changes in the stimulus. For example, receptors in our joints not only provide information that the joint has been

headings of exteroreceptors and enteroreceptors (including proprioreceptors).

Exteroreceptors

Exteroreceptors provide information about our
external environment and include light
(vision), sound (hearing), chemical (taste,
smell), temperature, touch, pressure, and pain
receptors. Clearly these must be located near to
the body surface. The 'special' senses of vision,
hearing, taste and smell are considered later
and this discussion will focus on cutaneous
(skin) receptors only.

Cutaneous receptors are distributed all over
the body surface but the density of receptors
present in an area varies according to needs.
They respond to a variety of stimuli and are of
three classes: mechanoreceptors, thermoreceptors, and nociceptors.

MECHANORECEPTORS

Mechanoreceptors are of relatively simple
structure. They consist of the terminal
dendrites of sensory neurons and are either
'free' or encapsulated in structures of connective tissue. Their membranes are sensitive to
physical deformation and the receptors
include:

1 Merkel's discs: disc-like arrangements of
dendrites in contact with epidermal cells,
which respond to touch.

2 Meissner's capsules: egg-shaped structures
in the dermis containing dendrites which
respond to touch.

3 Pacinian corpuscles: well-studied oval structures distinguished by their concentric
layers of connective tissue. Dendrites are
found within the layers, but the layers are
viscous and return to their original form
after deformation and so exhibit adaptation.
They are pressure receptors and are located
in deep subcutaneous tissues, submucosa,
around joints and in mammary glands.

4 Root hair plexus: nerve dendrites are
wrapped around the base of a hair root and
respond to deformation induced by
movement of the hair shaft when touched.

The same cutaneous receptors seem also to
be responsive to vibration in which the nerve
ending is repeatedly distorted at various
frequencies. Low frequency and high
frequency vibrations are discerned by the
involvement of different receptor types.

THERMORECEPTORS

These are thought to be 'free' nerve endings
which are sensitive to changes in temperature.
There are 'hot' and 'cold' receptors which
respond to different temperature ranges,
though the ranges overlap. Together they
provide information over a range of skin
temperature from 0 to 45 °C.

NOCICEPTORS

It is unclear as to what constitutes a 'pain'
receptor. Nociceptors are probably free nerve
endings, some of which at least are sensitive to
chemicals released from damaged cells in the
vicinity. Others may be those of other senses,
such as touch or temperature, which convey the
sensation of pain when stimulated excessively.

Enteroreceptors

Enteroreceptors provide information about our
internal environment and include pressure,
osmotic pressure, chemical, temperature, and
pain receptors. Those located in blood vessels
and in the viscera are referred to as viscero-
receptors.

Many enteroreceptors are of similar appearance and function as the cutaneous receptors
described above: mechanoreceptors, thermoreceptors and nociceptors are all present. Others
are chemoreceptors and stretch receptors,
which respond to specific alterations in the
internal environment of the body.

CHEMORECEPTORS

This is a diverse range of receptors which
monitor the concentrations of body fluid
constituents. Examples are those which

monitor plasma hydrogen ion concentration (pH) or plasma glucose concentration. Receptor cells usually carry surface chemicals that will specifically interact with the substance to be monitored. When activated these cells either promote electrical activity in associated nerve cells, as in the detection of increased blood acidity by the carotid bodies when carbon dioxide retention has occurred, or otherwise promote the release of a hormone, possibly from the receptor cell itself, as in the release of aldosterone from the adrenal gland when blood potassium is elevated.

STRETCH RECEPTORS

Stretch receptors are nerve endings in contact with tissues that undergo changes in tension. They include receptors which monitor arterial blood pressure (these are usually called baroreceptors), receptors responding to the presence of food in the gut, and those that respond to wall tension as the bladder fills with urine. These receptors are therefore types of mechanoreceptor.

Proprioreceptors

Proprioreceptors are a group of enteroreceptors that provide information regarding the position of parts of the body in space and so are the receptors of posture and movement.

Proprioreceptors are highly specialized types of mechanoreceptor responding to tension or movement induced by associated structures. They include muscle spindles, Golgi tendon organs, joint receptors, and the vestibular apparatus of the inner ear. All promote electrical activity when stimulated, and this is carried via sensory nerve cells to the central nervous system for processing.

MUSCLE SPINDLES

These spindle-shaped structures contain nerve endings in contact with modified skeletal muscle fibres. They respond to changes in length and their role in the control of muscle contraction is discussed in Chapter 16.

GOLGI TENDON ORGANS

Golgi organs are stretch receptors within the tendons and monitor the tension induced when the attached muscle contracts. They seem to have a protective role and cause muscle contraction to cease (i.e. 'give way') if the tension developed threatens injury.

JOINT RECEPTORS

Joint receptors provide information about the position of the joint and also about how rapidly the position is changing during movement. They consist of nerve endings associated with connective tissue within the joint.

VESTIBULAR APPARATUS

The structure of the inner ear includes three semicircular canals attached to a distended structure called the vestibule (Figure 14.3). Both contain modified mechanoreceptors in which hair extensions of the receptor cell are embedded in a gel-like substance. Any movement of the gel or receptor cell causes a distortion of the hairs and so stimulates the receptor cell.

The semicircular canals are placed at right-angles to each other and are filled with a viscous fluid called the endolymph. The base of each canal connects with the vestibule via a distended region called an ampulla (Figure 14.3) within which lies an elevated area called the crista. The crista contains the receptor cells, the hairs of which are embedded in a projection called the cupula. Movement of the head causes the endolymph to flow within the canals, and this deflects the cupulae in the ampullae which in turn stimulates the receptor cells. Associated sensory neurons are stimulated and activity passes to the brain via nerve fibres within the vestibulocochlear nerve (cranial nerve VIII), thus providing information that the head has moved. The arrangement of the three semicircular canals means that movement in all three planes can be detected.

The vestibule contains two sac-like areas called the utricle and saccule (Figure 14.3).

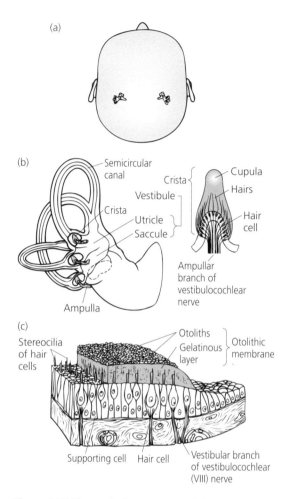

(a)

(b)
Semicircular canal
Crista
Vestibule
Crista
Utricle
Saccule
Ampulla

Cupula
Hairs
Hair cell
Ampullar branch of vestibulocochlear nerve

(c)
Stereocilia of hair cells
Otoliths
Gelatinous layer
Otolithic membrane
Supporting cell   Hair cell
Vestibular branch of vestibulocochlear (VIII) nerve

Figure 14.3 The vestibular apparatus of the inner ear. (a) Relative position in the head. (b) The vestibular structures: utricle, saccule, and semicircular canals. An enlarged crista is shown. (c) The macula of the utricle and saccule.

Both contain receptor cells with hairs projecting into a membrane; collectively this membrane and the receptor cells are called a macula. On the surface of this gel-like membrane lie small crystals of calcium carbonate called otoliths (hence the membrane is called the otolithic membrane), which slide over the membrane surface when the head is moved. This distorts the cilia of the receptor cells and generates receptor potentials. Once again, electrical activity passes to the brain via fibres within the vestibulocochlear nerve.

THE 'SPECIAL' SENSES

The complexity of the special senses is such that details of their functions are described separately in the next section. An overview is provided here in order to introduce them.

Vision requires the detection of light, the properties of which include brightness (intensity) and colour (wavelength). The receptor cells of the eye contain chemicals – visual pigments – which absorb light and consequently break down into component molecules. It is this process that activates the cell membrane and produces the receptor's generator potential which in turn stimulates action potentials in associated sensory nerve cells. The pigment chemical then re-forms.

The ratio of undissociated to dissociated pigment provides a means of monitoring light intensity, whilst different pigments which respond optimally to certain wavelengths convey a means of detecting colour. Light receptors therefore respond to electromagnetic stimuli, but only within the relatively narrow range of wavelengths determined by the pigments present. Electrical activity is conducted to the brain via the optic nerves (cranial nerve II).

Hearing requires the detection of sound intensity (loudness) and frequency (tone). Both are complex modalities but some generalizations can be made regarding the basis of their detection. The pressure waves which make up 'sound' are conducted through the ear and generate pressure waves of the same frequencies within the fluid-filled inner ear, or cochlea. Here receptor cells lie on the surface of a stiff membrane called the basilar membrane (see next section) which vibrates in response to the pressure waves and so the receptor cells are distorted by its movements. The receptors of hearing are therefore a type of mechanoreceptor. The pattern of distortion seems to be important in conveying information regarding sound intensity and frequency. Electrical activity from the receptors is conducted to the brain via sensory fibres within the vestibulocochlear nerve (cranial nerve VIII).

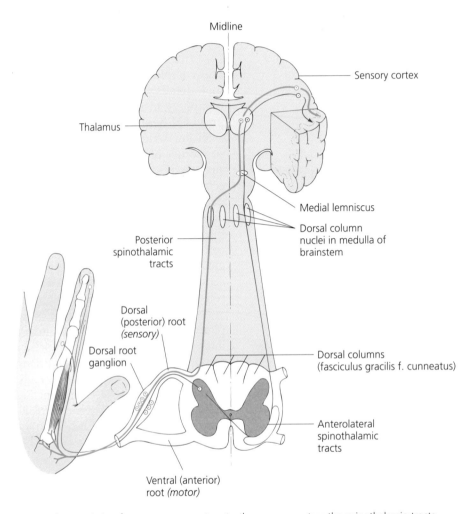

Figure 14.4 Routes of transmission from sensory receptors to the sensory cortex: the spinothalamic tracts.

Taste and smell receptors are highly specialized chemoreceptors. As with other chemical senses they are stimulated when molecules interact with other molecules on the surface of the receptor cells. Unlike other chemoreceptors, however, these receptors respond to an enormous range of molecules. Prior to detection the molecules must first be dissolved in water and this is provided by saliva and nasal secretions. Electrical activity from taste receptors on the tongue is conveyed to the brain via the facial and glossopharyngeal nerves (cranial nerves VII and IX) whilst that from the nose is conducted via the olfactory nerve (cranial nerve I).

INTERPRETATION OF RECEPTOR ACTIVITY

Electrical activity generated by receptors is conducted via sensory neurons to the central nervous system. Much eventually arrives in the brain for integration, coordination and, if appropriate, to convey conscious perception of the stimulus. The pathways along which sensory information travels is generally:

Receptor

↓

Thalamus of brain
(thalamos = inner body)

↓

Cerebral cortex
(sensory association area)

This plan is very simplistic, however, and pathways may involve other brain 'nuclei' before or after activity enters the thalamus. Similarly, information may be transmitted to parts of the brain other than the cerebral cortex, such as the cerebellum (see Chapter 13), and may not always involve transmission through the thalamus, although this usually is the case. Processing may not even involve the brain at all, information being integrated by the spinal cord.

Sensory activity from peripheral receptors enters the dorsal horn of grey matter within the spinal cord via the dorsal roots of the spinal nerves (Figure 14.4). There some of the nerve cells synapse with others which ascend the cord to the brain. Some of these ascending neurons are found in the lateral and anterior aspects of the cord and pass directly to the thalamus within the brain. Accordingly these pathways are called the lateral and anterior spinothalamic tracts, respectively. In general the lateral tract conveys information from nociceptors and thermoreceptors, whilst the anterior tracts carry information from touch and pressure receptors. One feature of these tracts is that the neurons within the cord that are stimulated by incoming sensory nerve cells actually cross through the cord before passing to the thalamus, i.e. information from these receptors passes to the opposite side of the brain.

In contrast, those sensory fibres which carry activity from deep touch receptors and proprioreceptors (especially those in joints) do not synapse immediately within the cord. Rather they ascend the spinal cord themselves, passing up the posterior aspects of the cord (Figure 14.4; note that the sensory fibre of single neurons must therefore extend from the receptor site all the way to the brainstem). Accordingly these pathways are called the posterior or dorsal columns of the cord. These neurons eventually synapse with nerve cells of nuclei within the brainstem, called the dorsal column nuclei, the fibres of which then cross over to the other side and thence pass to the thalamus. As with the spinothalamic tracts, the crossing over of neurons within the brainstem means that the left side of the brain receives information from the right side of the body and vice versa.

Proprioreceptor activity from muscles may also ascend the posterior spinocerebellar tract (which therefore lies in a posterior aspect and passes to the cerebellum at the back of the brain) of the spinal cord. The role of these receptors and the cerebellum are discussed in Chapter 16.

Electrical activity from the special senses passes either directly to the thalamus, and thence to the cerebral cortex, or passes via other nuclei particularly within the brainstem and hypothalamus. The exception is that from the olfactory receptors of the nose as these do not pass via the thalamus. The pathways are considered in more detail in the next section.

Details of the anatomy and physiology of the 'special senses'

VISION

General anatomy and function of the eye

The eye is basically a sense organ which focuses light waves onto receptor cells, but it also has the capacity to adjust the amount of light incident on the receptor region. Its anatomy is related to these functions.

The eye is approximately spherical, with a white-coloured fibrous protective and supportive layer called the sclera. Anteriorly a thin layer of modified skin, the conjunctiva, extends from the eyelids to the sclera (Figure 14.5a). Laterally the sclera is attached to the bone of the orbit of the skull by six extrinsic muscles (i.e. three antagonistic pairs) which produce lateral and vertical movement of the eye upon contraction and relaxation of the appropriate antagonistic muscle pairs and are controlled by the oculomotor and trochlear nerves (cranial nerves III and IV). At the rear of the eye the sheath of the optic nerve fuses with the sclera, whilst at the front of the eye the sclera becomes the delicate and transparent cornea.

Lubrication of the sclera and, in particular, the cornea is provided by secretions from the lachrymal or tear gland found at the top outer area of each eye. Secretions drain into the nasal cavity via the lachrymal duct which originates at the inner corner of each eye. Tears also provide a means of irrigating the eye when an irritant is present.

Below the sclera lies a vascular layer called the choroid which provides nutrients to it. The choroid extends to the corneoscleral junction where it forms the ciliary body, which in turn forms the iris (Figure 14.5b). The ciliary body also contains smooth muscle cells capable of altering the shape of the lens, which is suspended by the suspensory ligaments. Also lying within the choroid are parasympathetic and sympathetic nerve fibres that enter the iris.

The inner coat of the eye consists of the light-sensitive retina. This extends from the ciliary body around the inner surface of the rear of the eye and it is in this layer that the light receptor cells, the rods and cones, are found. The retina also has its own nerve elements which are associated with the receptor cells and aid in processing of the information. The receptors are considered in more detail below. Two features worth mentioning here, however, are that the inner surface of the retina contains the blood vessels which maintain the layer, and that the exit point of the optic nerve (the optic disc) is devoid of receptors, and so is called the blind spot. Thus, light must pass through the vessels before detection by most of the retinal receptors, and the light must not be incident on the optic disc. Not surprisingly the 'blind spot' is off-centre and incident light largely avoids it. The visibility of the retinal blood vessels, using an ophthalmoscope, is an important clinical aid in the diagnosis of, for example, cerebral hypertension.

The lens of the eye divides the eyeball into two fluid-filled compartments. The anterior compartment contains aqueous humour which is a thin, watery fluid that is constantly being formed by the ciliary body and then reabsorbed by the canal of Schlemm at the base of the ciliary body. The humour supplies the nutritive needs of the cornea and iris; these do not have blood vessels and this is useful from the point of view of corneal transplants as immune cells do not gain access and tissue rejection therefore presents less of a problem than elsewhere in the body. Behind the lens the compartment is filled with vitreous humour, a colourless fluid made jelly-like by the presence

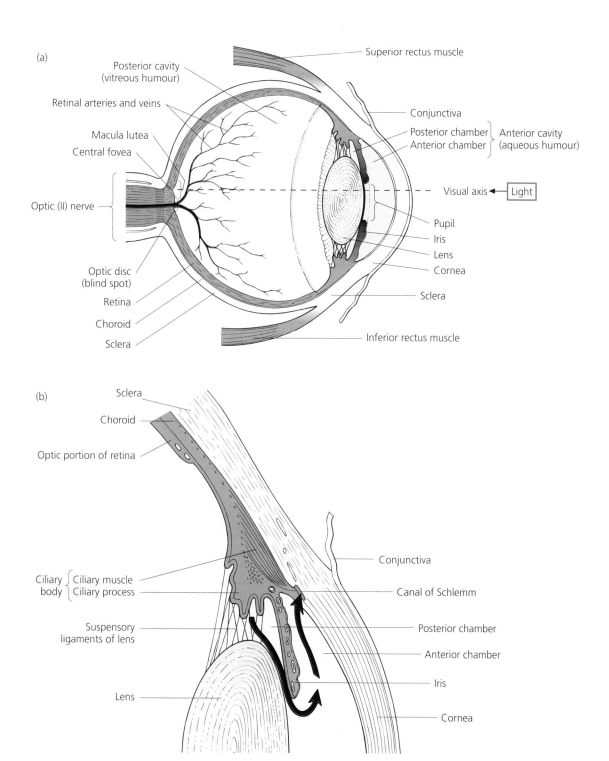

Figure 14.5 The eye. (a) General features and the visual axis. (b) Enlargement to show features of the ciliary body, and the circulation of aqueous humour.

of small amounts of mucoprotein. This is the largest compartment and the fluid, once formed, cannot be replaced if lost by injury.

Light enters the eye through the cornea, passes through the lens and ultimately arrives at the receptor cells of the retina. Although widespread in the retina, the receptor cells are particularly dense at the 'yellow spot' or fovea, an area devoid of blood vessels lying in line behind the lens. The fovea is packed with cone receptors which convey colour vision, though small numbers of these will also be found in other areas of the retina. Some rods will also be present in the fovea but they are mainly found outside it. Thus, the image of whatever is the centre of our attention can be focused onto the fovea for high definition, colour analysis and clarity, but peripheral images can still be discerned though not in such detail.

The ability to discern detail is called visual acuity and is illustrated by consideration of the size of the foveal cones. These are only 2–3 μm in diameter which means that the difference in angle of light incident on the fovea to stimulate a single cone cell, but not an adjacent one, is only 40 seconds of arc (1 second of arc = 1/3600 of a degree). In practice, acuity is measured by the reading of letters of different sizes, called Snellen tests. These include rows of letters that should be visible to an observer at certain distances away. The letters are designed so that their height will subtend an angle of 5 minutes of arc (= 1/12 of a degree) if it is read at the appropriate distance. Thus a person standing 6 metres (20 feet) away should be able to read the appropriate row of letters and this is called 6/6 or 20/20 vision. In contrast, if a person standing 6 metres distant can only read those letters which should normally be readable from further distances (e.g. 18 metres, called 6/18 vision), then he has an acuity defect.

The visual field observable with two eyes looking directly ahead is of the order of 210 degrees. Although the perimeter of such a wide field of view may not be observed in detail, any movement is easily detected. In fact, movement within the visual field is an extremely potent stimulus which causes a reflex movement of the eyes so that the moving object can be scrutinized. The control of eye movement is described later.

The light from an object which has attracted our attention must be focused if its image is to be formed at the fovea. In other words light rays are bent or refracted on entering the eye so that they fall onto that particular part of the retina. Vision, therefore, can be considered to involve four stages:

1 refraction of light waves onto receptor cells;

2 transformation of light energy into electrical energy;

3 interpretation of electrical signals generated in the eye; and

4 control of the amount, or intensity, of the light so that this is appropriate and does not under- or overstimulate the receptor cells.

Light refraction

Light is refracted when it passes from one medium into another. As light enters the eye it is refracted by the cells of the cornea. Most of the refractive power of the eye is in the cornea and little further refraction occurs through the humours. The lens provides the final focusing of light onto the retina.

The lens is basically a concentric series of transparent layers of lens fibre enclosed within a transparent capsule, and is held in position by the suspensory ligaments. The curvature of the lens capsule is flexible and can be distorted by contraction or relaxation of the muscle cells of the ciliary bodies attached to the suspensory ligaments. This in turn alters the focal length of the lens and therefore its capacity to refract light rays.

The degree to which light must be refracted depends upon the angle at which the light rays are incident on the eye. Light from a near object must be greatly refracted to bring it into focus on the retina whilst that from a distant object requires less refraction (see Figure 14.6).

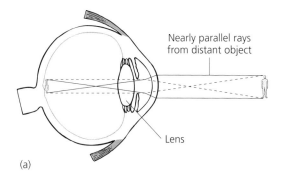

(a)

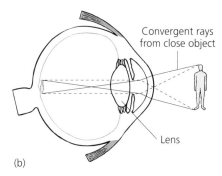

(b)

Figure 14.6 Accommodation: (a) objects 6 m (20 ft) or more away; (b) objects nearer than 6 m.
Note the refraction of light rays by the cornea and lens, the inversion of the retinal image, and the change in shape of the lens.

The curvature of the cornea and lens provides the flexibility necessary for comprehensive vision, that is, they allow accommodation to occur. After about 40–45 years of age the close focusing or accommodating ability of the lens declines as its structure and biochemistry changes.

Activation of the retinal receptor cells

A section through the retina is illustrated in Figure 14.7. It appears to be inverted in that the receptor cells lie below the associated nerve cells and, for much of the retina below, the blood vessels. This indicates that light is a powerful energy source and such barriers are of little consequence, although acuity is aided by the lack of vessels in the fovea. The receptor cells can be subdivided into those sensitive to wavelengths of light within the visible colour range (the cones) and those which are most sensitive to low light intensities and do not convey colour (the rods).

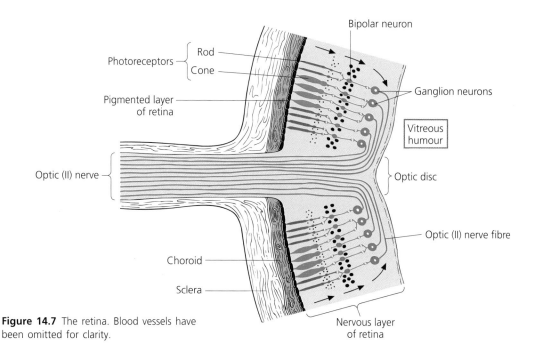

Figure 14.7 The retina. Blood vessels have been omitted for clarity.

A typical rod cell is shown diagrammatically in Figure 14.8. It contains the usual cell organelles but also contains light-sensitive pigment. This pigment, called rhodopsin, is comprised of two molecules, retinene (a derivative of vitamin A) and opsin. Light promotes the breakdown of rhodopsin into its constituents and, when this occurs, the receptor cell membrane is depolarized and a generator potential is produced. The two substances then recombine to reform the pigment.

The sensitivity of rod cells to light is determined by the amount of undissociated rhodopsin relative to dissociated pigment. In bright light most of the pigment is dissociated at any given time as it breaks down immediately upon re-forming. In contrast, much of the pigment is undissociated in poor light and so the eye is most sensitive. Thus, if a person enters a dark room from a bright one sensitivity increases 10-fold during the first 6 minutes as pigment re-forms. During the next 20 minutes or so the sensitivity increases by a further 1000-fold, although by this time only monochromatic vision will be possible as the cones require much greater light intensities to function. This increased sensitivity when light is poor is called visual adaptation and allows us to gain some vision even when there is very little light available. Of course if that person then re-entered a brightly lit room the effect would be dazzling as rhodopsin would dissociate in large quantities. Eventually adaptation would again occur as a new balance of dissociated to undissociated pigment becomes established and vision restored.

Cones behave in a similar fashion to rods but they contain slightly different pigments called visual purples. These exhibit peak sensitivity to light wavelengths corresponding to violet-blue (460 nm), bluish green-yellow (530 nm) and orange-red (590 nm) (Figure 14.9) and are therefore referred to as either blue, green, or red cones. On average they are sensitive to wavelengths of about 530 nm, which is about the wavelength of 'white' light produced by the correct proportions of colour wavelengths. Other wavelengths, such as those of infrared

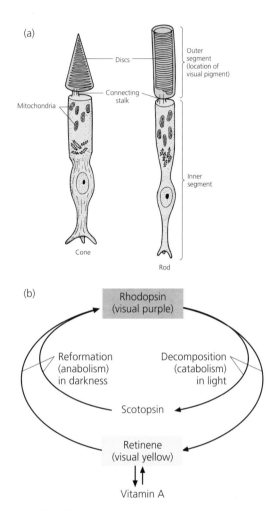

Figure 14.8 Rods, cones, and visual pigment. (a) Receptor cell types of the retina. (b) Behaviour of visual pigment (rhodopsin) in light and dark.

and ultraviolet, cannot be discerned by the human eye.

Available evidence suggests that 'colour vision' depends upon the proportions of blue, green and red cones that are stimulated. One criticism of this 'trichromatic' theory is that it does not explain why we are able to distinguish metallic colours. To see the full range of visible colours, however, does require the correct proportions of the three types of cone to be present. It is also clear that people who are deficient in particular cones have a colour 'blindness' appropriate to the deficit.

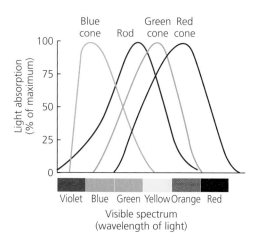

Figure 14.9 Light absorption by rods and cones.

Generator potentials of the rods and cones at threshold or above will promote depolarization of the sensory neurons they synapse with. The retina contains a complex arrangement of interacting nerve cells which have been given various names (Figure 14.7). The main type stimulated by the retinal receptors are called bipolar cells. These in turn synapse with other neurons, called ganglion cells, before action potentials are conducted into the optic nerve and thence to the brain. Other retinal neurons, called horizontal cells, are also involved and the interaction between the various nerve cells means that some processing of the information occurs before the action potentials even leave the eye.

Interpretation of the visual signals

Electrical activity passes from the retina to the optic nerve and thence to the brain. The pathway is of interest since activity from the left side of the retina of each eye passes to the right side of the brain and vice versa (Figure 14.10). This crossover of neural pathways from the left and right sides of the retinae occurs at the optic chiasma which lies just anterior to the pituitary gland at the base of the brain. The significance of crossover is that light from an object incident on, say, an area of the retina of the left eye, will stimulate a relatively different area of the retina of the right eye and comparison of the data enables us to perceive depth in the visual world.

After crossover the bundles of nerves cells pass to the dorsal lateral geniculate body of the thalamus but in doing so remain tightly packed into discrete nerves. Lesions of these nerves cause a profound loss of vision. After the thalamus, however, the neural pathways diverge (Figure 14.10) and so electrical activity from the retina eventually arrives at various parts of the brain for processing. These areas are involved in putting together a perceptional image of the objects within the visual field, and for controlling eye movements. The visual perceptional areas of the brain are comprised of virtually all of the occipital lobe of the cerebrum, of parts of the frontal/parietal motor cortex, and of parts of the brainstem. Interestingly, a blow to the back of the head causes us to perceive 'light' as nerve cells are mechanically activated. In addition, electrical stimulation of certain areas of the cerebrum produces hallucinatory effects.

One aspect of an image which is intensely examined by the brain are its edges. Patterns of cells within the visual area of the cerebral cortex have been shown to exhibit bursts of activity if the orientation of an object within the visual field is altered. Recognition of an object is clearly more complex than this but probably involves analysis of topographical features of the object, based at least partly on memory but also involving degrees of reasoning. The mechanism of the latter is still unclear.

Additional nuclei of the brain which also receive sensory input from the eye include the suprachiasmatic nucleus (i.e. it lies above the optic chiasma) of the hypothalamus. This is thought to control the sleep and wake circadian rhythmicity in response to light cues (see Chapter 23). The accessory optic nuclei and superior colliculi of the brainstem also receive inputs and are involved in controlling eye movement. The pretectum areas of the brainstem are involved in controlling pupil diameter.

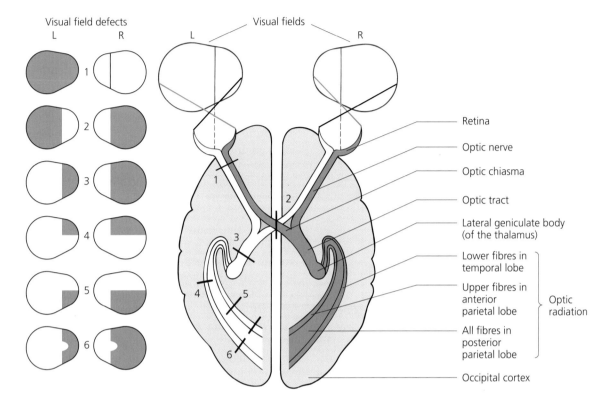

Figure 14.10 Visual pathways and field defects. Numbers 1–6 refer to neural lesions.

Control of the intensity of light entering the eye

The adaptation of retinal receptor cells to differences in light intensity was described earlier and is an important homeostatic response which enables us to maintain vision in both bright and poor light. The process is facilitated by the restriction of light entering the eye under bright conditions and by the admission of as much light as possible under poorly illuminated conditions.

On entering the eye, light must pass through the pupil of the iris. This contains pigmented cells but also antagonistic smooth muscle cells known as the radial and circular muscle fibres. As their names suggest, the former extend from the centrally located pupil to the periphery of the iris, and the latter extend circumferentially around the pupil. In bright light parasympa-thetic nerve activity stimulates contraction of the circular muscle fibres, and relaxes the radial ones, resulting in a constriction of the pupil. In dim light, sympathetic nerve activity contracts the radial fibres and relaxes the circular ones, resulting in pupil dilatation. The aperture of the pupil can therefore be reflexly altered accord-ing to light conditions.

The influence of sympathetic activity to dilate the pupil may also play a role in the all-out activity called the 'fight, flight, and fright' response in the alarm stage of the general adaptation syndrome (see Chapter 22), since pupil dilatation increases the illumination of peripheral areas of the retina and may even expand the visual field. Perception will there-fore be heightened. Sympathetic stimulation of pupil dilatation during times of excitement may even be a sexual attractant in the appro-priate setting!

Control of eye movement

The physiology of vision also includes the control of eye position in relation to focusing on near or distant objects, and in relation to following a moving object. Thus, if the attention is switched from a distant to a near object, the eyes must converge so that the image of the object still lands on the fovea of each eye. Continual assessment of the position of the image ensures that it is kept on the fovea; as the object moves toward the eyes then the image is returned to the fovea by further convergence (Figure 14.11). The processing involved in the control of these movements takes a fifth of a second and, to put this into context, it means that the last visual fixation that a batsman, for example, has on a cricket ball travelling at 90 mph will be when the ball is still more than 10 metres away from him. The delay, therefore, has implications in our ability to follow rapidly moving objects.

Movement within the visual field is a potent stimulus to attract attention. The eyes will usually reflexly focus on an unexpected moving object, which may be tracked as it moves across the visual field. Visual pursuit of a moving object is a complicated process and involves a 'programming' of the direction and speed of movement. Provided movement is not too rapid, tracking is very smooth (Figure 14.11). If the movement is rapid, the eyes must carry out extremely quick catching-up movements and this means that, for a fraction of a second, the object is not exactly where the brain perceives it to be! These rapid eye movements are called saccades and similar movements, without the 'programming', are also performed in, for example, scanning a piece of text or a painting. They are amongst the fastest movements which the body is capable of producing.

HEARING

'Sound' is the perception of small pressure waves generated in air or water by a vibrating

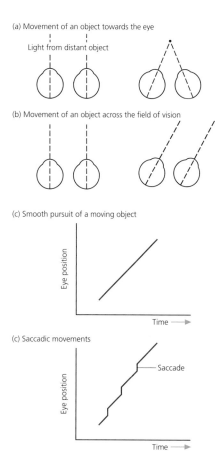

(a) Movement of an object towards the eye

Light from distant object

(b) Movement of an object across the field of vision

(c) Smooth pursuit of a moving object

Eye position

Time

(c) Saccadic movements

Saccade

Eye position

Time

Figure 14.11 Eye movements. (a) In tracking an object as it moves closer, the eyes must converge to maintain the image on both retinae. (b) Movement of an object across the visual field produces eye movements which keep the eyes parallel. Such tracking of an object may involve (c) smooth pursuit, although if the object is moving too rapidly (as in d), the eyes must make small, rapid adjustments called saccades to 'catch up' with the object.

object (e.g. the vocal cords of the larynx). Vibrations set up alternate compressions and decompressions of the air and the number of compressions per second (or cycles per second; 1 cycle/s = 1 Hertz or Hz) gives the sound its frequency and this is perceived as pitch. The amplitude of the compressions gives sound its intensity or loudness. Sound intensity is measured in decibels: rustling leaves have a decibel rating of 15, that of conversation 45. The ear can detect frequencies over a range of

20–20 000 Hz, and intensities almost as low as 0 decibels. A sound intensity of 115–120 decibels produces pain within the ear.

Hearing is basically a process by which pressure waves produced by the compression cycle are transmitted to, and detected by, receptor cells within the inner ear. Electrochemical activity from the receptors must, of course, be ultimately interpreted by the brain.

The ear

The ear is divided into three component parts: the external, middle, and inner ear (Figure 14.12). The visible external ear, or pinna, is deeply folded and this introduces minor perturbations in the sound pressure waves and helps in locating its source. Comparison of signals from both ears also facilitates the location of sound.

The aperture of the external ear penetrates the skull via the auditory meatus or external auditory canal, which terminates at the eardrum or tympanic membrane. This membrane is under a degree of tension and vibrates at the same frequencies as those of sound pressure waves incident upon it.

The vibrating membrane sets up similar vibrations in the transmission system of the middle ear, which is comprised of three small bones or ossicles (called the malleus, incus, and stapes) within an air-filled chamber (Figure 14.13a). The presence of a middle ear conveys four major advantages:

1 The force of vibration is greatly increased in the ossicles and this is essential as the tympanic membrane is considerably larger than the aperture of the inner ear, and also because the inner ear is fluid-filled.

2 The middle ear chamber connects directly with the nasopharynx via the Eustachian or auditory tube. Thus any major change in external air pressure (distinct from the small fluctuations produced by most sounds) can quickly be applied to the middle ear via the nasopharynx and so equilibrate the pressure on either side of the tympanic membrane. Swallowing facilitates this process by opening

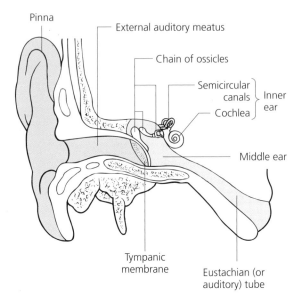

Figure 14.12 General anatomy of the ear.

the aperture of the Eustachian tubes in the nasopharynx. 'Ballooning' of the eardrum is therefore prevented, and this protects the membrane from damage. It will not protect against very sudden changes in air pressure, however, such as occur in explosions.

3 The middle ear chamber provides a means of dissipating the sound pressure waves after they have traversed the inner ear, thus making the receptor cells receptive to further stimulation.

4 The transmission of vibrations along the chain of ossicles means that if our external environment is extremely noisy, excessive amplitudes of vibration of the ossicles and inner ear produced by pronounced movement of the tympanic membrane can be reduced by altering the contact between the bones and the tympanic membrane and inner ear. This is achieved by small muscles (called the tensor tympani and the stapedius) which on contraction pull the malleus away from the tympanic membrane and pull the stapes away from the aperture to the inner ear. This mechanism, therefore, is analogous to the reflex reduction of the

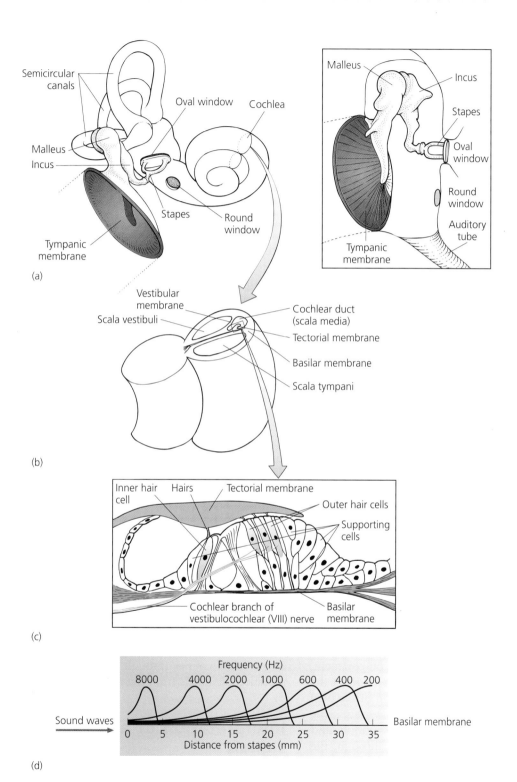

Figure 14.13 Hearing. (a) Middle ear and position of the cochlea. (b) Section through a 'turn' of the cochlea. (c) Receptor cells and associated structures in the cochlea (organ of Corti). (d) Deflections of the basilar membrane by sounds of different frequency.

pupil diameter in the eye in response to bright light in that excessive stimulation is prevented from entering the receptor area – another example of homeostatic adaptation.

The stapes has a flattened surface which makes contact with the membrane that occludes the aperture to the inner ear. This aperture, the oval window or fenestra ovalis, provides access to the fluid-filled cochlea in which the receptor cells are found, and so vibration is transferred from the ossicles to the cochlear fluid. Pressure waves within the fluid are eventually dissipated by being transmitted back into the middle ear via another membrane-enclosed aperture called the round window or fenestra rotunda.

The inner ear contains a number of structures: the cochlea involved in hearing and the components of the vestibular apparatus involved in balance. The latter were described earlier.

The cochlea

This structure is shaped like a snail shell, and the coils increase the surface area of the receptor membrane within them. A cross-section through the cochlea is shown in Figure 14.13b. The structure is very complex but can generally be described as one in which the receptor cells 'sit' on a membrane, called the basilar membrane, with their hair-like extensions projecting into a gel-like matrix, the tectorial membrane. The whole is bathed by a fluid, called endolymph, and the compartment (called the scala media) containing the endolymph is separated by a membrane (Reissner's membrane) from another fluid-filled compartment called the scala vestibuli, which contains perilymph (Figure 14.13b). The scala vestibuli connects with a lower perilymph compartment, called the scala tympani, via a small hole at the tip or apex of the cochlea. Vibration of the oval window produces vibrations within the endolymph and within the scala vestibuli, and these are eventually dissipated through the scala tympani and thence into the middle ear via the round window. Vibrations in the endolymph cause the basilar membrane to be

deflected and a wave of oscillations to pass along it. The hair projections of the receptor cells are distorted and this results in the generation of action potentials in sensory nerve endings.

The conduction of sound waves through water is highly efficient. Low frequency sounds travel easier than high frequency ones, however, and evidence suggests that low frequency components of sounds produce greatest oscillation of the basilar membrane at the further turns of the cochlea, where the membrane is less stiff, whilst high frequency sounds stimulate the earlier turns. This is illustrated in Figure 14.13d. Thus receptors at one end of the basilar membrane are stimulated by low frequency sounds and those at the other by high frequencies. The amplitude of vibration of the membrane provides information about the intensity of the sound waves. Thus, as with vision, some processing of the stimulus is provided by the sensory organ itself. The full process is extremely complex, however, and beyond the bounds of this book.

The sensitivity of the cochlea to sound depends upon frequency. The ear is most sensitive to the range of frequencies associated with human speech (1000–4000 Hz). Clinically an initial hearing test involves assessment of the intensity 'threshold' of sounds across a range of frequencies. An audiogram can then be produced which, when compared with norms, indicates any loss of hearing at given wavelengths (Figure 14.14). Tones generated via headphones are conducted to the inner ear by the usual route, but tones can also be conducted via bones of the skull. Conduction of sound through bone (by applying the tone to the mastoid process behind the ear) bypasses the middle ear and any hearing defect can then be narrowed down to an inner ear or middle ear deficit. Hearing difficulties may also arise, of course, through errors in the interpretation of signals from the ear by the brain.

Interpretation of auditory signals

Sensory nerve fibres from the cochlear receptors pass via the cochlear fibre bundles of the

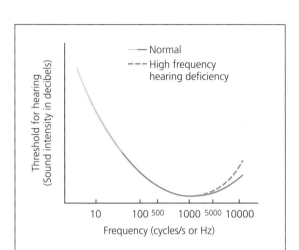

Figure 14.14 The audiogram.

vestibulocochlear nerve (cranial nerve VIII; sometimes called the auditory or acoustic nerve) to the cochlear nuclei of the brainstem (Figure 14.15). Here they synapse with other fibres which subsequently synapse with other neurons within various nuclei of the brainstem, including the inferior colliculi, before passing to a part of the thalamus called the medial geniculate body. Neurons then carry the signal to the auditory area of the cortex which is part of the cortex of each temporal lobe of the cerebrum. Sensory fibres from each ear interact within the brain and each temporal lobe receives input from both ears, and so damage to one temporal lobe normally has minimal effects on hearing. A further pathway within the brainstem also carries information to the reticular formation, a structure which, amongst various functions, is involved in the

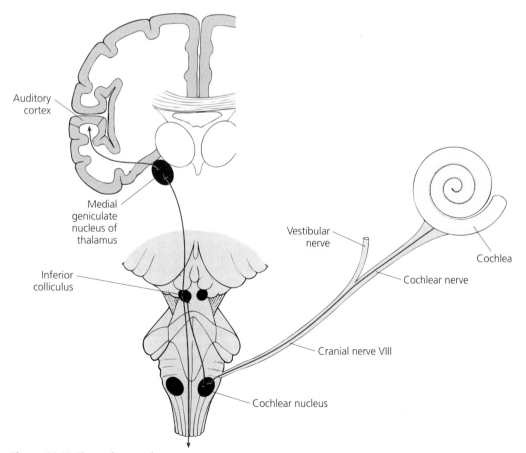

Figure 14.15 The auditory pathway.

sleep–wake cycle. Thus, sound is an effective waking stimulus even from deep sleep.

TASTE AND SMELL

The senses of taste and smell involve chemoreceptors which respond to the presence of molecules dissolved in the fluid layer which bathes them. The two are not mutually exclusive and stimulation of the olfactory receptors of the nose is an important aspect of taste, even though taste is looked upon as being a feature of the oral cavity.

Taste (gustation)

Taste is sensed by receptors present in 'buds' on the surface of the tongue, epiglottis, pharynx and palate. Each 'bud' consists of four types of cell, some of which are chemoreceptors, others being responsible for nutritive support (Figure 14.16). There are some 10 000 taste 'buds' on the tongue alone and these are clustered together in papillae. Each papilla may contain up to five taste 'buds' (these are called fungiform papillae because of their shape) or up to 100 buds (these are called vallate papillae). Smaller filiform papillae are also present but these contain few if any taste buds.

Four basic tastes have been identified: sweet, sour, bitter, and salt. The taste buds responsible for these modalities are arranged in particular areas of the tongue (Figure 14.16), but all four are 'tasted' to various degrees by the receptors of the palate, epiglottis, and pharynx. Tastes such as 'sweet' are obviously desirable as they imply a rich caloric value of the food present in the mouth. Bitter tastes may be offensive; if extreme the food may be rejected as potentially toxic. Salt and acidic foods may or may not be considered desirable. For example, salt depletion of the body fluids stimulates a 'salt' appetite and salty foods may then be chosen in preference to others.

The four kinds of taste buds do not appear to differ histologically and the ways in which the molecules generate action potentials is still

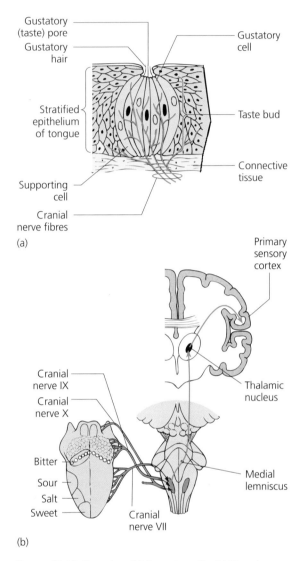

Figure 14.16 Gustation. (a) Receptor cells. (b) Neural pathways from receptors to sensory cortex.

debatable. Different cell membrane or metabolic pathways are presumably involved and this may explain why substances such as the dipeptide lysyltaurine tastes salty yet clearly does not contain sodium chloride, and why lead salts taste sweet yet do not contain sugars. Further phenomena which illustrate the complexity of taste are that a protein modifier (called miraculin) will make acidic substances taste sweet, and that genetic variation means

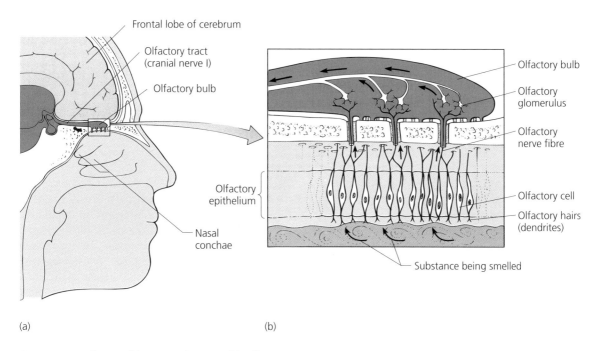

Figure 14.17 Olfaction. (a) Receptor location. (b) Olfactory receptors and neural pathway.

that only a proportion of people can taste the substance phenylthiocarbamide (PTC).

Interpretation of gustatory signals

Activity from the anterior two-thirds of the tongue pass via the facial nerve (cranial nerve VII) to the brainstem (Figure 14.16). The glossopharyngeal nerve (cranial nerve IX) conveys activity from the posterior third. Fibres from the pharynx, epiglottis and palate pass to the brainstem via the vagus nerve (cranial nerve X). Within the brainstem, all inputs pass to a collection of nerve cells within the medulla oblongata (the nucleus of the tractus solitarius) from which fibres pass to specific areas of the thalamus. They then synapse with other neurons which pass to the cortex of the parietal lobe.

Smell (olfaction)

The sense of smell depends upon receptors present within the mucous membrane of the nasal epithelium, an area measuring 5 cm² in the roof of the nasal cavity. There are some 10–20 million receptor cells here (with other supportive or secretory cells) which are in fact modified nerve cells. The nerve endings are expanded into olfactory rods from which cilia project into the bathing fluid layer and molecules dissolved within the mucus interact with surface molecules in the cilia membrane (Figure 14.17). Proteins present within the fluid are thought to facilitate the presentation of odour molecules to the receptors.

Odour-producing molecules are generally small but odour is more dependent upon molecular configuration than on size. The olfactory cells are particularly sensitive at detecting characteristic odours and humans can distinguish up to 4000 different odours. The detection of intensity of particular odours is not so well developed, however. How such a diverse range of odours can be detected is unknown but is unlikely to depend simply upon a similar range of complementary receptor molecules (i.e. 'lock and key'). For example, the chemicals camphor and hexachlorethane smell identical but are very different molecules with different chemical properties.

Attempts to classify smell modalities have suggested that odours can be separated into seven types: putrid, musky, floral, pungent, peppermint, ethereal, and camphoraceous. A combination of these is suggested to produce the range of odour perceptions of which we are capable. The diversity of odours goes beyond the limits of these modalities, however, and to call these 'primary' odours would be misleading.

Pain fibres also originate in the olfactory epithelium and are stimulated by irritative characteristics of odours, for example peppermint and chlorine. Sneezing and tear secretion are reflexly induced after stimulation of these fibres and these are clearly defensive mechanisms against a perceived noxious vapour.

Adaptation to a stimulus is also noticeable with smell, and may only apply to a single odour within a collection of odours; the 'thresholds' for other odours are unchanged. Adaptation allows us to remain within a particular environment without constantly perceiving a particular dominant odour, unless it is noxious. The mechanism is unknown but probably involves modulation of receptor function and also of central processing.

The presence of two nostrils helps in the determination of the direction from which a smell originates because they introduce a slight delay in the stimulation of one part of the olfactory epithelium relative to the other.

Interpretation of olfactory signals

Sensory fibres from olfactory receptors terminate in the olfactory bulb, a distended terminal of the olfactory nerve (cranial nerve I), where they synapse with other neurons in what are called the olfactory glomeruli (see Figure 14.17). These form synapses with other neurons within the vicinity, before neural activity passes via the olfactory nerve to various structures within the limbic system (see Chapter 13), including an area of the cerebral cortex. Smell is possibly unique amongst the senses in that afferent neural activity does not relay via the thalamus.

Initial processing of the activity probably occurs in the olfactory glomeruli but final processing occurs in the primary olfactory cortex located in the temporal lobe of the cerebrum. Pathways linking the limbic system with the hypothalamus provide the input to hypothalamic 'drive' centres associated with smells, for example autonomic arousal and sexual arousal.

Role of sensory receptors in homeostasis

How sensory function enables the body to monitor aspects of the internal and external environments was outlined at the beginning of this chapter. Physiological systems help to ensure that the intracellular environment is maintained appropriate to the functioning of a cell, and a coordination of systemic function is necessary, as described in Chapter 1. This is facilitated by the maintenance of individual systemic homeostasis. For example, the perfusion of tissues is dependent upon various factors including regulation of the (blood) pressure that provides the necessary driving force. Baroreceptors within the arterial system detect changes in blood pressure and resultant cardiovascular responses then restore the pressure within homeostatic limits.

Similarly, a decrease in the partial pressure of oxygen in blood will stimulate peripheral chemoreceptors, the primary effect of which is to promote respiratory function. It is also clear, however, that chemoreceptor stimulation also causes peripheral vasoconstriction, other than that of the heart and brain, which raises arterial blood pressure and facilitates the delivery of oxygen to these vital tissues.

These two examples illustrate the role of senses in systemic homeostasis, but the influence of hypoxia on arterial blood pressure also illustrates how systemic control overlaps, in this instance at the expense of a reduced perfusion to 'non-vital' tissues. Again we see how changes to one system influences others.

The predictive element of the special senses was described earlier. This has obvious advantages in the course and planning of actions, the consequences of which are that the internal environment is more likely to be optimal if threatening situations can be avoided. The special senses also facilitate our capacity to operate in the range of environments with which we come into contact each day, and help us to maintain independence of our actions. In so doing it could also be said that these senses play a role in our social and psychological well-being, in addition to the maintenance of physiological homeostasis.

Examples of homeostatic control system failures and principles of correction

The range of homeostatic disturbances induced by sensory failure is large. Many examples are covered in other chapters and this section will only include some of the commoner disorders of the special senses.

THE EYE

Blurred vision

Blurred or distorted vision results from a failure of the refraction of light rays to focus an image on the retina. Thus a thickened lens or elongated eyeball will cause the image to be focused at a point in front of the retina (a condition called myopia or nearsightedness), whereas a long slimmer lens or a shortened eyeball or poor accommodation, such as occurs with age, may cause the focal point to fall behind the retina (a condition called hypermetropia or longsightedness; Figure 14.18). An irregular curvature of the lens or cornea will disturb the focusing of central and peripheral aspects of an image and this is called astigmatism.

The capacity for a lens to accommodate to near objects diminishes with age, producing an inability to focus on near objects, or presbyopia.

All these disorders are correctable with appropriate spectacle lenses. For example a convex spectacle lens will cause convergence of light rays before they are incident on the cornea and this will correct a refractory deficiency as in longsightedness (Figure 14.18). Similarly a concave lens will cause divergence of light rays and correct excessive refraction produced by the eye, as in shortsightedness.

Cataract

Loss of lens transparency by a change in its structure (a cataract) will prevent the transmission of light, resulting in blindness. Correction of total vision loss is by implantation of an artificial lens.

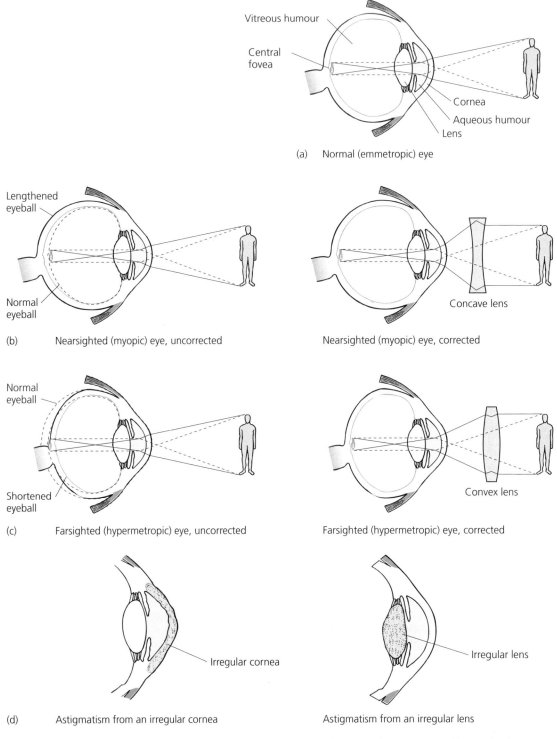

(a)   Normal (emmetropic) eye

(b)   Nearsighted (myopic) eye, uncorrected

Nearsighted (myopic) eye, corrected

(c)   Farsighted (hypermetropic) eye, uncorrected

Farsighted (hypermetropic) eye, corrected

(d)   Astigmatism from an irregular cornea

Astigmatism from an irregular lens

Figure 14.18 Abnormal focusing by the eye. (a) Normal. (b) Nearsighted vision and its correction. (c) Farsighted vision and its correction. (d) Astigmatism.

Glaucoma

If the rate of secretion of aqueous humour exceeds that of its resorption then an increased humour pressure will result, called glaucoma. The elevated pressure is transmitted to the vitreous humour which then crushes the retinal blood vessels. Blindness may result if it is untreated. Treatment is aimed at improving fluid drainage either by surgery or by pharmacological contraction of iris sphincter muscles to release the occluded duct.

Infection

Conjunctivitis is an inflammation of the conjunctiva caused by an infection or by the presence of irritants.

THE EAR

Nerve and conduction deafness

Impairment of cochlear nerve function will result in deafness, called nerve deafness, as will a disruption of the conduction pathway of the middle ear, called conduction deafness.

Nerve deafness frequently disturbs the vestibular apparatus, producing further symptoms of vertigo and nausea. Collectively this is called labyrinthine disease and commonly results from infection, trauma, local arteriosclerosis, allergies, or ageing. Tinnitus is a term given to a ringing in the ears and this is often present, particularly if the deafness arises from the production of excessive endolymph as this depresses the basilar membrane. This is called Ménière's syndrome.

Treatment depends upon cause and may include destruction of the semicircular canals using ultrasound, a reduction in endolymph secretion through the use of diuretics, local vasodilatation using an elevated blood CO_2 content or, in extreme cases, by surgical intervention.

Excessive ear wax

Excessive production of wax (cerumen) into the external auditory canal can impair hearing, especially if it becomes impacted on the tympanic membrane. Treatment is usually by periodic irrigation.

Infection

Abnormal Eustachian tube function may allow bacteria from the nasopharynx to enter the middle ear, causing inflammation, a condition called otitis media. Antimicrobial agents may prevent further progress of infection but rupture of the tympanic membrane and inner ear infection can still occur.

TASTE AND SMELL

Inflammation and mucous congestion of the nasal cavity as a consequence of infection will clearly interfere with the olfactory epithelium, resulting in a loss of sense of smell. Smell is also essential to taste and the loss of olfactory function will therefore also influence taste perception. Prevention of fluid drainage from the cranial sinuses into the nasal cavity may also lead to infection (sinusitis).

Summary

1 The homeostatic control of physiological systems and cellular function is dependent upon the facility to 'sense' changes in all aspects of the internal environment, and also of many elements of the external environment.

2 Senses depend upon receptor cells which have specializations, usually of the cell membrane, that enable them to respond to specific parameters. Some senses are polymodal in that they can detect more than one quality of a stimulus. These are the special senses of vision, hearing, taste, smell, and pain.

3 Information from peripheral senses including cutaneous receptors, proprioreceptors, and visceral receptors passes to the brain via tracts within the spinal cord. Numerous relays may be involved but almost all pass through the thalamus of the brain on the way to the sensory areas of the cerebral cortex.

4 The eye is a sense organ which causes light rays to be focused onto receptors of the retina. Biochemical features of the receptors allow us to perceive light of different wavelengths (colour) as well as intensity.

5 Information from the retinal receptors passes via the thalamus to various components of the brain, particularly the visual cortex of the occipital cerebral lobe. Processing produces 'vision' and is also important in controlling eye movement.

6 The ear consists of external, middle, and inner structures, the latter including organs of hearing and of balance. Transmission of sound to the fluid-filled inner ear occurs via small ossicles within the air-filled middle ear.

7 Pressure waves induced in the cochlea of the inner ear are converted into electrochemical signals which provide both intensity and frequency information. Electrochemical activity passes to various parts of the brain, but especially to the auditory cortex of the temporal lobes.

8 Taste and smell result from stimulation of chemoreceptors of the tongue and nasal cavities. Although involving an interaction between receptor molecules present on the receptor cell membranes and food or odour molecules, the process is more complex than a simple 'lock-and-key' mechanism. The actual mechanism is unknown, but it enables us to detect a wide variety of different molecules.

9 Information from the nose and tongue passes to various structures within the brain. Apart from the cerebral cortex, other important olfactory processing areas include structures of the limbic system.

Review Questions

1 Describe three different types of mechanoreceptors with their associated receptive stimuli.

2 Describe the anatomical structure of thermoreceptors.

3 Distinguish between unimodal and polymodal receptors.

4 Explain how muscle tendons help maintain posture.

5 Suggest why the location of Golgi tendon organs is associated with their function.

6 Describe the functions of the external, middle, and inner ears in formulating the sensation of hearing.

7 What are the roles of the following:
(a) Eustachian tubes; (b) ceruminous glands; (c) hairs in the external auditory meatus.

8 Using knowledge gained in Chapter 13 and this chapter, trace the pathway of visual impulses from the retina to the occipital cortex using the following terms:
(a) threshold; (b) generator potential; (c) action potential; (d) depolarization; (e) repolarization; (f) synaptic transmission; (g) excitatory post-synaptic potential; (h) inhibitory post-synaptic potential.

9 Describe the roles of the vestibular apparatus and the semicircular canals in proprioception.

10 Distinguish between superficial and deep receptors.

11 Describe how each extrinsic eye muscle is involved in movement of the eye.

12 What is the function of the lachrymal apparatus?

13 Describe the structure and function of the three layers of the eye.

14 Describe the function of the cornea and lens during accommodation.

15 How does light intensity affect the size of the pupil?

16 Compare and contrast the photoreceptors of the retina.

17 Trace the pathway of an olfactory impulse from a receptor to the auditory centre of the cortex.

18 Trace the pathway of gustatory impulses from the four taste receptors (describing their distribution) on the tongue to the gustatory centre of the cortex.

19 Briefly describe the role of the sensory receptors in homeostasis.

20 Name two homeostatic imbalances of each sensory modality.

15

Coordination III: Hormones

Introduction: relation of hormones to cellular homeostasis

Overview of the anatomy, physiology, and chemistry of the hormonal system

Details of the homeostatic functions of hormones

Examples of homeostatic control system failures and principles of correction

Summary

Review questions

Introduction: relation of hormones to cellular homeostasis

Cells are the basic functional units of life, and their activities vary considerably between tissues according to their role in the body. For cells and tissues to function at all they require an appropriate rate of delivery of specific nutrients and this is only achievable by the regulation of the functions of other tissues and organs. Such functions must also be compatible with the roles of these tissues, whether it be, for example, the acquisition of nutrients by digestion of food in the gut, or the degree of vasoconstriction necessary for the maintenance of an adequate arterial blood pressure to transport metabolites to the cells.

Physiological function cannot be static, since parameters are subject to change under the influence of extrinsic factors, and systemic function must also respond according to the needs of the individual at any given time. Although some tissues are able to exert limited intrinsic control of their activities, as in the effects of oxygen lack/carbon dioxide excess to alter tissue blood flow in muscle and brain, the overall regulation of tissues, and the integration of organ functions, are provided by the coordinating systems of the body: the nervous and hormonal systems.

Nerve cells and hormones each provide a means of communication between different parts of the body but, whereas nerve cells provide a physico-chemical route by which 'messages' can be conducted directly between tissues, hormones are purely chemical 'messengers' which are conveyed by the extracellular fluids to their target tissues. The principles of nervous function were described in Chapter 13, but it is worthwhile considering here the advantages and disadvantages of the two coordinating systems in order to highlight their different, but sometimes inter-relating and overlapping, roles.

General comparison of neural and hormonal systems

1 Hormones are released from specific secretory cells in one part of the body, dispersed in extracellular fluid (usually blood plasma), and interact with target cells elsewhere. In contrast, nerve cells extend from one tissue to another and provide a direct communication link. They too, however, depend upon the secretion of neurotransmitters into extracellular fluid (usually tissue fluid) at synapses and these must interact with receptors on target cells. The distances travelled by neurotransmitters are of course very small, and nerve cells have the advantage that they can convey 'messages' (i.e. impulses) very rapidly to the target cells. The disadvantages, though, are that this direct link must be established with every target cell within a tissue, and that link must be maintained; neural damage may irreversibly prevent communication.

2 The rapidity at which neural impulses are conducted means that target cells can quickly be induced to alter their activities. In contrast the time taken to induce the release of hormones from stores within secretory cells (or synthesize them in some cases), and to conduct them to targets, means that responses are much slower, of the order of several minutes or perhaps 1–2 hours if the hormone has to be synthesized first. Hormones, therefore, are important in regulating medium- or long-term functions of tissues, such as controlling body fluid composition or growth. Hormone operation would clearly be unsuitable, for example, in the rapid change in cardiac function that is necessary to control blood pressure when we stand up.

3 Both systems can act concurrently in the regulation of an organ. The rapidity of neural responses is advantageous, for example, in the moment-to-moment coordination of gut motility, but the slower response to hormones is more appropriate in the control of gut secretions, although neural activity can also alter these.

4 Some nerve cells in the hypothalamus also synthesize hormones and therefore represent an overlap between the systems. These cells are referred to as neurosecretory cells.

5 Nervous activity modulates the release of certain hormones, and some hormones influence neural activity. The two systems, therefore, may not always act in isolation.

6 From the clinical viewpoint, the fact that both systems utilize the release of a chemical, and its interaction with target receptors, means that many drugs have similar modes of action, either as receptor antagonists or agonists, or as agents which interfere with chemical synthesis, storage, or release.

Overview of the anatomy, physiology, and chemistry of the hormonal system

In order to understand how the hormonal system is activated, and the actions of hormones, it is necessary to consider (1) how secretory tissue is organized, (2) the nature and (3) chemistry of hormonal secretions, (4) how hormones induce a change in target cell activity, and (5) the general principles of how hormone release is regulated.

SECRETORY TISSUES: EXOCRINE AND ENDOCRINE GLANDS

The cells of many tissues secrete chemicals as part of their normal roles, but not all secretions can be called hormones. Cells which secrete chemicals are frequently collected into discrete areas of tissue that are collectively called glands.

Glands which release their secretions outside the body (including into the lumen of the gut, which strictly speaking is external) are called exocrine glands. Many, for example salivary glands and the pancreas, require ducts to transport their secretions. Not all exocrine glands are ducted, however. Many of the cells which secrete digestive enzymes, and those which produce mucus, release their secretions directly. Hormones are not usually produced as exocrine secretions.

Those glands which secrete the major hormones of the body are referred to as endocrine glands. The prefix endo- indicates that secretions are released into fluids within the body. This process does not require the presence of ducts to transport the secretion as it can be released directly into the extracellular fluid. Hence these glands are sometimes referred to as ductless glands.

In a few instances, a gland has both exocrine and endocrine functions. Thus the pancreas is an exocrine gland which releases digestive juices into the duodenum, but also has 'islets' of endocrine tissue which secrete the hormones insulin, glucagon, and somatostatin into the circulatory system. The pancreas, therefore, is a mixed gland. The gonads are also mixed glands.

WHAT IS A HORMONE?

By definition a hormone is a substance produced by cells in one part of the body, that is secreted into the blood in response to a specific stimulus and in amounts that vary with the strength of the stimulus, and has its actions some distance from the site of secretion known as the hormone's target tissue. Hormones are therefore endocrine secretions and the hormonal system is frequently referred to as the endocrine system (endocrinology is the study of hormones).

The term 'hormone' was coined almost 100 years ago, and since then numerous chemical messengers which influence the activity of tissues have been identified. Although they, too, are usually referred to as hormones, not all fit the conventional definition. Thus:

1 Autocrine secretions are those which are released into the interstitial fluid and influence the activities of the cell which secreted them. An example is the way in which oestrogen hormones secreted by ovarian follicle cells during the menstrual cycle stimulate those same cells to secrete further oestrogen.

2 Paracrine secretions are those which are released into interstitial fluid and influence the activities of other cells within the immediate vicinity. Delivery of the secretion to the target cells is by diffusion through the fluid; the secretion is not blood-borne. Prostaglandins are examples of paracrine secretions and these are synthesized by most, if not all, tissues. They provide an intrinsic modulation of tissue functions.

3 Pheromones are secretions that are released out of the body and change the behaviour of other organisms. There is considerable evidence for their presence in a variety of species, and it is thought that humans, too, produce pheromones as sexual attractants, probably via apocrine sweat.

These secretions are all chemical messengers and highlight the difficulty in defining the term 'hormone'. This chapter uses the term in its broadest sense, i.e. a chemical messenger released from secretory cells in response to a specific stimulus, in amounts which vary with the strength of that stimulus, and which

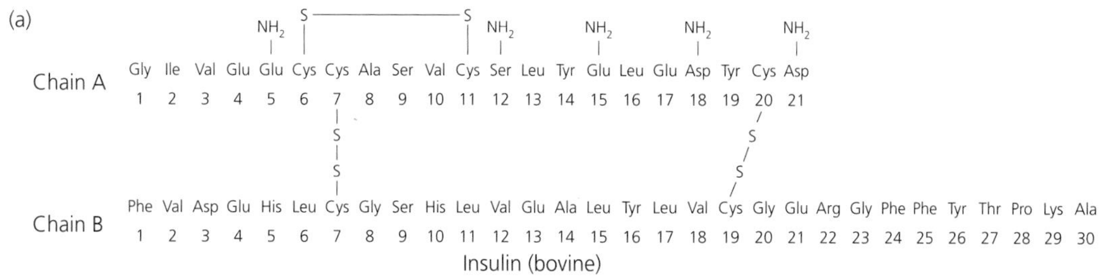

(a)

Chain A

Gly Ile Val Glu Glu Cys Cys Ala Ser Val Cys Ser Leu Tyr Glu Leu Glu Asp Tyr Cys Asp
1   2   3   4   5   6   7   8   9   10 11 12 13 14 15 16 17 18 19 20 21

Chain B

Phe Val Asp Glu His Leu Cys Gly Ser His Leu Val Glu Ala Leu Tyr Leu Val Cys Gly Glu Arg Gly Phe Phe Tyr Thr Pro Lys Ala
1   2   3   4   5   6   7   8   9   10 11 12 13 14 15 16 17 18 19 20 21 22 23 24 25 26 27 28 29 30

Insulin (bovine)

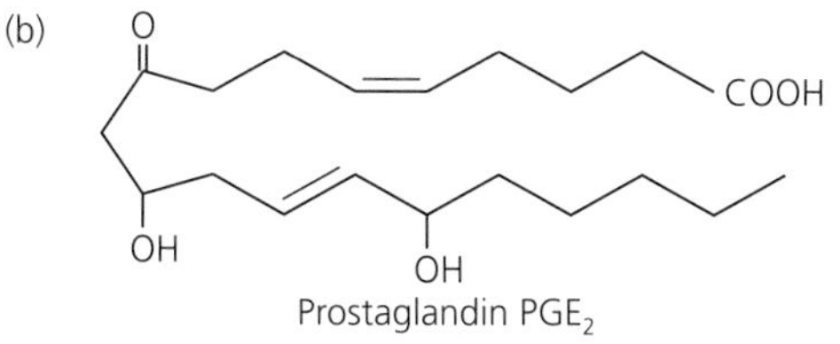

(b)

COOH

OH   OH
Prostaglandin PGE$_2$

Figure 15.1 Molecular structures of (a) a representative peptide hormone and (b) a prostaglandin.

influences the activities of other cells (whilst recognizing that this still omits autocrine secretions).

Regarding the types of target cell, hormones can be classified as being tropic or non-tropic. Tropic hormones are those which stimulate other endocrine tissues to release their hormones (trop- = to turn on). Non-tropic hormones promote the activities of non-endocrine tissues. Names of tropic hormones frequently, but not always, end in the suffix -tropin.

Hormonal chemistry

Hormones are a diverse range of substances but can basically be divided into four types: peptides, catecholamines, steroids, and prostaglandins. Examples are given later, but some general features of their functional chemistry are noted here:

1 Peptides are small chains of amino acids (Figure 15.1a), although interaction between the amino acids produces a precise three-dimensional shape. Other molecules might be attached to the peptide, for example glucose in glycopeptides. They are soluble in water but are only poorly soluble in lipid, and after synthesis can be stored in membrane-bound vesicles within the secretory cells. Release necessitates exocytosis following fusion of the vesicles with the plasma membrane of the cell and this usually involves an influx of calcium ions into the cell. Hormonal interaction with target cells requires the presence of specific receptors on the surface of those cells. Examples of peptide hormones include insulin, vasopressin and oxytocin.

2 Catecholamine hormones are derivatives of the amino acid tyrosine, and are therefore of similar chemical structure (Figure 15.2). They, too, are only slightly soluble in lipid, are stored in intracellular vesicles, and require the presence of surface receptors on target cells. The similarity of their chemical structure may result in overlap in their actions, though receptor subtypes are found in certain tissues and these enable each hormone to have specific actions in those tissues. Adrenaline and noradrenaline are examples of catecholamines.

The hormones produced by the thyroid gland (thyroxine and tri-iodothyronine) are also modified amines, and are synthesized as required from tyrosine stored within the thyroid gland. They, too, require the presence of surface receptors on target cells.

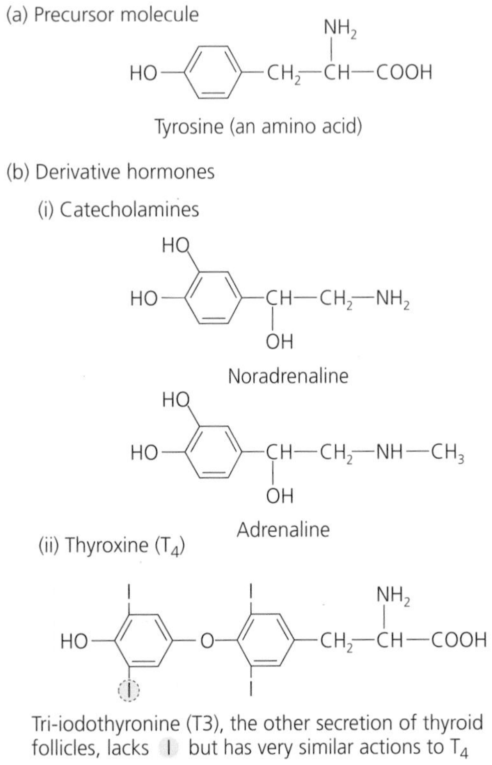

(a) Precursor molecule

Tyrosine (an amino acid)

(b) Derivative hormones

(i) Catecholamines

Noradrenaline

Adrenaline

(ii) Thyroxine (T_4)

Tri-iodothyronine (T3), the other secretion of thyroid follicles, lacks I but has very similar actions to T_4

Figure 15.2 Molecular structure of (a) tyrosine (b) derivative amine hormones.

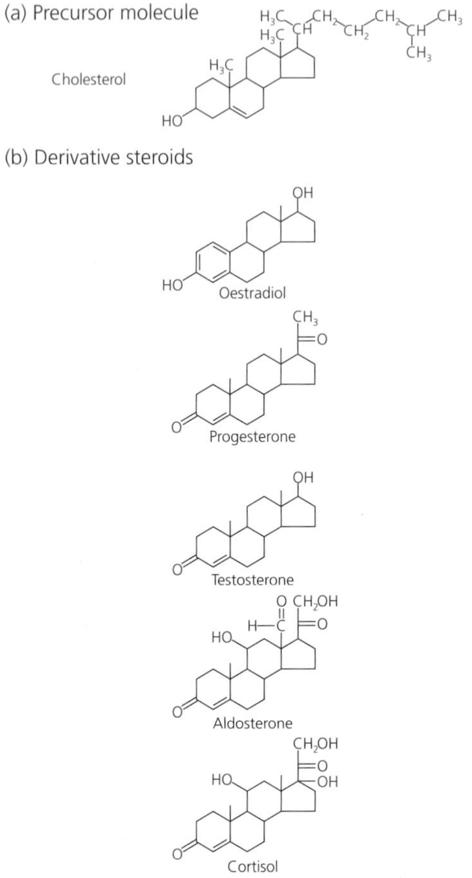

(a) Precursor molecule

Cholesterol

(b) Derivative steroids

Oestradiol

Progesterone

Testosterone

Aldosterone

Cortisol

Figure 15.3 Molecular structures of (a) cholesterol and (b) derivative steroid hormones.

3 Steroid hormones are all derivatives of cholesterol and are therefore modified lipids. Examples include testosterone, the oestrogens, cortisol, and aldosterone. They cannot be stored as they are highly lipid-soluble and so must be synthesized as required. This delay is one factor in the relative slowness of responses to stimuli which promote steroid release. Being lipid-soluble, steroids readily diffuse into target cells and the hormone receptors are intra-cellular.

Steroids have similar molecular structures (Figure 15.3), and overlap in their actions can occur. For example, the influence of oestrogens on fluid balance during the menstrual cycle includes a stimulation of aldosterone receptors in the kidney.

4 Prostaglandins (Figure 15.1) are derivatives of 'essential' unsaturated fatty acids such as linoleic acid and gamma-linolenic acid. They are lipid-soluble, are synthesized as required, and act intracellularly in target cells.

MECHANISM OF HORMONE ACTION: SECOND MESSENGER CHEMICALS

Responses to hormonal action involve an amplification of the signal until it is sufficient to produce an effective change in target cell activities. This is necessary because the amount of hormone released is considerably diluted in extracellular fluid and so interactions with target cell receptors are of a relatively low key. This difficulty is overcome by the generation of other 'messenger' chemicals within the cytoplasm of the cell following combination between the hormone molecule and cell receptor.

Peptide hormones and catecholamines interact with membrane receptors of target cells and this interaction activates chemicals which collectively are referred to as second messengers, the hormone itself being the first messenger. There are a number of examples of second messenger depending upon cell type: cyclic adenosine monophosphate (or cyclic-AMP), cyclic guanosine monophosphate (cyclic-GMP), calcium ions (complexed with a protein called calmodulin), and modified membrane lipids (inositol triphosphate in particular).

Second messengers in turn promote the activation of protein kinases present within the cell (Figure 15.4). These are enzymes which activate further enzymes, called phosphorylases because they incorporate phosphate groups into the molecules of yet other enzymes/proteins and activate them. The effect of having numerous stages of chemical activation is that a 'cascade' is produced. Just as the blood clotting cascade produces amplification in the amount of fibrin produced in response to the initial release of small quantities of platelet factor, the second messenger/ protein kinase system results in the activation of large numbers of enzymes following receptor activation. Thus one molecule of the hormone glucagon, which promotes glycogenolysis in liver and skeletal muscle cells, induces the generation of more than 100 molecules of glucose. Hormones are therefore potent substances.

Apart from amplification, a second messenger system also has the advantage that a cell can easily be induced to respond identically to different hormones or stimuli, provided that the different receptors are in place on the cell membrane. Figure 15.5 illustrates the release of glucose from a liver cell by the hormones glucagon (a peptide) and adrenaline (a

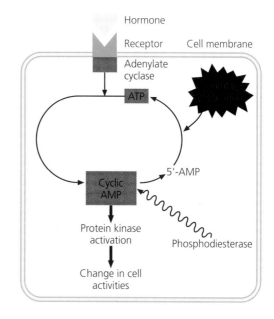

Figure 15.4 Second messenger (= cyclic-AMP) activation following interaction between a peptide or catecholamine hormone and its receptor. Note that the process is dependent upon enzyme activation; the hormone/receptor interaction activates *adenylate cyclase* which converts ATP to cyclic-AMP, which in turn activates *protein kinases*. Responses cease when the hormone is enzymatically removed from the receptor, and/or when cyclic-AMP is catalysed to 5'-AMP by *phosphodiesterase*.

catecholamine). Both hormones promote the mobilization of glucose from glycogen stores, but under different circumstances.

For thyroid hormones the entire membrane receptor/hormone combination is internalized by the cell, and cell activation then results from a very different sequence of events from that observed during activation by peptides and catecholamines. Thus thyroid hormones trigger gene transcription (expression) and so promote enzyme synthesis; it is these enzymes which alter cell activity (Figure 15.6). The principle of amplification, and 'second messengers' still applies, but this mode of action is generally slower than that of peptide hormones and catecholamines.

The mode of cell activation by steroids is similar to that of thyroid hormones, except that receptors to them are actually found within the

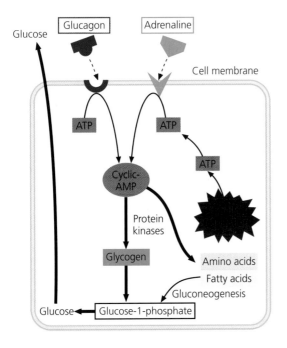

Figure 15.5 Promotion of glycogenolysis and gluconeogenesis by cyclic-AMP, generated in response to receptor activation by the hormones glucagon and adrenaline.

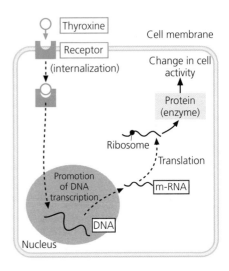

Figure 15.6 Mode of action of thyroid hormones (T_3, T_4). Note that stages will all involve enzyme activation, but result in a promotion of protein synthesis by the cell. Action of steroid hormones is similar, except that the hormone receptor is already internal (the hormone can diffuse across the cell membrane). Compare with cell activation by peptides and catecholamines, shown in Figures 15.4 and 15.5.

cytoplasm of target cells, rather than on the cell membrane, because steroids are lipid-soluble.

To summarize, second messengers and subsequent chemicals provide the means to amplify the stimulus resulting from the interaction between a hormone and its receptor. They also provide the diversity of responses necessary for the maintenance of homeostasis under a variety of circumstances. Enzymatic deactivation of the second messenger, and of the phosphorylated enzymes, and enzymatic separation of the hormone molecule from its receptor result in cessation of the target cell response.

REGULATION OF HORMONE RELEASE: STIMULI AND PRINCIPLES OF CONTROL

Details of stimuli for the release of individual hormones, and the control of that release, are given in the next section. As an introduction, however, it is worthwhile to consider here general aspects of (1) the stimulus required, and (2) the regulation of secretion.

Features of the stimulus

Many hormones have essential roles in the homeostatic regulation of physiological systems. The stimuli for their release therefore relate to a diverse range of parameters, including the composition of body fluids, blood pressure, blood volume, body temperature, and nutrient content of digestive chyme. For example, it was described in Chapter 12 how antidiuretic hormone (ADH) plays a vital role in the maintenance of body water content. It is therefore appropriate that the release of this hormone is in direct response to the increased osmotic pressure of body fluids that occurs when we are dehydrated. As the osmotic pressure is corrected, the stimulus declines and

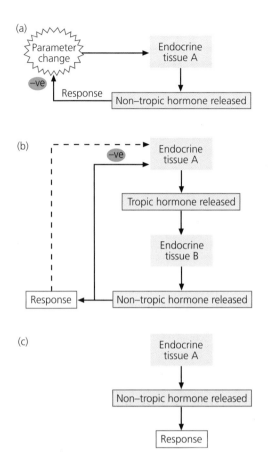

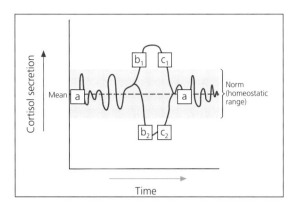

Figure 15.8 Graphic illustration of the homeostatic control of hormone release using cortisol as an example.
a Release of cortisol, within its homeostatic range, appropriate to the needs of the body at a particular time.
b_1 Excessive release (hypersecretion) of cortisol so that plasma concentrations exceed normal values.
b_2 Inadequate release (hyposecretion) of cortisol so that plasma concentrations are lower than normal values.
c_1 Decreased cortisol release as a consequence of negative feedback on the release of corticotropin from the anterior pituitary. Plasma concentration of cortisol declines to within homeostatic range.
c_2 Increased release of cortisol as a consequence of reduced negative feedback on the release of corticotropin from the anterior pituitary. Plasma concentration of cortisol increases to within homeostatic range.

Figure 15.7 (a) Short-loop feedbacks and (b) long-loop feedbacks in the control of hormone secretion. Note that in (b) feedback can arise from the response or from the non-tropic hormone itself. (c) Open-loop system is illustrated in which no negative feedback is evident.

hormone release is reduced accordingly. The amount of ADH released is directly related to the magnitude of the change in osmotic pressure.

In contrast to the role of hormones in the maintenance of a constant environment, some hormones are released in order to induce change relative to the needs of the body at that time. Thus adrenaline has an important role in the heightening of cardiovascular responses during exercise; once the exercise has finished, the release of the hormone declines again. Adrenaline, and others, also induce metabolic change and such hormones will have widespread effects throughout the body.

Principles of control

In the examples given of the actions of antidiuretic hormone during dehydration, and of adrenaline in exercise, removal of the stimulus directly reverses the change in hormone release. This is a simple negative feedback loop, and is called a short loop since there is only one stage to the process (Figure 15.7a).

The number of stages involved in the eventual secretion of some hormones, for example cortisol, utilize a long-loop feedback system. This is frequently observed when the initial stimulus for the release of a non-tropic hormone must act through intermediary tropic hormones (Figure 15.7b). Negative feedback effects of each intermediary ensure that the final release of cortisol is rigorously regulated. Negative feedback principles are illustrated diagrammatically in Figure 15.8 and throughout this book.

In contrast, there are occasions when certain hormones are released which do not appear to have a negative feedback mechanism to control their secretion. For example, growth hormone promotes a variety of metabolic actions, none of which could be envisaged as providing a stimulus to decrease its secretion. This is called an open-loop system (Figure 15.7c), although it might just be the case that the feedback mechanism remains to be discovered!

Details of the homeostatic functions of hormones

Feedback loops and the regulation of the secretory activities of individual endocrine glands are described in detail in the next section. The major known hormones have essential roles in physiological homeostasis. Although hormonal actions are diverse there is a degree of overlapping, and examples have been given throughout this book in which interactions between secretions are important for the overall control of some parameters. For example, blood pressure regulation involves a number of vasoconstrictor hormones of different chemistry and origin. For clarity, though, this section will take a systematic approach and describe the secretions of individual endocrine tissues (Figure 15.9).

The secretion of hormones frequently involves others which directly antagonize or promote (agonize) the process. Where appropriate, this section also highlights how this interaction helps to regulate a particular parameter, or helps control the release of a particular hormone.

THE HYPOTHALAMIC–PITUITARY AXIS

The hypothalamus at the base of the brain, and the pituitary gland attached to it by a 'stalk', form a functional unit. To describe those functions it is convenient to consider the elements separately.

Hypothalamus

This collection of brain 'nuclei' has a diverse range of functions including controlling the 'drives' of human nature: feeding, drinking, and sexual behaviour. It shares some functions with other parts of the brain, particularly with those areas of the limbic system that are responsible for emotion, anxiety and aggression (see Chapter 13). Neurons also project between the hypothalamus and structures of the brainstem, and through these projections the hypothalamus exerts a control on the autonomic nervous system. The hypothalamus, therefore, mediates many of the psychological influences on physical function including those of stress (see Chapter 22).

Another means by which the hypothalamus acts to change physical function is via its influence on the pituitary gland. Although the hypothalamus is comprised of neural tissue, some of its neurons act as endocrine cells, by synthesizing and secreting hormones. Accordingly, these secretions are referred to as neuroendocrine. Most of these hormones are released into small portal blood vessels which form a direct link between the hypothalamus and pituitary (Figure 15.10). The hormones are conveyed to cells within the anterior and intermediate lobes of the pituitary which themselves produce hormones; such hypothalamic hormones are therefore tropic hormones which promote or inhibit the release of secre-

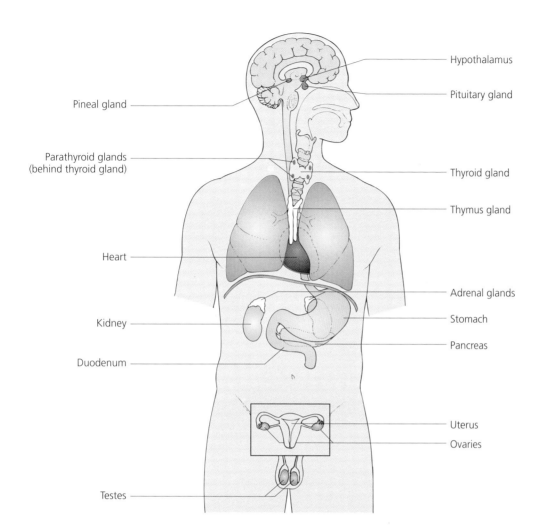

Figure 15.9 Location of major endocrine glands and associated structures.

tions from the anterior and intermediate lobes of the pituitary. According to their actions they are referred to as either releasing or inhibiting hormones, or factors, and are usually named after the pituitary hormone which they influence (see Table 15.1).

Other hypothalamic hormones are actually secreted directly from the posterior lobe of the pituitary, and the secretory 'cells' in this part of the pituitary are really the axon terminals of hypothalamic neurons. The hormone, having been synthesized in the neuronal cell body in the hypothalamus, is transported along the axon to the terminals where it is stored in vesicles ready for release. The posterior lobe of the pituitary therefore consists of neurosecretory tissue and its secretions are considered below.

The secretion of hypothalamic hormones occurs in response to either the stimulation of specific receptor cells within it, or in response to stimulation from higher brain centres. The homeostatic role of hypothalamic secretions, and the control of their release, are considered under the relevant part of the pituitary gland.

Table 15.1 Summary table of the secretions, actions, and regulation of some of the major endocrine glands

Gland	Hormone	Target	Action	Homeostatic regulation
Hypothalamus	*Releasing hormones	Anterior/middle pituitary	Release of various hormones (see text)	Negative feedback from target endocrine secretions. Neural input to hypothalamus
	*Inhibitory hormones	Anterior/middle pituitary	Inhibit release of various hormones (see text)	Unclear. Neural input includes hypothalamus
Anterior pituitary	Corticotropin (ACTH)	Adrenal cortex	Release of glucocorticoids	Negative feedback from glucocorticoids. Hypothalamic regulatory hormones
	Thyrotropin (TSH)	Thyroid follicles	Release of thyroxine	Negative feedback from thyroxine. Hypothalamic regulatory hormones
	Gonadotropins (luteinizing hormone, follicle stimulating hormone)	Gonads	Oestrogens and progestins (female). Testosterone (male)	Negative feedback from gonadal hormones
	†Growth hormone (somatotropin)	Various tissues	Metabolic (see text)	Unclear. Hypothalamic regulatory hormones
	Prolactin	Breast.	Lactation (role in male unclear)	Unclear. Hypothalamic regulatory hormones
	†Melanocyte-stimulating hormone (MSH)	Skin melanocytes	Promotes melanin synthesis	Unclear. Hypothalamic regulatory hormones
Posterior pituitary	Vasopressin (antidiuretic hormone)	Kidney and arterioles	Water retention, vasoconstriction (BP regulation)	Negative feedback from plasma osmotic pressure, and from arterial blood pressure
	Oxytocin	Breast and uterus	Lactation. Labour (role in male unclear)	Negative feedback after suckling. Positive feedback from uterus in labour
Thyroid	Thyroxine (T_4)	Various tissues	Metabolic, especially role in basal metabolism	Hypothalamic regulatory hormones, thyrotropin from pituitary
	Calcitonin	Bone	Promote calcium deposition	Negative feedback from plasma calcium concentration
Parathyroid	Parathyroid hormone (PTH)	Bone, kidney	Promote calcium resorption from bone, activation of vitamin D in kidney	Negative feedback from plasma calcium concentration

Table 15.1 (Continued)

Gland	Hormone	Target	Action	Homeostatic regulation
Adrenal cortex	Glucocorticoids (e.g. cortisol)	Various tissues	Metabolic, permissive influence on other hormones	*Hypothalamic regulatory hormones, corticotropin from pituitary
	Mineralocorticoids (e.g. aldosterone)	Kidney	Promote sodium reabsorption and potassium excretion	Negative feedback from effects on blood volume and plasma potassium concentration
Adrenal medulla	Catecholamines (adrenaline, noradrenaline)	Heart and circulation, also various other tissues (see text)	Promote cardiac function, vasoconstriction (BP regulation)	Sympathetic nervous system activity
Duodenum	Secretin CCK-PZ	Digestive glands, gall bladder, pancreas, stomach	Promote secretion of pancreatic enzymes, bile and regulate gastric emptying	Presence of food products in the duodenum
Pancreas	Insulin (B-cells)	Liver, skeletal muscle	Promote glucose utilization (hypoglycaemic agent)	Negative feedback from blood glucose concentration, plus others (see text)
	Glucagon (A-cells)	Liver, skeletal muscle	Promote glucose mobilization (hypoglycaemic agent)	Negative feedback from blood glucose concentration, plus others (see text)
	Somatostatin (D-cells)	A- and B-cells of pancreas	Modulate release of insulin and glucagon	Presence of insulin or glucagon
Gonads Ovaries	Oestrogens (e.g. oestriol). Progestins (e.g. progesterone)	Reproductive tract, breast + secondary sexual characters	Regulation of menstrual cycle. Behaviour	Hypothalamic hormones, plus gonadotropins from pituitary
Testes	Androgens (e.g. testosterone)	Reproductive tract + secondary sexual characters	Regulation of spermatogenesis and accessory glands of reproductive tract. Behaviour	Hypothalamic hormones, plus gonadotropins from pituitary

*Hypothalamic regulatory hormones include releasing and inhibitory hormones.
†Also produced in middle lobe of the pituitary gland.

The pituitary gland (or hypophysis)

The pituitary is of mixed embryological origin: the anterior part is formed from an upgrowth of the oral cavity of the embryo, whilst the posterior part is a downgrowth from the overlying brain. This helps to explain how the anterior lobe is comprised of non-neuronal secretory cells, whilst the posterior lobe is

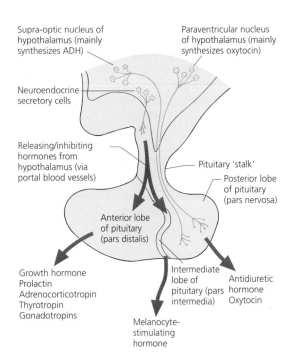

Supra-optic nucleus of
hypothalamus (mainly
synthesizes ADH)

Paraventricular nucleus
of hypothalamus (mainly
synthesizes oxytocin)

Neuroendocrine
secretory cells

Releasing/inhibiting
hormones from
hypothalamus (via
portal blood vessels)

Pituitary 'stalk'

Posterior lobe
of pituitary
(pars nervosa)

Anterior lobe
of pituitary
(pars distalis)

Growth hormone
Prolactin
Adrenocorticotropin
Thyrotropin
Gonadotropins

Intermediate
lobe of
pituitary (pars
intermedia)

Antidiuretic
hormone
Oxytocin

Melanocyte-
stimulating
hormone

Figure 15.10 The hypothalamic–pituitary axis and the main
secretions.

comprised of axon terminals from hypothalamic neurons (plus supporting cells).

Anterior lobe (or adenohypophysis)

Most of the anterior lobe of the pituitary consists of that part called the pars distalis. The pars intermedia is a small piece of tissue which lies between the pars distalis and the posterior lobe of the gland (Figure 15.10). Most hormones of the anterior lobe are secreted from the pars distalis. They are all peptides and most are tropic secretions which influence a variety of other endocrine tissues in the body; for this reason the anterior lobe has been called the 'master' gland.

The anterior lobe produces a number of hormones which are identified, together with their main actions, in Table 15.1. To maintain an appropriate rate of hormone release that is adequate to sustain homeostasis, most secretory cells are subject to negative feedback inhibition from the secretions of their target endocrine tissues (details are given when the individual target glands are discussed). This places a high degree of control on the pituitary gland, and reflects the potency of the actions of secretions from it.

Most anterior lobe hormones are released in response to the presence of hypothalamic releasing factors. Some, namely the peptides growth hormone, melanocyte-stimulating hormone (MSH) and prolactin, are primarily controlled by hypothalamic inhibitory factors, although releasing hormones are also present. Why the control should be different for these hormones is unclear. One suggestion is that their actions do not alter parameters that are easily monitored. Growth hormone has widespread metabolic effects: it promotes lipolysis, glycogenesis, protein synthesis, and cartilage production, and is essential for childhood growth, and for sustaining tissue function in adults (another name for growth hormone is somatotrophin; soma = body; troph = nutrition). MSH (which is the main secretion of the pars intermedia) promotes pigmentation of skin melanocytes. Prolactin promotes milk production during lactation.

In other words it is suggested that these three hormones operate via an 'open-loop' secretion and their secretion is continuously inhibited unless the hypothalamus reduces the secretion of inhibiting factor. This is in contrast to pituitary hormones controlled by hypothalamic releasing factors as these will stimulate the pituitary unless they themselves are inhibited via negative feedback.

This view may be simplistic, however. For example, some of the actions of growth hormone are mediated by secretions from the liver called somatomedins. It is feasible that these and other as yet unknown substances could provide a negative feedback signal.

Posterior lobe (or neurohypophysis)

The posterior lobe of the pituitary, sometimes called the pars nervosa, secretes two hormones

– vasopressin and oxytocin. Axon terminals contain vesicles of just one hormone and the cell bodies of the different neurons lie primarily in different parts of the hypothalamus (Figure 15.10). The hormones have very different actions. Vasopressin is involved in the control of blood pressure, via its vasoconstrictor actions, and water balance via its retentive actions in the kidney (hence its alternative name antidiuretic hormone; ADH) whereas oxytocin is involved in labour and lactation. Some studies indicate that oxytocin may also be involved in regulating fluid balance, perhaps by acting with vasopressin. Though debatable, such actions could help to explain the presence of oxytocin in males!

Vasopressin is released following the stimulation of osmoreceptors in the hypothalamus (responding to the effects of dehydration), or of arterial baroreceptors (responding to hypotension). Correction of the changed parameter removes the stimulus and provides the negative feedback which causes secretion to decline. Oxytocin is reflexly released during labour (when positive feedback operates – see Chapter 19) and during suckling. In the latter case its release declines when the baby stops feeding, another negative feedback response.

THE THYROID GLAND

The thyroid gland has four lobes which straddle the lower end of the trachea. It secretes two very similar substances called tri-iodothyronine and tetra-iodothyronine (abbreviated T_3 and T_4 respectively), and also a peptide hormone called calcitonin.

T_3 and T_4

These are modified amines, derived from the amino acid tyrosine (Figures 15.2 and 15.11b). Their names reflect the number of iodine atoms that are incorporated into each hormone molecule. They are released together and have similar actions although T_4 is the main secretion and is commonly called thyroxine.

Incorporation of iodine into the molecules of thyroid hormones is one of the main reasons why iodine must be included in our diet. The iodide ion is actively taken up by the gland and initially incorporated into tyrosine residues attached to a protein called thyroglobulin, which is stored in extracellular spaces within the lobules of the gland (Figure 15.11a,b). The uptake of administered radioisotopic iodine is a clinically useful means of monitoring thyroid function, and is also detectable following accidental exposure to emissions from nuclear explosion.

When required, T_3 and T_4 are generated from thyroglobulin and released into the blood. Release is promoted by thyroid-stimulating hormone (TSH; increasingly known as thyrotropin) from the anterior pituitary gland, which in turn is released in response to TSH-releasing hormone from the hypothalamus (Figure 15.11c). Both thyroxine and TSH have negative feedback actions and there is, therefore, a tight control on thyroid hormone release (using both short- and long-loop feedbacks). The need for this is clear when one considers that the main function of thyroxine is to determine basal metabolic rate.

Calcitonin

Calcitonin is secreted by diffuse groups of cells within the thyroid gland (Figure 15.11a). Its main role is to promote the uptake of calcium ions by bone cells when plasma calcium concentration is elevated. As the concentration declines, the release of calcitonin is reduced (i.e. a short-loop negative feedback). Plasma calcium concentration is determined by the balance between calcitonin release, vitamin D activation, which promotes calcium uptake from the gut, and the release of parathyroid hormone, which promotes the release of calcium from bone. The interactions are summarized in Figure 15.12.

THE PARATHYROID GLANDS

The parathyroid glands are four small areas of tissue found on the posterior surface of the

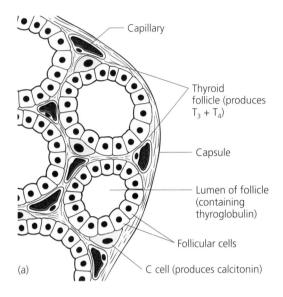

(a)

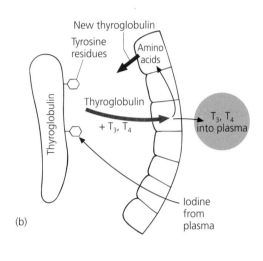

(b)

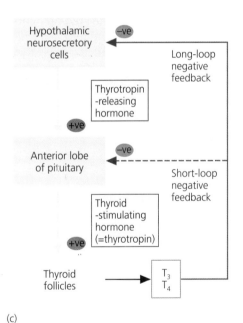

(c)

Figure 15.11 (a) The thyroid gland. (b) The synthesis of T_3 and T_4 from iodine/tyrosine, and thyroglobulin. (c) The feedback control of T_3 and T_4 secretion.

lobes of the thyroid. They secrete the peptide parathyroid hormone (abbreviated PTH). This hormone is released when plasma calcium ion concentration is below its homeostatic range, and stimulates bone resorption accordingly (Figure 15.12). It also promotes activation of vitamin D, which is now recognized to be a

hormone, and this increases calcium absorption from the gut. Thus, by directly stimulating the release of calcium from bone and indirectly enhancing the absorption of calcium from the gut, PTH rapidly corrects any deficiency in calcium concentration. Its release is inhibited as the calcium concentration begins to rise

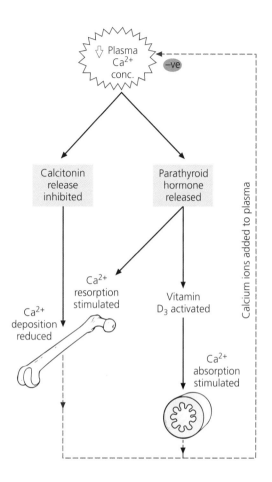

Figure 15.12 Hormonal responses to a decreased ionized calcium concentration in plasma. Note that the calcium concentration is largely a balance between calcium deposition in, or resorption from, bone, and uptake from the gut. The latter must also compensate for urinary losses.

above its homeostatic range; there is a short-loop feedback via the calcium concentration.

THE ADRENAL GLANDS

As their name suggests, the adrenal glands lie adjacent to the kidneys. In fact they lie on top of them, hence their alternate name – suprarenal glands. Each can be subdivided into

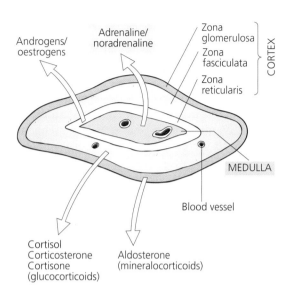

Figure 15.13 Cross-section through an adrenal gland to illustrate cortical zones, medulla, and associated hormones.

the cortex (outer) and medulla (inner) areas; cortical cells secrete steroid hormones, medullary cells secrete catecholamine hormones (Figure 15.13).

The adrenal cortex

The cortex secretes a range of steroids which collectively can be divided into the glucocorticoids, with gluconeogenic actions, and the mineralocorticoids, with effects on the electrolyte composition of plasma. The sex steroids (androgens/oestrogens) are also synthesized but amounts are small when compared with gonadal steroid production.

Glucocorticoids

Glucocorticoids are produced by the outer layers of the cortex, called the zona reticularis and zona fasciculata (see Figure 15.13). There are a number of these steroids, with similar molecular structure and actions. The two main ones are cortisol and corticosterone and these hormones have a variety of actions. In particular they promote protein catabolism in skeletal muscle, the synthesis of glucose (from the released amino acids) and glycogenesis (from the synthesized glucose) in the liver. They therefore have a role in the maintenance of glycogen. The hormones also mobilize free fatty acids from adipose tissue, and inhibit the uptake of glucose by many tissues. The net effect is to increase plasma glucose and free fatty acid concentrations.

Glucocorticoids also exert 'permissive' effects on the activities of other tissues and on the actions of other hormones. Other effects are to stimulate red blood cell production, and to reduce inflammation. Clearly they have wide ranging effects on the body and it is perhaps not surprising that they are released when the body is under stress, including during surgical trauma. They have been called the 'hormones of stress' and our capacity to cope with demands is markedly reduced in their absence (Chapter 22).

The release of glucocorticoids is stimulated by adrenocorticotropic hormone (ACTH; increasingly called corticotropin) from the anterior pituitary gland (Figure 15.14). This in turn is released in response to the secretion of corticotropin-releasing hormone from the hypothalamus. The glucocorticoids exert an inhibition on the release of both hormones via short- and long-loop feedbacks and therefore provide a high degree of control.

Mineralocorticoids

Mineralocorticoids are steroids secreted by cells of the zona glomerularis of the adrenal cortex (Figure 15.13). The main one is called aldosterone, the release of which is stimulated by sodium deficiency and by an increased plasma potassium concentration. It has an important role in the maintenance of sodium (and hence water) and potassium balance. Its main action is on the kidney where it stimulates sodium uptake in exchange for potassium or hydrogen ions, thus conserving sodium but increasing the excretion of potassium/hydrogen ions. It also promotes sodium reabsorption from sweat and

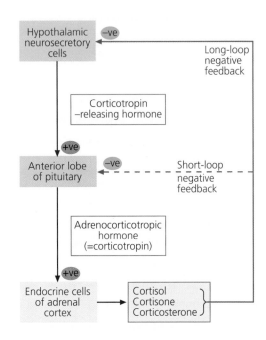

Figure 15.14 Glucocorticoid release and its feedback control.

saliva, and stimulates sodium absorption from the gut.

The effects of sodium deficiency on aldosterone release are mediated by the hormone angiotensin (Figure 15.15). This peptide hormone is produced from a precursor (angiotensinogen) found in plasma, although final activation is produced by the actions of angiotensin converting enzyme as blood passes through the lungs. The initial conversion of angiotensinogen is induced by the enzyme renin, released from cells close to the renal glomeruli (in the juxtaglomerular apparatus) during sodium deficiency. The complex link between these hormones is referred to as the renin–angiotensin–aldosterone axis. The axis has a role in blood pressure control (see Chapter 9). Reversal of the disturbance causes the activation of angiotensin to decline, leading to reduced aldosterone secretion (i.e. a long-loop feedback mechanism).

The stimulation of aldosterone release when plasma potassium concentration is elevated is

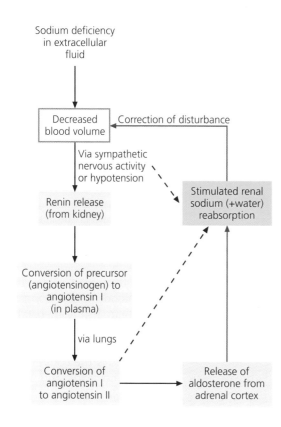

Figure 15.15 The renin–angiotensin–aldosterone axis and the regulation of sodium balance. Note that aldosterone is only one of the components to influence renal function.

reversed by a short-loop feedback control when the actions of the hormone correct the disturbance. Whereas a number of hormones influence sodium excretion (Chapter 12), aldosterone is the only one known to have a major influence on potassium balance.

Sex corticoids (androgens/oestrogens)

The secretion of these hormones by the adrenal gland is slight when compared with that from the gonads. Their actions in adulthood are probably of little consequence but they have important influences on fetal development, and on prepubertal growth during childhood. The release of adrenal androgens can, however, induce facial hair growth and voice deepening in post-menopausal women.

The adrenal medulla

The adrenal medulla secretes the catecholamine hormones adrenaline (epinephrine) and noradrenaline (norepinephrine); adrenaline is the main secretion. These hormones are synthesized and released by cells which are neuronal in embryological origin, and which are the equivalent of post-ganglionic nerve cells of the sympathetic nervous system (see Chapter 13).

The hormones are released when sympathetic nerves to the adrenal glands are activated, and their actions support the activities of this branch of the autonomic nervous system. Particular effects are to promote cardiac function, induce selective vasoconstriction and vasodilatation, increase sweating, reduce salivation, induce bronchodilatation, decrease gut motility, and mobilize glucose and fatty acids. All these actions equip the body for physical activity. Sympathetic stimulation is usually transient, and its activity declines once the demand for activity has passed. Hormone release is then reduced. Sympathetic activity, and catecholamine secretion, may be sustained in severe distress, however, as a consequence of the limbic/hypothalamic modulation of autonomic nuclei in the brainstem (Chapter 22).

THE GONADS

The testes and ovaries produce steroid and peptide hormones, steroids being the major ones. The steroids produced by males are collectively called androgens, the main one being testosterone. Females produce oestrogens, the main ones being oestriol, oestradiol, and oestrone, and also progestins, the main one being progesterone. These steroids are essential for the regulation of the female menstrual cycle, and breast development, and for spermatogenesis and sperm capacitation in males (Chapter 18). The testes also produce the peptide inhibin which, though poorly understood, seems to modulate spermatogenesis.

Control of hormone release is via the gonadotropic hormones of the anterior pituitary – follicle-stimulating hormone and luteinizing hormone. These are named after their effects in the female, but are chemically identical in both sexes. They are released in response to the presence of hypothalamic gonadotropin-releasing hormone. Regulation is exerted by negative feedback effects of the gonadal steroids on the hypothalamus and pituitary (i.e. short- and long-loop feedbacks) and is described in more detail in Chapter 18.

THE GUT AND PANCREAS

The gut

The gut produces a wide variety of hormones which mediate digestive functions. The main hormones are the peptides gastrin, secretin and cholecystokinin-pancreozymin (abbreviated CCK-PZ). Gastrin is mainly produced in the stomach, and the other two in the duodenum.

Gastrin release is stimulated by the presence of food in the stomach and has a role in gastric acid secretion. Gastrin also stimulates gastric motility to mix the chyme, and the emptying of gastric contents into the duodenum. Its release is inhibited, however, if the acidity of the chyme becomes intense.

Secretin is of historical interest because it was the first hormone identified, and the term 'hormone' was coined after its discovery. It is secreted by duodenal mucosal cells in response to the presence of acid in the duodenal chyme and acts to neutralize, and then alkalinize, the chyme by stimulating the secretion of a bicarbonate-rich fluid from the pancreas. As the

acidity falls, the release of secretin declines (i.e. a short-loop feedback).

CCK-PZ is released from duodenal mucosal cells in response to the presence of chyme and promotes the secretion of digestive enzymes by the pancreas. It also has other actions in relation to fat digestion in that it promotes the release of bile from the gall bladder and reduces gastric emptying, which increases the time that chyme remains in the duodenum.

The pancreas

The endocrine tissue of the pancreas is found as discrete clusters of cells, called the islets of Langerhans, which produce the peptide hormones insulin, glucagon, and somatostatin (Table 15.2).

Insulin release from the B- or beta-cells of the islets is promoted when blood glucose concentration is elevated beyond its homeostatic range, and acts to stimulate the uptake of glucose by liver and skeletal muscle cells. Glycogenesis is promoted, as is the conversion of glucose into certain amino acids and fatty acids, and these actions maintain intracellular glucose homeostasis. Insulin release decreases as plasma glucose concentration declines. Insulin is the only known hormone which reduces blood glucose concentration.

Insulin release is also stimulated by the presence of the duodenal hormone gastric-inhibitory peptide (GIP), released in response to the presence of monosaccharides in the digestive chyme. Its effect on insulin release is seen as being anticipatory of a glucose load entering the circulatory system.

Glucagon release from the A- or alpha-cells is stimulated by a decrease in the glucose concentration of plasma below its homeostatic range, and also by insulin itself. Its actions are the opposite of those of insulin, promoting the mobilization of glucose by glycogenolysis and gluconeogenesis. Glucagon release declines as the plasma glucose concentration increases.

Somatostatin release from the D- or delta-cells is stimulated by both glucagon and insulin. Its actions are not fully understood but

Table 15.2 Factors which influence the release of the pancreatic hormones (a) insulin and (b) glucagon

Excitatory influences	Homeostatic relevance	Inhibitory influences	Homeostatic relevance
(a) Insulin			
Direct influence of elevated blood glucose concentration	Increased glucose utilization after food intake. Promotes glycogenesis	Blood glucose deficit	Reduction of glycogenesis, leaving more glucose available for cellular respiration
Increased parasympathetic nervous activity from hypothalamus to pancreatic B-cells (in response to elevated blood glucose)	Increased glucose utilization after food intake. Promotes glycogenesis	Increased sympathetic nervous activity from hypothalamus to pancreatic B-cells (in response to stress or exercise)	Reduction of glycogenesis, leaving more glucose available for cellular respiration
Duodenal hormones (e.g. CCK-PZ) in response to glucose present in digestive chyme	Feed-forward release of insulin in preparation for glucose load from gut	Somatostatin (released by direct stimulation of pancreatic D-cells by insulin)	Fine control of insulin release in presence of stimulatory factors
(b) Glucagon			
Direct influence of blood glucose deficit	Promotion of glycogenolysis and gluconeogenesis to provide glucose for cellular respiration	Direct influence of elevated blood glucose concentration	Decreased glycogenolysis/ gluconeogenesis. Increased glucose utilization (via promotion of insulin release)
Increased parasympathetic nervous activity from hypothalamus to pancreatic A-cells (in response to blood glucose deficit)	Promotion of glycogenolysis and gluconeogenesis to provide glucose for cellular respiration	Somatostatin (released by direct stimulus of pancreatic D-cells by glucagon)	Fine control of glucagon release in presence of stimulatory influences

it seems to act as a paracrine secretion and modulates the release of the other two hormones, thus preventing excessive secretion.

The interaction between these three hormones in relation to the regulation of blood glucose concentration is illustrated graphically in Figure 15.16.

THE THYMUS GLAND

The thymus is a lymphoid gland found in the neck which has an important role in the differentiation of T-lymphocytes in immune responses. Differentiation is incompletely understood but is promoted by peptide hormones, released from the thymus, called thymin, thymosin, and thymopoietin. The mechanism of their control is unknown.

THE PINEAL GLAND

The pineal is an outgrowth of neural tissue situated in the roof of the third cerebral ventricle, deep within the brain. Its main secretion is the peptide melatonin. Documented actions of this hormone include the induction of sleep. It also prevents ovulation via an inhibition of the release of gonadotropin-releasing hormone from the hypothalamus (its overproduction can delay puberty). Links with the human menstrual cycle have not been established, however.

There is some evidence that melatonin influences the secretion of other pituitary hormones, and the rich innervation of the pineal by sympathetic neurons would seem to suggest further roles. One role, though not directly endocrine, is that of a mediator of circadian rhythms. The gland receives impulses from the eyes and is postulated to be involved in the light/dark synchronization of the rhythmicity observed for some physiological parameters, presumably via its neural links with the hypothalamus and thence the pituitary gland.

The gland is also of interest for other reasons. It has for many years been postulated to be the 'spiritual' centre of the brain, conveying conscience as a human faculty. There is no evidence for this, however, although it could also be argued that 'conscience' is an indeterminate faculty!

OTHER HORMONES

Various other hormonal secretions have been identified, and the numbers continue to grow. Many are secreted by cells which do not form identifiable glands. Rather they are cells which

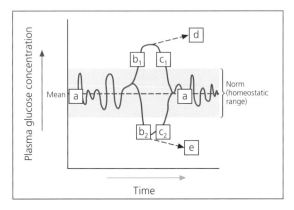

Figure 15.16 Homeostatic regulation of plasma glucose concentration by insulin and glucagon.
a Fluctuations of plasma glucose concentration within the homeostatic range. Release of insulin and glucagon is basal, perhaps as a consequence of the actions of somatostatin.
b_1 Elevated plasma glucose concentration following a carbohydrate meal, *or* after mobilization of glucose from stores.
b_2 Declining plasma glucose concentration as a consequence of fasting, *or* elevated utilization.
c_1 Restoration of glucose concentration to the homeostatic range as a consequence of increased glucose utilization including transfer into stores. These actions are promoted by the release of insulin and inhibition of glucagon secretion.
c_2 Restoration of glucose concentration to the homeostatic range as a consequence of glucose mobilization from stores or by glucose synthesis. These actions are promoted by glucagon.
d Persistent elevation of plasma glucose concentration as a consequence of inadequate utilization (failure to release insulin, or of its actions) leading to hyperglycaemia and the mobilization of fatty acids and amino acids for energy (as in diabetes mellitus).
e Persistent reduction of glucose concentration as a consequence of reduced intake of carbohydrate (as in starvation) leading to hypoglycaemia and mobilization of fatty acids and amino acids for energy.

have roles other than that of being secretory, and this function of such cells may only recently have been identified. In addition to those substances now accepted as being hormones, a host of others are putative ones. A comprehensive list of all these secretions is not possible, but some of those recognized as hormones are given below.

Atrial natriuretic factor is a peptide hormone that originates from cells lining the atria of the heart (particularly the right atrium) and was identified as recently as the early 1980s. The hormone is named because of its actions to increase renal sodium excretion (directly and via an inhibition of aldosterone release), but it also has an important role in promoting vasodilatation, particularly of veins. It is released when an increase in blood volume stretches the atrial wall. Although this could occur transiently, for example when venous return is increased during exercise, the main role of the hormone is probably in the longer term regulation of blood volume. Its vasodilatory actions help the circulatory system to accommodate any increase in volume (and therefore avoid arterial hypertension) whilst the renal actions help to reduce blood volume (by excreting sodium chloride and water).

Prostaglandins are local hormones, and were named after they were first identified as prostatic secretions in seminal fluid. They are paracrine secretions produced by most, if not all, body tissues, and probably only influence cells in the vicinity of their secretion. There are various kinds of prostaglandin (E_2, F_{2alpha}, being the main ones) and their role varies with the tissue. For example, prostaglandins help to maintain blood flow to tissues such as the stomach, they influence transport mechanisms in the kidney, they contract the cervix after coitus, and the uterus during birth, and they are pain-producing substances when tissues are damaged (Chapter 21). They act either directly or by modulating the actions of other hormones.

Erythropoietin is a hormone produced by conversion of a precursor (erythropoietinogen) in plasma by the enzyme erythrogenin, released from the kidney when blood perfusing the organ is deficient in oxygen. The hormone promotes red blood cell production by bone marrow (Chapter 8).

Endothelium-derived relaxing factor (EDRF) is a substance produced by capillary endothelial cells and has an important role in the intrinsic regulation of vascular resistance in tissues. Its actions are to stimulate the production of nitrous oxide by the cells, and this in turn causes vasodilatation.

A host of peptide growth factors have been identified, for example epidermal growth factor. Although these promote mitosis in tissues, their precise role and the control of their secretion are unknown.

Examples of homeostatic control system failures and principles of correction

In view of the essential role of hormones in the coordination of physiological function, it is not surprising that failure of the homeostatic control of hormone release can have pronounced effects on the health of an individual. The number of hormonal disorders is very large, and new research into, for example, the role of nitrous oxide in mediating the actions of endothelium-derived relaxing factor in hypertension, suggests that the range is likely to increase further. Some of the major disorders are identified in Table 15.3.

Causes of hormonal disorders can arise from excessive or inadequate secretion, illustrated in Figure 15.17. Alternatively they may arise from an inadequate response of target tissues to what could be normal or even elevated plasma concentrations of the hormone.

ALTERED SECRETION

Disturbances of hormonal secretion can result in either (1) an excessive release of hormone

Table 15.3 Homeostatic disturbance as a consequence of inappropriate secretion of selected hormones

Hormone	Hyposecretion	Hypersecretion
Growth hormone	In children, retards growth (pituitary dwarfism)	In children, promotes growth (pituitary gigantism). In adults promotes growth of selective tissues (acromegaly)
Vasopressin (ADH)	Dehydration (diabetes insipidus)	Overhydration, hypo-osmolality. Hypervolaemia (syndrome of inappropriate ADH)
Thyroxine	In childre, reduced mental development (cretinism) and dwarfism. In adults, facial oedema, slow heart rate, low body temperature, lethargy (myxoedema)	High metabolic rate, tachycardia, weight loss, insomnia, nervous tremors, oedema behind the eye (e.g. Graves' disease – exophthalamic goitre)
Parathyroid hormone	Decreased plasma calcium concentration leading to increased neural excitability (leading to tetany)	Demineralization of bone
Insulin	Elevated blood glucose leading to polyuria, glucosuria and circulatory disorder. Excessive fat/protein metabolism (diabetes mellitus)	Decreased blood glucose leading to overstimulation of sympathetic nervous system. Hypoglycaemic coma due to brain cell dysfunction
Cortisol	Decreased blood glucose concentration leading to lethargy and muscle weakness. Low blood pressure (Cushing's syndrome)	Redistribution of fat (e.g. 'moon face' and 'buffalo hump'). Excessive oedema including ascites). Bruising, poor wound healing (Addison's disease)
Aldosterone	Elevated plasma potassium concentration leading to disorder of nerve/muscle function.	Decreased plasma potassium concentration leading to disorder of nerve/muscle function. Sodium retention (aldosteronism)

(called hypersecretion) or (2) an undersecretion of hormone (called hyposecretion).

Hypersecretion

Hormones induce a response which changes a parameter within a physiological system (that parameter could of course be another hormone). The change in parameter value usually provides the feedback necessary to regulate hormonal release. Hypersecretion commonly results from a failure of the feedback mechanism. For example, the feedback controls of cortisol and thyroxine release depend upon their effects to inhibit the secretion of those hypothalamic and pituitary hormones necessary for their release. Failure of

the hypothalamus or pituitary to respond will result in a persistent release of the hormone and this is a common cause of excessive cortisol release (Cushing's syndrome) and thyroxine release (Grave's disease).

The feedback failure usually results from a lack of receptors on the cells, but what makes these receptors decline is unclear. Autoimmune responses are thought to be a frequent cause, and immune responses also appear to be responsible for the enlargement of the thyroid gland (called a goitre) that is observed in hyperthyroidism.

Gland hypertrophy, and overactivity of its cells, is also seen when there is a tumour present as tumour cells may 'escape' negative feedback processes. Alternatively, elevated

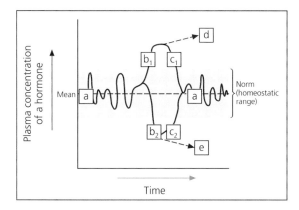

Figure 15.17 The homeostatic control of hormone concentration, and its failure.
a Plasma concentration of hormone fluctuating within its basal range, sufficient to maintain basal functions.
b_1 Elevated hormone concentration as a consequence of stimulated release, or a mismatch between hormonal secretion, metabolism, and excretion.
b_2 Decreased hormone concentration as a consequence of a mismatch between hormonal secretion, metabolism, and excretion.
c_1 Return of hormone concentration to homeostatic range via negative feedback, leading to decreased secretion.
c_2 Return of hormone concentration to homeostatic range via diminished negative feedback, leading to increased secretion.
d Persistently elevated hormone concentration due either to hypersecretion by the gland or to inadequate metabolism and/or excretion (for example in liver or kidney disease).
e Persistently decreased hormone concentration due to hyposecretion by the gland, as a consequence of inadequate hormone synthesis or inadequate release as in insulin-dependent diabetes mellitus and hypothyroidism.

plasma concentrations of a hormone might reflect non-glandular secretion of the hormone. Thus the actual gland might continue to be closely regulated via a negative feedback, but tumours elsewhere, which do not have the appropriate receptors and are unresponsive to feedback control, could produce the hormone even when this is inappropriate. In this case the necessary genes are expressed by the tumour cells and induce synthesis of the appropriate cellular enzymes (remember that differentiation of cell type depends upon which genes within the genome are activated).

Principles of correction relate to either reducing the release of the hormone or to antagonism of its actions. The latter is generally unsuccessful as a long-term control, and surgical ablation of glandular tissue is usually used, if it is feasible.

Gland ablation is not without problems, however. The major endocrine glands secrete more than one hormone and so contain cells of different secretory function. Thus, ablation of gland tissue to remove, for example, thyroid follicle cells, will also remove tissue which secretes calcitonin and parathyroid hormone, and may therefore induce disorders of calcium metabolism.

Hyposecretion

Inadequate secretion of hormone can have a number of causes. First, the glandular cells may lack receptors and so fail to respond to the activating stimulus. For example, Hashimoto's disease, a form of hypothyroidism, results from an inability of the thyroid follicle cells to respond to thyrotropin from the pituitary gland. The cause of receptor loss is unclear, but commonly seems to be associated with autoimmune responses, or the consequences of ageing.

Hyposecretion might also reflect an inability of glandular cells to synthesize the hormone, as in insulin-dependent (or early onset, or juvenile) diabetes mellitus. Lack of synthesis usually results from genetic mutation and may be inherited, congenital, or arise from the effect of ageing.

Another cause of inadequate synthesis is a deficiency, usually dietary, of the precursor molecule. For example, a lack of iodine in the diet can cause thyroxine deficiency, and goitre as the gland 'attempts' a corrective response. Dietary deficiencies as causes of hormonal disorder are rare in Western societies however.

The principles of correcting a hyposecretory disorder is either to promote release of the hormone using drugs, or to administer the hormone or an agonistic analogue.

LACK OF TARGET TISSUE RESPONSE

Inadequate target response might alter the secretion rate of a hormone if that target cell was glandular, as outlined above. This section is more concerned with non-glandular target tissues.

Inadequate target tissue response might result from a lack of receptors to a hormone as this prevents the tissue from 'recognizing' the hormone when it is present. Examples are the disturbance of water homeostasis called diabetes insipidus, in which the collecting duct cells of the kidney do not respond to vasopressin, and that of glucose metabolism called insulin-independent (or maturity-onset) diabetes mellitus, in which tissues either do not respond to insulin or there is hyposecretion of the hormone.

Clinical intervention is directed at either using alternative means to control the parameter which the hormone regulates (e.g. controlling the dietary intake of glucose in insulin-independent diabetes mellitus) or pharmacologically enhancing tissue function (e.g. the use of metabolism-promoting drugs in diabetes mellitus).

Finally, it might be that target cells fail to respond to a hormone because of an underlying disorder of the tissue itself. This would not be considered as an endocrine disorder, although improving hormonal actions might be part of the treatment.

Summary

1 Hormones are chemical 'messengers' which provide a means of communication between tissues in different parts of the body, and therefore are part of the coordinating mechanisms of the body.

2 The process of hormone synthesis/release, transportation in extracellular fluid and interaction with target cells means that responses are slower when compared with those of nerve stimulation, and so hormones are generally not involved in responses which must occur rapidly, i.e. within seconds.

3 Hormones are secreted by glands, though not all glandular secretions can be considered to be hormones. Hormone-secreting glands are generally referred to as endocrine glands.

4 Hormones are able to produce a large response by target cells because the cell activation is amplified through the 'cascade' effect of 'second messenger' activation (hormones are the first messenger chemical).

5 Many hormones are tropic, that is they promote the release of further hormones from target gland tissue. Others are released in response to non-hormonal stimuli, and promote a change in those parameters.

6 Hormone release is usually controlled by negative feedback mechanisms.

7 Hormones are either peptides, catecholamines (modified amino acid), steroids (modified lipid), or prostaglandins (modified fatty acid). Their diverse actions help to regulate the range of physiological parameters vital for health.

8 Disorders of hormone function arise from a failure to control hormonal secretion, or from a lack of response of target tissues to the hormone after it is released. Clinical intervention is directed at correcting the secretory defect, at replacing the hormone (if it is deficient in blood), at preventing/promoting hormone action with appropriate antagonistic/agonistic drugs, or stimulating tissue function by other pharmacological means.

Review Questions

1 Distinguish between endocrine, exocrine and mixed glandular tissues.

2 Explain how the hypothalamus controls the actions of the pituitary gland.

3 Why is the pituitary referred to as the 'master' gland?

4 Distinguish between tropic and non-tropic hormones.

5 Identify the site of action of local and systemic hormones, giving appropriate examples of each.

6 List six types of endocrines secreted by the anterior pituitary gland.

7 Give examples of the following:
(a) peptide hormone; (b) steroidal hormone; (c) amine hormone.

8 Discuss the mechanism of hormonal action at the target cell level.

9 How does the structure and function of the posterior pituitary differ from that of the anterior pituitary?

10 Using the following terms discuss negative feedback principles:
thyroid-stimulating hormone releasing factor (TSHRF); thyroid-stimulating hormone (TSH); thyroxine; hypothalamus; anterior pituitary gland; thyroid gland; negative feedback, high levels; normal levels and low levels.

11 Describe the locations of the thyroid, parathyroid, and adrenal glands.

12 Describe the importance of iodine in the diet for the manufacture of thyroxine.

13 Discuss the importance of parathyroid hormone (PTH) and calcitonin in the homeostatic regulation of calcium in the blood.

14 Describe the mechanisms which control the release of adrenal medullary and adrenal cortical hormones.

15 Name the hormones released from the adrenal glands and give the primary function of each hormone.

16 The pancreas is an example of a mixed gland. Name the secretions from its endocrine and exocrine tissues.

17 The pineal gland releases a hormone in the dark phase of the day/night period. Name the hormone and its function associated with this phase.

18 List the functions of atrial-natriuretic factor and prostaglandins.

19 Endocrine homeostatic imbalances are due to an overactive or an underactive gland, discuss in general terms what are the possible aetiological factors associated with each condition.

20 Discuss in general the underlying principles of correction of hypersecretory and hyposecretory endocrine glands.

16

The skeletomuscular systems: Control of posture and movement

Introduction: importance of posture and movement in health

Overview of the anatomy of the skeletal system I: bone

Overview of the anatomy of the skeletal system II: the skeleton

Overview of skeletal muscle anatomy and muscle contraction

The skeletomuscular system and support of the body

Details of the control of posture and movement

Examples of homeostatic failures and principles of correction

Summary

Review questions

Introduction: importance of posture and movement in health

The skeletomuscular systems enable us to maintain a posture against gravity, and to move in a coordinated way. Failure to maintain the contraction of appropriate muscles, the flexibility of joints, or adequate bone strength rapidly induces inadequate mobilization. This might be an inability to cope with, say, stairs or distance walking, or an inability to withstand gravity and therefore maintain an upright posture.

Lack of mobility can lead to a dependency upon mobility aids, or on other individuals, in order to perform basic activities of daily living. Postural problems can become exacerbated with time compounding the difficulty, and may lead to further problems; for example

difficulties in breathing may be experienced, and changes in cardiovascular and digestive functions become apparent. Dependency, and its accompanying effect on body image, can also have a severe influence on 'psychological' well-being.

The control of posture and movement involves the contraction and relaxation of appropriate skeletal muscles, but also requires adequate support provided by the skeletal system. It is not the intention of this book to provide a detailed anatomy of the skeletomuscular systems, but overviews of the skeleton and muscles are necessary in considering how posture and movement are maintained.

Overview of the anatomy of the skeletal system I: bone

Bone is a connective tissue, i.e. it consists of a matrix of ground substance, secreted by specialized cells. Its supportive strength comes from the deposition of mineral salts (a mixture of calcium phosphate and calcium carbonate called hydroxyapatite) in the matrix. The matrix does, however, convey a certain degree of flexibility to bones.

Although strong, bones are also light and this is facilitated by the presence of internal 'spongy' bone tissue, and by cavities. The cavities may be filled with marrow tissue, adipose tissue, or even air in the facial sinuses. The main strength of bone arises from the outer layers of 'compact' bone tissue.

SPONGY AND COMPACT BONE

Spongy bone

As its name implies, spongy bone consists of a meshwork of calcified 'beams', or trabeculae (Figure 16.1). The meshwork is constructed along the lines of greatest pressure exerted on the bone and these minute 'archways' and 'beams' provide considerable strength. The spaces within the meshwork help to reduce bone weight.

Spongy bone, and the marrow tissue and adipose tissues within the spaces, are supplied with nutrients by arteries which penetrate the outer compact bone via small openings called the nutrient foramina.

Compact bone

Compact bone is the very hard and dense material which people normally associate with bone. Close examination of a cross-section reveals it to have a complex structure and it actually consists of minute cylindrical structures (<0.5 mm in diameter) called osteons or Haversian systems (Figure 16.1). Osteons are comprised of concentric layers, or lamellae, of bone which enclose a central, or Haversian, canal. This canal runs along the axis of the bone, and conveys blood vessels, lymphatic vessels and neurons into the bone tissue. Side canals radiate into the lamellae and so enable blood to perfuse the entire compact bone structure.

Nutrients from the blood vessels within the side canals diffuse via other, even smaller, channels called canaliculi. The canaliculi are filled with interstitial fluid, and expansions (called lacunae) contain the bone cells (or osteocytes; osteo- = bone; -cyte= cell).

The blood vessels of bone originate from the outer covering of bone which is a fibrous membrane called the periosteum. This membrane can be converted into bone (i.e. ossified) if underlying bone is damaged.

BONE CELLS

Bone cells are of various types according to their role in bone.

OSTEOCYTES AND OSTEOBLASTS

Osteocytes are the main cells of fully developed bone and are derived from osteoblast cells which produced the bone. Osteoblasts are responsible for the maintenance of bone structure, including calcium deposition/resorption according to body calcium balance.

OSTEOCLASTS

These large cells are responsible for bone resorption during bone shaping.

OSTEOGENIC CELLS

These are cells found in the periosteum and bone marrow. They are 'stem' cells capable of differentiating into osteoblasts or osteoclasts during times of mechanical stress or injury.

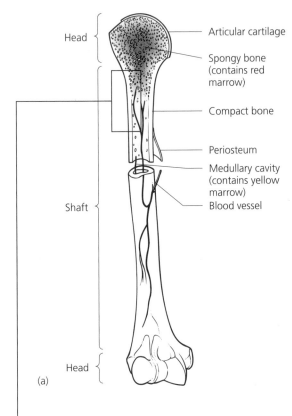

Head
Articular cartilage
Spongy bone (contains red marrow)
Compact bone
Periosteum
Medullary cavity (contains yellow marrow)
Blood vessel
Shaft
Head

(a)

BONE SHAPE AND EXTERNAL FEATURES

Bones are present in various shapes and sizes according to function, but some generalizations can be made. They are classified as long, short, flat, irregular, or sesamoid bones.

LONG BONES

Bone length is greater than bone width. Long bones are found in the limbs and provide a wide scope for body movement, but also help to absorb the stresses of body weight.

SHORT BONES

These bones are of nearly equal width and length. They are generally not strong but produce flexible structures, such as the wrist and ankle.

Figure 16.1 Bone tissue. (a) Longitudinal section of a long bone. (b) A magnified view of compact bone.

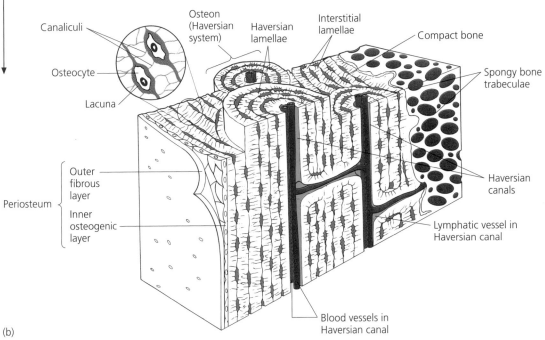

Canaliculi
Osteocyte
Lacuna

Osteon (Haversian system)
Haversian lamellae
Interstitial lamellae
Compact bone
Spongy bone trabeculae

Periosteum
Outer fibrous layer
Inner osteogenic layer

Haversian canals
Lymphatic vessel in Haversian canal
Blood vessels in Haversian canal

(b)

FLAT BONES

These are thin, plate-like bones. Their roles are to provide protection (e.g. the skull) and to provide an extensive surface area for the attachment of large muscles (e.g. the shoulder blade or scapula).

IRREGULAR BONES

These are bones which have complex shapes that are related to their functions, for example the bones of the backbone or vertebral column.

SESAMOID BONES

The kneecap, or patella, is the main example of this type of bone. Sesamoid bones strengthen tendons.

Bones have many irregular external features, arising because of the need for muscle/ligament attachment, for articulating joints between bones, and (sometimes) for the passage of blood vessels, nerves, and lymphatic vessels.

Protrusions that serve primarily for muscle attachment are frequently named as processes, tubercles (tuberosities), or trochanters. Condyles are protrusions which form an articulating surface and so have a smooth area which in life is lined with joint cartilage. Some bones, particularly the flat bones, are strengthened by ridges of bone called crests or spines.

The passage of blood vessels directly through a bone necessitates the presence of a perforation, usually called a foramen (= 'window'; plural foramina). In some bones the passage of vessels/nerves is facilitated by a notch or groove on the bone.

Overview of the anatomy of the skeletal system II: the skeleton

SKELETAL STRUCTURE

The skeleton is comprised of 206 bones, and can be divided into two parts: the axial and appendicular skeletons.

Axial skeleton

The axial skeleton consists of the skull, vertebral column (backbone), ribs and sternum (breastbone) and the hyoid bone, in other words bones which form the vertical axis of the body (Figure 16.2).

The skull

The skull consists of 8 bones of the cranium and 14 facial bones.

The cranium basically forms a bony 'box' which surrounds and protects the brain. The bones are smooth on the outside but uneven internally as a consequence of brain shape and the presence of blood vessels. Vessels and nerves gain access to the cranial cavity via openings in the skull; for example the spinal cord enters via the foramen magnum (see Figure 16.3c). The cerebral lobes and the cerebellum of the brain produce three distinct 'bulges', called fossae, on the bones of the cranium.

The facial bones provide attachment for facial muscles, form the mandible (lower jaw), protect cavities such as those of the nose, eyes, and sinuses, and form the palate of the mouth. The nomenclature of facial bones is complex, sometimes referring to associated tissues (e.g. the nasolachrymal ducts, which conduct tears from the eye orbit to the pharynx, pass through

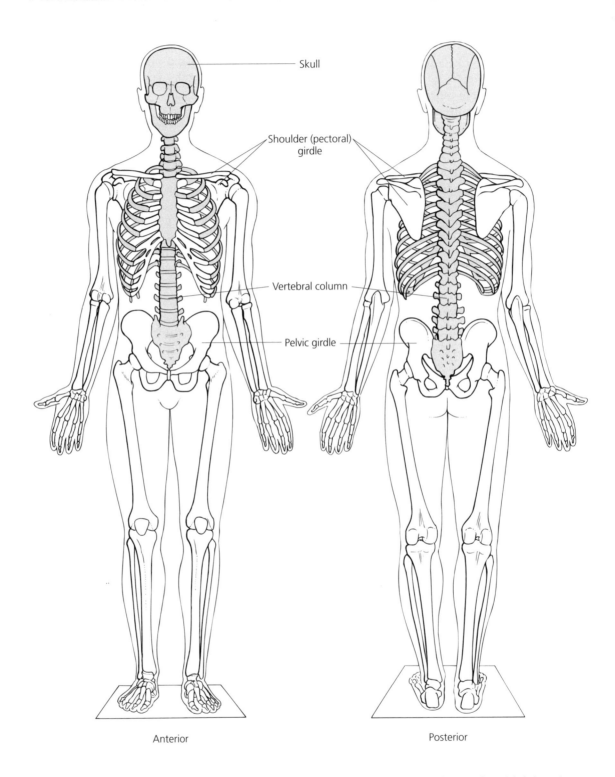

Figure 16.2 The two major divisions of the skeletal system: the axial and appendicular skeletons. The axial skeleton is shown in colour.

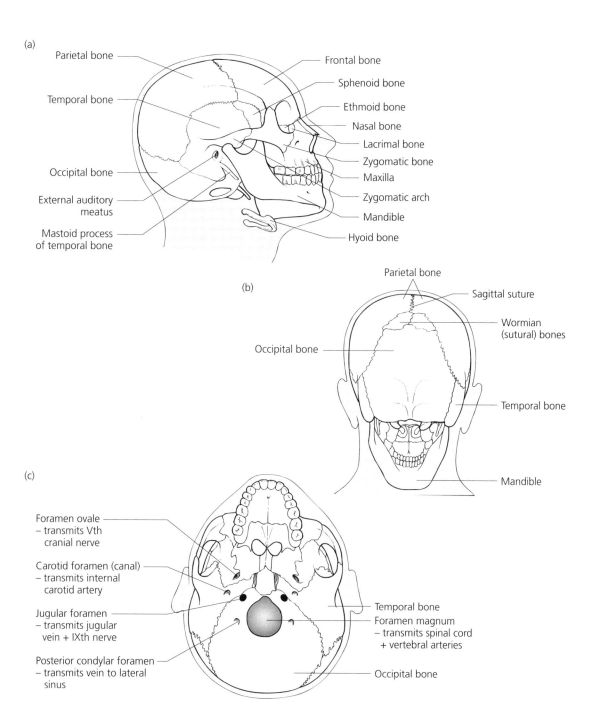

Figure 16.3 Principal bones of the skull. (a) Lateral view. (b) Posterior view. (c) Inferior view (also includes the larger foramina features).

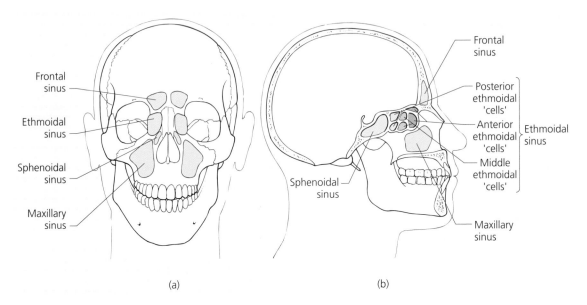

Figure 16.4 Paranasal sinuses: (a) anterior view (b) median view.

the lachrymal bones of the orbit), but usually referring to the classical names of facial anatomy (e.g. the zygomatic bones form the prominences of the cheeks or zygoma).

The major bones of the skull are identified in Figure 16.3. Most of the joints between them are fixed, i.e. they are held tightly by cartilage as they do not perform any kind of movement. These are the sutures. Cranial sutures do not fully form until some time after birth and allow for skull distortion at birth and also for rapid brain growth (see Chapter 19). In contrast the mandibular joint between the mandible and the temporal bone of the cranium allows a wide range of movement: mouth opening, closing, protrusion, retraction and side-to-side movement. The range of articulation aids food chewing and facial expression.

The paranasal sinuses are air-filled cavities within the frontal, maxillary, ethmoid, and sphenoid bones (Figure 16.4). The cavities help to lighten the bone and their association with the nose gives resonance to the voice.

The vertebral column

The vertebral column supports the upright or bipedal posture of the body, and protects the spinal cord, but provides flexibility of movement. Flexibility is provided by the column consisting of 33 individual bones (Figures 16.5 and 16.6): 7 cervical (i.e. neck); 12 thoracic (i.e. upper trunk, or thorax); 5 lumbar (i.e. lower trunk); 5 sacral (i.e. of the sacrum, a component of the pelvis); 4 coccygeal (i.e. of the coccyx or 'tail'). The individual bones of the sacrum and coccyx are usually fused together, although the coccyx articulates with the sacrum.

The vertebrae articulate with their neighbours, and muscle attachment is provided by bony processes. Thoracic vertebrae also have articular surfaces which form joints with the ribs.

The main body, or centrum, of the vertebral bone provides strength and also acts as a shock absorber during postural changes. A large central cavity called the vertebral foramen accommodates the spinal cord, and spaces between adjacent bones, called the intervertebral foramina, allow access/exit for blood vessels and spinal nerves. The first two cervical vertebrae (abbreviated C_1 and C_2) are modified to form a joint with the base of the skull. C_1 (also called the atlas) has articulating surfaces on the upper aspect which allow

(a)

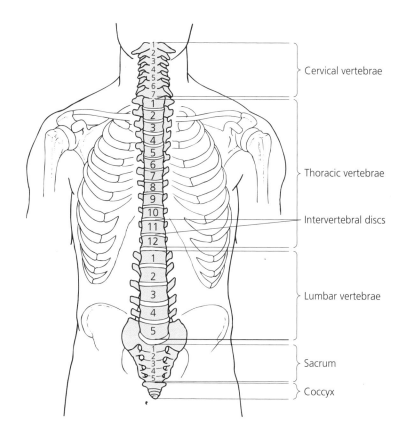

(b)

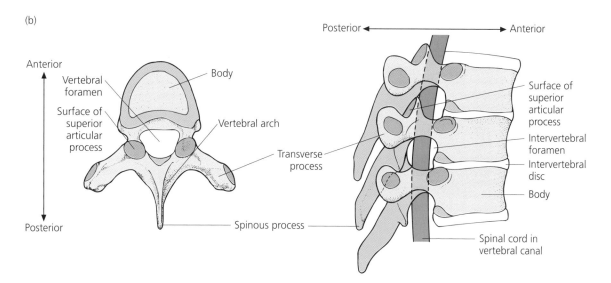

Figure 16.5 The vertebral column. (a) General structure. (b) General structure of a vertebral bone.

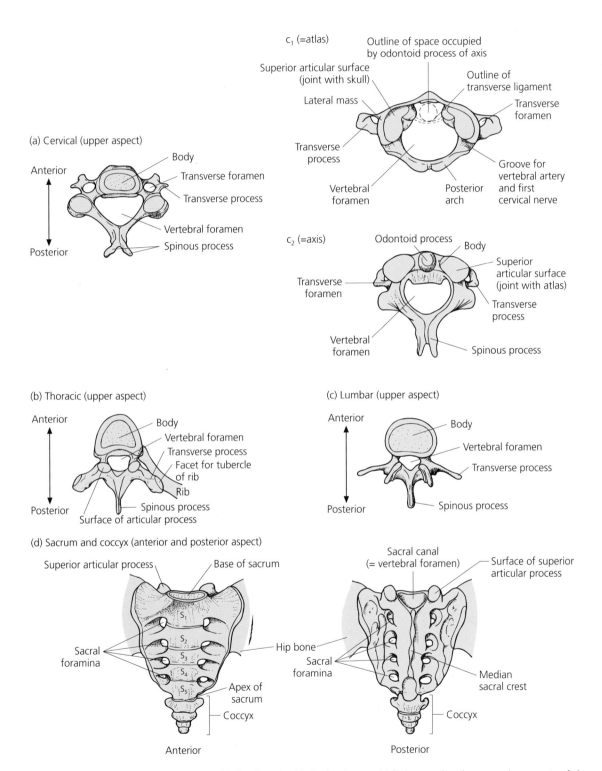

Figure 16.6 Vertebrae of (a) the cervical, (b) the thoracic, (c) the lumbar, and (d) the sacral and coccygeal segments of the vertebral column.

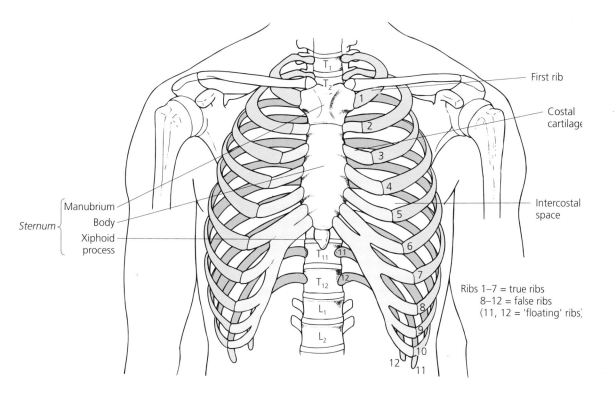

First rib

Costal cartilage

Intercostal space

Sternum {
Manubrium
Body
Xiphoid process

Ribs 1–7 = true ribs
8–12 = false ribs
(11, 12 = 'floating' ribs)

Figure 16.7 The ribs and sternum (anterior view).

forward and backward movement of the head. C_2 (also called the axis) has an upper vertical process, the odontoid process, which projects from the body of the bone into the modified vertebral foramen of the atlas, and this allows rotational movement of the head (Figure 16.6a).

The centrum of a vertebral bone is separated from its neighbour by an intervertebral disc (inter- = between), which is comprised of an outer fibrocartilage layer and an inner semi-solid core. The discs contribute to vertebral column flexibility, and also help in absorbing shock during movement. Should the tough outer layer rupture, then the core distends through the fissure and exerts pressure on nearby spinal nerves, producing pain. This is a 'slipped' or prolapsed disc.

The individual vertebral joints provide only limited movement and are very supportive.

Collectively, however, the column has a high degree of flexibility, particularly in bending forwards – sideways and backward movements are limited. The supporting aspect of the vertebral column in relation to posture is considered again later.

Ribs and sternum

The sternum is a flat, dagger-shaped bone situated in the anterior midline of the chest (Figure 16.7). There are three parts, called the manubrium, the body and the xiphisternum, which articulate and facilitate chest expansion during breathing. The xiphisternum is cartilaginous until well into adulthood, when it ossifies, and provides attachments for some abdominal muscles and for the diaphragm. The manubrium and body have pairs of articular surfaces which form joints with the rib bones.

(a)

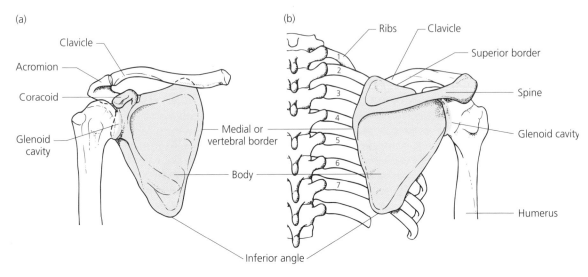

(b)

(c)

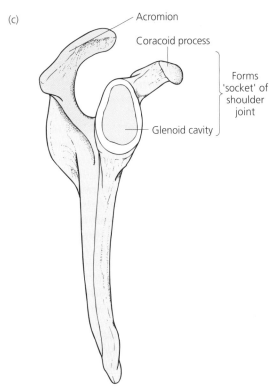

Figure 16.8 The pectoral girdle and shoulder joint. (a) Anterior view. (b) Posterior view. (c) Scapula in lateral view.

These are referred to as true ribs. Of the five pairs of false ribs, three are attached to the costal cartilage of the last true rib and two have no sternal attachment; these latter are the floating ribs.

The rib cage provides protection for the underlying organs of the chest (lungs, heart, and associated vessels), provides attachment for postural and respiratory muscles, and helps support the shoulder girdle of bones. The floating ribs extend far enough down the back to provide some protection for the kidneys.

Hyoid

The hyoid is a U-shaped bone found at the base of the tongue (see Figure 16.3a). It does not articulate with any other bone or cartilage, but forms an attachment for several muscles involved in chewing and swallowing. It is held in place by various other muscles.

Appendicular skeleton

The appendicular skeleton consists of the limb bones and the bones of the limb girdles, and is

The manubrium also articulates with the clavicle or 'collar bone'.

Seven pairs of ribs articulate directly with the sternum via costal cartilages (Figure 16.7).

so named because these bones are 'appended' onto the axial skeleton (see Figure 16.2).

Pectoral girdle, arm and hand

The pectoral or shoulder girdle consists of the two collar bones and shoulder blades, called clavicles and scapulae respectively (Figure 16.8). The clavicle is a slender bone which articulates with the sternum at one end and the scapula at the other. The clavicles provide a site for muscle attachment, but also help to brace the shoulder.

The shoulder blades are large, flat triangular bones. The blade is strengthened by a ridge or spine on its posterior surface. Although a large bone, the blade articulates at just one end, with the clavicle and humerus of the arm, and much of it is held in place by many muscle attachments and ligaments. Its structure and mode of attachment facilitates the rotational movement of the shoulder.

The bones of the arm consist of the humerus of the upper arm, and the ulna and radius of the forearm. The humerus is a long bone which articulates with the scapula and with the radius and ulna at the elbow (Figure 16.9a). The joint with the scapula is a 'ball and socket' joint (see below) which provides a wide range of movement. At its distal end, at the elbow, the humerus is flattened to form the articular surfaces. The bone is strengthened at this point by condyles, one of which (the medial epicondyle) is crossed by the ulnar nerve. It is this nerve which is pinched against the humerus when the elbow is knocked.

The radius of the forearm is found on the outer, or lateral, side, whilst the ulna is found on the inner forearm, or medial side. They are joined together along their length by a membrane and articulate with the humerus as a 'hinge' joint at the elbow, and with the carpal bones of the wrist.

The olecranon process of the ulna forms the elbow 'bone' and helps to prevent overextension of the arm when the elbow is straightened. The radius forms a more substantial wrist joint than does the ulna.

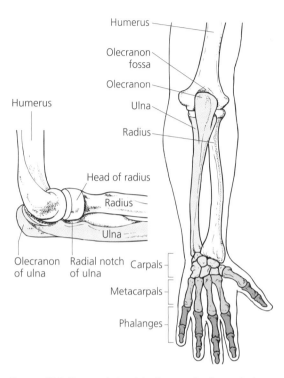

Figure 16.9 Bones of the right forearm (radius and ulna with elbow detail).

WRIST AND HAND

The wrist bones are called carpals, of which there are eight in each wrist (Figure 16.9b). They are short bones arranged roughly in two rows, and are connected by ligaments. One row articulates with the radius and ulna, whilst the other articulates with the five metacarpal bones of the palm. The latter articulate with the proximal finger bones, or phalanges; there are three phalanges in each finger and two in the thumb.

Pelvic girdle, leg and foot

The hip or pelvic girdle consists of two 'innominate' bones and the sacral bones of the vertebral column. The innominate bones are each actually comprised of three bones, the ilium, ischium and pubis, that have fused together to

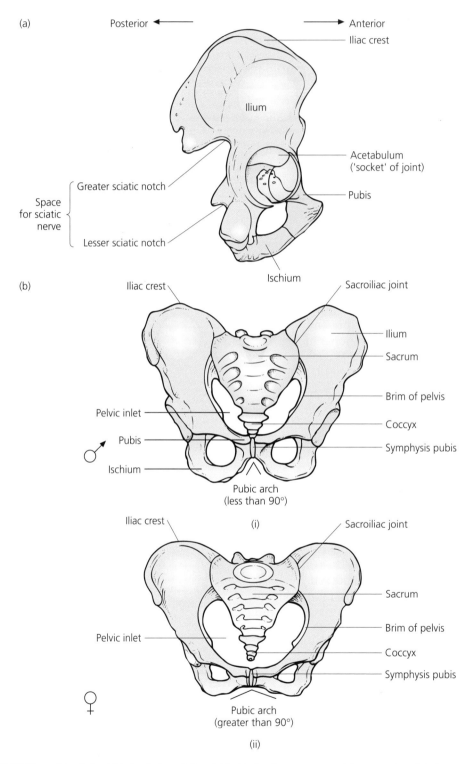

Figure 16.10 The pelvic girdle. (a) Lateral view of the right side to show component bones and acetabulum. (b) Anterior view of (i) male pelvic girdle, (ii) female pelvic girdle.

form a strong bowl-shaped structure (Figure 16.10). The junction of the three bones forms a deep depression called the acetabulum and this acts as a receptacle for the head of the thigh bone or femur (Figure 16.10a).

The ilium is the larger of the three bones. It is a large, flattened bone, strengthened by bony ridges or spines, and forms attachments with the large postural muscles of the thigh and buttock. It articulates with the sacrum, though movement is very limited. The ischium is also a substantial bone, and supports the weight of the body when sitting. The pubis extends to the front of the lower abdomen; the right and left pubic bones unite at the symphysis pubis, a joint which ordinarily has very limited movement but becomes lax in the female prior to childbirth under the actions of the hormone relaxin.

The bowl-shaped structure provided by these bones protects the organs of the lower or inferior abdomen, including the reproductive tract. Not surprisingly, the shape of the pelvic cavity is different between the sexes, being wider and shallower in the female to accommodate the fetus during pregnancy (Figure 16.10b).

The thigh bone, or femur, is a strong long bone which articulates at the hip and at the knee. The large head of the femur forms a 'ball and socket' joint with the acetabulum of the hip (Figure 16.11a). Bony protrusions at the knee end (called the medial and lateral condyles of the femur) articulate with the kneecap, or patella, and with the tibia of the lower leg. The patella is secured in position by extensive cartilages and serves to protect the knee joint and to strengthen the ligaments of that joint (Figure 16.11).

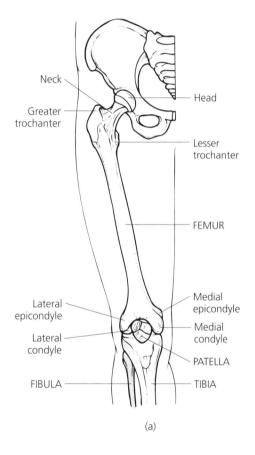

(a)

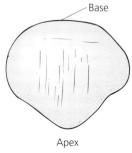

(b)

Figure 16.11 Bones of the upper leg and kneecap (patella). (a) The femur, anterior view. (b) The right patella: left, anterior view; right, posterior view.

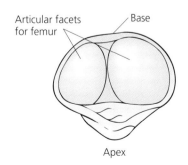

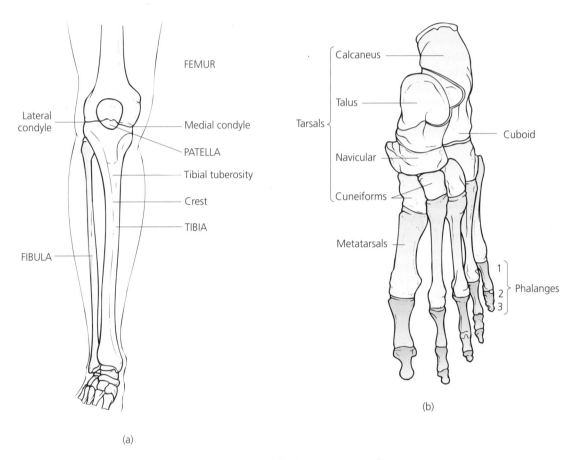

(a)

(b)

Figure 16.12 Bones of the lower leg and foot. (a) Tibia and fibula, anterior view. (b) Foot.

The bones of the lower leg are called the tibia and fibula. The tibia forms the shin bone (the prominent crest running along the front of the bone can easily be felt), and articulates with the femur at the knee and with the bones of the ankle (Figure 16.12a). The fibula is a more slender bone (it is not weight-bearing) and articulates with the tibia at the knee end and with ankle bones.

The seven ankle and heel bones are collectively called tarsals; the talus is the main tarsal bone of the ankle joint whilst the calcaneus is the heel bone (Figure 16.12b). The instep of the foot is formed from five longer, more slender bones or metatarsals, and these in turn articulate with the proximal bones of the toes (like the fingers, these too are called phalanges).

There are three phalanges in each toe, except for the big toe which has only two.

JOINTS

Strictly speaking, a joint is simply the point of contact between bones or between cartilage and bone, and its presence does not always imply movement. Those between bones which provide little or no movement are called fixed joints, whilst those between bone and cartilage are called cartilaginous joints. Joints which allow movement are called synovial joints and the forms of such joints present enable the body to have a wide diversity of movement.

Fixed and cartilaginous joints

Fixed joints include the sutures of the skull, in which a thin layer of dense fibrous connective tissue unites the bones (during life some sutures are replaced by bone so that there is complete fusion). The joint between the shafts of the ulna and radius of the forearm, and that between the tibia and fibula near the ankle, are other examples of fixed joints. These, however, have more connective tissue present than is found in sutures and the joint is slightly movable.

Cartilaginous joints include the symphysis pubis between the anterior surfaces of the pubis bones of the pelvic girdle, and the discs between the bodies of vertebrae. They differ from fixed joints in that the fibrocartilage present makes the joint slightly more movable. The joint between the cartilaginous tip of a growing bone, called the epiphysis, and the underlying bone matrix is also a cartilaginous joint.

Synovial joints

Synovial joints are characterized by the presence of a joint, or synovial, cavity (Figure 16.13a). The cavity contains synovial fluid, enclosed within a capsule. The fluid is viscous because of the presence of hyaluronic acid (a constituent of cartilage) but is basically secreted from the blood plasma. Its role is to provide lubrication, and to provide nutrients for cartilage cells within the joint. An important property of the fluid is that the viscosity reduces as the joint is used, thus increasing the lubricative effects. Phagocytic cells within the fluid keep the joint free of debris.

The capsule consists of a tough, but flexible, outer layer of dense connective tissue which unites the articulating bones and helps prevent dislocation. The connective tissue fibres of the capsule are frequently arranged in parallel bundles, which are orientated to provide maximal strength to the joint. Such bundles are called ligaments. The inner layer of the capsule consists of loose connective tissue, elastin, and adipose tissue. This is the synovial membrane and it is this which secretes the synovial fluid.

The joint surface of the articulating bones is smoothed by a covering of hyaline cartilage. Additional cartilaginous discs (or menisci) may be present to ensure a tight fit between joint surfaces of very different shapes.

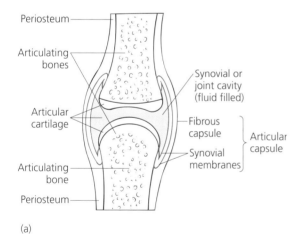

(a)

Figure 16.13 Synovial joints. (a) General form. (b) Subtypes of joints and their movements.

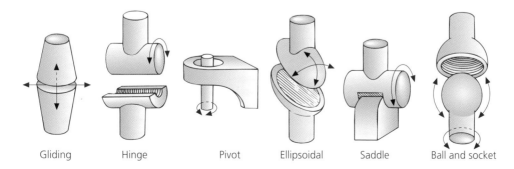

(b)   Gliding   Hinge   Pivot   Ellipsoidal   Saddle   Ball and socket

Although the general structure of synovial joints is similar, there are wide variations in the articulation produced. Various subtypes of joint are recognized, according to structure and to the movements allowed (Figure 16.13b) as follows:

BALL AND SOCKET

This consists of a ball-shaped surface on one bone fitted into a cup-like socket in another. The advantage of this type of joint is that it permits movement in three planes, including rotation. Examples are the shoulder and hip joints.

HINGE

In hinge joints a convex surface of one bone fits into the concave surface of another. This structure provides movement in one plane only. Examples are the elbow, knee, and ankle.

PIVOT JOINT

In this joint a protrusion from one bone articulates within a ring (partly of bone, partly ligament) structure on another. The joint provides rotational movement. Examples include the joint between the first two vertebrae (atlas and axis) which allows rotation of the head, and between the proximal ends of the ulna and radius of the forearm, which allows rotation of the forearm and hence of the hands.

ELLIPSOIDAL JOINTS

In these joints an oval-shaped condyle on one bone articulates with an elliptical-shaped cavity on another. The joint permits up and down and back and forth movement. Saddle joints are modified ellipsoidal joints which allow a greater range of movement in the two planes. Unlike the ball and socket joint, ellipsoidal joints do not allow rotation. An example is the joint between the radius and the carpal bones of the wrist.

GLIDING JOINTS

In these joints the articulating surfaces are flat and permit movement from side to side, and from back and forth. Though twisting and rotation might be expected to be possible by this structure, they are normally prevented by ligaments, or by adjacent bones. Examples are those between the carpals of the hand, between the tarsals of the foot, between the sternum and clavicle, and between the scapula and clavicle.

Bursae

Where skin, tendons or muscle rub on the surface of bone as a joint moves, small sacs of fluid called bursae (singular = bursa) prevent friction. These sacs are made of synovial membrane and the fluid is of similar composition to that of synovial fluid. Inflammation of the bursae produces bursitis.

Overview of skeletal muscle anatomy and muscle contraction

Muscles consist of cells that are capable of changing their length and shape. Three types of muscle cell are found in the body: smooth, cardiac, and skeletal (see Chapter 4). Smooth muscle cells are essential for the functioning of many tissues. For example, it provides the capability to change the diameter of blood vessels and airways, to alter gut motility, to empty the urinary bladder, and to reduce the size of the uterus during birth. Cardiac muscle produces the movement and shape change necessary for the pumping action of the heart. Skeletal muscle is associated with the movement or prevention of movement, of the skeleton, as appropriate, and it is this type of muscle that is considered in detail in this chapter.

Skeletal muscle lies immediately below the skin. In fact there are over 600 muscles in the body, arranged to support the skeletal system for the maintenance of posture and to facilitate movement. It is beyond the scope of this book to consider all muscles individually, and the interested reader is referred to the many available texts which do so. There are some aspects, however, which must be described if the role of muscle in determining posture and movement is to be understood. These are (1) muscle nomenclature, (2) muscle architecture and general anatomy, (3) muscle histology, and (4) the mechanism of muscle contraction.

MUSCLE NOMENCLATURE

To study fully labelled diagrams of the body musculature can fill the reader with trepidation as he is confronted with muscle names such as the levator palpebrae superioris! The nomenclature of muscles is classical and relates to various features of the muscle, i.e.:

- Muscle shape (e.g. the deltoid muscle of the shoulder is delta- or triangular-shaped).

- Muscle size (e.g. the gluteus maximus muscle of the buttock)

- Muscle location (e.g. the tibialis anterior lies in front of the tibia bone of the shin).

- Muscle attachments (e.g. the sternohyoid muscle is attached to the sternum and hyoid bones).

- Number of 'heads' of muscle origin (e.g. the biceps muscle of the upper arm has two 'heads').

- Movement type (e.g. levator indicates a muscle lifts something).

- Axis of muscle fibres relative to bone (e.g. transversus).

Frequently the nomenclature of muscles relates to one or more of these features. In the example given earlier:

> Levator palpebrae superioris
> = lifter   lip   upper

i.e. the name indicates its position and action.

MUSCLE ARCHITECTURE AND GENERAL ANATOMY

Muscle attachments

Generally speaking each muscle has a wide central region, or belly, and two ends which attach to other tissues, usually bone or cartilage (Figure 16.14a). The connection is provided by means of tough cords of connective tissue called tendons. These are extensions of the connective tissue which forms an integral part of the structure of the muscle and bone, and the tendons therefore provide a continuity between muscle and bone.

The 'achilles' tendon is the largest tendon in the body and attaches the large muscle of the calf (the gastrocnemius) to the heel bone (calcaneus). In some parts of the body, however, the tendons of muscles combine to form a sheet-like structure called an aponeurosis. Such structures are, for example, found in the abdominal wall and in the palms of the hands.

Muscles are covered in layers of dense connective tissue, called the deep fascia (the superficial fascia, or subcutaneous layer, between muscle and skin is described in Chapter 17). For many muscles the deep fascia acts to separate them and so facilitates them to function independently (Figure 16.15a).

Below the deep fascia lies another connective tissue sheath called the epimysium, from which more connective tissue extends into the muscle itself. This latter is called the perimysium (peri- = around) and encloses bundles of muscle fibres, which are elongated cylindrical cells that lie parallel to each other (Figure 16.15b). Each bundle of fibres is called a

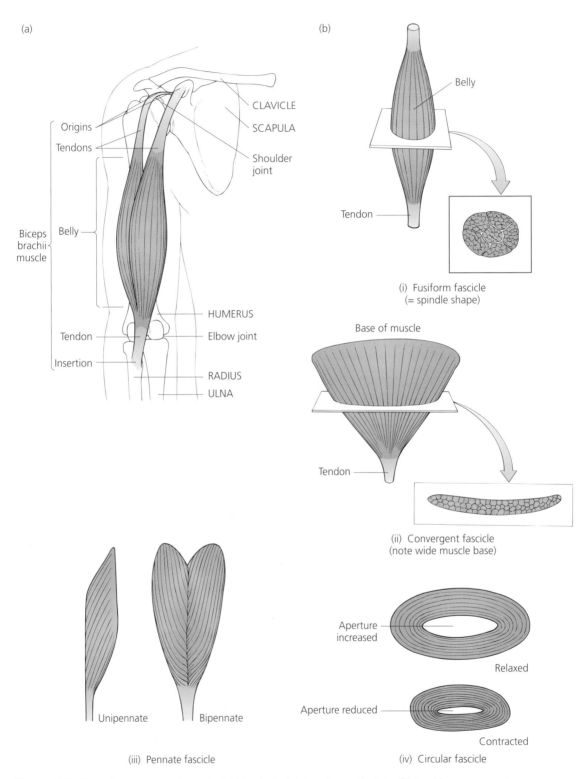

Figure 16.14 General appearance of muscle. (a) Muscle 'belly', insertion and origin. (b) Fascicle arrangements.

fascicle. Each muscle fibre is itself covered in a further extension of connective tissue, called the endomysium (endo- = inner). The three sheaths of connective tissue provide support for the muscle fibres and muscle, and also convey blood vessels, lymphatic vessels, and nerves into the muscle structure.

Muscle size and fascicle organization

Muscles vary considerably in size, according to how many fascicles, or bunches of muscle fibres, are present and to the length of the muscle belly. Fascicle and tendon arrangement also influence muscle appearance (Figure 16.14b). For example, the fascicles may run in parallel to the long axis of the muscle. Such muscles are referred to as fusiform (or spindle-shaped if a belly is present) or strap types. Fusiform types such as the biceps of the upper arm are generally able to generate a greater force of contraction than strap types of muscle like the rectus abdominus muscle of the anterior abdomen wall.

Fascicles may also be arranged obliquely to the long axis of the muscle and give the muscle a feather-like appearance. These are referred to as pennate-type muscles (penna = feather) and are generally stronger than strap or fusiform types. An example is the deltoid muscle of the shoulder, which is particularly important in maintaining the position of the shoulder girdle.

Finally fascicles may be arranged in a circular pattern around an aperture (Figure 16.14b). Contraction of these muscles causes a change in aperture size and they are found, for example, around the mouth and also around the anus and urethra (to form the external sphincters).

Muscle arrangement in relation to associated bones

When a muscle contracts it tends to cause a bone to move, but normally only the bone

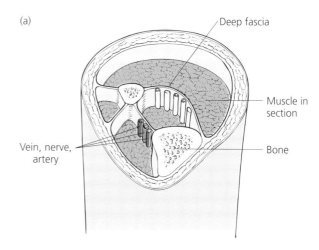

(a)

Deep fascia

Muscle in section

Bone

Vein, nerve, artery

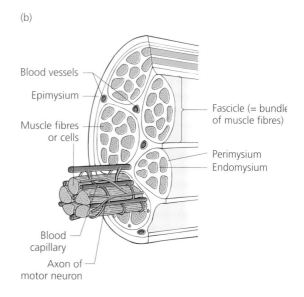

(b)

Blood vessels

Epimysium

Muscle fibres or cells

Fascicle (= bundle of muscle fibres)

Perimysium
Endomysium

Blood capillary

Axon of motor neuron

Figure 16.15 Connective tissue sheathing of muscle. (a) Deep fascia between muscles. (b) Sheaths within a muscle.

attached to one end moves. This is called the insertion end of the muscle; the stationary end is called the origin. The mode of movement, however, varies according to the particular situation and sometimes the origin end becomes the insertion end. In other words such terms are relative but are useful when considering disorders of specific movements.

MUSCLE FIBRE HISTOLOGY

Muscle fibres are muscle cells (Figure 16.16). Many are as long as the muscle itself; if one imagines the size of muscles, such as the quadriceps femoris of the thigh, then some fibres may be as long as 30 cm! Each fibre is surrounded by a plasma membrane which, in order to distinguish it from that of other cells, is called the sarcolemma (sarco- = flesh). Below this is a layer of cytoplasm (the sarcoplasm) within which can be seen organelles. Muscle fibres have numerous nuclei, however, and a muscle 'cell' is actually derived from numbers of cells that have fused to form a long structure, or syncytium, which functions as though it were a single cell.

The advantage of this differentiation is that whole muscles comprised of large numbers of muscle fibres can be induced to contract rapidly and efficiently. The high degree of complexity of the muscle fibre, however, means that skeletal muscle is largely a 'stable' tissue in that it cannot divide mitotically once the fibres have formed. Small numbers of undifferentiated stem cells are present but not enough to compensate for damage to the tissue.

Many of the organelles within the muscle fibre are identical to those found in cells elsewhere: many of the metabolic activities of the fibre are common to other cells. Some are modified, however (Figure 16.16c). For example the sarcoplasmic reticulum is analogous to the endoplasmic reticulum but extends into the protein filaments of the fibre (see below). It helps convey calcium ions into the interior of the cell for activation of the contractile process. Similarly, the sarcolemma produces tubular invaginations of the fibre, called transverse or T-tubules, which also convey membrane events into the interior.

The inner core of the muscle fibre is comprised of numerous minute fibrils, called myofibrils (myo- = muscle), which run longitudinally along the fibre in close association with the sarcoplasmic reticulum. Each fibril consists of a precise arrangement of smaller, thread-like structures of protein called myofilaments (Figure 16.16b). Microscopically the filaments

(a)

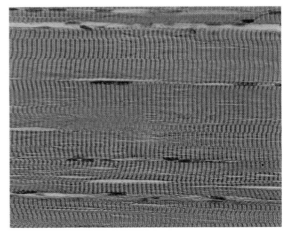

(b)

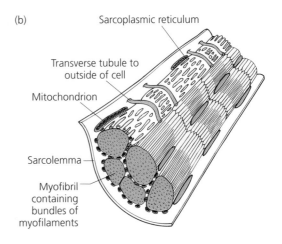

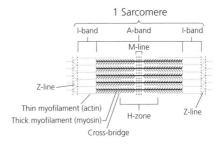

Figure 16.16 Muscle histology and microfilament arrangement. (a) Light microscopy photograph of a muscle fibre to show striations. (b) Intracellular features. (c) Filament arrangement. I-band, striation due to actin filaments only; H-zone, striation due to myosin filaments only (M-line, striation due to central area of myosin); A-band, striation due to myosin and myosin/actin overlap.

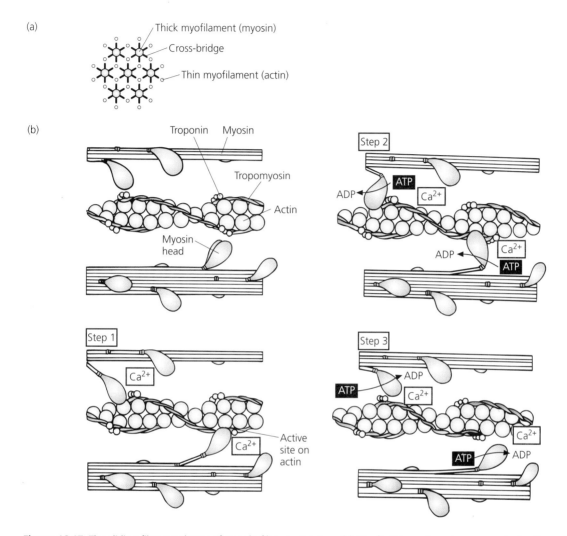

Figure 16.17 The sliding filament theory of muscle fibre contraction. (a) Myofibril in section. Arrangement of actin and myosin filaments in a myofibril. (b) Myofilament interaction. Step 1, distortion of troponin/tropomyosin by calcium ions. Formation of bond between myosin head and active site on actin. Step 2, splitting of ATP by myosin to provide energy to move myosin/actin cross-bridges (actin is pulled along myosin), and then to break cross-bridge for new actin/myosin interaction. Step 3, movement of myosin heads to interact with next active site on actin.

appear as thick and thin threads: thick ones are composed of a protein called myosin, thin ones of one called actin. Viewed microscopically the arrangement of myosin and actin filaments within the muscle fibre makes the fibre appear to have stripes or striations of light and dark areas and skeletal muscle is frequently referred to as striated muscle (Figure 16.16). The shade of the stripe reflects the protein type present in that particular part of the fibre. The bandings

repeat in sequence along the fibre, indicating that the fibre has distinct functional segments; each segment of banding is called a sarcomere (meros = part).

MUSCLE CONTRACTION

The contraction of a muscle necessitates the contraction of the large numbers of muscle fibres of which it is comprised. Although common processes are involved in contracting the individual fibres, the behaviour of the muscle, and the actual tension developed within the muscle as a consequence of contraction, can vary.

Contraction of muscle fibres

Muscle fibre contraction results from an interaction between the myosin and actin protein filaments within the fibre, promoted by neural stimulation.

The sliding filament theory of muscle fibre contraction

Figure 16.17 illustrates how this process is thought to operate. The interaction between myofilaments is initiated when calcium ions are released into the sarcoplasmic reticulum. When these ions reach the area of the filaments they have two important actions.

First, calcium ions cause a protein called troponin associated with actin filaments to distort its molecular shape and this in turn distorts another associated protein called tropomyosin. This latter response exposes sites on the actin molecule that interact with complementary sites on the myosin filaments, called the myosin 'heads'. The interaction between myosin and actin filaments thus forms cross-bridges which act to 'pull' the actin filament over that of the myosin. The myosin heads then detach and move to the next active sites on the actin, and the actin is pulled further along the myosin in a process analogous to a ratchet mechanism. The whole process is so rapid that as many as 100 repeat interactions can occur per second.

The actin filaments are attached to a proteinaceous structure (the Z-line) which lies transversely across the muscle fibre and marks the boundary of each sarcomere. As a consequence of the myosin/actin interaction the sarcomere reduces in length; multiplied up and the whole muscle fibre will shorten (Figure 16.18).

The second action of calcium is to stimulate myosin to act as an enzyme which splits ATP

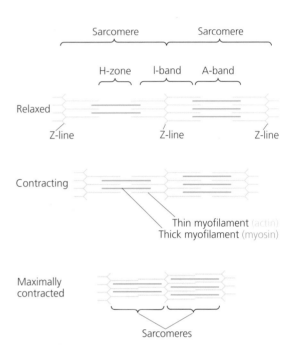

Figure 16.18 Shortening of sarcomere length during myofibril contraction. Note that myofilament lengths do not change, but the overlap between actin and myosin increases (with resultant narrowing of the A- and I-bands).

(adenosine triphosphate) and cause the release of energy. It is this energy which is used to move the myosin heads to the exposed active actin sites, and also to break the myosin/actin cross-bridges.

Clearly the reservoir of ATP within the fibre is limited and, as it is utilized, more must be synthesized to sustain the contractile process. Cellular respiration of glucose will be promoted, but in order to maintain a contraction lasting for several seconds an alternative source is required. Muscle cells contain a substance called creatine phosphate which, when combined with ADP produced during muscle contraction, generates new ATP and creatine (using the enzyme creatine phosphokinase). Breakdown of excess creatine produces creatinine, a 'waste' substance which is excreted in urine.

The calcium necessary to initiate muscle contraction largely comes from stores within distended areas of the sarcoplasmic reticulum

(a)

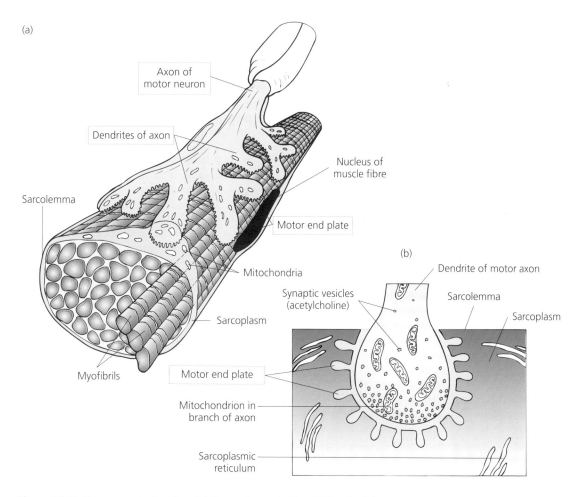

Figure 16.19 Neuromuscular junction. (a) The motor end plate. (b) Detail of the synapse.

called terminal cisternae that are found close to the transverse tubules of the sarcolemma. The cisterns are induced to release their calcium when the muscle fibre is stimulated by an associated motor nerve cell. Active uptake of the ions back into the cisterns after nerve stimulation has ended stops the contraction.

The neuromuscular junction or motor end plate

The muscle fibre synapses at numerous points along its length with dendrites from the same neuron. The synaptic structure at the neuron/muscle fibre interface (called a motor end plate to distinguish it from neuron–neuron synapses) is illustrated in Figure 16.19. Synaptic function was described in Chapter 13 and the neuromuscular end plate acts in similar fashion, utilizing acetylcholine as a neurotransmitter chemical. When released from the nerve cell by arrival of an electrical impulse, the acetylcholine causes a depolarization of the sarcolemma which is then transmitted into the muscle fibre by the transverse tubules.

Contraction of whole muscles

Observation of the contraction of whole muscle identifies a variety of forms of contraction (see Figures 16.20 and 16.21).

(a)

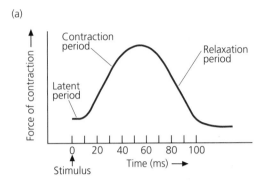

(b)

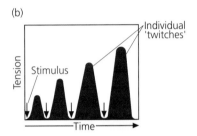

(c)

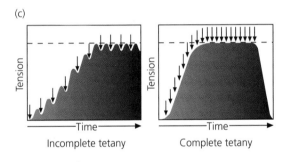

Incomplete tetany   Complete tetany

Figure 16.20 Relationship between stimulus frequency and muscle tension. (a) Twitch produced by a single stimulus. (b) Treppe produced by continued activation/relaxation. (c) Tetany induced by continued activation.

TWITCH

This is a momentary, spasmodic contraction produced by a brief, single stimulus.

TREPPE

If a muscle is repeatedly stimulated, but is allowed to relax between stimuli, the contraction induced by each stimulus increases in intensity to a maximum. This principle is used by athletes in 'warm ups'.

TETANY

If a muscle is repeatedly stimulated but is not allowed to relax fully between stimuli, the contractions induced by each stimulus are additive so that each twitch summates to produce an intense, continuous contraction called a tetanic contraction.

ISOTONIC

Consider if an object is lifted. Muscles of the arm must generate the force, or tension, necessary to move the load. Once the object is moving, however, further tension need not be developed (even though the muscle is shortening as the skeletal joint moves). The contraction is then said to be isotonic (iso- = equal; tonos= tension).

ISOMETRIC

In lifting an object, tension must be developed before the object can be moved. During this time the skeletal joint is stationary and muscle length will therefore remain constant. The contraction is then said to be isometric (metros = length). For very heavy loads the tension generated by isometric contraction can be considerable.

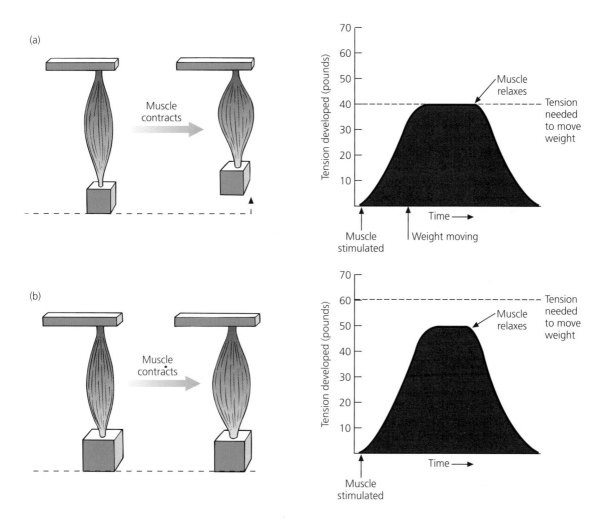

Figure 16.21 (a) Isotonic and (b) isometric contractions. In (a) muscle tension increases until the weight moves and then remains constant even though the contraction continues. In (b) the weight cannot be moved; muscle tension increases during the contraction but the muscle does not shorten.

The skeletomuscular system and support of the body

'Posture' is the position of the body in space and includes whole body orientation and also the relative positions of body parts. Movement results in a change of posture which may involve propulsion of the body from one point to another. The maintenance of posture, and the control of postural changes during movement, depends upon five factors: (1) the strength of bone to support the body; (2) skeletal adaptations to withstand the forces applied during standing, running and walking; (3) the ability of muscles to withstand fatigue; (4)

Figure 16.22 Curvatures and arches in the skeletal system which aid an upright posture. (a) Vertebral column. (b) Femur. (c) Foot.

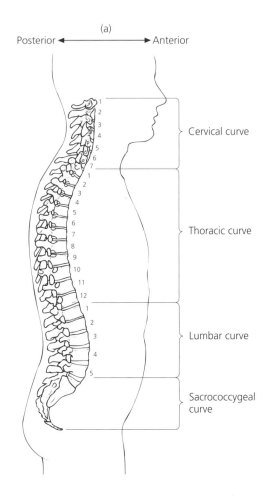

anatomical relationships between muscle, bone, and nerve supply; and (5) the control of individual muscle tension or tone. The latter involves a complex integration of sensory and motor activity by the central nervous system and is described in detail later in a separate section.

BONE STRENGTH: REMODELLING

Although heavily mineralized, bone is not an inert tissue. Calcium salts are deposited or removed as required by the body (e.g. in the regulation of plasma calcium ion concentration). Similarly, the selective deposition of mineral results in the changes in bone shape that are observed during growth, and this may involve the removal of mineral from one part of the bone and deposition in another. This redistribution of mineral is called bone remodelling.

Remodelling of bone occurs throughout life as 'old' bone is renewed, or if bones are fractured by injury. Once a bone has basically healed after injury, the individual should be encouraged to undertake light exercise, because this promotes an increase in bone density. Thus, physical stress placed on bone is another important stimulus to promote bone remodelling, with calcium deposition in the 'stressed' areas being favoured. This process ensures maximum strength at the most load-bearing points within the skeleton, such as the femur head.

Bone, then, is a dynamic tissue, yet the control of bone density and shape is little understood. Certainly the hormones parathyroid hormone, calcitonin and vitamin D have an influence, but their release and actions relate to the homeostatic control of plasma calcium concentration (Chapter 15) and not to modelling and remodelling of bone. Growth hormone and the sex steroids also have an influence during childhood and puberty but much remains to be discovered.

SKELETAL ADAPTATIONS

Humans are the only species which can sustain an upright posture for long periods and various skeletal adaptations help to overcome the influence of gravity. In addition, the forces exerted on the foot during walking are equivalent to a

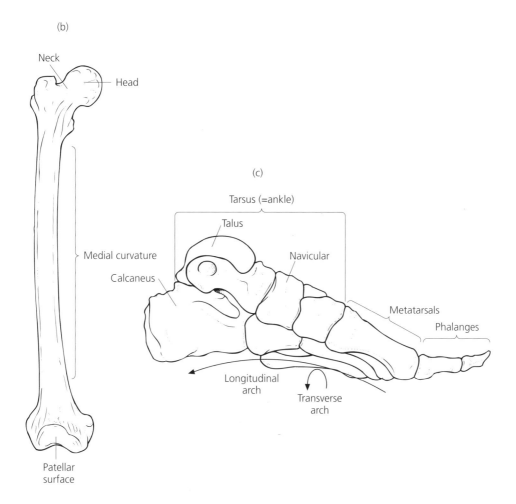

(b)

Neck

Head

Medial curvature

Patellar
surface

(c)

Tarsus (=ankle)

Talus

Navicular

Calcaneus

Metatarsals

Phalanges

Longitudinal
arch

Transverse
arch

sudden three-fold increase in body weight, and even more so during running; the skeleton must absorb the resultant shock.

The main skeletal adaptations involve the vertebral column, pelvis, limb bones (especially the femur), joints, and the foot skeleton.

Vertebral column

The vertebral column is a major determinant of the vertical axis of the body. Curvatures give it a distinct S-shape in side view (Figure 16.22a). Although babies are born with thoracic and sacral curvatures the development of the

cervical curvature after about 3 months is necessary if the head is to be held erect, and the development of the lumbar curvature during the later part of the first year is necessary if the baby is to sit up and eventually stand.

The curvatures are therefore essential for an upright posture. They result from contraction of the muscles of the back and a tightening of ligaments, and also provide a spring-like structure which helps to absorb the forces applied to the skeleton during walking/running (this is also facilitated by the intervertebral discs). They also ensure that the body's centre of gravity, i.e. the point in the body through which most of the weight acts, lies over the

pelvis. The lumbar curve is especially important in this respect, and its curvature may
increase if weight distribution in the body
alters, for example during pregnancy. The
additional stresses placed on the lumbar curve
during pregnancy are responsible for the lower
back pain that is frequently experienced.

Pelvis

The pelvic girdle is the site of the body's
centre of gravity and is an extremely robust
structure that is strengthened by fusion of its
composite bones and by inflexible joints with
the vertebral column (Figure 16.10). The bones
also have large attachment areas for the
postural muscles of the back, buttocks, and
thigh.

Femur

The human femur has an inner curvature
which distinguishes it from the femur of other
animals (Figure 16.22b). When standing, the
curvature brings the knee joint, shin bones, and
foot close to the vertical axis of the body and
so almost in line with the centre of gravity. In
females, the wider pelvis necessitates an even
more pronounced curvature.

Apart from facilitating weight-bearing, the
femur curvature also means that the centre of
gravity is not thrown widely out of position
during walking, and so helps maintain balance.
The femur curvature also provides a spring-
like action which enables it to absorb some of
the forces applied to it during walking. This
helps to reduce the 'jarring' effect on the pelvis
and vertebral column.

Joints

Joints subjected to physical stresses must be
reinforced if they are not to be dislocated.
Those joints which have to support the body
weight are reinforced with substantial
ligaments and cartilage, and are associated
with powerful muscles. The knee is a good
example of such a joint.

The structure of the knee joint (which is
actually an aggregate of three joints) is shown
in Figure 16.23. Note the presence of extensive
ligaments and muscle tendons, and also how
the orientation of the fibres of these connective
tissues stabilize the joint. Cruciate ligaments
within the joint capsule between the tibia and
the femur help to reduce any twisting motion
of the knee. The arrangement of ligatures
generally supports the knee during normal
standing or walking. Forces applied from an
unexpected direction, for example on the side
of the knee, may overcome the resistance
provided and result in dislocation. Torn
ligaments weaken the joint considerably and
such injuries, frequently observed in sport, can
be very disabling.

Foot skeleton

The weight-supporting and stress-absorbing
properties of the foot are provided by the
bones of the heel and ankle, and by the foot
arches (Figure 16.22c).

On standing, the body weight is exerted on
each ankle, and the weight is then distributed
between the heel bone (calcaneus) and the
metatarsal bones. The weight is therefore
directed to the ground via the calcaneus and
the distal heads of the metatarsals. The
relatively large size of the calcaneus was noted
earlier. Its shape helps give it strength, and
also provides a site of attachment for the large
calf muscles via the Achilles tendon.

The articulation between the tibia/fibula
bones of the lower leg and the main bone of
the ankle (the talus) is most stable in the standing position or, especially, when the foot is
flexed in the crouching position. Extending the
foot causes the articulation to occur with the
narrower part of the talus, resulting in instability when standing on tip-toe.

During walking the strength of the calcaneus
enables it to withstand the impact with the
ground. The body weight is then quickly
distributed to the lateral border of the foot
along the metatarsals, and eventually across

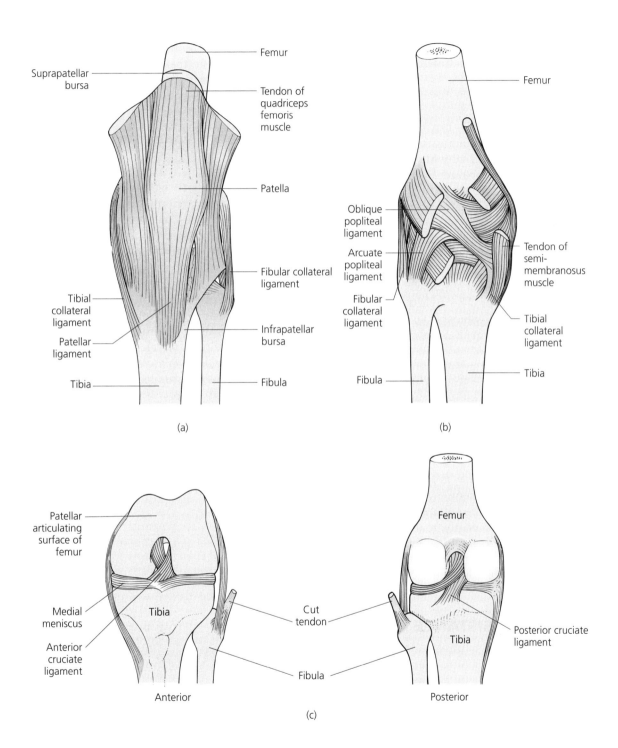

Figure 16.23 The knee joint: detail of ligaments and tendons: (a) anterior view; (b) posterior view. In (c) flexed and posterior views are shown to illustrate the cruciate ligaments and menisci within the joint.

the heads of the metatarsals to that of the first metatarsal bone at the base of the big toe (= the ball of the foot). By this time the heel will have left the ground.

Running increases the forces applied and the distal heads of the metatarsals distribute the weight more evenly. The role of the toes during walking/running is to provide stability at this point of contact with the ground, but also to impart a forward thrust which facilitates the movement.

The metatarsals and associated heel/ankle bones form the foot arches (Figure 16.22c). The first three form the high arch, called the medial longitudinal arch, on the inside of the foot, whilst metatarsals IV and V form the lower arch, called the lateral longitudinal arch, on the outside of the foot. The arched structures are maintained by ligaments and by attached muscles. The main ligament is called the plantar (i.e. underside of foot) calcaneonavicular ligament (i.e. it attaches to the calcaneum and to the navicular bone of the ankle, which articulates with the talus). A weakening of this ligament causes a failure to maintain the relative positions of these bones and therefore of the high arch, and causes a 'fallen arch' or 'flat foot'.

The role of the arches is to absorb the forces applied to the foot, especially during walking/running; they flatten slightly during impact of the foot on the ground and spring back into shape once the foot is lifted. The arches also help to prevent blood vessels and nerves in the foot from being crushed.

FATIGUE RESISTANCE OF MUSCLES

The maintenance of posture and physical activity requires muscles either to maintain a degree of contraction or to contract repeatedly, for perhaps long periods of time. Such muscles must therefore be fatigue resistant. In contrast, some movements involve very rapid contractions maintained for only a small period of time. Types of muscle fibre have been identified that are best suited to these roles, but it is important to note that muscles will contain a mixture of fibre types; only the relative proportion of fibre types varies.

'Slow' and 'fast' muscle fibre types

A single muscle twitch requires a contraction followed by a relaxation. The time required for these two processes to occur varies between muscle fibres and accordingly these are classified as 'slow' twitch (or type I) and 'fast' twitch (type II) fibres (although subtypes, particularly of fast fibres, are recognized which have intermediate rates of contraction).

'Slow' fibres are relatively more frequent in those muscles that are unlikely to have a large role in activities which necessitate rapid contraction/relaxation cycles. Postural muscles are therefore 'slow' muscles. The fibres have an excellent blood supply, and also have a rich store of myoglobin, a haemoglobin-like pigment which provides an oxygen store. The fibres therefore appear red in colour, as does the muscle, and have the capacity to maintain ATP production by aerobic metabolism (Figure 16.24). They are therefore resistant to fatigue.

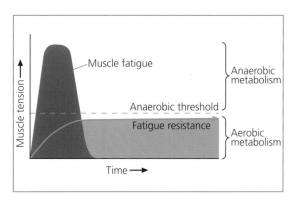

Figure 16.24 Fatigue resistance in muscles. 'Fast' twitch muscles rapidly exceed the anaerobic threshold during contraction. 'Slow' twitch muscles can maintain contraction below anaerobic threshold for long periods of time (but can exceed threshold during, say, exercise).

'Fast' fibres increase in proportion in those muscles that are responsible for producing rapid movements, as in the movement of the eye or hand. The rapid contraction is facilitated by large numbers of mitochondria and an extensive sarcoplasmic reticulum. The rapidity of the contraction/relaxation cycle, however, is such that ATP supplies are rapidly exhausted and the diffusion of oxygen from blood is inadequate to maintain the degree of metabolism. These fibres have little myoglobin (oxygen would rapidly be depleted even if it was present) and are not so well vascularized as 'slow' muscles. They therefore appear pale in contrast to 'slow' muscle, and so are called white muscle. They are capable of anaerobic metabolism, which supports the contractile activity, but the accumulation of metabolic products such as lactic acid rapidly causes fatigue.

ANATOMICAL RELATIONSHIPS BETWEEN MUSCLE, BONE, AND NERVE

Muscle and bone relationship

Some aspects of the attachment of muscle to bone were considered earlier, but simply forming an attachment is not necessarily sufficient for a muscle to move a skeletal structure. The force of contraction developed by the muscle must be sufficient to move the load placed upon it, i.e. the weight of the bone and the weight associated with the bone (tissues, body weight, or an object to be lifted). The generation of adequate power is facilitated by the arrangement of fascicles within the muscle, and by the leverage provided by the position of muscle insertion relative to the joint to be controlled. Fascicle arrangement was considered in the earlier section on general muscle architecture.

Levers

By causing bones to move, skeletal muscles are utilizing a system of levers (Figure 16.25).

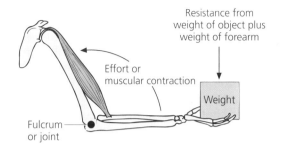

Figure 16.25 An example of a skeletomuscular lever.

Thus the bone to be moved acts as the 'arm' of the lever, which will move about the joint or fulcrum. The resistance to be overcome is the load. The arrangement of muscle, lever arm, and fulcrum varies but a general feature is that the further the muscle insertion is away from the fulcrum the greater the leverage will be. Thus more power can be generated when the insertion is some distance from the joint, than if the same muscle was inserted close to the joint. The movement will be slower, however.

Levers enable considerable forces to be generated. Without leverage it would, for example, be difficult to stand from a squatting position without considerably increasing our muscle bulk.

Muscle and its innervation: the motor unit

A muscle fibre will contract once it has been stimulated by its motor neuron, but the extent of the contraction induced can be varied by the time interval between the arrival of nerve stimuli (see 'treppe' and 'tetany' phenomena mentioned earlier). In practice, however, the resultant force of contraction of the whole muscle produced by nerve stimulation will usually depend upon how many fibres have been stimulated; the greater the contraction required, the more fibres will need to be stimulated.

For those large muscles which must develop a considerable force, for example the major postural muscles of the buttocks, the process would clearly be most efficient if stimulation of a motor neuron could induce the simultaneous contraction of large numbers of fibres, otherwise large numbers of nerve cells will be required. In fact a single nerve cell may innervate hundreds of muscle fibres in such muscles.

In contrast, muscles which are small, such as pupillary muscles inside the eye, may have fibres that are innervated by individual neurons. The number of fibres innervated by a single nerve cell is called a motor unit and to increase the force of contraction of a muscle requires the recruitment of appropriate numbers of motor units by activating further neurons.

Details of the control of posture and movement

The control of posture and movement depends upon the regulation of the tension of individual muscles appropriate to the desired joint position, or to the movement to be induced. Some features of muscle anatomy (viz. muscle architecture, size, shape, motor unit size) pertinent to the strength and type of contraction to be induced have already been described. This section is concerned with the regulation of motor neuron activity to muscles, and considers the kind of sensory information required, reflex responses, and the central nervous system centres involved in coordinating motor output. First, however, the relationship between those muscles associated with the movement of a single joint must be considered.

MUSCLE ACTION

The degree of tension observed in individual muscles will be appropriate for the maintenance of position of the associated joint. Changes in the tension of muscles relative to others produces movement.

A muscle which primarily produces a movement is called an agonist, whilst that which opposes the movement is called an antagonist. The latter only opposes contraction sufficient to protect the joint involved, and it does not normally prevent the movement from occurring (note the difference in usage of these terms in pharmacology in which agonistic drugs promote an action, antagonistic ones prevent or reverse it).

The actions of an agonist could adversely influence additional joints nearby, and these are stabilized by the simultaneous contraction of synergistic muscles. Once a movement is induced, its potentially disruptive effect on posture and balance has to be counteracted by the contraction/relaxation of other muscles. The joints controlled by these muscles may be some distance away from those directly affected by the agonists and are distinguished by the term fixator or postural muscles.

For example, consider the movement of the knee joint during walking. A number of muscles in the leg are involved, but the main ones are the quadriceps femoris (quad- = four; there are four parts to this muscle) of the thigh, and those which comprise the hamstring muscles at the back of the thigh (Figure 16.26). Both sets of muscles have attachments with the top of the femur or bones of the pelvis, and with the tibia of the lower leg. The quadriceps is an extensor muscle in that its contraction extends the leg; the hamstrings are flexors and cause the joint to bend or flex during contraction.

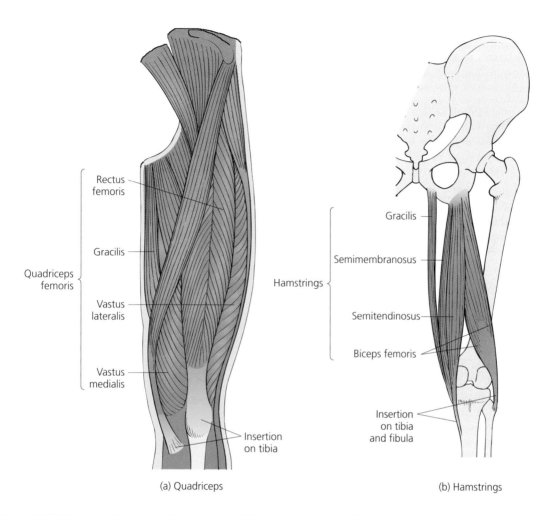

(a) Quadriceps

(b) Hamstrings

Figure 16.26 Muscles which control the knee joint: (a) flexors, anterior view; (b) extensors, posterior view.

During walking the knee extensor muscles will be agonistic as the leg is extended, the flexors antagonistic. When the knee is flexed, the situation is reversed. The movement therefore requires cyclical stimulation/relaxation of the muscles involved. Other synergistic muscles associated with the knee, ankle or hip must also be contracted or relaxed as appropriate. Any tendency for the body to be unbalanced by the disturbance in posture promoted by walking must be counteracted by contraction or relaxation of postural muscles elsewhere, for example in the opposite leg, the back, and the shoulders. Thus, what appears to be a relatively simple movement, and one which we would normally take for granted, requires complex responses throughout the muscular system.

The coordination of muscle contraction/relaxation is described later; the next section considers the sensory information that is required for the nervous system to exert that control.

PROPRIORECEPTION

The brain must be 'aware' at all times of the spatial positions of the body parts, and of the orientation of the body in general, although we are not usually consciously aware of this information, nor of its integration to produce moment-to-moment corrections and alterations of posture.

The senses were described in Chapter 14, and many are involved in the monitoring of posture. Vision is clearly of use in monitoring spatial positioning, yet closing our eyes or looking away does not prevent us from being aware of our posture, the position of our hands, etc., and blind people fare at least as well as visually able people in this respect. Other, perhaps less obvious, receptors are involved.

For example, the mechanoreceptors of the skin convey tactile information, and so the contact between, say, foot and ground, can be monitored. Most postural information, however, is produced by a variety of receptors collectively called proprioreceptors (or proprioceptors; proprio- = position). These receptors are the vestibular receptors, joint receptors, tendon receptors, and the muscle 'spindles'. To be effective, they must not only have static properties to monitor position, but must also be capable of monitoring position change, the rate of change, direction of change, and any acceleratory component (called dynamic properties).

Vestibular (or equilibrium) receptors

The vestibular receptors are found within the vestibular apparatus of the inner ear (Figure 16.27a). They can generally be divided into two: the otolithic organs and the semicircular canals.

The otolithic organs (the utricle and saccule) contain masses of small calcium carbonate crystals lying on top of a jelly-like otolithic membrane (otolith = ear stone, Figure 16.27c). Receptor hair cells project into this membrane. The rest of the utricle/saccule is filled with endolymph fluid. If the position of the head alters, the fluid moves but the denser otolithic membrane moves more slowly. As fluid moves

over the membrane it distorts the hair cells and generates electrical activity which is transmitted to the brain via the vestibulocochlear nerve (cranial nerve VIII). These receptors, then, provide information regarding the orientation of the head. The response is too slow to convey dynamic information, and so these are concerned with static equilibrium.

Dynamic equilibrium is monitored by receptors of the semicircular canals (Figure 16.27b). There are three canals in each ear, arranged at right-angles to one another in three planes. At the base of each canal there is a distended region, called the ampulla, in which lies the crista, an elevated structure containing the receptor cells. The hair-like projections from these cells are inserted into a jelly-like covering, called the cupula. When the head moves, fluid movement within the canals causes a deflection of the cupula and activates the receptors. Impulses generated pass to the brain via the vestibulocochlear nerve. Comparison of the information from each crista, and each ear, gives information regarding the direction and plane of head movement, if it is rotational, and how rapidly it is moving. These receptors are therefore important if head position changes rapidly.

Joint receptors

Joint receptors are nerve endings found within the cartilage and synovial capsule of the joint. They respond to distortion of the joint and provide information regarding the position or change of position of the joint (a 'static' property), and the rate of change and acceleration during joint movement ('dynamic' properties)

Tendon receptors (or Golgi tendon organs)

Receptors within the tendons of muscles are composed of small bundles of collagenous fibres enclosed in a capsule and supplied with

(a)

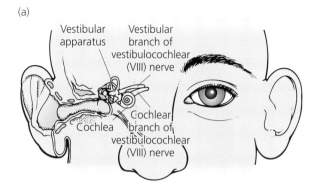

(b)

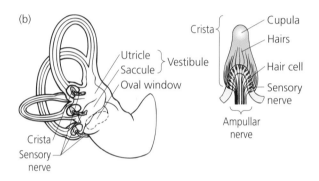

(c)

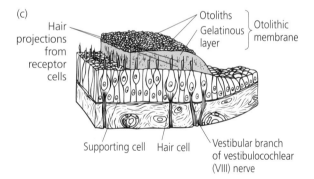

Figure 16.27 The vestibular apparatus. (a) General position. (b) Crista of the semicircular canals. (c) Otolithic membrane of the utricle/saccule.

nerve endings. They are arranged in line with the muscle fibres and provide information regarding fibre tension. Their role in posture and movement is unclear, however, as muscle 'spindle' receptors are more important in monitoring muscle length. It is likely that tendon receptors provide a protective function by prompting a sudden cessation of muscle contraction if excessive tension is being applied to the tendons. In this way the tendons are prevented from damage, or even separation from the bone. This action is observed, for example, when muscles apparently 'give way' if a too-heavy object is being lifted.

Muscle spindles

These receptors are named because of their spindle shape. The receptor is actually a collection of modified muscle fibres enclosed within a connective tissue capsule (Figure 16.28). The fibres are said to be intrafusal (intra- = inside; fusiform = spindle-like), to distinguish them from the other muscle fibres, which are said to be extrafusal. The spindle fibres are joined by connective tissue to adjacent extrafusal fibres, and so any stretching or shortening of the latter will also cause distortion of the spindle, and a change in intrafusal fibre length.

The length of intrafusal fibres is monitored by sensory nerve endings (Figure 16.28). Primary afferent endings spiral around the centre of the spindle fibres, whilst the secondary afferents are 'flower-spray' endings which innervate the ends of the spindle fibres. The primary sensory neuron is of the type IA (i.e. large diameter, myelinated and very rapidly conducting; see Chapter 13). The secondary sensory neuron is slower conducting and is classified as a type II neuron.

Both types of sensory nerve ending respond when the length of the intrafusal fibre is altered, and continue to do so for a period of time after. The nerve activity therefore conveys static information regarding spindle, and hence muscle, length. The primary endings also impart information regarding the rate of change, and so provide a dynamic component.

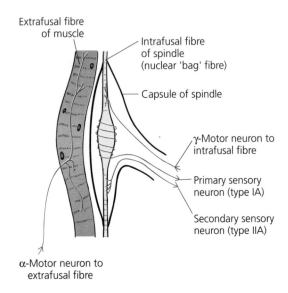

Figure 16.28 A muscle spindle fibre and its innervation. See text for details.

The spindles also have a motor efferent innervation (classified as gamma-neurons, or gamma-efferents; see Chapter 13) which causes the intrafusal fibres to contract in the same way that nerve activity contracts the extrafusal fibres of the muscle. This has implications for the control of muscle length, as the next section illustrates.

MUSCLE SPINDLES IN POSTURE CONTROL: REFLEXES

A reflex response is extremely rapid and involves neural pathways which are integrated within the spinal cord, thus removing the necessity to process information by the brain, which would introduce a delay before the response was initiated. The importance of reflexes in postural control cannot be over-emphasized.

Some reflexes are apparent soon after birth, including the feeding reflex, the grasping reflex, and the 'positive supporting reaction' seen as an extension of the legs when firm

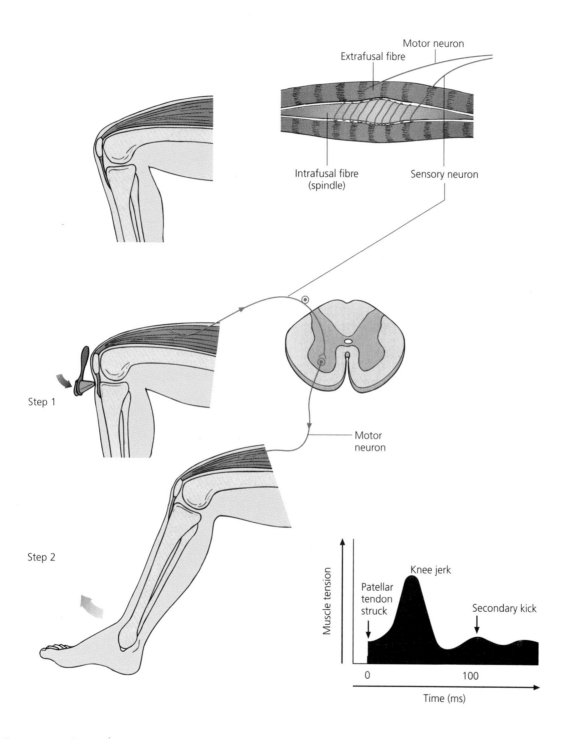

Figure 16.29 The 'stretch' reflex as illustrated by the 'knee jerk'. Step 1: when a reflex hammer strikes the patellar tendon, the muscle spindle fibres stretch, resulting in a burst of activity in the afferent fibres that synapse on motor neurons inside the spinal cord. Step 2: an immediate reflexive kick is produced by the activation of motor units in the stretched muscle. A small secondary kick may occur if the leg rebounds past its resting position. This can be seen in the graph.

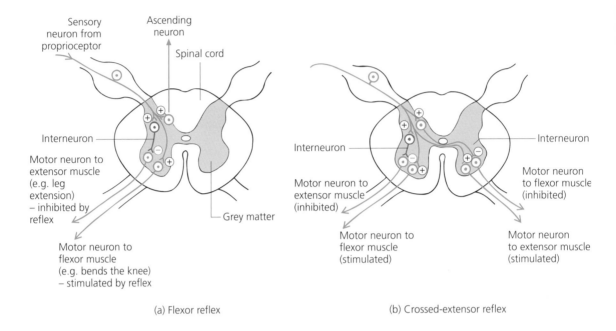

(a) Flexor reflex   (b) Crossed-extensor reflex

Figure 16.30 (a) Flexor reflex. Influence of a stimulus to promote a flexor response, and a relaxation (inhibition) of limb extensors. This promotes leg withdrawal. (b) Crossed-extensor reflex. Influence of same stimulus to promote flexor response on same side, and to stimulate extensors on the opposite side. Opposite leg will be extended to support the change in body position.

contact is made on the soles of the feet. Many reflexes become modified as the baby grows. For example, the reflex changes in position of body and limb, induced by stimulating the vestibular apparatus of the ear, must remain operative during involuntary head movement but must be suppressed during voluntary movement of the head.

A reflex change in muscle contraction results from the stimulation of a receptor, the conduction of sensory activity to the central nervous system via sensory neurons, and the activation of motor neurons which promote contraction of the appropriate muscle. The fundamental elements of a reflex are illustrated by the 'stretch' reflex observed in stimulating a 'knee jerk'.

The 'knee-jerk' is induced by tapping the patellar tendon, which attaches the extensor muscle of the knee (the quadriceps femoris) to the tibia (Figure 16.29). Tapping the tendon therefore stretches the fibres of the quadriceps,

and increases the length of the spindles within it. The sensory nerve endings of the intrafusal fibres are activated and impulses pass along the sensory neurons to the spinal cord. Here the afferent neurons synapse directly with rapidly conducting motor nerve cells which convey impulses to the extrafusal muscle fibres of the quadriceps, causing them to contract. As a consequence the muscle shortens and the knee is extended. The presence of only one synapse in the sensory neuron–motor neuron pathway means that this is a monosynaptic reflex arc. Other reflexes may utilize interneurons in the pathway, thus increasing the number of synapses and the time taken to initiate a response.

The role of the 'stretch' reflex is to keep muscle length constant. Thus if the muscle spindle receptors are stretched, the muscle contracts. The significance of this can be seen in two commonplace examples:

1 Consider a situation in which an individual is standing by a supermarket shelf, contemplating what to buy, when he is bumped into by another shopper. The unexpected change in posture causes involuntary changes in the length and tension of various muscles and reflex responses of spindle activation play an important role in the quick return to stability. Other synergistic and postural muscles will also be activated partly because of the stimulation of other proprioreceptors, and partly because of synapses between spindle sensory neurons and other motor neurons in the spinal cord.

The interactions of spindle sensory neurons and motor neurons in the spinal cord are schematically shown in Figure 16.30. By involving interneurons the reflex response can simultaneously promote contraction of the muscle which was stretched, contraction of appropriate muscles in another limb, and relaxation of antagonistic muscles (which facilitates the shortening of the agonistic muscle). The stretch reflex thus makes a powerful contribution to the maintenance of posture.

2 When an object such as a ball is thrown for us to catch, or when we intend to lift an object, we unconsciously appraise the forces required, based on object size, composition, etc. An appropriate muscle tension is generated but if we have under- or overestimated, then control of the situation is lost. If the object was heavier than anticipated then muscles in the arm will be stretched, activating the spindles and reflexly stimulating further muscle contraction. In this example, the spindles are providing a servocontrol, and can be directly linked into homeostatic theory (Figure 16.31).

The muscle spindle, then, has an important role in determining muscle length. The actual length induced can be altered by the activation of the gamma-efferent neurons to the spindle fibres. Stimulation of these motor neurons by the central nervous system alters intrafusal fibre length independent of the length of extrafusal fibres. The spindle will be stimulated,

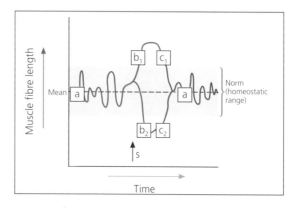

Figure 16.31 Muscle spindles providing servocontrol when an object is caught or lifted (S, stimulus, i.e. object impact on hand or lift begun).
a Setting of muscle length by muscle spindle activation following mental assessment of weight of object.
b_1 Extension of muscle due to weight of object being *greater* than anticipated. Stretch applied to muscle spindles.
b_2 Decrease of muscle length due to weight of object being *less* than anticipated. Muscle spindles shorten.
c_1 Restoration of muscle length following spindle activation, as a result of reflex activation of muscle contraction.
c_2 Restoration of muscle length due to spindle deactivation, as a result of reflex decrease in muscle tone.

however, and the muscle will reflexly contract accordingly (or relax if efferent activity is reduced so that intrafusal fibres relax). The spindle, therefore, can act to restore muscle length if it is suddenly altered by external forces, as in the 'stretch' reflex, but can also modify the muscle length at any moment in time as a consequence of gamma-efferent stimulation by the brain.

Apart from synapsing with motor neurons, spindle afferents will also synapse with ascending neurons within the cord, conveying information to appropriate areas of the brain, and so maintaining the constant awareness of spatial positioning.

MUSCLE SPINDLES DURING MOVEMENT

The role of muscle spindles to regulate muscle length means that they could potentially act to

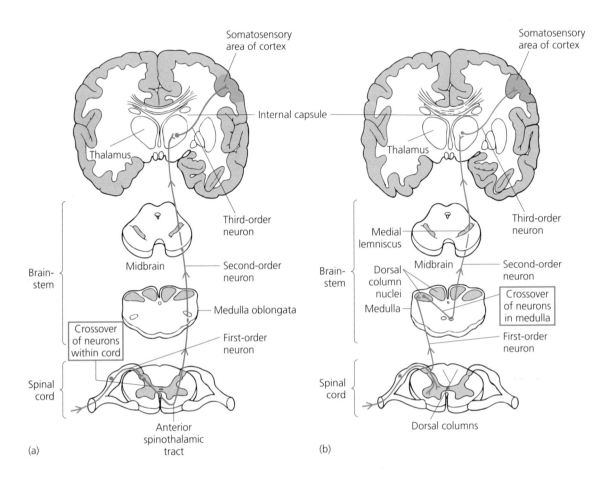

Figure 16.32 Sensory input from proprioceptors (other than vestibular) to the sensory cortex. (a) Anterior spinothalamic pathway. (b) Posterior spinothalamic pathway.

restrict movement by preventing the necessary muscular changes. A mechanism is therefore required to vary the length of muscle maintained by the spindle, and this is due to the efferent motor innervation of the intrafusal fibres of the spindles.

Individual muscles are contracted during voluntary movement via activation of their motor neurons as a consequence of activity generated in the brain and transmitted to them. Contraction of the extrafusal fibres will, of course, tend to shorten the intrafusal fibres of the spindles and reduce their length also; the reflex response to the reduced tension would be to cause muscle relaxation. In fact this is prevented by the simultaneous co-activation of the gamma-efferent neurons to the spindles, which causes the intrafusal fibres to contact simultaneously with the extrafusal fibres. In this way spindle tension is maintained and the sensory nerve endings do not detect any change in intrafusal fibre stretch.

INTERIM SUMMARY

It is clear from the preceding discussions that the control of individual muscle contraction involves a complex integration of sensory information and the activation of appropriate motor neurons. The brain receives a bewildering array of information regarding every aspect of posture, and also moment-to-moment updates on how the position of body parts and body orientation is changing. Motor neuron output must strike a balance between that produced by reflex responses to changes in muscle/tendon activity, and that produced by motor output from the brain. Apart from simultaneously controlling the motor activity to each of the 600+ muscles of the body, the brain must also control the co-activation of muscle spindle fibres. Clearly the control of posture and movement is of a complexity of the highest order, and much of the brain is concerned with that control. The next section considers some of the parts of the brain involved.

NEURAL INTEGRATION IN THE CONTROL OF POSTURE AND MOVEMENT

Brain architecture was described in Chapter 13, and readers are referred to that chapter for supplementary material.

Sensory input

Sensory information from the muscles, tendons, and joints, together with that from various touch and vibration mechanoreceptors, pass to the somatosensory (soma = body) areas of the cerebral cortex or to the cerebellum. The main tracts of spinal cord neurons which convey this information are the posterior spinothalamic tracts (i.e. in the posterior aspect of the cord and passing to the thalamus), and the spinocerebellar tracts (from cord to cerebellum).

Neurons of the spinothalamic tracts ascend the cord and synapse with neurons in the dorsal column nuclei of the medulla oblongata (Figure 16.32). From here projections cross over to the other side of the medulla and thence pass to the thalamus via the brainstem tract

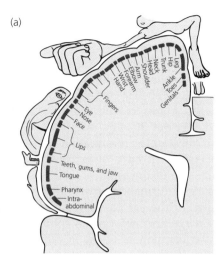

(a)

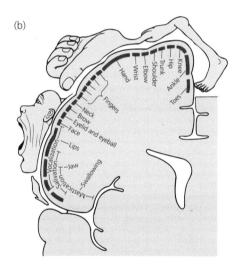

(b)

Figure 16.33 Topographical analysis of the sensory and motor areas of the cerebral cortex. (a) Somatosensory cortex, right hemisphere. (b) Motor cortex, right hemisphere.

called the medial lemniscus, and then they are relayed to the cerebral cortex. The crossover in the medulla means that information from one side of the body passes to the opposite side of the brain.

Areas of the somatosensory cortex can be identified which receive information from particular parts of the body (Figure 16.33a). More grey matter is devoted to the face and hands than, say, to the entire trunk, and this relates to the complexity and volume of information from those parts.

The spinocerebellar tracts ascend the lateral aspects of the cord to the medulla where they pass to the cerebellar cortex via the cerebellar peduncles. Many of the neurons will have crossed over but this time within the cord, and so again most of the information from one side of the body will have been conveyed to the opposite side of the brain.

Sensory information from the vestibular apparatus of the ear passes to the brain via a cranial nerve and not via the spinal cord: the vestibular component of the vestibulocochlear nerve sends fibres to the vestibular nuclei of the medulla, and to the cerebellum. Some information is conveyed from the medulla to the superior colliculi of the midbrain, which are areas involved in coordinating eye movement. In this way, head movement detected by the vestibular receptors induces appropriate changes in eye position (these are called vestibulo-ocular reflexes).

Table 16.1 Principal forebrain and midbrain nuclei, or basal ganglia, involved in the control of voluntary and involuntary movement

Cerebral nuclei
  Caudate nuclei (cauda = tail)
  Lentiform nuclei (lenticula = lens)
  Putamen (= shell)
  Globus pallidus (= pale ball)
  Amygdaloid nuclei (amygda = almond)

Midbrain nuclei
  Substantia nigra (= black substance)
  Red nuclei
  Subthalamic nuclei
  Reticular formation (rete = net)

Motor output

The mass of sensory information received by the brain is constantly monitored, integrated and relayed to those areas which determine the motor output from the brain. This output originates from various parts of the brain: the motor

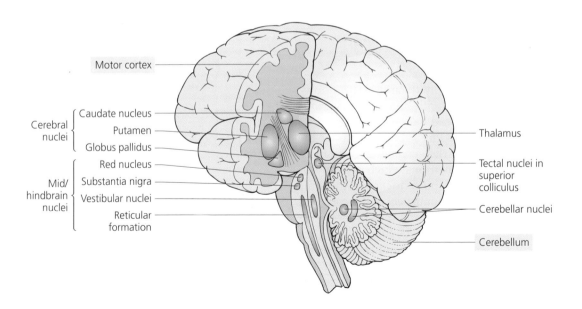

Figure 16.34 Some of the structures of the brain involved in the control of movement.

cortex, the basal ganglia, and the cerebellum.

The motor cortex is an extensive area of grey matter which occupies parts of the frontal and parietal lobes of the cerebral hemispheres, and lies immediately anterior to the somatosensory cortex (Chapter 13). The motor cortex can also be 'mapped' (Figure 16.33b). The complexity of controlling hand and facial movements is reflected in the disproportionate areas involved in their coordination.

The basal ganglia are a number of paired masses of grey matter within the cerebral hemispheres; these are collectively called the cerebral nuclei. Some midbrain nuclei, however, are functionally linked with the cerebral nuclei and are usually considered as components of the basal ganglia. The names of the nuclei reflect their appearance to early anatomists, or their position. Major ones are identified in Table 16.1 and Figure 16.34.

The presence of identifiable structures in the control of posture and movement has enabled research to determine some of their roles. In general terms the motor cortex appears to be involved in the production of precise movements, whilst the basal ganglia seem to be involved in the subconscious production of gross intentional movement, rhythmic movements such as walking, and the positioning of the body prior to producing an intended movement. This compartmentalization of the control of muscle contraction is too simplistic, however, and the cortex and basal ganglia exhibit numerous interconnections (excitatory and inhibitory), some of which even form 'circular' pathways so that neural activity feeds back onto the grey matter whence it came.

Further connections are present between the cortex, the basal ganglia and the cerebellum. Observations indicate that the cerebellum 'assists' the other areas by controlling the timing and sequence of contractions. The cerebellum therefore has a vital role in the precise control of fine movements necessary for writing, for hitting a tennis ball, or for placing the foot during walking (i.e. without stamping!), for example.

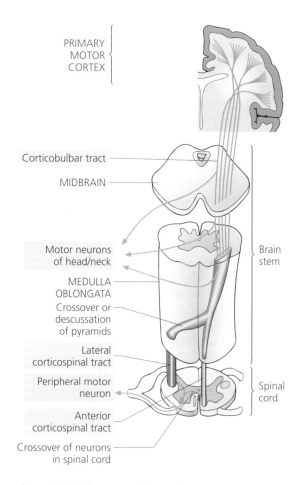

Figure 16.35 The pyramidal tracts from the motor cortex to muscles. The major tracts of neurons are identified in colour.

Once integrated, motor output passes to the skeletal muscles via two major pathways: the pyramidal and extrapyramidal systems.

Pyramidal pathways

The pyramidal pathway originates from the motor cortex. Nerve fibres descend through the brain and either pass down the spinal cord (via corticospinal tracts) to synapse in grey matter with the appropriate peripheral motor neuron, or pass to the nuclei of various cranial nerves within the brainstem (via corticobulbar tracts). Neurons of the tracts which lie within the brain or cord are referred to as upper motor neurons, whilst peripheral fibres are lower motor neurons.

The lateral and anterior corticospinal tracts are the main ones of the pyramidal pathway (Figure 16.35). The lateral tracts are characterized by the crossing over, or decussation, of the upper motor neurons within the medulla, where the tracts are actually called the pyramids. The anterior tract fibres cross over within the grey matter of the cord, where they synapse with the lower motor neurons. The crossing over means that the muscles of one side of the body are controlled by the opposite side of the brain.

The corticobulbar tracts do not project to the spinal cord at all and are involved in the control of movements of the head and neck, via the various cranial nerves.

Extrapyramidal pathway

The extrapyramidal pathway includes all those motor tracts that are not part of the pyramidal system. They normally originate in the brainstem components of the basal ganglia and are named according to their site of origin:

RUBROSPINAL TRACTS (RUBRO = RED)

These originate from the red nuclei of the midbrain. Fibres cross over and descend in the lateral aspects of the cord.

TECTOSPINAL TRACTS (TECTUM = ROOF)

These originate from the superior colliculi of the tectum area of the midbrain, which receive input from the eyes. This tract is therefore part of the pathway which controls movement in response to visual stimuli.

VESTIBULOSPINAL TRACTS

These derive from the vestibular nuclei of the medulla, and are influenced by input from the vestibular receptors of the inner ear.

Examples of homeostatic failures and principles of correction

The failure of the skeletomuscular system to provide anti-gravity support, with consequences for posture and/or movement, results from a variety of skeletal and muscular disturbances.

SKELETAL DISTURBANCES

Skeletal disorders can be divided into those resulting from a loss of bone strength and those from joint disorder (Figure 16.36).

Bone strength

One of the most common mobility problems is that caused by bone fracture. This may result from accidental application of excessive physical stress on a bone, but can also arise during normal activity if bone density and/or flexibility are compromised.

Loss of bone mineral and matrix are observed in osteoporosis, a common problem of ageing. The high incidence of the condition in elderly women reflects the role of oestrogens in bone maintenance prior to the menopause.

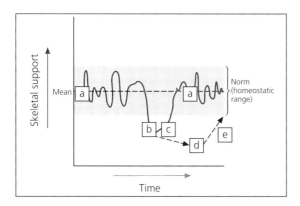

Figure 16.36 Skeletal support as a homeostatic mechanism.
a Combined strength of bone and skeletal structure sufficient to maintain body weight, as a result of adequate bone density, and joint support and flexibility.
b Decreased capability to maintain posture against gravity due to loss of bone density or joint support.
c Restoration of posture maintenance due to improved bone density or joint repair or joint replacement.
d Persistent failure to maintain skeletal support due to sustained bone weakness (e.g. by irreversible PTH-secreting tumours or advanced age) or to sustained joint failure.
e Restoration of capability to support body weight via the use of aids.

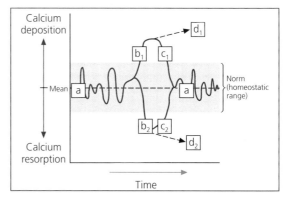

Figure 16.37 Schematic representation of the deposition/resorption of calcium into/from bone.
a Balance between the release of calcium from bone (= resorption) and calcium deposition.
b_1 Enhanced calcium deposition in response to the release of the hormone calcitonin (when plasma Ca^{2+} is elevated above normal) or when the bone is regularly stressed, as in physical exercise, or during bone growth.
b_2 Enhanced calcium resorption in response to parathyroid hormone (when plasma Ca^{2+} is lower than normal) or during enforced bed-rest.
c_1, c_2 Restoration of balance when plasma calcium concentration is normalized or (for c_1) when growth slows, or (for c_2) if bed-rest ends.
d_1 Persistent bone deposition in, e.g. osteopetrosis ('brittle' bones).
d_2 Persistent bone resorption due to PTH-secreting tumour, or (in females) oestrogen withdrawal following the menopause.

Compression fractures of the vertebrae and fractures of the neck of femur are frequent consequences of the loss of bone strength. Conversely, brittle bones are also produced if the mineral : matrix ratio is excessive, i.e. when bones are too dense and flexibility is lost. This is called osteopetrosis.

Loss of mineral alone, with maintenance of the protein matrix, produces weakened but pliable bones. This is called osteomalacia and is observed when calcium resorption from bone is in excess of calcium deposition, as in vitamin D deficiency (or rickets). Osteomalacia is also observed as a secondary effect of certain tumours which secrete parathyroid hormone and promote excessive calcium resorption from bone.

Inflammatory disease of bone (osteitis or Paget's disease), as distinct from osteomyelitis, an inflammatory disease of the marrow cavity promotes the development of cysts within bone and so reduces bone density.

Bone calcification homeostasis is depicted in Figure 16.37. Correction of a disorder is directed at removing the underlying cause. The onset of age-related osteoporosis in women is markedly slowed by early post-menopausal oestrogen-replacement therapy.

Joint disorders

Weight-bearing joints must be strong but must also remain flexible. Inflammatory disease (osteoarthritis) results in the loss of joint cartilage and calcification of the joint capsule, and drastically reduces joint flexibility. The frictional contact between bones exacerbates the inflammation, causes bone erosion and induces pain. Joint inflammation is also observed in rheumatoid disease. Inflammation specifically of the vertebral joints is called spondylitis, and ossification of the joint tissue is referred to as ankylosing spondylitis. Both conditions reduce vertebral flexibility and restrict mobility.

Torn joint ligaments are often observed in sports injuries, in which excessive physical forces are applied, and may be secondary to joint dislocation.

Correction of joint disorder may involve a reconstruction of the joint structure (called arthroplasty), or surgical removal/repair of torn cartilages. Total joint replacement with artificial joints may be necessary in advanced inflammatory disease.

Joint disorder may also be secondary to muscle problems. For example, scoliosis is a misalignment of vertebrae which produces a lateral curvature of the vertebral column, and is caused by unbalanced muscle strength on either side of the column, or by a laxity of ligaments.

MUSCLE DISTURBANCES

Postural and movement disorders resulting from failure to maintain an appropriate muscle contraction arise because of (1) a defect of the muscle fibre itself; (2) inappropriate fibre activation by the motor neuron; or (3) a disorder of the central nervous system (Figure 16.38).

Muscle fibre defect

Muscle weakness due to fibre defect usually occurs when the fibre is deficient in protein filaments or if the sarcolemma structure prevents it from being electrically stimulated. Fibre protein is adversely affected in malnutrition, and diabetes mellitus, when the protein is utilized as an energy substrate, and in prolonged bed-rest when the lack of physical stress removes the need for muscles to produce a large force of contraction.

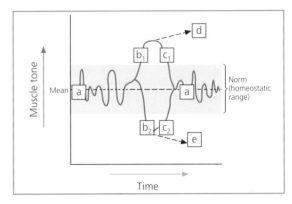

Figure 16.38 Maintenance of appropriate muscle tone as a homeostatic function.

a Degree of muscle contraction, at any given time, sufficient to maintain appropriate joint support.

b_1 Excessive muscle contraction, resulting in decreased muscle spindle tension.

b_2 Deficient muscle contraction, resulting in muscle spindle stretch.

c_1, c_2 Reflex restoration of muscle tone, mediated by the muscle spindles.

d Persistent muscle contraction due to persistently elevated motor neuron activity (e.g. some time after spinal cord section or excessive output from the brain) or due to over-excitability of sarcolemma (e.g. during an alkalosis, or tetanus). Spasticity results.

e Persistently deficient muscle contraction due to muscle fibre defect (e.g. muscular dystrophy), neuromuscular synapse defect (e.g. myasthenia gravis), or inadequate motor neuron activity (e.g. multiple sclerosis, polyneuritis, motor neuron disease). Muscle weakness or paralysis ensues.

The contraction of a muscle fibre requires the induction of an action potential, or electrical change, in the sarcolemma. In Duchenne's muscular dystrophy a structural protein of the sarcolemma, called dystrophin, is deficient. The role of dystrophin is still poorly understood but its lack causes the muscle weakness and eventual wastage typical of this inherited disorder.

Correction of muscle fibre disorder is directed at removing the underlying cause, and physiotherapy to maintain existing muscle. In the case of Duchenne's dystrophy, the gradual development of genetic therapies raises some hope that the underlying gene mutation can be corrected.

Inappropriate neuromuscular excitation

Providing that the central nervous system is intact, the excitation of muscle depends upon the properties of the sarcolemma itself, the neuromuscular synapse, and the peripheral motor neuron.

Excitation of the sarcolemma involves an influx of sodium ions (i.e. electrical current) which depolarizes the membrane. The 'threshold' at which the action potential is induced depends upon the ease at which ionic influx can be activated. The threshold is susceptible to calcium ion concentration in the extracellular fluid (not the calcium released intracellularly following stimulation) and acute reductions in calcium concentration induced by an alkalosis, which alters the ratio of free calcium ions : calcium bound to plasma protein, can result in such a lowering of the threshold that a maximal muscle contraction is produced (i.e. tetany). Another cause of tetany is the release of toxins by certain micro-organisms, and thus is referred to as tetanus.

Excitation also requires a functional neuromuscular synapse. Inadequate acetylcholine production or release, or an inadequate number of receptors in the post-synaptic membrane (i.e. the sarcolemma) will prevent activation. The antagonism of acetylcholine by curare-like drugs is used clinically to relax muscles prior to surgery. Similar effects of synaptic dysfunction are observed in the muscle weakness disorder myasthenia gravis.

Disorder of the motor neurons supplying the muscles may result from a deterioration of the neuron itself (as in the inherited spinal muscular atrophies), inflammation of the neuron (polyneuritis) as a consequence of infection, or from a loss of myelin from the neuron (e.g. in multiple sclerosis, and poliomyelitis).

Crushing the nerve, for example when an intervertebral disc has prolapsed, or if muscles of the lower back undergo spasm contractions, will affect associated muscle function and also induce severe pain.

Correction of neuromuscular disorders is limited as many are inherited disorders, or result from autoimmune responses, and cause considerable damage to the tissues. Therapies are usually directed at maintaining/improving remnant muscle strength using physiotherapy and exercise to increase the physical stresses on those muscles. Postural changes may require certain muscle groups to be targeted to restore normal joint function.

CENTRAL NERVOUS SYSTEM DISORDER

This chapter has described the complex anatomical structures required for the maintenance of posture and mobility, but also has highlighted the degree of control exercised by the central nervous system. Disorders of those control areas have pronounced effects on the ability to maintain posture or to produce precise, or even gross, movement.

Loss of sensory input, or the prevention of the transmission of neural activity to peripheral motor neurons, reduces the capacity of the brain to control movement. Thus spinal cord injury, neuron inflammation (polyneuritis), loss of myelin (multiple sclerosis, poliomyelitis) and motor neuron degeneration (motor neuron disease) have severe effects.

Although protected by the cranium, the position of the cerebral cortex and cerebellar cortex at the surface of the brain make these structures susceptible to damage from head trauma, or from subarachnoid or subdural haemorrhage. Both cortices have central roles in the coordination of movement.

Deeper structures, such as the basal ganglia, are less susceptible to physical trauma but will be affected by localized hypoxia resulting from cerebrovascular haemorrhage (stroke), circulatory restriction (e.g. at birth leading to cerebral palsy), or restricted respiration (e.g. asphyxia, drug-induced dyspnoea). Glucose deficiency during hypoglycaemic episodes may also induce temporary disorder as energy requirements of neurons are not met.

Disturbance in the balance of excitatory : inhibitory neuronal pathways will disrupt the integration necessary to produce controlled movement. This may be caused by loss of myelination (as in multiple sclerosis) or by neurotransmitter disorder. Thus, Parkinson's disease produces movement disorder because of a deficiency of the inhibitory transmitter dopamine in tracts from the substantia nigra to other basal ganglia. Similarly, the movements characteristic of Huntington's chorea, or St Vitus' dance, result from a deficiency of the inhibitor transmitter gamma aminobutyric acid (GABA) from other tracts.

Summary

1 The skeletomuscular system provides the support and mobility required for the performance of basic activities of living.

2 The skeleton consists of spongy and compact bone, the strength of which is determined by the density of mineral and by the structural organization of the tissue.

3 Skeletal joints vary in their degree of flexibility. Those essential for movement are called synovial joints, and enclose a lubricant-filled space. Where joints are subjected to considerable physical stresses, the structure is strengthened by extensive ligaments and by powerful postural muscles.

4 The strength of certain joints, particularly the knee joint and the joints of the pelvis, facilitate support of the body weight during standing. Curvatures within the skeleton, namely of the vertebral column, femur and foot arches, help to absorb the physical forces applied to the skeleton during standing, walking, and running.

5 Muscles support the skeleton and provide the capacity to move joints. They are comprised of bundles of muscle fibres, called fascicles, and are activated by associated motor nerves. Muscle fibres are a functional syncytium of cells which became fused together during differentiation. Each fibre acts as one cell and stimulation contracts the entire fibre.

6 Under the microscope, muscle fibres exhibit a striated pattern which repeats along the fibre. Each 'segment' is called a sarcomere, and the striations result from the arrangement of protein filaments within it.

7 Muscle fibre contraction involves an interaction between the actin and myosin protein filaments. Molecular cross-bridges between the proteins cause the actin to 'slide' over the myosin, thus pulling the ends of the sarcomere together and so shortening the fibre. The process requires the presence of calcium ions, released into the cytoplasm of the muscle fibre as a consequence of nerve stimulation.

8 The neuromuscular junction exhibits the properties of a synapse, utilizing the release of the neurotransmitter acetylcholine, which induces a change in the electrical property of the muscle fibre. Each muscle fibre within a muscle is innervated, but the numbers of fibres, called a motor unit, that are innervated by branches from a single motor neuron varies from muscle to muscle. Large postural muscles in particular have large 'motor units' and this aids the efficiency of maintaining protracted periods of contraction.

9 Muscle fibres capable of maintaining contraction for long periods must utilize aerobic metabolism in order for them to withstand fatigue. These are called 'slow' fibres. In relative terms, 'fast' fibres produce a much faster contraction and relaxation but rapidly exceed aerobic capacity and therefore fatigue quickly.

10 The arrangement of muscles in relation to joints provides a system of levers which facilitates movement by reducing the force of contraction necessary to move the joint.

11 The degree of contraction produced by a muscle must be appropriate to the situation, and this means that all of the 600+ muscles of the body must be individually controlled. Control is provided by reflex action and by coordination of the neural output from the brain.

12 Sensory information is provided by proprio-ceptors, or positional receptors. These are found in the joints, tendons of muscles, in the muscles themselves, and in the inner ear (balance or equilibrium receptors) and provide continuous information regarding the position and movement of joints, of tension in muscles, of muscle length, and of head position in relation to gravity.

13 Muscle spindle receptors are of particular importance as these not only monitor muscle length but can also act to control that length. This is possible because they consist of modified muscle fibres and can be induced to contract or relax according to activity of their own motor innervation. Thus spindle length can be varied independently of the rest of the muscle, and in doing so can reflexly induce muscle contraction or relaxation. Muscle length, therefore, is determined by the neural activity in the motor nerve cells which inner-vate its fibres, and also by the motor nerve cells which innervate the spindles. This dual innervation provides a high degree of control, and also emphasizes the complex nature of motor coordination provided by the brain.

14 Much of the brain is involved in receiving sensory information from around the body, and in motor control. The latter areas are the motor cortex of the cerebrum, the basal ganglia), and the cerebellum of the hindbrain. Interactions between these areas occur, involv-ing complex excitatory and inhibitory neural pathways, before the final activity is conveyed to the appropriate peripheral motor neurons.

15 Disturbances of skeletal and muscle structure, of the innervation of muscle fibres and of the control of motor nerve activity from the central nervous system, are responsible for many mobility disorders. Their occurrence emphasizes the combined role of the skeleton and associated muscles in posture and movement control.

Review Questions

1 Discuss the importance of movement and posture to health.

2 How do compact and spongy bone differ in structure?

3 Name the specific osteocytes involved with the following functions:
(a) bone formation; (b) bone reabsorption.

4 Distinguish between axial and appendicular skeletons, listing the bones associated with each skeletal system.

5 How are joints classified?

6 What are the general rules applied to nomenclature of muscles?

7 Describe a neuromuscular junction.

8 Describe the molecular machinery of muscle contraction.

9 Define the following terms with reference to contraction of the whole muscle:
(a) twitch, (b) isotonic, (c) isometric.

10 List the adaptations of the human skeleton which enable bipedal posture.

11 Distinguish between 'slow' and 'fast' muscle fibres.

12 Distinguish between the origin and insertion of a muscle.

13 What is the function of the following muscles:
(a) an agonist (prime mover); (b) a synergist; (c) an antagonist.

14 Name the proprioreceptors found in the human body and briefly describe their location and function.

15 Describe the role of muscle spindles in the reflex response.

16 List the reflexes that are present at birth.

17 Consider the neural integration of sensory input and motor output in the control of posture and movement.

18 Distinguish between the pyramidal and extrapyramidal pathways.

19 How can sense organ malfunction affect posture and movement?

20 List the homeostatic imbalances of posture and movement associated with the following:
(a) skeletal disorders, (b) muscle disorders.

The skin: Regulation of body temperature

17

Introduction: influence of temperature on cellular homeostasis

Overview of the anatomy and functions of the skin

Details of the physiology of temperature regulation

Role of the skin in homeostasis

Examples of homeostatic control system failures and principles of correction

Summary

Review questions

Introduction: influence of temperature on cellular homeostasis

The rate at which metabolic reactions proceed within a cell generally depends upon four factors:

1 the provision of appropriate substrate;

2 the presence of appropriate enzymes;

3 the chemical environment within the cell;

4 the prevailing temperature.

Genes and integrated systemic functions are responsible for ensuring that conditions are conducive for functional optima. The optimum temperature for metabolic processes to occur in man is 36–37°C and values lower than this will reduce the rate of chemical reaction. In contrast, although higher temperatures might be expected to increase the rate of reaction as more energy is put into the process, the reverse is usually observed. This is because the additional heat energy breaks the weak hydrogen bonds between amino acids within protein molecules (including enzymes) and this disturbs their three-dimensional shape. The denaturing of enzymes results in the loss of specific binding sites (see Chapter 3) with the consequence that their activities as catalysts are diminished. The temperature optimum is therefore a balance between the effects of heat to promote chemical reactions, and the rate at which enzymes are denatured (Figure 17.1).

Cells, and hence physiological systems, will function most efficiently if temperature is held virtually constant at or close to the optimum. This means homeostatically balancing the rate of heat production by metabolism with the rate of heat transfer across the skin and respiratory surfaces. At rest some 70–75% of metabolic

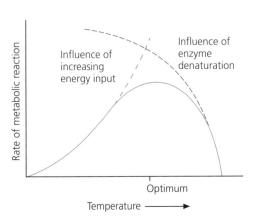

Figure 17.1 Influence of temperature on metabolic processes. Optimal reaction rate is determined by the balance between the effect of energy (heat) input into the reaction, and the thermal denaturation of enzyme (catalyst) structure.

heat is generated by the brain and organs of the chest and abdomen (which comprise the body 'core'), reflecting the extent of metabolic activities of these organs. As we shall see later only the temperature of this 'core' is held constant.

The importance of the skin as the major site of heat transfer between the body and external environment means that the temperature of the peripheral tissues (which comprise the body 'shell') is more variable. Peripheral tissues such as the skin and skeletal muscles are therefore subjected to the effects of variable temperatures, though this usually means cooling and not overheating. The easier it is for heat loss to occur across an area of skin, the lower its temperature will be in relation to other skin areas. The limbs provide the main sites for heat loss as they have a large surface area relative to their volume and will generally have lower temperatures than the skin of the chest and abdomen.

Controlling the rate of heat transfer across the skin is an essential component of the thermoregulatory process, and the skin must be considered to be an organ in its own right. The skin also has other roles, however, and these, together with the anatomy of the skin, are reviewed in the next section.

Overview of the anatomy and functions of the skin

ANATOMY OF THE SKIN

The skin consists of two principal parts: the outer epidermis and the inner dermis (Figure 17.2a). Below the dermis lies a subcutaneous layer (sub- = below; cutaneous = of the skin), sometimes called the superficial fascia. Strictly speaking, this layer does not develop embryologically as part of the skin but it is functionally linked with it.

Epidermis

Cell layers

The epidermis is a stratified squamous epithelium (see Chapter 2) and consists of four layers of cells: a basal layer (= stratum basale), a 'prickly' layer (= stratum spinosum), a granular layer (= stratum granulosum) and a tough cornified layer (= stratum corneum – Figure 17.2b). Areas of skin, such as the soles of the

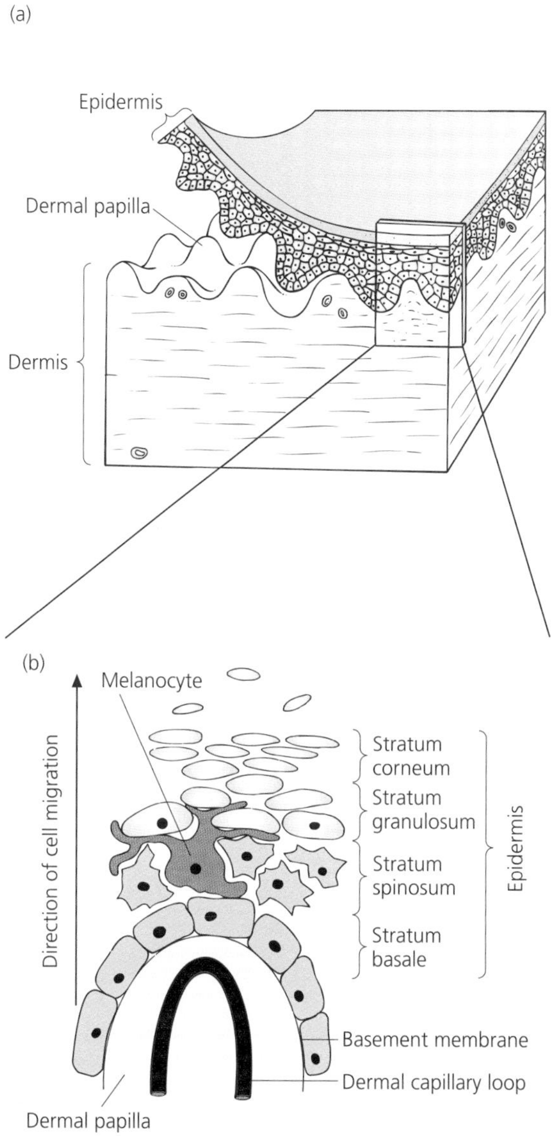

(a)

(b)

Figure 17.2 The epidermis. (a) General plan and relation to the dermis. (b) Cell layers.

feet, that are exposed to considerable frictional stress have a fifth layer, and this is a 'clear' layer called the stratum lucidum that lies between the granular and corneal layers.

Cells of the epidermis are generated by mitotic division of cuboidal/columnar cells of the basal layer, and this layer is often referred to as the germinal layer of the skin. Some of the daughter cells maintain this layer whilst others ascend toward the surface of the skin. Within the stratum spinosum the cells become irregularly shaped and may even appear 'prickly', hence the name of this layer. Tactile nerve endings, called Merkel's disc (see Chapter 14), may also be present in this layer.

Cells continue to ascend and begin to flatten. They also begin to produce keratohyalin, which will eventually be converted to the tough, waterproofing protein keratin. The compound is stored in the cells, and this layer is therefore called the 'granular layer'. Whilst within this layer, the nuclei of the cells begin to degenerate and consequently metabolism declines.

In the skin of the palms and soles the cells may produce a substance which is intermediary between keratohyalin and keratin. This is called eleidin and is a translucent substance. The cells therefore appear clear, and so this layer is called the stratum lucidum.

Cells continue their ascent and eventually become completely filled with keratin. By this time the cells are dead. This is the corneal layer and provides a physical barrier against external physical stresses, and environmental agents such as bacteria and chemicals. The latter include water as the epidermis is impervious.

In total the epidermis is from 0.5–3 mm thick depending upon site. Although its thickness relates to the physical stresses placed on that area of skin, it is ultimately determined by the rate of cell division in the basal layer. Division must be maintained at a rate similar to that of cell attrition from the corneal layer. As mitosis declines with age, therefore, it is not surprising that the epidermis becomes thinner. Epidermal growth factor is a peptide which has been isolated from salivary glands and has been found to promote mitosis in epithelia, including the epidermis, though its precise role in the maintenance of the skin is unclear.

Epidermal coloration: melanocytes

Interspersed amongst cells of the basal and 'prickly' layers are cells called melanocytes

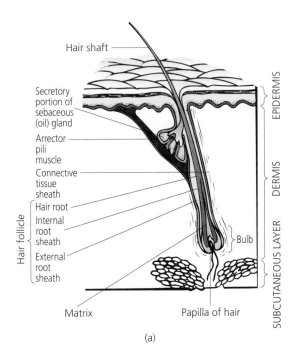

(a)

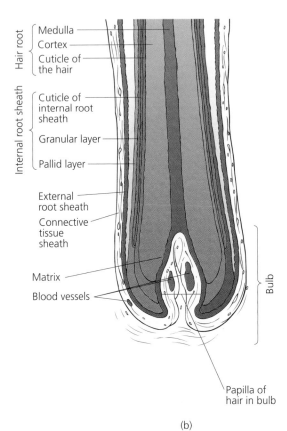

(b)

Figure 17.3 Hair. (a) Principal parts of a hair and associated structures. (b) Longitudinal section of a hair root.

which contain the pigment melanin (Figure 17.2b). These cells have extensive processes. When melanin production is stimulated, pigment released from the processes will be taken up by other epidermal cells and so will pigment most areas of skin. Skin pigmentation primarily relates to the amount of pigment present and there is little racial difference in the numbers of melanocytes present. Melanin protects the underlying basal layer, and dermis, from the harmful effects of ultraviolet radiation from the sun. The pigment is synthesized from the amino acid tyrosine, a process stimulated by the actions of ultraviolet light and by melanocyte-stimulating hormone (MSH), which is released from the anterior and intermediate lobes of the pituitary gland. Albinism, which is characterized by pigment-free melanocytes and hair, occurs when a genetic deficiency prevents the synthesis of those enzymes necessary for the conversion of tyrosine to melanin. People who are albino therefore have a skin which lacks the protection provided by melanin against excessive ultraviolet light.

In the absence of large amounts of pigment the skin is pinkish-white and its coloration is mainly determined by the visualization of blood within it. There are no blood vessels within the epidermis, however, and the demands of the cells are met by vessels within the dermis.

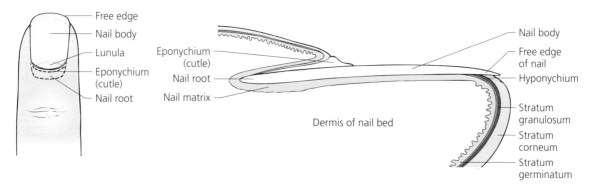

Figure 17.4 Structure of nails. (a) Fingernail viewed from above. (b) Sagittal section of a fingernail and nail bed.

Other epidermal cells

Further cell types are found scattered within the epidermis and these have the forbidding name of non-pigmented granular dendrocytes (dendrite = branch; the characteristics of these cells is that they are granulated and have branching processes). They are cells of the immune system and interact with helper and suppressor T-lymphocytes in assisting immune responses.

Hair and nails: epidermally derived structures

HAIR

The primary function of hair, or pili, is to protect underlying skin or structures. For example, head hair helps to prevent the heating effect of the sun on brain function, and to reduce heat loss in the cold, whilst eyebrows protect the eyes from direct sun and from particulate matter in the air. Touch receptors are also associated with hairs and so hair also has a sensory role.

The shaft of a hair is visible externally and consists of an inner structure of granulated cells and air spaces, a cortex of melanin-pigmented cells (with extensive air spaces in those people with white hair) and an outer cuticular layer of heavily keratinized cells

(Figure 17.3). All cells are of epidermal origin, although the root of the hair penetrates the dermis.

The hair root consists of the growing region of the hair and also a protective sheath. The outer sheath originates from the basal and 'prickly' layers of the epidermis, whilst the inner sheath derives from clusters of germinative cells, called the matrix, which produce new hairs after old ones are shed. A papilla of connective tissue is present below the matrix and contains blood vessels which supply the matrix cells. Collectively the root, matrix and papilla comprise the hair follicle (Figure 17.3).

Ducts of sebaceous glands are associated with hair follicles, although some are also found in hairless skin, such as the lips and eyelids. The secretory portion of the gland lies in the dermis. These glands produce sebum, which is an oily mixture of fats, cholesterol, protein, and salts, that helps to maintain the suppleness of hair and skin, and aids water-proofing of the epidermis. It also contains bactericidal chemicals.

Small arrector muscles within the dermis of the skin are also associated with follicles (Figure 17.3a) and cause the hairs to stand erect, when stimulated. This is an important thermoregulatory mechanism (see below) but also occurs during moments of anxiety and alarm.

About 70–100 hairs are shed from the scalp each day and will be replaced by growth from the matrix. Rates of replacement may be reduced by various stressors, however, ranging from excessive anxiety to the effects of fever.

NAILS

Finger- and toenails consist of extremely hard keratinized epidermal cells. They provide protection for the tips of the fingers and toes and also aid the manipulation of small objects.

The root of the nail is hidden within the nail groove at its base, and largely consists of a germinative matrix which produces cells that will comprise the main nail body (Figure 17.4). The proximal border of the nail and the epidermal cells of the nail groove are lined by a narrow band of epidermis called the cuticle or eponychium.

The nail body typically appears pink because the underlying epidermis is thin and so the vascularized dermis is visible. The white crescent, or lunula, at the nail base is produced by the obscuring of the dermal blood by the thickened epidermal layer below this part of the nail body.

Dermis

The dermis is the subepidermal layer of the skin and is basically composed of connective tissue, including collagen and elastin fibres. These fibres provide the skin with durability and elasticity. The spaces between the fibres contain many of the structures associated with the skin, such as blood vessels, nerves, sensory receptors (including touch and pressure receptors, thermoreceptors and nociceptors) hair follicles, arrector muscles, and the ducts of subcutaneous glands (Figure 17.5). The orientation of collagen fibres within the dermis is useful during surgery since damage is limited if fibres can be prised apart rather than cut across. In this way scarring is reduced.

The upper region of the dermis has small projections called dermal papillae which project into the epidermis. Such papillae contain touch-sensitive receptors (Meissner's corpuscles), and also loops of blood capillaries that supply the active layers of the epidermis. These loops are vertically orientated and are visible as small pin-pricks of blood when the epidermis is grazed. The papillae, which in the fingertips produce the 'fingerprints', are genetically determined and hence have a unique pattern in individuals.

Subcutaneous layer and glands of the skin

This layer consists of areolar connective tissue and adipose tissue, and attaches the dermis to the underlying tissues. Being 'loose' connective tissue, the subcutaneous layer is an ideal site for injection since the volume of injectate is more easily accommodated, and therefore less painful! The presence of relatively few collagen fibres means that the subcutaneous layer allows flexibility of movement of skin across the underlying tissue, and this helps to prevent shearing injuries due to friction.

The subcutaneous layer contains various glandular structures, and the ducts of these pass to the skin surface via the dermis and epidermis. The skin contains three types of gland that produce secretions onto the surface. The sebaceous glands lie within the dermis, but are associated with hair follicles, and were mentioned earlier. The other two types are found in the subcutaneous layer, and these are the sweat (or sudoriferous) glands and the ceruminous glands.

Sweat glands

Sweat, or perspiration, is a mixture of water, salts, and products of metabolism (e.g. urea, uric acid, amino acids, ammonia, lactic acid). The composition can be varied, however, particularly in relation to water and salt content. Most of the sweat produced by the skin is thin and watery, but in some areas it is viscous. Sweat

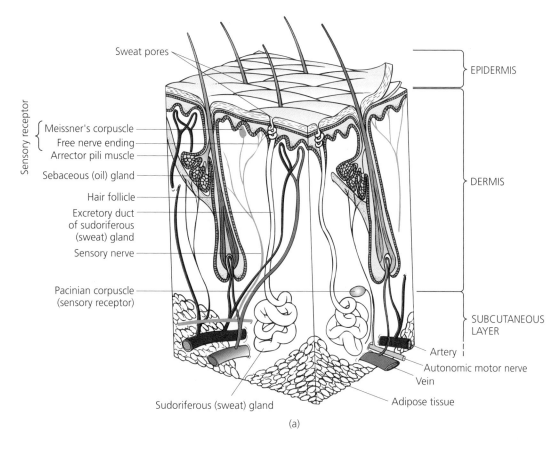

Figure 17.5 Structures of the dermis and subcutaneous layer. Note that hairs are epidermally derived and that sweat glands are actually present in the subcutaneous layer. Not shown are the collagen/elastin fibres which form the matrix of the dermis.

glands can therefore be subdivided into two types, according to the type of sweat they produce and therefore to their structure. These are called the apocrine and eccrine glands.

Apocrine glands are simple tubular structures and are found in the skin of the axillae (armpits), pubic areas, and the areolar areas of the breast. Their secretion is viscous. It has been suggested that apocrine secretions contain pheromones, particularly those which are sexual attractants.

Eccrine glands are more widely distributed, though they are absent from lip margins, penis, labia minora and outer ear. They are simple coiled tubular glands and produce a watery secretion.

Ceruminous glands

These are modified sudoriferous glands and are found within the skin of the auditory canal. The mixture of sebum (from sebaceous glands) and secretions from ceruminous glands forms a sticky wax-like substance called cerumen or ear wax. This provides a barrier to particulate matter and so protects the tympanic membrane. Occasionally the secretion of cerumen may be excessive and induces conditions which promote troublesome bacterial growth. Hearing will also be impeded if excessive wax is present.

Mammary glands are also specialized sudoriferous glands and are described in Chapter 18.

FUNCTIONS OF SKIN

The skin has a major role in the regulation of body temperature, but other roles can be ascribed to it.

Temperature regulation

The importance of skin in the regulation of body temperature was identified earlier and is explained in more detail in the next section. Its vital role stems from it being the main interface between the body and the external environment (its surface area in the adult is some 1.8 m²).

Protection from infection

Being in contact with the external environment, the skin is the first line of defence against potential pathogenic organisms. Apart from being a physical barrier, the bactericidal constituents of sebum and the acidic nature of skin secretions also provide a degree of chemical protection.

Excretion

Sweat contains various substances, including metabolic products. Although normally a relatively minor route for the excretion of 'wastes' and excess substances, nevertheless the amount of substance lost from the body via sweat must be considered a component of total excretion. This is particularly the case for water and salts. For example, even in cool, temperate conditions sweat accounts for almost 10% of the water output from the body, whilst in very hot weather sweat secretion may rise to as much as 4 litres per day and exceed the total excreted by other routes, including urine.

Prevention of tissue dehydration

The exposure of underlying 'wet' tissues to the environment produces extensive loss of water by evaporation, and is a concern during surgical procedures, or when burns are extensive. A skin which is impervious to water when it is intact (note that sweat secretion via ducts is a physiological process) is therefore essential for existence.

Support and shape

This is an obvious role of the skin. Support of the viscera is provided by muscles of the body wall but is facilitated by the tough, durable nature of the overlying skin. Muscles, skin, and adipose tissues also give rise to the body shapes associated with sexual dimorphism.

Details of the physiology of temperature regulation

BASIC PRINCIPLES OF HEAT TRANSFER

Heat can be transferred to or from the environment by three main processes (see Figure 17.6).

Radiation

Any physical body at a temperature above absolute zero (0° Kelvin or –273°C) will radiate energy. The wavelength of energy emission is determined by the actual temperature of the

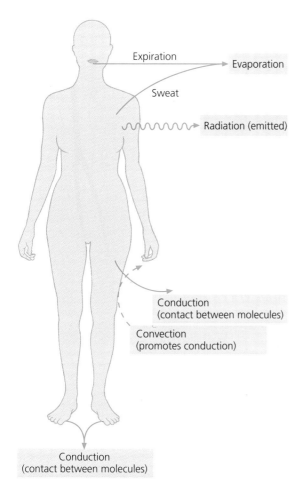

Expiration

Evaporation

Sweat

Radiation (emitted)

Conduction
(contact between molecules)

Convection
(promotes conduction)

Conduction
(contact between molecules)

Figure 17.6 Routes of heat loss from the body. Note that heat *gains* by conduction and radiation will be promoted in hot environments.

body. In humans this is in the infrared region of the spectrum and can be visualized using appropriate aids. Radiation is usually the main way in which heat is lost or gained by the body.

Conduction

Conduction is the direct transfer of energy between molecules which have made physical contact. This will include contact between molecules within the skin and those of air or objects in contact with the skin.

Evaporation

Converting water into vapour requires energy (584 calories or 2450 Joules per ml) and the evaporation of sweat from the skin, or water from the oral cavity and respiratory tract, are effective means of removing heat from the body.

The rate of transfer of heat by radiation and conduction is determined by the temperature gradient which exists between the skin and air. If the skin is warmer than the surrounding air then heat will be lost from it. If it is cooler then heat will be gained from the environment. Convectional currents may replace air warmed at the skin surface with cooler air and so continue to promote heat loss. This is the basis of 'wind chill' factors in weather reports.

TEMPERATURE REGULATORY MECHANISMS IN COLD CLIMATES

Temperature gradients when the environment is cold or cool favour heat loss from the body. The temperature of the body 'core' can only be held constant, therefore, if the production of heat by metabolism matches the rate at which heat is being lost. The homeostatic regulation of the 'core' temperature in cold conditions can therefore utilize two strategies: to lower the temperature gradient between skin and air and so reduce the rate of heat loss, or to increase the rate of metabolic heat production to compensate for the enhanced heat loss (Figure 17.7).

Decreasing the skin–air temperature gradient

The temperature gradient between skin and air can be reduced by either warming the air in contact with the skin, or by reducing the temperature of the skin itself.

Air warming can be widespread (e.g. by raising the central heating or by moving to a warm area!) or local to the skin surface. The

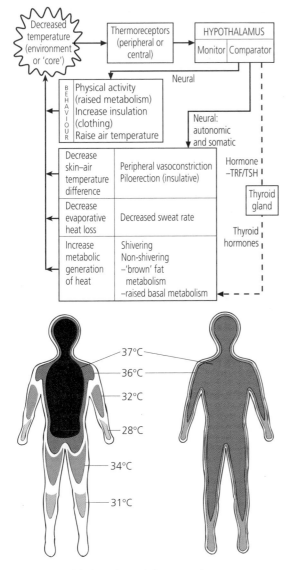

Figure 17.7 (a) Flow chart of thermoregulatory responses to cooling. Note the range of effector mechanisms and tissues employed in the response. See text for details. (b) Temperature distribution in the body of a man at room temperatures of 20°C (left) and at 35°C (right). At 35°C room temperature, a core temperature of 37°C (shaded area) extends almost to the surface of the body. At 20°C room temperature, the core temperature is restricted to the trunk and head.

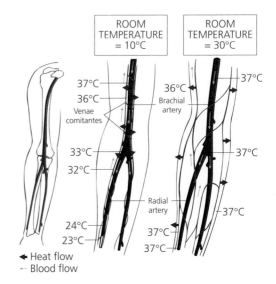

Figure 17.8 Countercurrent heat exchange in the arm during cold conditions. At 10°C room temperature, venous blood draining from the arm passes in close proximity to the arterial blood entering the arm. Heat passes from the warm arterial blood to the cooler venous blood, thus facilitating its retention in the body. At a room temperature of 30°C, the venous blood is shifted to more superficial vessels and so negates the heat exchange mechanism.

insulating the body or by physiologically stimulating arrector muscles that cause hairs to stand erect (called piloerection). Both will trap an unstirred layer of air against the skin; this will rapidly warm up as air has a low specific heat (i.e. the heat required to raise the temperature of 1 g by 1°C). The effect is reduced by air currents which dislodge the layer. In water, warming the water close to the skin is expensive as water has a high specific heat and requires a lot of energy to raise its temperature. Once warmed, however, the layer cools very slowly, and can form an effective insulation layer if there are no currents to disturb it. This is the basis of the 'wet suit' in aquasports.

Reducing skin temperature is achieved by reducing the rate of blood flow to the skin through cutaneous sympathetic nerve activation. If conditions are extreme then underlying tissues will also vasoconstrict and the 'core' of tissue which is thermoregulated will contract

latter involves the warming of air close to the skin irrespective of what the surrounding air temperature is. This is achieved by externally in size (Figure 17.7b). Heat conservation is also facilitated by 'heat exchange' mechanisms in the limbs. In this way venous blood, having cooled near the skin surface (blood supply to the skin cannot be stopped entirely), is warmed by incoming arterial blood. This is aided by the close anatomical arrangement of veins and artery, and their countercurrent flow, within the limbs (Figure 17.8). Much of the heat from the arterial blood entering the limb is therefore returned to the body via this mechanism and so is conserved. The loss of heat from skin can be reduced still further by the deposition of fat in subcutaneous adipose tissue, which acts as an internal insulator.

Increasing the metabolic rate

Most of the energy generated by cellular respiration is unharnessed by the cell. Raising the metabolic rate is therefore an efficient means of generating heat in response to enhanced heat loss in cold conditions. The means of generating heat can be placed into two categories: shivering and non-shivering thermogenesis.

Shivering is a series of small, repeated muscular contraction/relaxation cycles, which increase the metabolic rate of the tissue. The coordination of these involuntary muscle movements involves the hypothalamus, cerebral cortex, and cerebellum and requires considerable integrative neural activity. Shivering is impractical and of limited use as a long-term mechanism, but as a rapid response to the cold it is extremely effective and, if severe, can double a person's total metabolic rate. Similarly, exercise is another excellent short-term measure to generate additional heat.

Non-shivering thermogenesis involves an elevation of the basal metabolic rate, i.e. the rate at which cells generate energy in the absence of extrinsic stimulation (see Chapter 6). In neonates, in whom temperature regulatory processes are immature, 'brown' fat is thought to be utilized to provide additional heat. This adipose tissue is found mainly between the shoulder blades and is 'coloured' by the presence of extensive blood vessels (the more familiar 'white' fat has a poor vascularization). The tissue is innervated by sympathetic nerves which promote metabolism of the stored lipid, when stimulated. Little of this energy is incorporated into ATP and so almost all is released from the adipocytes into the circulation and the heat carried into the 'core'. The heat generated will help to compensate for the relatively high heat losses experienced by neonates as a consequence of a large body surface area : volume ratio.

The capacity to generate additional heat metabolically without the inconvenience of shivering is an attractive mechanism for cold adaptation. Adults do not have 'brown' fat reserves, however, and the evidence for non-shivering thermogenesis in adults in cold or cool climates is controversial. Some findings have implicated an increased release of thyroid hormones in the cold, which would alter basal metabolism throughout the body.

THE 'COMFORT ZONE'

Although heat is conserved by the body when air temperature is considerably lower than that of the core temperature, an air temperature similar to that of the core would also cause major difficulties. This is because heat is continually generated by metabolism and its removal from the body would be difficult in the absence of a temperature gradient. An air temperature of 24–25°C constitutes a comfort zone in which physiological mechanisms to conserve heat (or promote its loss – see below) are little stimulated.

TEMPERATURE REGULATORY PROCESSES IN HOT CLIMATES

An air temperature above the comfort zone means that the rate of heat loss to the environment will begin to decrease, and so the balance between heat gained from metabolism and that lost from the body will be disturbed. This will

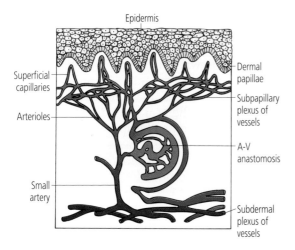

Figure 17.9 Arrangement of blood vessels in skin of the finger. Note the arterial–venous anastomosis; when patent this will substantially increase the rate of blood flow through the skin.

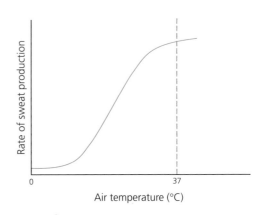

Figure 17.10 Influence of air temperature on the rate of sweat production.

Table 17.1 The relative rates of heat loss via evaporative and non-evaporative means

	Air temperature (°C)				
Heat loss	20	25	30	35	40
Evaporative (% of total)	15	30	50	95	100
Non-evaporative (% of total)	85	70	50	5	0

Note the importance of sweat as a heat loss mechanism in hot environments.

especially be the case if metabolism is increased by physical activity. Heat loss from the body must now be promoted, through mechanisms which elevate the temperature gradient between skin and air, and promote sweat production. Metabolic rates are little changed in hot spells, although appetite may be reduced.

Elevating the skin–air temperature gradient

The air temperature close to the skin may be cooled by reducing insulation (i.e. removing clothing, reducing piloerection) and by introducing air convection. Skin temperature is raised by vasodilatation within the skin, which effectively expands the 'core' area into the periphery (Figure 17.7b). A diagram of cutaneous vasculature in areas effective at promoting heat loss, that is the limbs, is shown in Figure 17.9. One feature is the presence of arterial–venous anastomoses which, via dilatation of certain arterioles, shunt blood directly into the venous system, bypassing capillaries. This means that more blood per unit time can perfuse these areas.

The heat exchange mechanism in the limb is also less effective in warm weather as venous blood returning from the limbs is directed away from deep veins (which lie adjacent to incoming arteries) to more superficial vessels (Figure 17.8).

Sweat production

The evaporation of sweat from the body surface is an effective means of removing heat from the body. Indeed, when air temperature is so high that changes in cutaneous blood flow can no longer sustain a temperature gradient that favours heat loss (and may even promote heat gain) then evaporation is the only physiological response available for temperature regulation (Figure 17.10 and Table 17.1). The secretion of eccrine sweat is observed to increase as air temperature rises, and this is mediated by autonomic nervous activity. Secretion rates may be as high as 4 litres per day and can have consequences for water and electrolyte (especially sodium) balance. The importance of sweat as a temperature regulatory mechanism is illustrated by the difficulties of the elderly to maintain a constant 'core' temperature in hot environments as a consequence of decreased numbers of sweat glands and reduced effectiveness of autonomic activity.

SUMMARY OF TEMPERATURE HOMEOSTASIS

Temperature homeostasis is illustrated diagrammatically in Figure 17.11. The receptors necessary to detect a change in the 'core' are located within the hypothalamus, and nuclei within this area of the brain provide the monitoring process and determine the 'set-point'. Other temperature receptors are found within the skin, and also provide afferent input into the hypothalamus. These receptors (called Ruffini organs and Krauss end-bulbs) will detect a change in conditions at the body surface, and so homeostatic processes can be instigated before consequential changes in 'core' temperature have occurred. Together the central and peripheral thermoreceptors provide an efficient means of ensuring 'core' temperature does not markedly change.

FACTORS WHICH INFLUENCE 'CORE' TEMPERATURE

Assuming that temperature regulatory mechanisms are intact then 'core' temperature is extremely well regulated near to the 'set-point'. The actual 'set-point', however, is subject to

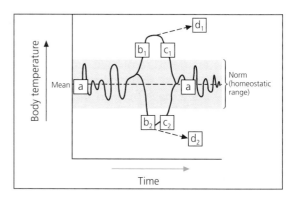

Figure 17.11 Temperature homeostasis.
a Body (core) temperature dynamically fluctuating about the set-point.
b_1 Elevated body temperature as a consequence of *either* increased metabolism (e.g. exercise, or following a meal) *or* decreased heat loss (e.g. excessive insulation, or high ambient temperature).
b_2 Decreased body temperature as a consequence of either reduced metabolism (e.g. in sleep) *or* increased heat loss (e.g. inadequate insulation, or low ambient temperatures).
c_1 Restoration of normal body temperature via behavioural or physiological processes to promote heat loss (e.g. cutaneous vasodilatation, removal of clothing) or to decrease metabolic heat generation (e.g. lethargy and inactivity).
c_2 Restoration of normal body temperature via behavioural or physiological processes to promote heat conservation (e.g. cutaneous vasoconstriction or increased clothing) or to increase metabolic heat production (e.g. shivering, non-shivering thermogenesis).
d_1 Persistently elevated body temperature (= hyperthermia) as a consequence of inadequate heat loss (e.g. extremely hot weather) or excessive heat production (e.g. in hyperthyroidism).
d_2 Persistently reduced body temperature (= hypothermia) as a consequence of excessive heat loss (e.g. very cold weather, exposure) or deficient heat production (e.g. in hypothyroidism). Inefficient homeostatic processes make the elderly and very young particularly susceptible to hypo- and hyperthermia.

slight changes within and between individuals and core temperature changes accordingly.

Circadian rhythmicity

Body temperature displays a 24-hour rhythmicity, linked into the day–night cycle, but which can be synchronized to match activity–rest cycles (see Chapter 23). The fluctuation is of the order of ±0.5°C.

Sex differences

Generally speaking there is little difference between the temperature of men and women. In women there is a slight decrease in body temperature a few days prior to menstruation and this is maintained during the pre-ovulatory phase of the menstrual cycle. The change is less than 0.5°C and appears to be associated with the low secretion of progesterone during this period. After ovulation body temperature rises again to 'normal'.

Age

Temperature regulatory mechanisms in the neonate and infant are immature and are compounded by the relatively large surface area : volume ratio which favours heat loss. Indeed the newborn, and premature babies, are very susceptible to environmental changes and require a protected environment. Heat loss is compensated for by a relatively high metabolic rate and the core temperature (37.5–38°C) is actually higher in young children than in adults.

Fever

Fever, or pyrexia, is an indication that pathogenic infection has occurred. The elevated temperature observed is, in fact, a physiological response to the presence of substances (pyrogens) released by the pathogens themselves, and/or by certain cells of the immune system. The hypothalamic 'set-point' is altered from 37°C to 39°C or so and even a 'normal' body temperature is then recognized as being too low. Hence mechanisms such as shivering and cutaneous vasoconstriction are

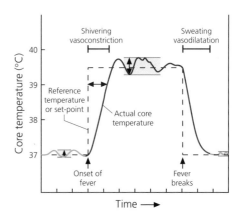

Figure 17.12 Time course of a typical febrile episode. The actual body temperature lags behind the rapid shifts in set-points. Note that regulation is maintained during the fever but is less precise, so that temperature fluctuations are generally greater than normal.

implemented which raise 'core' temperature to the new homeostatic mean (Figure 17.12). The individual therefore appears pale and expresses feelings of being cold. As the pathogen is destroyed a point is reached when pyrogen release cannot sustain the new hypothalamic set point, and this then reverts to normal. The pyrexic temperature is now in excess of the homeostatic mean and heat loss is promoted by cutaneous vasodilatation and sweating. The individual will report feeling hot, and the skin will appear 'flushed' and clammy. The advantage of such a process is that the pyrexia interferes with the metabolic enzymes of · the pathogen, reducing its reproductive activities and making it more susceptible to attack by the immune system. The disadvantage is that our own metabolic processes are also affected and make us feel 'ill'.

Role of the skin in homeostasis

The excretory function of the skin has been mentioned and usually acts to support other, more significant excretory routes. The involvement of skin is most apparent if certain

substances are secreted in much greater loads than usual. For example, sweat volume in hot environments will rapidly induce dehydration, and result in hypovolaemia and a disturbance

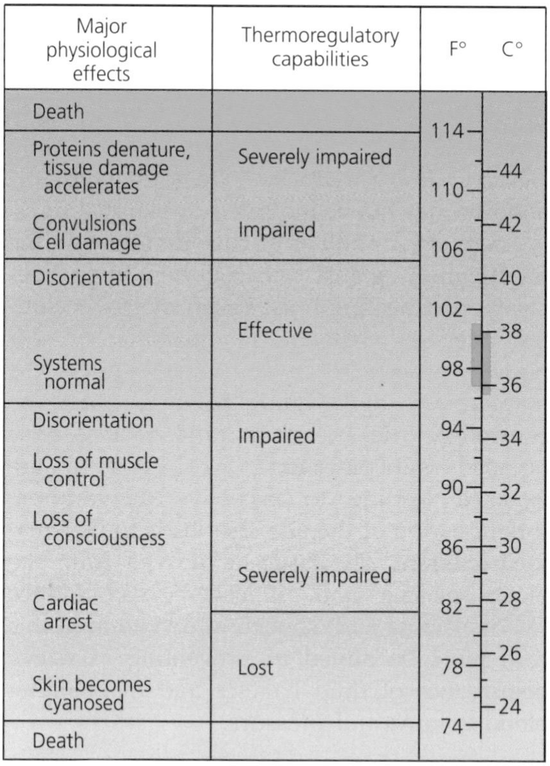

Major physiological effects	Thermoregulatory capabilities	F°	C°
Death		114	
Proteins denature, tissue damage accelerates	Severely impaired	110	44
Convulsions Cell damage	Impaired	106	42
Disorientation		102	40
	Effective	98	38
Systems normal			36
Disorientation	Impaired	94	34
Loss of muscle control		90	32
Loss of consciousness		86	30
	Severely impaired	82	28
Cardiac arrest			26
	Lost	78	
Skin becomes cyanosed		74	24
Death			

Figure 17.13 Normal and abnormal body temperatures, and their physiological effects.

in body fluid electrolyte composition if uncompensated. The consequences are potentially life-threatening. Insufficient excretion of various substances via the urine may also result in increased losses via the skin. For example, renal failure causes an increased excretion of uric acid in sweat, and this may crystallize, leading to an intense itching (pruritis).

The major way in which the physiology of the skin integrates with the functioning of other systems is through its role in the regulation of 'core' temperature. Vital core tissues function optimally within a very narrow temperature range. Disturbances in temperature will result in a change in function (Figure 17.13).

Neural tissues are most susceptible to a change in core temperature and nerve conduction velocity decreases at high temperatures as enzymes denature. The consequences are headache, mental confusion, delirium, and lethargy. Disruption of integrative neural processes will also affect the control of other tissues, themselves already disturbed by the hyperthermia. Lower than normal temperatures induce similar neurological symptoms but this time as a consequence of a reduced metabolic rate.

The effect of hypothermia on metabolic rate is comparable to that of reduced thyroid activity (hypothyroidism; note that thyroxine influences the basal metabolic rate). Symptoms of hypothyroidism include a reduced heart rate, slowed reflexes, lethargy, and poor mentation.

Examples of homeostatic control system failures and principles of correction

Skin structure is susceptible to damage by physical trauma (including burns and radiation), by infection and by dietary deficiency of substances, particularly certain vitamins, which are essential for epithelial maintenance. The capacity of the skin to facilitate temperature regulation may also be compromised under certain circumstances.

SKIN STRUCTURE

Changes in skin structure can be extensive, as in burns, ulcers or inherited disorders, or may be localized as in acne, warts, cold sores, and melanoma.

Burns

Burns have been traditionally classed as first-, second- or third-degree injuries according to the visible extent of damage to the skin. This is now considered too simplistic. For example, an assessment must also take into account the depth of injury, if there is facial injury, if there are breathing difficulties, or if the site is prone to infection, for example in the perineal area.

Depth of injury is important because it influences the capacity for tissue regeneration. Thus, 'partial thickness' injury may be superficial and influence only the epidermis (also called first-degree burn), or may be deep and affect some of the dermis (called second- or third-degree burn). Wound healing and a degree of regeneration is likely, though some scarring may occur, if the area damaged is not too extensive. 'Full thickness' (or fourth-degree burn) injury includes the epidermis, dermis, and subdermal tissues such as muscle. This depth of damage will have destroyed any germinal cells and will require skin grafting.

Burns are also now classed as being major, moderate, or minor. Assessment is via various charts but also includes recognition that children under 10 years have proportionately larger heads than adults (and very young children have immature immunity responses) and that adults over 40 years exhibit poorer homeostatic control as a consequence of the ageing process.

Major burns are those in which (1) more than 25% of the body surface area (BSA) is damaged (more than 20% in children under 10 years and adults over 40 years) or (2) more than 10% of BSA is full thickness injury, or (3) the face, hands, feet, or perineal area are badly damaged, or (4) there is inhalation injury, or (5) there is pre-existing disease such as poor peripheral circulation.

Moderate burns are those in which (1) 15–25% of BSA is damaged (10–20% in children under 10 years and adults over 40 years), or (2) less than 10% of BSA exhibits full thickness injury.

Minor burns are those in which less than 15% of BSA is damaged (10% in children under 10 years and adults over 40 years), or (2) less than 2% of BSA exhibits full thickness injury.

A further complication of assessment is that electrical burns may be extensive internally, and this may not be indicated by external signs.

There are a number of considerations in the intervention against burn injuries. In particular, wound healing must be promoted (including infection control), the flexibility of scar tissue, especially over joints, must be maintained, and fluid balance must be controlled. The effects on fluid balance arise because subepidermal 'wet' tissues are exposed leading to excessive dehydration. Inflammation of the site also leads to oedematous exudate. The latter is derived from the blood plasma and, if severe, can induce hypovolaemia and 'shock'. Intervention in this case must be aimed at preventing excessive disturbance of fluid balance and maintaining blood volume and pressure.

Ulceration including decubitus ulcers (pressure sores)

Ulceration of the skin occurs when areas are subjected to prolonged ischaemia, leading to cell death (necrosis) and tissue atrophy. Pressure sores are commonly observed in people confined to bed-rest in whom body weight acting on a point of skin, frequently the buttocks, sacrum or heels, induces the ischaemia. The problem is exacerbated if cutaneous circulation is poor anyway, as in the elderly, or people with diabetes mellitus. In such cases the skin may even ulcerate without an additional effect of weight. Intervention is aimed at preventing prolonged ischaemia, and by promoting wound healing should ulceration occur.

Acne, warts, and cold sores

These are all produced by infection. Acne is an inflammation of sebaceous glands in response to bacterial infection. The problem is particularly noticeable during puberty when gland activity increases. Warts are produced by a focus of cells which divide excessively in response to infection by a kind of virus, called a papovavirus. Cold sores are lesions produced by infection of skin with herpes simplex virus (type 1). The virus is one which may lay dormant for long periods, with cold sores appearing only when the virus is 'triggered'. This activation may be in response to factors such as ultraviolet light, or the release of sex steroids.

Psoriasis

Psoriasis is perhaps the best known example of an inherited skin condition, although most cases do not appear to have a familial link. Skin eruptions occur because mitotic divisions proceed too rapidly.

Melanoma

Melanoma is a cancer of the skin. As its name implies it is a cancer of the pigmented melanocytes. The main cause seems to be overexposure of melanocytes to ultraviolet radiation, leading to genetic mutation which prevents control of the cell cycle.

HYPOTHERMIA AND HYPERTHERMIA

Clinical disturbance of body thermoregulation results in a core temperature which is elevated (hyperthermia) or reduced (hypothermia) outside the homeostatic range. Fever is considered a hyperthermia even though it results from a deliberate resetting of the temperature set-point by the hypothalamus. Most disturbances, however, result from inappropriate changes in metabolic heat production and/or the capacity to control heat gain or loss via the skin (Figure 17.11). Intervention is directed at removing the cause of the altered metabolic rate, or to facilitate heat conservation or exchange.

Summary

1 The skin is the largest organ of the body, the functions of which are closely associated with it being the physical barrier between the body and external environment. It is protective but also has a vital role to play in the regulation of body temperature.

2 In structure the skin consists of three layers – the epidermis, dermis, and subcutaneous layers.

3 The epidermis forms the outer layer and consists of cells which eventually form the tough keratinized outer surface. Nails and hair are modified epidermal structures that project into the dermis, a layer of connective tissue which contains blood vessels, neurons, and various other structures. The subcutaneous layer contains the sweat glands, the ducts of which project through the dermis and epidermis.

4 Body temperature regulation is essential if the functioning of vital tissues is to be optimal. Constancy of body temperature can only be achieved if heat generation from metabolism is balanced by appropriate rates of heat loss, particularly across the skin. Changes in heat exchange with the environment are the main responses to adverse environments, but changes in the metabolic rate may also play a role, particularly in the cold.

5 The temperature of the body 'core' is tightly controlled. There is a circadian rhythmicity, however, and values may also decrease slightly in women during the pre-ovulatory phase of the menstrual cycle. Fever is a physiological response to infection and results from a resetting of the homeostatic set-point. It probably helps to reduce the metabolic activity of the invading pathogen and so reduces the rate of spread of infection.

6 Skin function is adversely affected by factors which alter its structural integrity. In addition, factors such as age and metabolic disorders limit the capacity to regulate body temperature.

Review Questions

1 List four factors which determine the rate of metabolic reactions.

2 Name the three layers of skin.

3 List the general functions of skin.

4 Which layer of skin is referred to as a stratified epithelium? Name the subdivisions of the layer.

5 Which skin components help prevent loss of body fluids through the skin?

6 Which cells produce melanin? What is the function of this pigment?

7 Which tissues constitute the dermis and what are their functions?

8 List the functions of the subcutaneous adipose tissue.

9 Describe the structure and functions of hair.

10 List the three glands associated with skin.

11 Differentiate between apocrine and eccrine sweat glands.

12 The sweat glands and sebaceous glands contribute to the skin's acidic surface (pH5.5). How is this regarded as an external defence mechanism?

13 The skin is referred to as a 'labile' tissue due to its repair capabilities. What does this mean?

14 Discuss what is meant by the following terms with reference to heat transfer:
(a) radiation; (b) conduction; (c) evaporation.

15 Describe the homeostatic regulation of the 'core' temperature when the body is subjected to cold environmental conditions.

16 Describe the homeostatic regulation of the 'core' temperature when the body is subjected to hot environmental conditions.

17 Describe the physiological changes associated with pyrexia (fever).

18 Discuss the homeostatic imbalances associated with the following:
(a) burns; (b) pressure sores; (c) acne; (d) melanoma.

Reproduction

Introduction: relation of reproduction to homeostasis

Overview of the anatomy and physiology of the human reproductive systems

Details of reproductive physiology

Examples of homeostatic system control failures and principles of correction

Summary

Review questions

Introduction: relation of reproduction to homeostasis

All organ systems of the body operate as homeostatic controls to maintain the psychophysiological well-being of the individual. At the cellular level of organization, reproduction may be regarded as a homeostatic process in which cells divide by mitosis once they have reached their optimal size. Cellular reproduction is necessary to maintain the appropriate growth, development, specialization, and repair of human tissues, thus contributing to an individual's well-being.

At the organism level of organization, reproduction may be regarded as a homeostatic control adapted for the survival of the species (Figure 18.1). The human reproductive system is 'dormant' until puberty, when there seems to be a trigger which activates the genetic code responsible for the production and secretion of hormones responsible for the initiation and continuation of this developmental stage.

Although the common purpose of both sexes is to produce offspring, their functional roles are quite different. The male gonads (gono = seed; in the male these are the testes) manufacture up to half a billion gametes (sperm) per day, which are mixed with glandular secretions, creating a mixture called semen. This fluid is routed from the male system by the process of ejaculation. The complementary role of the female gonads (the ovaries) is to manufacture and mature female gametes ('eggs' or 'ova') and subsequently release, or ovulate, one potential ovum per month, although sometimes two ova are released simultaneously from both ovaries. These gametes travel to the Fallopian tubes, sometimes called the oviducts. Upon sexual intercourse, the male and female gamete may fuse at fertilization, and this fusion produces a new cell called the zygote. This cell contains all the genetic information required to produce a human. A pregnancy is initiated if the zygote-derivative implants into the the lining of the uterus, or womb. Thus, although the female and male are equal partners in the fertilization

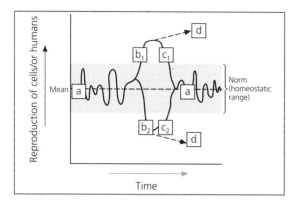

Figure 18.1 Cellular and sexual reproduction: homeostatic devices.
a Reproductive function fluctuating within its homeostatic range. On a cellular level, this reflects that cellular reproduction matches cellular loss. On an organism level, this reflects that the population size is sustainable, for example by its food supplies.
b_1 Increased reproductive capacity. On a cellular basis, this

reflects that cell reproduction is greater than cellular losses, as occurs following injury when cells are reproducing to replace lost or damaged cells. Alternatively, it could indicate some underlying pathology, such as tumour growth *or* hypertrophied organs. On an organism basis, this reflects that the human population number has increased beyond its capabilities of maintaining such a population explosion.
c_1 Homeostatic 'controls' which correct the cellular disturbance, as occurs normally during post-healing periods and when cancers are destroyed by the body's anti-cancer agents *or* via clinical interventions using chemotherapy, radiotherapy, surgery, and/or laser therapy. Homeostatic 'controls' which correct the 'population explosion', for example limited food supplies accompanied by the survival of the fittest.
b_2 A decreased cellular reproduction as occurs normally, with the ageing process, or abnormally, in pathological wasting conditions, such as anorexia nervosa. A severe decrease in the population as occurs in natural disasters, such as war, famine, etc.
c_1 and c_2 Correction of underlying 'pathology' or natural changes. d Irreversible imbalances, for example, certain cancers.

process, it is the female's uterus that provides a life-support system until birth for the developing embryo/fetus. During this period, called gestation, the female's homeostatic parameters are reset to provide a suitable environment for prebirth development, and nutritional support via breast milk for the newborn until it is able to take a mixed diet.

The intentions of this chapter are to present an overview of the anatomy and physiology of the male and female reproductive systems, and a detailed account of the physiological processes and hormonal mechanisms responsible for the homeostatic regulation of reproductive function. The physiology underpinning birth control will also be discussed, and common male and female homeostatic imbalances, with their principles of correction identified.

Overview of the anatomy and physiology of the human reproductive systems

The human reproductive system consists of:

1 A pair of primary sex organs, collectively called the gonads, which produce, store, and nourish the developing sex cells, or gametes, and are involved in the initial transport of the gametes (i.e. sperm and potential ova), and which function as endocrine tissue to

synthesize hormones that coordinate activities peculiar to the different sexes.

2 A diverse range of other structures, such as ducts that transport gametes, accessory glands that secrete fluid into ducts, and external genitalia associated with the sexes.

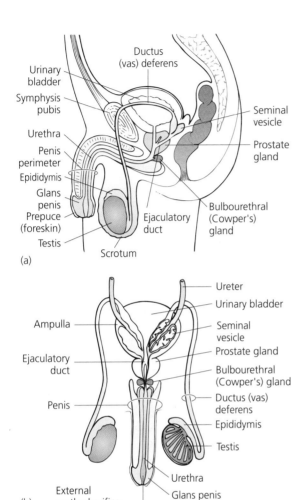

(a)

(b)

Structure	Function
Testis	Produce sperm and sex hormone
Accessory organs	
VAS deferens, urethra	Carry sperm out of the body
Glands–seminal vesicles, prostate, Cowper's	Contribute the majority of fluid within semen
Scrotum	Houses the testis outside the pelvic cavity–essential for viable sperm production
Penis	Organ of copulation and excretion

Figure 18.2 The male reproductive system: (a) sagittal view and (b) posterior view of male reproductive organs.

The various functions of the male and female reproductive tracts are summarized in tables accompanying Figures 18.2 and 18.9, and an outline of the structure and function of the male and female reproductive tracts now follows.

THE MALE REPRODUCTIVE SYSTEM

The male reproductive system is adapted for the production of spermatozoa, the transportation of sperm to the female reproductive tract, and for producing hormones which control the development of the secondary sexual characteristics, such as enlargement of the larynx, the development of the male form, and body, pubic, and facial hair.

The primary sex organs are called the testes (testis, singular). These produce the male gamete, the spermatozoa, in a process called spermatogenesis. This process is controlled by the release of a gonadotropin hormone, called follicle-stimulating hormone (FSH), from the anterior pituitary gland. The testes store sperm until they are either released from the body, or are broken down into their component parts and then recycled to contribute to intracellular homeostatic mechanisms. They also contain endocrine cells which produce and secrete the male hormones, the androgens. This process is again regulated by the release of a gonadotropin, luteinizing hormone (LH), from the anterior pituitary. Testosterone is the main androgen produced by the testes.

The accessory reproductive organs consist of the scrotum, ducts, glands and penis, and these protect the sperm and aid its transport outside the body (Figure 18.2).

Structure of the testes

The paired oval-shaped testes, or testicles, originate from close to the posterior abdominal wall of the embryo. They develop from the embryonic tissue which also gives rise to the

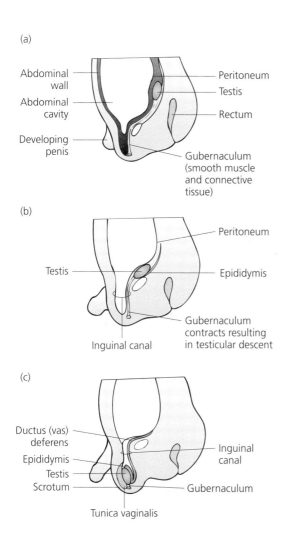

(a)

Abdominal wall

Abdominal cavity

Developing penis

Peritoneum

Testis

Rectum

Gubernaculum (smooth muscle and connective tissue)

(b)

Testis

Peritoneum

Epididymis

Gubernaculum contracts resulting in testicular descent

Inguinal canal

(c)

Ductus (vas) deferens

Epididymis

Testis

Scrotum

Inguinal canal

Gubernaculum

Tunica vaginalis

Figure 18.3 Descent of the testes. The testes descend from the posterior abdominal wall into the scrotum during fetal development. (a) Six-month fetus. (b) Seven-month fetus. (c) At birth.

urinary system, indeed the urethra of the male provides a common route for the exit of sperm and urine from the body. The testes descend through the inguinal canal into their sac-like scrotum during the seventh month of gestation following contraction of specialized muscular tissue, called the gubernaculum (Figure 18.3). The testes are thus suspended outside the abdominal pelvic cavity and this means that their temperature is 2–3°C below the core body temperature of 37°C. The testicular venous plexus also contributes to the cooler temperature of the testes since it coils around the testicular artery and functions to absorb heat from arterial blood, thus cooling it before it enters the testes. Sperm development will only progress normally at this cooler temperature.

Each testis is surrounded by the tunica albuginea, a connective tissue capsule which extends inwardly, dividing it into compartmenting lobules. Each lobule contains one to four seminiferous tubules which produce sperm. These sperm-producing factories are continuous with other tubules (the ductus efferentia, epididymis, vas deferentia, and urethra), that provide the distribution route for sperm exiting from the body (Figure 18.4a). A cross-section of the seminiferous tubules reveals that it contains immature sperm cells at various stages of development (Figures 18.4b–d). That is, the most immature cells, called the spermatogonia, are located peripherally whereas the fully mature spermatozoa are located centrally within the tubule lumen. In between these two locations the cells are of advancing maturity, and are called primary spermatocytes, secondary spermatocytes, and spermatids, respectively.

Embedded between the developing sperm cells are the Sertoli, or sustentacular cells. Their homeostatic functions are to:

1 Support, nourish and protect developing spermatogenic cells.

2 Phagocytose degenerating spermatogenic cells.

3 Control the movement of spermatogenic cells.

4 Control the release of sperm into the lumen of the seminiferous tubules.

5 Secrete chemicals which maintain testicular homeostasis. For example, inhibin is a hormone which depresses FSH production, and hence spermatogenesis, and androgen-binding protein helps prevent androgen

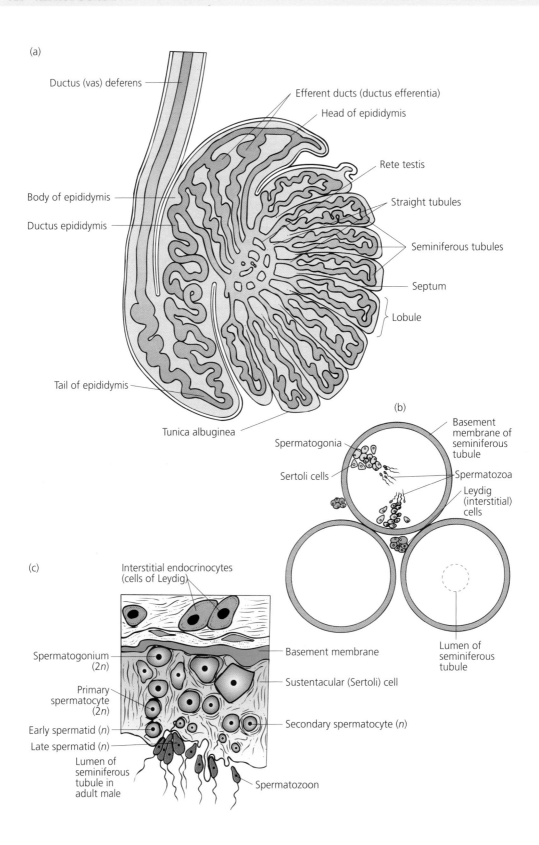

(a)

Ductus (vas) deferens

Efferent ducts (ductus efferentia)

Head of epididymis

Rete testis

Body of epididymis

Straight tubules

Ductus epididymis

Seminiferous tubules

Septum

Lobule

Tail of epididymis

Tunica albuginea

(b)

Spermatogonia

Basement membrane of seminiferous tubule

Sertoli cells

Spermatozoa

Leydig (interstitial) cells

Lumen of seminiferous tubule

(c)

Interstitial endocrinocytes (cells of Leydig)

Spermatogonium (2n)

Basement membrane

Primary spermatocyte (2n)

Sustentacular (Sertoli) cell

Early spermatid (n)

Secondary spermatocyte (n)

Late spermatid (n)

Lumen of seminiferous tubule in adult male

Spermatozoon

hormones (i.e. testosterone) from going beyond their homeostatic parameters, and also facilitates the actions of the androgens. These secretions provide negative feedback loops which maintain reproductive function within its homeostatic parameters (see later text and Figure 18.14).

Accessory organs of the male reproductive system

Accessory organs of the male system comprise the duct system, various secretory glands, and the penis.

The duct system

Once produced, the sperm are moved from the seminiferous tubules to the straight tubules (Figure 18.4a). The latter lead to a network of ciliated ducts, called the rete testis (rete = net), which empty into the ductus efferentia. From here the sperm are transported through a duct system averaging 8 metres in length. In order of transit the sections of duct are called the epididymis, the vas, or ductus, deferens, and the urethra (Figure 18.2b).

EPIDIDYMIS

From the rete testes the spermatozoa enter the head, body and then the tail of the epididymis via the ductus efferentia. It takes about 2 weeks for the sperm to transit the epididymis. The homeostatic functions of this region are:

1 To absorb excess fluid from the lumen, and secrete nutrients into the lumen, so as to provide a suitable environment for sperm maturation, i.e. ensuring motility and fertility.

2 To act as a temporary storage site for sperm until they are either released into the vas deferentia when the male is sexually aroused and ejaculates, or are catabolized and their constituents recycled.

THE VAS DEFERENS (DUCTUS DEFERENS)

The vas deferens is approximately 40–45 cm long. It begins at the epididymis and ends behind the urinary bladder, where it expands to form the ampulla region from which the ejaculatory ducts emerge. These ducts penetrate the muscular wall of the prostate gland and upon contraction empty their contents into the urethra (Figure 18.2b).

THE URETHRA

The urethra extends for a distance of about 15–20 cm from the urinary bladder to the tip of the penis. This terminal portion of the male system, together with the penis, serve both the urinary and reproductive systems as it conveys urine and semen to the exterior. Thus, these structures form a common part of the urogenital tract. Figure 18.5a illustrates that the urethra has three anatomical regions:

1 The prostatic urethra which passes through the prostate gland.

2 The membranous urethra. This is a short segment that passes from the prostatic urethra to the penile urethra, and which penetrates the urogenital diaphragm and the muscular floor of the pelvic cavity.

3 The penile urethra which extends from the distal border of the urogenital diaphragm to the external orifice at the tip of the penis.

Accessory sex glands

The accessory glands of the male reproductive tract include paired seminal vesicles, paired

Figure 18.4 The testes. (a) Internal structure, sagittal section illustrating internal anatomy. (b) Diagram representing seminiferous tubules. Spermatocytes in turn give rise to sperm cells by meiosis. (c) Microscopic cross-section of a portion of a seminiferous tubule, showing the stages of spermatogenesis. Cells increase in maturity as they move towards the lumen: n = haploid; $2n$ = diploid.

(a)

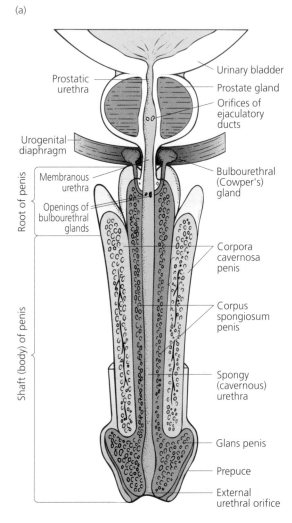

(b)

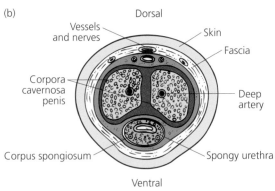

Figure 18.5 Structure of the penis. (a) Longitudinal section. (b) Transverse section.

bulbourethral (Cowper's) glands, and a single prostate gland (Figure 18.2). They contribute approximately 95% of the fluid contained in semen (note: semen is the fluid conveyed and expelled from the urethra via peristalsis during ejaculation). The seminiferous tubules and the epididymis produce secretions that contribute a small percentage to semen. Collectively the secretions activate sperm in the semen by providing nutrients for their motility, and buffers to counteract the acidic environments of the urethra and the female tract.

The seminal vesicles

The seminal vesicles are located on the posterior wall at the base of the bladder and secrete a viscous alkaline fluid which accounts for approximately 60% of semen volume. It contains chemicals, such as fructose, prostaglandins, and ascorbic acid, that contribute to the viability of the sperm. Fructose provides the essential fuel necessary to initate and maintain the beating of the sperm flagella. Prostaglandins are thought to:

1 decrease the viscosity of the mucus plug which guards the entrance to the uterus of the female (i.e. the cervix);

2 stimulate anti-peristalsis of the female reproductive tract and so aid transportation of sperm to the Fallopian tubes;

3 stimulate the release of the hormone relaxin, and of certain enzymes that enhance sperm motility;

4 stimulate seminal plasmin which has bactericidal properties. Together with other unidentified chemicals with antibiotic properties, this action may help to prevent urinary tract infections and thus must be considered a part of the homeostatic external defence mechanisms;

5 stimulate clotting factors (e.g. fibrinogen) in semen which cause its coagulation after ejaculation;

6 stimulate fibrinolysin which liquefies the coagulant mass approximately 5–20 minutes

after it clots, so that the sperm can swim out and begin their journey within the female tract.

Ascorbic acid acts as a cofactor in some metabolic reactions within the sperm's cytoplasm.

The prostate

The prostate, a large gland positioned just below the bladder, secretes a thin, milky, alkaline secretion which accounts for approximately 14–30% of semen. It contains fibrinolysin, and acid phosphatase, two enzymes important in promoting maximum motility of the sperm.

The bulbourethral (Cowper's) glands

The bulbourethral glands are inferior to the prostate and are so called because of their shape, and because they secrete their fluid directly into the urethra. They release a thick clear alkaline mucus just prior to ejaculation, and this neutralizes traces of acidic urine that reside in the urethra, and lubricates the end of the penis prior to, and during, sexual intercourse. Most lubricating fluid for intercourse, however, is provided by the female reproductive organs.

The average volume of semen ejaculated is 2.5–6 ml, and contains approximately 50–120 million spermatozoa per millilitre. A sperm count lower than 20 million per ml is likely to indicate male sterility. The vast number of sperm is required since only a small percentage survive and eventually reach the site of fertilization, and, although only one sperm fertilizes an 'ovum' (or more precisely a secondary oocyte – see later), fertilization requires the combined action of large numbers of them to digest the barrier produced by the follicular cells surrounding the ovum.

Structure of the penis

The cylindrically shaped penis is a urogenital organ. It is the male organ of copulation and its shape facilitates the introduction of sperm into the female reproductive tract during sexual intercourse; therefore the structure is a necessity for the perpetuation of the species. It is also the male organ of urinary excretion since it conveys urine through the urethra to the external environment.

The penis and the scrotum constitute the male external genitalia. The penis consists of an attached root and a free body or shaft that ends in an enlarged sensitive tip, called the glans penis, over which the skin is doubly folded to form a loosely fitted retractable case, the prepuce or foreskin (Figure 18.5a).

Internally, the penis comprises the spongy urethra and three cylindrical masses or bodies (corpora) of spongy erectile tissue. All three masses are enclosed by a fibrous connective tissue (fascia) and loose-fitting skin (Figure 18.5b). The two larger uppermost cylinders are the corpora cavernosa; the smaller lower one which contains the urethra is the corpus spongiosum.

The male sexual act

During sexual arousal, increased parasympathetic nerve activity causes vascular spaces or sinuses within the spongy erectile tissue of the penis to vasodilate and become engorged with blood. The expansion compresses the veins draining the penis, and so most blood is retained, enlarging the penis and causing it to become rigid. The resultant erection permits the penis to perform a penetrating role during sexual intercourse. Ejaculation is a sympathetic reflex which also causes the bladder sphincter to close and so prevents the mixing of urine and semen in the urethra (which could immobilize the sperm), and prevents semen entering the bladder. Ejaculation occurs when peristaltic contractions from the testes spread to the epididymis, vas deferens, and accessory glands simultaneously to the closing of the bladder sphincter; muscles in the penis contract and the semen is discharged. The penile flaccid state returns when the arteries constrict and pressure on the veins is relieved.

THE FEMALE REPRODUCTIVE SYSTEM

The female reproductive system is adapted for:

1 Oogenesis, i.e. the production of eggs or ova.

2 Receiving sperm.

3 Providing a suitable environment for fertilization and for prebirth development (Chapter 19).

4 Producing hormones which control the development of secondary sexual characteristics, such as pubic hair, and the provision of the feminine form.

The female reproductive system, therefore, has a greater variety of tasks in comparison to the male system, which is only involved in sperm production and ejaculation. This is reflected in the increased complexity of the female reproductive organs.

The primary sex organs are the paired ovaries. These produce oocytes (i.e. cells that develop into mature ova following fertilization), and also contain endocrine cells which produce and secrete the hormones progesterone, oestrogens, and relaxin.

The accessory reproductive organs consist of the uterine (Fallopian) tubes, the uterus (womb), the vagina, and the external genitalia that comprise the vulva (Figure 18.6a). In addition, the mammary glands have a significant role in female reproduction (see later and Chapter 19).

Ovaries

The paired ovaries are structures about twice the size of almond nuts. One lies on each side of the pelvic cavity. Their position is supported by ovarian ligaments which anchor them medially to the uterus, whilst suspensory ligaments anchor them laterally to the pelvic wall, and broad ligaments anchor them to the posterior wall of the pelvis (Figure 18.6b).

Each ovary contains a hilus where nerves, blood, and lymphatic vessels enter/exit and, just as the testes are adapted for sperm and hormonal production in the male, the ovaries are adapted for the production of ova (ovarian = egg receptacle) and hormones. Therefore they contain germ cells, distributed as a germinal epithelium found as a surface layer of cuboidal cells in the outer cortex of this organ (Figure 18.7). Other structures include the tunica albuginea, a capsule of connective tissue immediately encloses the general epithelium, and a stroma, a region of connective tissue deep to the tunica albuginea in the outer cortical and inner medullary regions.

The cortical region of the ovary contains the ovarian follicles. Each follicle consists of an immature egg, or oocyte, enclosed by one layer of follicle cells and many layers of granulosa cells. As the menstrual cycle proceeds, the follicles progressively change their structure, as follows.

1 Primary follicles consisting of a couple of layers of cuboidal or columnar epithelial cells are formed in the early stages of the menstrual cycle. The inner layers comprise the granulosa cells.

2 Secondary follicles develop fluid-filled spaces around the granulosa cells; the spaces unite to form a centrally fluid-filled cavity or antrum.

3 A Graafian follicle is observed just prior to the release of the oocyte at ovulation. It is the most mature stage of follicular development. The oocyte is referred to as a secondary oocyte.

4 A corpus luteum (= yellow body) develops after ovulation. This consists of the Graafian follicle minus its oocyte and encasing granulosa cells. The corpus luteum degenerates into the corpus albicans (= white body) unless fertilization takes place, when it is retained for a while as the corpus luteum of pregnancy.

Like the testes, the ovaries originate from embryonic tissue close to the posterior abdominal wall, near the developing kidneys. During development they descend to locations just below the pelvic brim, where they remain attached to the lateral pelvic wall.

(a)

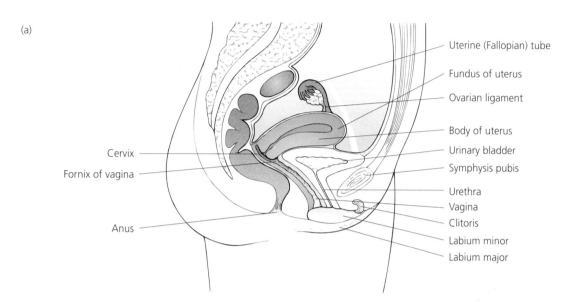

(b)

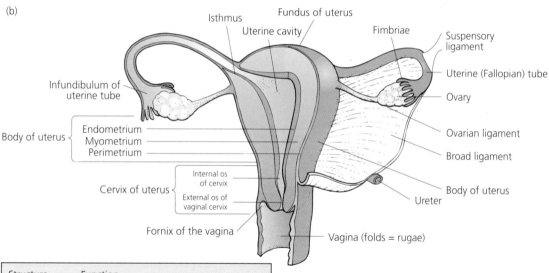

Structure	Function
Ovaries	Produce ova and sex hormones
Uterine tubes	Carry ova from ovary to uterus
Uterus	Houses and nourishes developing embryo
Vagina	Receives sperm during intercourse, exit point for menstrual flow, birth canal
Vulva	Protection, sexual arousal
Mammary glands	Produce milk

Figure 18.6 The female reproductive system. (a) Sagittal section. (b) Female organs in frontal section.

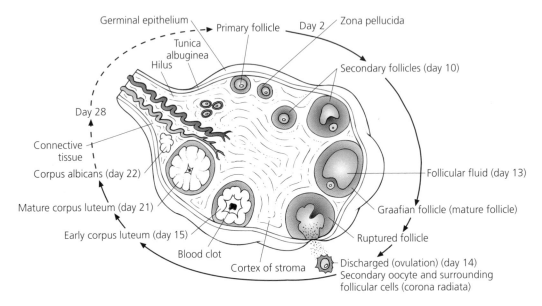

Figure 18.7 Diagram of an ovary. Time approximations indicated in parentheses are for a menstrual cycle averaging 28 days.

Fallopian tubes

The two Fallopian tubes (or oviducts or uterine tubes) transport the secondary oocyte, or fertilized ovum if fertilization has taken place, to the uterus. The oviducts are attached to the uterus at its superior outer angles, which lie in the upper margins of the broad ligaments. Each tube is approximately 10 cm long and has three distinct regions:

1 the isthmus is the narrow, thick walled portion that joins the uterus;

2 the ampulla is the intermediate, dilated portion that makes up about two-thirds of its length; and

3 the infundibulum is the funnel-shaped, terminal component that opens into the peritoneal cavity surrounding the ovary; the opening has a fringe of finger-like projections, called the fimbriae (Figure 18.8).

The wall of the Fallopian tube consists of three layers:

1 The internal mucosa is a ciliated columnar glandular epithelium adapted to aid the

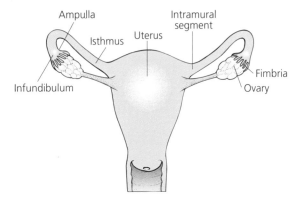

Organ	Function
Ovary	Production of egg cells and female sex hormones
Uterine tube	Conveys egg cell toward uterus; site of fertilization; conveys developing embryo to uterus
Uterus	Protects and sustains life of embryo during pregnancy
Vagina	Conveys uterine secretions to outside of body; receives erect penis during sexual intercourse; transports fetus during birth process

Figure 18.8 The Fallopian (uterine) tubes and uterus.

movement of the ovum and to provide it with nutritional support. This layer is in direct contact with the peritoneum of the pelvic cavity and is continuous with the cavity of the uterus, and hence with the vagina. Thus, it is an area which may become infected by pathogens (for example, gonococcal bacteria) introduced into the vagina. Spreading of inflammation is also a common occurrence. Salpingitis (inflammation of the Fallopian tubes), for example, readily spreads and causes peritonitis (inflammation of the peritoneum), a serious problem.

2 The muscularis layer. This middle region comprising inner circular, and outer longitudinal, muscle sublayers is responsible for the peristaltic movements that move the ovum into the uterus.

3 The serosa is an outer serous connective tissue membrane.

Approximately once a month a secondary oocyte, or immature ovum, ruptures from the surface of the ovary near the infundibular region of the Fallopian tube in a process called ovulation. The ovum is swept into the tube by suction pressure generated by the ciliated epithelium of the infundibulum. It is then propelled along the Fallopian tube by ciliary action, supplemented by peristaltic contractions of the muscularis layer. Fertilization usually occurs in the ampulla of the uterine tube (at this point the secondary oocyte becomes an ovum) and may occur at any time up to 24 hours post-ovulation. The resultant zygote, divides by mitosis, producing a specialized structure, the blastocyst, which descends into the uterus over the next few days. If unfertilized, the secondary oocyte disintegrates and the remains leave the female tract. The details of fertilization are discussed in Chapter 19.

UTERUS

The uterus is located between the bladder and rectum, and is the site of menstruation (if fertilization has not occurred), implantation, embryo–fetal development, and labour.

A female who has never been pregnant has an inverted pear-shaped uterus, approximating to 7.5 cm, and 5–3 cm at its widest and narrowest parts respectively (Figure 18.8). Anatomically, it is divided into an expanded superior body, called the fundus, a constricted isthmus, and an inferior narrow neck region called the cervix which opens into the vagina at its external orifice, the cervical os (Figure 18.6b). The cervix can be readily felt by inserting a finger into the vagina; it feels like the tip of the nose. The space within the uterus is called the uterine cavity. Three pairs of suspensory ligaments stabilize the position of the uterus and limit its range of movement.

Histologically the uterine wall can be divided into three main layers: an inner endometrium, a muscular myometrium and an outer serosa or perimetrium. The endometrium is a mucous membrane and consists of three distinctive layers:

1 Stratum compactum, a compact surface layer of ciliated, columnar epithelium.

2 Stratum spongiosum, a spongy middle layer of loose connective tissue.

3 Stratum basale, a dense inner layer that is attached to the underlying myometrium.

The superficial functional zone of the endometrium (layers 1 and 2, sometimes collectively referred to as the stratum functionalis) nourishes the developing embryo, and is sloughed off following delivery, or during menstruation if fertilization has been unsuccessful, in response to low levels of the sex hormones oestrogens and progesterone.

The thick myometrium layer forms the bulk of the uterine wall, and its thicker upper fundic and thinner lower cervical regions are good examples of structural adaptations to function. That is, to expel a fetus the fundic region contracts more forcibly than its cervical counterpart, dilating the cervix to encourage childbirth. The myometrium contains three layers of involuntary muscle fibres which extend in all directions giving the uterus great strength.

The uterine cavity is directed downwards and opens at the cervical canal at the internal os. The lower region of the cervical canal (or external os) opens into the vagina.

Vagina

The vagina is a thin-walled, muscular, tubular organ lying between the urinary bladder and the rectum, and extends from the cervix to the external genitalia. On average its length is between 7.5 and 9 cm. The fornix, that is, the region where the vagina attaches itself to the cervix, is an important anatomical landmark for the positioning of the contraceptive diaphragm (see Figure 18.17). The vagina is a distensible organ which serves as a passageway for the menstrual flow and for childbirth, hence it is often called the birth canal. It is the receptacle for the penis (and semen) during sexual intercourse, thus its wall is mainly composed of smooth muscle and its folded lining is lubricated with mucus to aid its role during copulation. The vaginal secretions are acidic (pH 3.5–4.0) and provide a hostile environment for microbial growth and for sperm. Although the alkaline semen acts to neutralize the acidity and ensure sperm survival, this is only partly successful since most sperm die due to the effects of the acidic pH on their enzyme systems.

External genitalia (vulva)

The vulva lies immediately external to the vagina and is comprised of a number of components: the mons pubis, labia majora, labia minora, the components of the vestibule and the clitoris (Figure 18.9).

The mons pubis is an elevated rounded fatty tissue area which cushions the underlying pubic symphysis during sexual intercourse. During puberty it becomes surrounded by pubic hair. From the mons pubis two elongated pigmented fatty folds of skin, called the labia majora (the homologue of the male scrotum), extend downwards enclosing and protecting other external genitalia. On the outside, these folds contain numerous hairs, sweat and sebaceous glands; inside there are two delicate hair-free skin folds, the labia

minora. These contain sebum producing cells and function to protect the opening of the urethra and vagina. They also enclose the vestibule which comprises:

1 The hymen. A folded mucous membrane which partly closes the vaginal orifice in young girls and those who have not had penetrative sex.

2 The vaginal orifice.

3 The external urethral orifice.

4 The opening of the mucus-secreting paraurethral (Skene's) glands (the homologue of the male prostate).

5 The mucus-secreting greater vestibular (Bartholin's) glands (the homologues of the male bulbourethral glands).

The role of the mucous glands is to lubricate the area, thereby facilitating intercourse. They are of clinical importance since they are sites of infection, particularly by gonococcal bacteria. These bacteria are especially difficult to eradicate if they become lodged in the paraurethral glands.

Clitoris

The clitoris, a small pea-shaped protruding organ composed of two layers of erectile tissue (i.e. corpora cavernosa), is the homologue of the male glans penis. Its hood, a layer of skin called the prepuce or foreskin, is formed by the junction of the labia minora folds. The clitoris is richly innervated with sensory nerve endings, and thus, like the penis, it is capable of enlargement upon tactile stimulation; this contributes to female sexual arousal.

Perineum

The perineum is a diamond-shaped, muscular region found in both sexes between the external genitalia and the anus. Clinically the area is of importance to females because of the danger of it being torn during childbirth. To avoid this, a small incision (called an

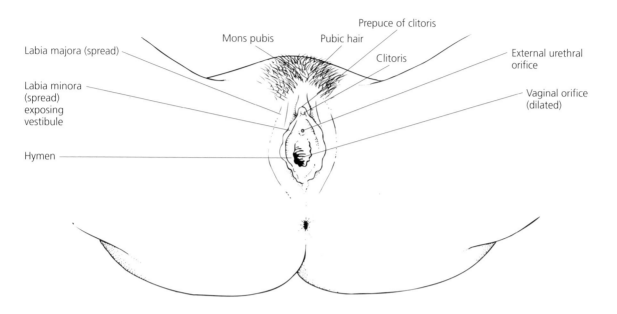

Figure 18.9 External genitalia of the female (the vulva).

Structure	Function
Mons pubis	Cushions the pubic symphysis during sexual intercourse
Labia majora	Enclose and protect other external reproductive organs
Labia minora	Form margins of vestibule; protect openings of vagina and urethra
Clitoris	Gland is richly supplied with sensory nerve endings
Vestibule	Space between labia minora that includes vaginal and urethal openings
Vestibular glands	Secrete fluid that moistens and lubricates vestibule

cation, and orgasm. During arousal, parasympathetic activation leads to the erectile tissue of the clitoris and other parts of the female genitalia becoming engorged with blood. Parasympathetic impulses also cause the lubrication of the vagina which facilitates coitus. During coitus, rhythmical contractions of the clitoris and vaginal walls produce stimulation that eventually leads to orgasm. Female orgasm is accompanied by peristaltic contractions of the uterine walls, vaginal walls, and the perineum muscles. The pleasurable sensation experienced with the contractions is analogous to that produced by male ejaculation.

episiotomy) may be made in the perineal skin and underlying tissues just prior to delivery. After delivery the incision is sutured.

The female sexual act

The phases of female sexual arousal resemble those of the male, i.e. involving erection, lubri-

MAMMARY GLANDS

The mammary glands are accessory organs present in both sexes. When a child reaches puberty, the male glands remain underdeveloped, whilst the surge of ovarian hormones (oestrogens and progesterone) in the female

(a)

(b)

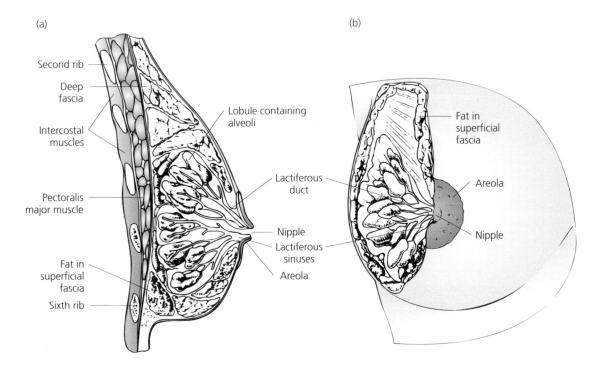

Second rib

Deep fascia

Intercostal muscles

Pectoralis major muscle

Fat in superficial fascia

Sixth rib

Lobule containing alveoli

Lactiferous duct

Nipple

Lactiferous sinuses

Areola

Fat in superficial fascia

Areola

Nipple

Figure 18.10 The anatomy of the mammary glands: (a) sagittal section; (b) anterior view (partially sectioned).

stimulate further gland development (Chapter 19). However, they only become functional following pregnancy, since their role is to produce and secrete milk in order to provide a source of nourishment to the newborn. The size of the breast is determined by the amount of fat around this glandular tissue and is not related to its functional capacity.

Developmentally these glands are modified sudoriferous, or sweat, glands and they are actually a part of the skin. The breast extends from the second to the sixth rib, and from the sternum to the axillae. It overlies, and is connected to, the pectoralis major muscles (Figure 18.10). Slightly below the centre of each breast is a ring of pigmented skin, the areola, which surrounds a central protruding nipple. Large areolar sebaceous glands give this region a slightly bumpy appearance; these glands secrete sebum to lubricate the areola and nipple during breast feeding. Exposure to cold, tactile or sexual stimuli stimulates the smooth

muscle fibres in the areola and causes the nipple to become erect.

In Caucasians (other than those with very dark complexions) the areola changes colour from a delicate pink to brown early in the first pregnancy, a fact of value in diagnosing a first pregnancy. Although it never returns to its original colour, the colour intensity decreases after lactation has ceased. In darker skinned women no noticeable colour change occurs in the first pregnancy.

Internally each breast consists of 15–25 irregular-shaped lobes radiating around the nipple, each of which is separated from one another by a sector or wall of connective tissue that forms the suspensory ligaments of the breast. In each lobe smaller lobules, called alveoli, are present in which are found milk-secreting cells. During lactation milk is passed from the alveoli glands to the lactiferous ducts. These enlarge as the lactiferous sinuses just before their openings on the surface of the nipple. The milk accumulates in the sinuses during nursing, whilst in non-pregnant, non-nursing females the breasts are underdeveloped and the duct system is rudimentary. The homeostatic control of lactation is described in Chapter 19. Suffice-to-say from puberty onwards, and especially during pregnancy and for a short time after delivery, oestrogens stimulate the development of the duct system and progesterone the development of the alveoli regions. Initiation and maintenance of lactation, however, involves two pituitary hormones, prolactin and oxytocin, which stimulate milk production and control milk let-down, respectively.

Details of reproductive physiology

GAMETOGENESIS

'Gametogenesis' is a general term which refers to the production of gametes by the gonads. 'Spermatogenesis' and 'oogenesis' are specific terms which refer to the production of the spermatozoa and ova by the male testes and female ovaries respectively. Gametogenesis involves mitotic and meiotic divisions of cells. The reader should therefore review the mechanism of cell division discussed in Chapters 2 and 20, since it is our intention at this point only to review a few key concepts:

1 Humans reproduce sexually by producing gametes by meiosis, a reduction division which ensures that the chromosome number in the gametes is halved to 23 (called the haploid number).

2 The fusion of male and female gametes produces a zygote, containing 23 pairs of chromosomes (called the diploid number), one partner of each pair from the sperm cell, the other from the ovum.

3 The zygote divides by a duplication division, called mitosis, to ensure that cells derived from it contain the diploid number of chromosomes. Consequently, just prior to cell division, the zygote and subsequent daughter cells must duplicate their DNA.

Spermatogenesis

Spermatogenesis is the sequence of events that occurs in the seminiferous tubules of the testis and lead to the formation of spermatozoa, the male gamete. It involves mitosis, meiosis, and a process called spermiogenesis. As discussed previously, histological investigation of the seminiferous tubules reveals that the majority of the cells comprising the tubule walls are at various stages of cell division (see Figure 18.4d). These cells, collectively called spermatogenic ('sperm-forming') cells develop into mature spermatozoa via a number of cell divisions and transformations briefly explained below.

Mitotic division of spermatogonia

The undifferentiated spermatogenic cells in direct contact with the germinal epithelium of the testis are called the spermatogonia. These stem cells divide continuously by mitosis until puberty; consequently all the spermatogenic cells in a young male are undifferentiated spermatogonia, and each contains 23 pairs of chromosomes, the usual number for human cells. During early adolescence certain hormones (gonadotropins and steroidal androgens) stimulate mitotic divisions of the

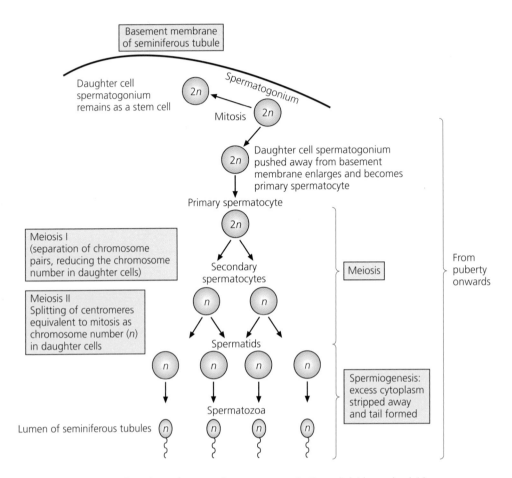

Figure 18.11 Spermatogenesis. Flow chart of events of spermatogenesis: 2n = diploid; n = haploid.

spermatogonia. Some of the new cells give rise to daughter cells to provide a reserve supply of the germ cell line, whilst others migrate towards the lumen of the tubule, where they enlarge and become primary spermatocytes. The latter are destined to become mature sperm via the processes of meiosis and spermiogenesis (Figure 18.11).

Meiosis

Meiosis involves two successive divisions. During the first meiotic division the chromosome pairs of the primary spermatocytes separate so that each forms two haploid secondary spermatocytes. Each secondary spermatocyte in turn give rise to two spermatids via the second meiotic division. The chromosomes during this second stage act much as they do in mitosis, that is the DNA is duplicated to ensure that daughter cells have an identical number of chromosomes as did the parent cell.

Spermiogenesis

Spermiogenesis is the final stage of spermatogenesis when spermatids differentiate into mature spermatozoa. This transformation involves streamlining the non-motile spermatid by shedding most of its superfluous cytoplasmic baggage and by providing a tail.

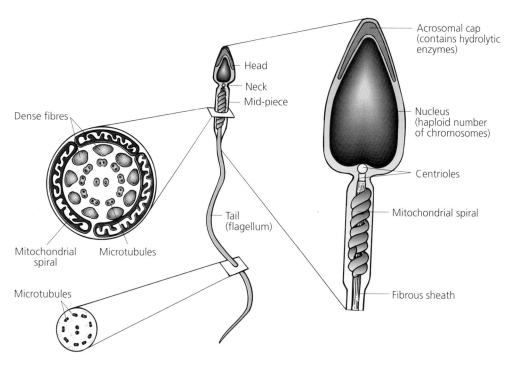

Figure 18.12 Human spermatozoa. Schematic diagram of a sperm cell, showing its internal structure and parts, including the head, mid-piece, and tail.

Each day spermatogenesis produces several thousand spermatozoa. Subsequent to their production they migrate to the epididymis stores, whereby over the next 18 hours to 10 days they undergo further maturation, a process called capacitation. After this the sperm are either expelled via ejaculation or they are catabolized and their constituents recycled. Sperm are also stored in the vas deferens, where they can retain their fertility for up to several months. Once ejaculated, however, they have a life expectancy of about 48 hours within the female reproductive tract.

The structure of spermatozoa

The mature spermatozoon is a tiny (approximately 60 μm long) tadpole-shaped structure consisting of three distinct regions: a flattened head, a cylindrical body or mid-piece and an elongated tail (Figure 18.12). The head is composed primarily of a nucleus which contains 23 densely packed chromosomes. Its anterior tip forms the acrosomal cap and this contains hydrolytic enzymes (e.g. hyaluronidase) which have a role in fertilization. A very short neck attaches the head to the mid-piece. The latter contains a central filamentous core with a large number of mitochondria arranged in a spiral and these organelles provide energy (ATP) for the contraction of protein filaments in the tail; the resultant propulsive forces move the sperm at a rate of 1–4 mm/min. The flagellated tail consists of several longitudinal fibres enclosed by a fibrous sheath.

A mature spermatozoon lacks many of the usual cell organelles including endoplasmic reticulum, Golgi body, lysosomes, and inclusions. It also does not contain glycogen or other energy reserves, and so must absorb nutrients, primarily fructose, from the surrounding seminal fluid.

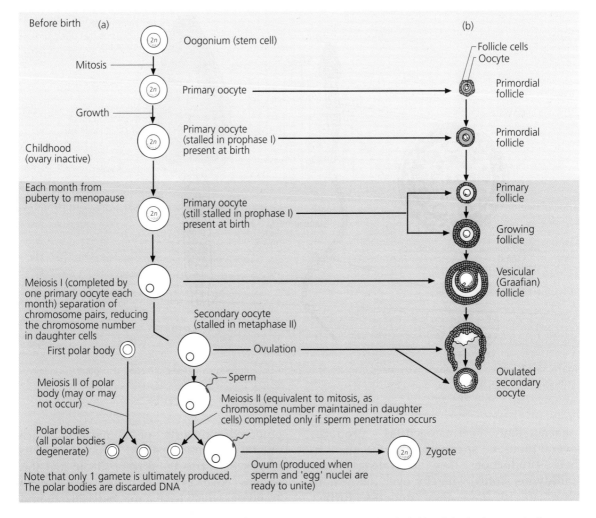

Figure 18.13 Oogenesis. (a) Flow chart of events of oogenesis: $2n$ = diploid; n = haploid. (b) Follicle development in the ovary.

Oogenesis

The female homologue of spermatogenesis is called oogenesis. As previously discussed, sperm production in males begins at puberty and generally continues throughout life. Gamete production in the female, however, is quite different. The first meiotic division of the undifferentiated oogonium (or stem cell) which produces the primary oocytes begins prior to birth.

Figure 18.13 illustrates how the female fetal oogonia, which are diploid at this stage, multi-

ply rapidly by mitosis to produce a reserve of germ cells. Subsequently, oogonia enter a growth phase and gradually primordial ovarian follicles appear, and the oogonia are transformed into primary oocytes. The latter become surrounded by a single layer of flattened follicle cells, the corona radiata. Many primordial follicles deteriorate before birth, and those remaining occupy the cortical region of the immature ovary. By birth a female's life supply of primary oocytes is approximately 750 000. These cells are 'stalled' in the early stages of the first meiotic division, and will not complete meiosis and produce functional 'ova' until stimulated to do so by hormonal changes following puberty.

Once the menstrual cycle is established, a small percentage of the primary oocytes begin their growth and developmental cycles each month. Only one oocyte per month (or perhaps one from each ovary) completes the first meiotic division, which ends when two haploid daughter cells, called a secondary oocyte and the first polar body, are produced. The secondary oocyte only undergoes the second meiotic division following fertilization by a sperm cell, and this division produces a haploid ovum and the second polar body. The first polar body may or may not divide again. The ovum, then, is only one of the daughter cells produced from the primary oocyte, and the mature ovum occurs only as a brief stage of oogenesis, as the haploid nuclei of ovum and sperm soon combine to restore the normal diploid number of chromosomes. The polar bodies are often referred to as the nuclear 'dustbins', since their DNA is catalysed. Details of conception, and embryonic and fetal development, are given in Chapter 19.

Within the woman's reproductive lifespan (i.e. from menarche to menopause) typically only one ovulation occurs each month, therefore only about 400–500 of the 750 000 primary oocytes present at birth are released during her lifetime. Thus, as in the male, nature has provided a generous supply of sex cells.

HORMONAL REGULATION OF GAMETOGENESIS IN THE MALE

The production of sperm clearly does not require the refinement associated with ova production. Nevertheless the control of spermatogenesis has two important aspects:

1 Development of spermatozoa from spermatogonium cells must be stimulated.

2 The spermatozoa must undergo a 'maturation' process without which they are inviable.

Spermatogenesis is controlled by an interplay between testosterone and the gonadotropin hormones, a relationship sometimes called the hypothalamic–pituitary–testicular axis. Another gonadal hormone, inhibin, may also be involved.

Clusters of interstitial cells between the seminiferous tubules (called cells of Leydig) secrete the male sex steroid testosterone in response to luteinizing hormone (LH) from the anterior pituitary gland (Figure 18.14). Testosterone is essential for the growth and maintenance of the testes and also for the 'capacitation' of spermatozoa in the epididymis. The other gonadotropin, follicle stimulating hormone (FSH), and also to a degree LH, stimulates Sertoli, or sustentacular, cells. These cells lie amongst the developing spermatogonia and secrete nutritive substances and chemicals that promote spermatozoa development. For example, an androgen-binding protein is released, and this facilitates the binding of testosterone to spermatogenic cells. In this way, FSH helps to make the spermatogenic cells receptive to the stimulatory effects of testosterone.

The whole process of spermatogenesis, therefore, is dependent upon the presence of appropriate concentrations of the pituitary gonadotropins and of the male sex steroid. The release of these hormones is kept in check by negative feedback. Thus, as testosterone is released beyond its homeostatic range it inhibits the release of LH and FSH by acting on the hypothalamus to suppress the secretion of gonadotropin-releasing hormone (Figure 18.14). As LH release declines, the secretion of testosterone will consequently be reduced. Testosterone already present in the blood is metabolized, the concentration of the hormone decreases, and so inhibition by negative feedback becomes less effective. Consequently, when the blood concentration of this steroid is below its homeostatic range, LH release increases again, and so on.

A second control component is present, however, in that the Sertoli cells also exert a degree of control on the rate of spermatogenesis. These

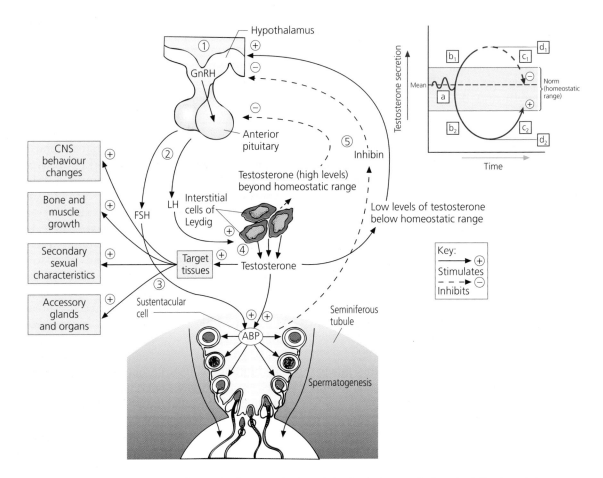

Figure 18.14 Hormonal regulation of testicular function, the hypothalamic–pituitary–testicular axis. 1 The hypothalamus releases gonadotropin-releasing hormone (GnRH). 2 GnRH stimulates the anterior pituitary to release gonadotropins – follicle-stimulating hormone (FSH) and luteinizing hormone (LH). 3 FSH acts on the sustentacular cells, causing them to release androgen-binding protein (ABP). 4 LH acts on the interstitial (Leydig) cells, stimulating their release of testosterone. ABP binding of testosterone then enhances spermatogenesis. 5 Rising levels of testosterone and inhibin exert feedback inhibition on the hypothalamus and pituitary.

a Testosterone fluctuating within its homeostatic parameters.
b_1 hypersecretion of testosterone.
c_1 Correction of imbalance via 'natural' negative feedback (e.g. inhibin) or via clinical removal of the underlying pathology causing the imbalance (e.g. removal of testicular cancer).
b_2 Hyposecretion of testosterone.
c_2 Correction of imbalance via 'natural' negative feedback stimulated by LH.
d_1 Irreversible clinical hypersecretion, e.g. hypothalamic and pituitary tumours.
d_2 Irreversible genetic disorders which result in low levels of testosterone.

cells release another hormone, called inhibin (a peptide), when the sperm count goes beyond its upper homeostatic limit. It directly inhibits the release of FSH from the pituitary, and probably also inhibits the hypothalamic secre- tion of gonadotropin-releasing factor. When the sperm count falls below its lower homeostatic limit (i.e. 20 million/ml semen), inhibin secre- tion is prevented and spermatogenesis is stimu- lated again.

Spermatogenesis is thus controlled by tight negative feedback loops involving the following hormones:

1 Gonadotropin-releasing factors from the hypothalamus, which stimulates the release of gonadotropins from the pituitary.

2 Pituitary gonadotropins (FSH and LH) which stimulate spermatogenesis, and the secetion of testosterone and inhibin.

3 Testicular hormones (testosterone and inhibin) which exert negative feedback controls on the secretion of hypothalamic releasing factors and the pituitary gonadotropins.

The names of the gonadotropins are actually derived from their functions in the female, and the hormones are chemically identical in the two sexes. In males, luteinizing hormone is sometimes called interstitial cell-stimulation hormone (ICSH), in recognition of its role in promoting testosterone secretion from the interstitial cells of the testes.

Testosterone exerts a number of actions, in addition to the capacitation of spermatozoa. These include:

1 Promoting the descent of the testes in the fetus towards the end of gestation.

2 Regulating the development of the male accessory sex organs.

3 Controlling the development and maintenance of the secondary sexual characteristics, such as the growth of facial, axillary, and pubic hair, enlargement of the larynx, and provision of masculine muscular development (Figure 18.14).

4 Being partly responsible for promoting a number of behavioural characteristics associated with adolescence.

Removal of the testes does not usually lead to a loss of secondary sexual characteristics, however, since there is an increased output of androgenic steroids from the adrenal cortex. The testes also produce female sex hormones, but their function in males is unclear.

Table 18.1 summarizes the major male reproductive hormones.

HORMONAL REGULATION OF THE FEMALE REPRODUCTIVE CYCLE

Changes occur periodically in the female between the onset of menses (menarche) and its cessation (menopause or climacteric). Menstruation, for example, is the visible external sign that cyclical changes to the endometrium are occurring. This section discusses the hormonal regulation of the menstrual and ovarian cycles.

The menstrual cycle involves cyclical changes within the endometrium and mammary glands in a non-pregnant female in response to changing levels of ovarian hormones (Figure 18.15). That is, each month the endometrium is prepared to receive a fertilized ovum; the development of this lining is essential for embryonic and fetal development during the gestatory period. If fertilization does not occur, part of the endometrium is shed as the menstrual flow. The ovarian cycle involves changes that occur in the ovaries during the menstrual cycle, and these include the maturation of a secondary oocyte, its release at ovulation, and the development and degeneration of the corpus luteum (Figure 18.15). The hormonal control of the events of both cycles is influenced by hormones of the hypothalamic–pituitary axis: the gonadotropin-releasing factors from the hypothalamus, the gonadotropin hormones (LH and FSH) from the anterior pituitary, and the steroidal oestrogens and progestins from the ovary (Figure 18.16).

The occurrence of the first menstrual flow is an indication that the uterus has begun to undergo cyclical development of its endometrium. The complete menstrual cycle becomes established with the eventual onset of ovulation. The menstrual cycle, therefore, is a sequence of changes to the reproductive tract

Table 18.1 Major reproductive hormones

Hormone	Functions	Source
Male		
GnRH (gonadotropin-releasing hormone)	Controls pituitary secretion of FSH and LH	Hypothalamus
FSH (follicle-stimulating hormone)	Increases testosterone production, aids sperm maturation	Pituitary gland (controlled by hypothalamus)
LH (luteinizing hormone)	Stimulates testosterone secretion	Pituitary gland (controlled by hypothalamus)
Testosterone	Increases sperm production, stimulates development of male primary and secondary sex characteristics, inhibits LH secretion	Interstitial endocrinocytes (Leydig cells) in testes (controlled by LH)
Female		
GnRH	Controls pituitary secretion of FSH and LH	Hypothalamus
FSH	Causes immature oocyte and follicle to develop, increases oestrogen secretion, stimulates new gamete formation and development of uterine wall after menstruation	Pituitary gland (controlled by hypothalamus)
LH	Stimulates further development of oocyte and follicle, stimulates ovulation, increases progesterone secretion, aids development of corpus luteum	Pituitary gland (controlled by hypothalamus)
Oestrogen	Stimulates thickening of uterine wall, stimulates oocyte maturation, stimulates development of female sex characteristics, inhibits FSH secretion, increases LH secretion prior to ovulation	Ovarian follicle, corpus luteum (controlled by FSH)
Progesterone	Stimulates thickening of uterine wall, stimulates formation of mammary ducts	Corpus luteum (controlled by LH)
hCG (human chorionic gonadotropin)	Prevents corpus luteum from disintegrating, stimulates oestrogen and progesterone secretion from corpus luteum	Embryonic membranes, placenta
Prostaglandin F_{2x}	Initiates parturition (labour)	Endometrium
Relaxin	Relaxes symphysis pubis and dilates uterine and cervix	Corpus luteum
Prolactin	Promotes milk production by mammary glands after childbirth	Pituitary gland (controlled by hypothalamus)
Oxytocin	Stimulates uterine contractions during labour, induces mammary glands to eject milk after childbirth	Pituitary gland (controlled by hypothalamus)

of a non-pregnant female, and is controlled by an interplay of the ovarian steroids and gonadotropin hormones. From a functional viewpoint, the uterus is anatomically most suited to carry one developing fetus, though multiple births are not uncommon. The cycle normally promotes the release of a secondary oocyte from an ovary and this becomes a mature ovum if it is fertilized. The product of fertilization (the zygote) develops into the early embryo, which must implant in the endometrium for a pregnancy to occur. The hormones involved in controlling these events, therefore, must:

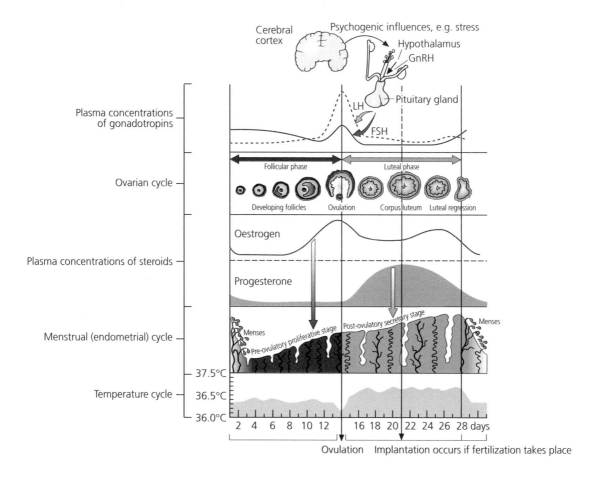

Figure 18.15 The female reproductive organs. Diagram illustrates the interrelationship of cerebral, hypothalamic, pituitary, ovarian and uterine functions throughout a usual 28-day cycle. Note: the LH surge causes ovulation. The low levels of steroids initiate menstruation.

1 Promote the development of a new endometrium.

2 Promote ovulation at a time when the endometrium is sufficiently developed for implantation to occur.

3 Promote further nutritive development of the endometrium, and prevent its 'shedding', in order to support the early embryo should implantation occur.

The processes involved are illustrated in Figure 18.15. The menstrual cycle typically has a duration of 28 days, although there is individual variation and it is subject to many environmental influences. Conventionally, timing begins at the onset of menstrual bleeding, when the endometrium that developed in the previous cycle begins to be shed, which lasts about 5 days. During this time (and just prior to it) the release of ovarian steroids is diminished and it is the lack of these which causes the endometrium to be shed. Thus, as ovarian steroid release is reduced, the negative feedback they exert on the anterior pituitary weakens and gonadotropins are secreted in increasing amounts.

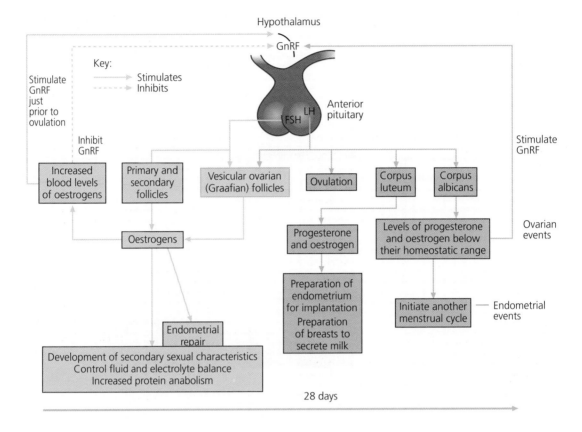

Figure 18.16 Functional aspects of the hypothalamic–pituitary–gonadal axis in females during the menstrual and ovarian cycles.

Pre-ovulation

The pre-ovulatory phase of the menstrual cycle involves the maturation of a (normally) single ovarian follicle and growth of a new uterine endometrium. The two gonadotropins (FSH and LH) are released concurrently. As its name implies, follicle-stimulating hormone promotes the development of ovarian follicles, which basically consist of an immature ovum surrounded by a mass of follicle cells. Perhaps 20 or so of these primary follicles will be stimulated in this way but there is normally one which is more advanced than the others. As the follicles develop, the gonadotropins stimulate the follicular cells to secrete oestrogens which then feed back and inhibit gonadotropin release

by the pituitary. Thus, further development for most of the follicles (now called secondary follicles) is retarded, and they atrophy and die. The most advanced one, however, will have become independent of the need for FSH by this stage and so continues to grow, as follicular cells proliferate. In addition to regulating this part of the cycle, the oestrogens released by the follicles also promote the growth of a new endometrium; that is a new stratum functionalis (functional layer) develops from the stratum basalis (basal or germinative layer).

The role of the follicular oestrogens is reflected in the name sometimes given to this part of the cycle – the follicular or proliferative phase (although this is better termed the pre-ovulatory phase).

Note that 'oestrogens' is a collective term used to describe six different steroids. The three most abundant oestrogens are 17-beta-oestradiol, oestrone, and oestriol.

Ovulation

Ovulation requires the transient release of luteinizing hormone in a 'surge' which is sufficient to prompt the shedding of the secondary oocyte from the mature Graafian follicle.

Ovulation occurs at about 14 days into the cycle, but again timing is variable between individuals. As Figure 18.15 shows, oestrogen released up to about 11–12 days powerfully inhibits the secretion of the pituitary gonadotropins. By an unknown mechanism, however, this negative feedback switches to a positive feedback with the result that secretion of pituitary stores of LH (and FSH) is stimulated by the presence of high concentrations of oestrogens in the blood. The resulting surge of LH release triggers events that cause the mature ovarian follicle to rupture and shed its secondary oocyte. The positive feedback influence on LH release is transient and quite soon reverses to negative feedback again.

Oestrogen secretion by the remnant follicle decreases slightly once the ovum has been released, but soon picks up again. The release of LH prior to ovulation also triggers the further proliferation and development of follicular cells within the follicle and these form the corpus luteum (= yellow body). The importance of luteinizing hormone in this respect is reflected in its name.

Post-ovulation

The post-ovulatory phase is marked by the continued development of the endometrium under the influence of progestins, principally progesterone, from the remnants of the Graafian follicle (the corpus luteum). The corpus luteum secretes increasing quantities of oestrogens and progesterone. Up to this point, progesterone release from the ovary has been only slight. The significance of its release after ovulation is that it promotes the secretory activity of glands within the endometrium, the vascularization of the superficial layer of the endometrium, and glycogen storage within the endometrial cells. These actions basically prepare the endometrium to receive the embryo, should the secondary oocyte be fertilized. The activities peak about 1 week after ovulation, which is about the time an embryo could be expected to arrive in the uterus after passage along the Fallopian tube. The importance of the corpus luteum and progesterone is reflected in the names for this phase of the cycle – the luteal or secretory phase (perhaps more correctly termed the post-ovulatory phase).

The release of progesterone has an additive effect on the negative feedback actions of oestrogens on the anterior pituitary gland. LH (and FSH) release eventually decreases to levels at which the hormone is incapable of maintaining the corpus luteum. If pregnancy has not occurred, this degenerates into the corpus albicans (= white body) and secretion of oestrogens and progesterone declines sharply. Consequently the endometrium cannot be sustained and it is shed and so the next menses begins. As ovarian steroid release diminishes, the secretion of gonadotropins increases once more and further ovarian follicles begin to develop and a new cycle is initiated.

Should the secondary oocyte be fertilized, and the early embryo implant in the endometrium, then the release of the ovarian steroids increases and initiates the maternal physiological changes associated with pregnancy. In this instance the functional integrity of the corpus luteum must be maintained for a few weeks in the absence of adequate LH. This is brought about by a hormone called human chorionic gonadotropin (hCG) which is released from the implanted embryo. By the time that secretion of hCG has diminished the developing placenta will be secreting steroids at a rate appropriate to maintain the pregnancy. In addition to maintaining the endometrium, progesterone

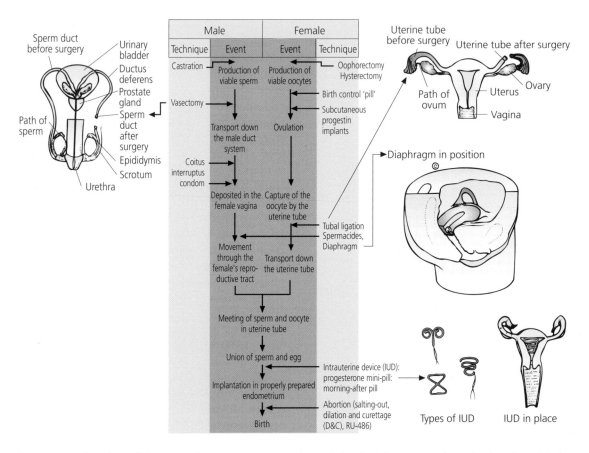

Figure 18.17 Flow chart of the events that must occur to produce a baby. Techniques or products that interfere with the process are indicated by coloured arrows at the site of interference and act to prevent the next step from occurring.

and oestrogens also prepare the mammary glands for lactation. Relaxin, a hormone secreted by the placenta towards the end of pregnancy, relaxes the pelvic ligaments and the pubic symphysis so as to aid the dilatation of the uterine cervix to facilitate delivery. Pregnancy, therefore, is an altered state of health in which the homeostatic set-points are reset. The changes to maternal physiology are discussed further in Chapter 19.

The female gonadal steroids (oestrogens and progesterones) clearly have potent physiological actions and their release cannot continue unchecked. The secretion of gonadotropins and

steroids therefore fluctuates with time, and utilizes negative feedback to establish a physiologically appropriate range of values. The onset of menopause is signalled by the climacteric when the release of steroids is insufficient to maintain the usual menstrual cycles, which therefore become less frequent. The climacteric typically begins between the ages of 40 and 50 years and occurs because of a failure of the ovary to respond to the pituitary gonadotropin hormones. The details of menopause are discussed in Chapter 19.

Table 18.1 summarizes the major female reproductive hormones.

PHYSIOLOGY OF BIRTH CONTROL

For physiological, logistic, financial, and/or emotional reasons most adults practise some form of birth control during their reproductive years. Methods of birth control include removal of the gonads and the uterus, sterilization, and mechanical and chemical contraception. Although research is making progress in its search for a male chemical contraceptive, so far the burden of birth control predominantly lies with women since most methods are female-directed (Figure 18.17). All methods are used to avoid unwanted pregnancies, and each has potential risks and benefits which must be carefully analysed on an individual basis. The interested reader is directed to other texts to consider the pros and cons of such methods as it is only the intention of this section to provide a brief overview.

Surgical methods

The surgical removal of the testes (castration), the ovaries (oophorectomy), and the uterus (hysterectomy) are all absolute and irreversible methods, and are performed only if the organs are diseased. The removal of the gonads (testes and ovaries) has adverse effects because of their important endocrine roles.

In contrast, sterilization in either sex also denies the provision of functional gametes for fertilization, but maintains the endocrine function of the gonads. One means of male sterilization is a vasectomy, whereby segments of the vas deferens (sperm tube) are removed or cauterized, thus making it impossible for spermatozoa to pass from the epididymis to the distal portions of the male reproductive tract. The cut ends do not reconnect and scarring eventually forms a permanent seal; such vasectomies are irreversible, making them unsuitable for individuals who still plan to have children but want to select the time. Vasectomies, however, can be reversible in a modified procedure that involves blocking the cut ends of the vas deferens with silicone plugs, which can later be removed.

Vasectomies do not impair normal sexual function since the epididymal and testicular secretions only account for approximately 5% of semen. Spermatozoa continue to develop in the epididymis until they are catabolized and recycled.

Female sterilization is generally achieved by performing a ligation of the Fallopian tube which prevents the secondary oocyte and sperm meeting. The procedure may be reversed, although this cannot be guaranteed. There is no impairment of sexual performance or enjoyment.

Natural and mechanical methods

Natural, and mechanical, contraceptive methods prevent fertilization without altering fertility. Natural methods include:

1 Coitus interruptus, which involves the withdrawal of the penis just prior to ejaculation. The voluntary control of ejaculation, however, is never assured since involuntary premature ejaculations are quite common.

2 Rhythm or fertility awareness methods. These take advantage of the fact that a secondary oocyte is fertilizable for a period of about 3 days during each menstrual cycle; a couple therefore avoids intercourse during this fertile period. The period is recognized by noting changes in the consistency of vaginal mucus, since the mucus changes from a sticky to a clear and stringy consistency during the fertile period, and by noting body temperature, since this rises slightly (0.2–0.6°F) after ovulation (see Figure 18.15).

The effectiveness of these techniques is limited, since few women have perfectly regular cycles, and some occasionally ovulate during the so-called safe period of menstruation.

Mechanical (barrier) methods of contraception include:

1 The condom: this prevents the deposition of sperm in the vagina.

2 The diaphragm: this stops sperm from passing into the cervix.

3 The intrauterine devices (IUDs): these are thought to change the uterine lining so that it produces a substance which destroys either the sperm, thus preventing fertilization, or the products of the fertilized ovum by preventing implantation. The use of IUDs is not widespread since they have been associated with pelvic inflammatory diseases, uterine perforations, and infertility.

Chemical methods

Chemical methods of contraception include spermicidal agents (foams, creams, jellies, suppositories) which kill spermatozoa, and oral contraceptives based on reproductive hormones.

Oral contraceptives manipulate the female cycle so that ovulation does not occur. Many contraceptive pills are now available and these are in widespread use. The most commonly used is the combination pill which contains both progesterone and oestrogens (with the former in higher concentrations). The combined effect of these hormones is to decrease the secretion of gonadotropins by inhibiting the secretion of hypothalamic gonadotropin-releasing hormone. Accordingly the levels of gonadotropins (FSH and LH) are not adequate to initiate follicular maturation or to induce ovulation, and the absence of the secondary oocyte means that pregnancy cannot occur. The mini-pill, or progesterone-only pill, has proven to be less effective in preventing pregnancy as the negative feedback response is weaker than that of oestrogens. The hormone does promote the formation of a mucus 'plug' in the cervix but this is not a perfect barrier to sperm.

Contraceptive pills are administered in a cyclical fashion, beginning 5 days after the start of the menses and continuing over the next 3 weeks. Placebo pills, or no pills, are taken in the fourth week of the cycle, to promote shedding of the endometrium. Despite their popularity, the use of the oral contraceptive pill is not without potential risks. Approximately 40–45% of women taking it experience side-effects ranging from minor problems, such as nausea, weight gain, irregular periods, and amenorrhoea, to life-threatening conditions, such as thrombosis (and its associated risks of heart attacks or strokes), liver tumours, and gallbladder diseases. Refinement of pill composition and health checks have now made the major problems rare, although women who combine this form of contraceptive with smoking and/or other risk factors associated with heart attacks and strokes are obviously increasing their chances of developing these conditions.

'Norplant' is a revolutionary contraceptive for women that was launched in 1993. The method involves administering a potent synthetic progesterone-related hormone (levonorgestrel) via six flexible tubes, each about the size of a match-stick, inserted under the skin of the upper arm. 'Norplant' has a 98.5% reliability, second only to the combined contraceptive pill. It provides reversible protection for up to 5 years, after which the capsules have to be removed and replaced with new ones if contraception is still required. 'Norplant' operates by:

1 preventing 50% of ovulations (i.e. negative feedback suppression of LH/FSH release is incomplete);

2 thickening the cervical mucus so sperm cannot swim through;

3 slowing down the transport of the successfully ovulated secondary oocytes so that fertilization becomes less likely;

4 thinning the endometrial lining so that the fertilized ovum cannot develop.

As previously discussed, the secretion of FSH by the pituitary is also inhibited by another gonadal hormone, inhibin (Figure 18.14). Inhibin may eventually prove to be an ideal contraceptive for both women and men.

Abortion

Abortion refers to the expulsion of the products of conception from the uterus. There are many forms of abortion broadly classified as either spontaneous or naturally occurring abortions, or induced or intentionally performed abortions.

Induced abortions may be performed as a form of contraception when the above birth control methods are not practised or have failed, although this is a highly controversial method. Procedures include vacuum aspiration (suction), surgical evacuation (scraping), or the use of saline solution or drugs. The latter interfere with the hormonal actions necessary to maintain pregnancy. For example, RU-486 (mifepristone) acts by blocking the quieting effects of progesterone on the uterus and is taken in the first 7 weeks of pregnancy in conjunction with prostaglandins to induce uterine contractions and a miscarriage. The drug has a 96–98% success rate. Similarly, anti-hCG vaccine inhibits the actions of chorionic gonadotropin and therefore stimulates a menstrual flow, instead of maintaining pregnancy.

Examples of homeostatic system control failures and principles of correction

Broadly speaking homeostatic failures of the reproductive system can be divided into:

1 Sexually transmitted diseases and inflammatory conditions which may be present in both sexes or specific to just one.

2 Conditions associated with infertility and sterility. The former refers to an abnormally low ability to reproduce; the latter refers to a complete inability to reproduce. Figure 18.18 summarizes the homeostatic failures responsible for infertility or sterility in either sex.

As with any organ system failure, imbalances include a vast number of conditions many of which are outside the scope of this textbook. Our intentions are to focus briefly on common imbalances. For further information the reader should refer to other texts, of which there is an abundance in well stocked libraries.

SEXUALLY TRANSMITTED DISEASES

Sexually transmitted diseases (STDs) are infectious and spread via direct sexual contact. They include the traditionally known bacterial venereal diseases – syphilis and gonorrhoea – previously the most common STDs. However, during the 1980s they have been superseded by non-specific urethritis and the viral infections of sexual herpes and acquired immune deficiency syndrome (AIDS). The latter is a consequence of infection by human immune deficiency virus (HIV) which may be transmitted during sexual contact.

The use of the contraceptive condom provides a physical barrier to prevent the spread of sexually transmitted diseases: however, their use has only been strongly advised since the discovery of HIV infection

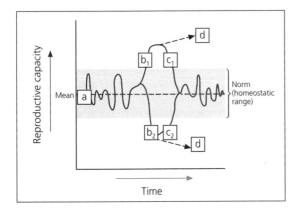

Figure 18.18 Reproductive capacity, a homeostatic function.
a Reproductive capacity fluctuating within its homeostatic range. This corresponds to the acquisition of 'normal' requirements for gametogenesis and the absence of factors (e.g. emotional) which may diminish the desire to have sexual intercourse.
b_1 Increased fertility as accompanies increased spermatogenesis (high sperm counts), or increased monthly ovulations. The latter can occur naturally, as in the case of twinning, or artificially, as a result of the IVF programme, producing 'superovulation'.
c_1 Contraception (either reversible or irreversible) encouraged to decrease the number of conceptions and potential offspring.
b_2 Decreased fertility, as occurs: (i) temporarily in females, accompanying distress, or anaemia; in males accompanying high testicular temperatures, fatigue, or increased alcohol intakes; and in both sexes accompanying malnutrition, fever, radiation or infections (STDs); (ii) permanently, as occurs in developmental structural abnormalities (e.g. male and female hermaphroditism, cryptorchidism) and physiological neural and hormonal mechanisms (e.g. hyposecretion of the gonadotropins).
c_2 Correction of the underlying pathology i.e. surgical removal of tumours, surgical correction of hermaphroditism, hormone administration in hyposecretion imbalances.
d Irreversibility of homeostatic imbalance as occurs with certain cancers.

and the fatal outcome of AIDS. HIV, and its progression into AIDS, is discussed further in Chapter 10, whilst this section discusses other infections.

Syphilis

Syphilis is caused by the bacterium *Treponema pallidum*, acquired through sexual contact or via placental transmission. Infected fetuses are usually stillborn or die shortly after birth. Sexually transmitted syphilis can affect any system of the body as the bacteria easily penetrate intact mucosal membranes, and skin abrasions, from which they then have easy access to local lymphatics and the circulation. Within a few hours of exposure a body-wide infection is in progress and if the disease is untreated it advances through primary, secondary, latent, and sometimes tertiary stages.

During the primary stage, an open sore (chancre) occurs at the point of contact. In the male this is typically the penis and thus is easily identifiable. In females, however, vaginal or cervix lesions are often undetected. The lesion persists for one to a few weeks, in which time it ulcerates, becomes crusty, heals spontaneously and disappears. Approximately 6–24 weeks later symptoms such as a skin rash, fever, and aching joints and muscles are indicative of the secondary stage. The symptoms then disappear and the disease ceases to be infectious. During this symptomless latent stage the bacterium may invade body organs; the signs of organ degeneration (such as brain changes) marks the appearance of the tertiary stage. The antibiotic penicillin interferes with the ability of dividing bacteria to synthesize new cell walls and is still the treatment of choice for all stages of syphilis.

Gonorrhoea

Gonorrhoea is caused by the bacterium, *Neisseria gonorrhoeae*. This STD primarily affects the mucous membranes of the urogenital tract, the rectum, and occasionally the eyes, throat, and lower intestines. Transmission is by direct contact, usually sexual. Symptoms vary depending upon sex of the individual concerned. Most women infected experience few symptoms and medical treatment is not sought. Consequently, these carriers spread the infection. The most common symptom in males is urethritis (see later), accompanied by painful urination and pus discharge from the penis. If untreated, gonorrhoea in males can lead to urethral constriction and inflammation of the entire duct system; in females it may lead to sterility. Correction involves antibiotic therapy, although strains are becoming increasingly resistant to these antibiotics, and thus, gonorrhoea is becoming increasingly prevalent.

Genital herpes

Many people are unaware that they suffer from genital herpes. It is caused by herpes simplex virus 2, an organism responsible for most herpes infections below the waist, including genital blisters on the prepuce and glans penis in the male, and the vulva and sometimes the vagina in females. Herpes simplex virus 1 is responsible for the majority of infections above the waist, for example, cold sores.

The painful lesions of the reproductive organs observed in genital herpes are usually more of a nuisance than a threat to life. If a pregnant woman suffers symptoms at the time of birth, a caesarean section is strongly advised to prevent complications in the newborn, since congenital herpes can cause severe malformations. Unlike syphilis and gonorrhoea, genital herpes is viral and incurable. The virus remains inside the body and so the person is subjected to recurrent symptoms. Treatment involves the administration of antiviral agents, analgesia and saline compresses. Sexual abstinence for the duration of eruption prevents sexual transmission.

Non-specific urethritis

Non-specific urethritis (NSU) is a condition in which the urethra becomes inflamed. This impedes the flow of urine, and urination is accompanied by a burning pain; there may also be a pus-containing discharge. NSU affects both sexes and can result from trauma (e.g. the passage of a catheter), chemical agents (e.g. alcohol), and non-specific microbes. Bacterial agents can pass from mother to infant during birth and so infect the eyes of the infant.

Many infections remain untreated as symptoms in the male are mild and females are usually asymptomatic. Bacterial NSU responds to tetracycline treatment.

Pelvic inflammatory diseases

Pelvic inflammatory diseases (PID) is a collective term used to include any extensive bacterial infection of the pelvic organs, especially the uterus, Fallopian tubes, or ovaries. The infection may spread to other tissues including the blood, where it may cause septic shock and death. Early treatment with antibiotics (tetracycline or penicillin) is essential to stop the PID spreading.

PHYSIOLOGICAL HOMEOSTATIC FAILURES

Homeostatic imbalances associated with infertility or sterility are common and most are attributed to problems with the female reproductive system. An infertile female has a low ability to produce functional ova and/or support a developing embryo/fetus; an infertile male, however, is incapable of producing a sufficient number of motile sperm for successful fertilization. Physiological, or functional, infertility and sterility have multifactorial aetiologies. Sexually transmitted diseases, for example, may damage reproductive structures, and thus abolish one's reproductive capacity. In addition, developmental structural abnormalities of the reproductive system and physiological problems affecting hormonal and neural regulation of reproductive function can cause sterility.

Male homeostatic failures

A reduced reproductive capacity in males may be due to factors that cause a decreased sperm production, structural abnormalities of the sperm, or an obstruction of the reproductive ducts.

Disorders of the testes

A decreased sperm production (called oligospermia) can result from disruption of seminiferous tubule function. The decrease may be temporary, as occurs with acute infections (the leading cause of infertility), or permanent, as occurs occasionally when a baby is born with undescended testes (cryptorchidism), or has a physical deficiency or obstruction (the leading cause of sterility). Cryptorchidism may cause hormonal imbalances; therefore such infants require early treatment by surgery or by testosterone injections which stimulate the descent of the testes. If untreated, spermatogenesis is permanently inhibited. Testicular cancers are associated with those with a history of late descended or undescended testes and most cancers arise from the sperm-producing cells. As with all cancers, correction is most effective when diagnosis is made early in the development of the tumour, and necessitates removal of the cancerous tissue.

Disorders of the prostate

The prostate gland is susceptible to infection, enlargement, and benign and malignant tumours. Benign prostatic enlargement, or hypertrophy, is a common problem in older men. Since the prostate surrounds the urethra, its enlargement can obstruct the flow of urine, resulting in secondary homeostatic imbalances of the bladder, uterus, and kidneys. Correction involves partial or total removal of the gland.

Prostatic cancer is a common and leading cause of cancer death in men, and since testosterone stimulates an increased growth rate of the cancer and oestrogens inhibit growth, treatment may involve surgical removal of the testes, or the administration of drugs that are testosterone antagonists or oestrogenic. Although drug administration does not stop the cancer, it may slow growth.

Disorders of the penis and scrotum

As discussed earlier the penis may be subjected to numerous sexually transmitted infections and structural abnormalities. Paraphimosis is a condition in which the foreskin fits so tightly over the glans penis that it cannot retract, thus correction involves circumcision. Mild paraphimosis causes the accumulation of dirt or organic matter under the foreskin, resulting in severe infections. Severe paraphimosis can result in urinary flow obstruction, and possibly result in the death of an infant born with this condition. After puberty failure to achieve a penile erection occurs and, although this does not affect spermatogenesis, it may cause infertility since normal intercourse may not be possible.

A common cause of scrotal swelling is the accumulation of fluid called a hydrocele which may result from an inguinal hernia. The latter occurs because the intestines are pushed through a weakened area of the abdominal wall that separates the abdominal pelvic cavity from the scrotum. Such hernias usually occur upon lifting heavy objects, although they can also be congenitally formed. Correction involves external supports that prevent organs from protruding into the scrotum, but the more serious hernias require surgical repair.

Homeostatic failure of the female reproductive system

Menstruation reflects the health of the endocrine glands that control the process. Imbalances of the female reproductive system frequently involve menstrual disorders. Amenorrhoea, the absence of menstruation, can be caused by endocrine disorders, abnormal congenital ovarian and uterine development, a change in body weight, or continuous rigorous athletic training. Correction involves treating the underlying disorder or condition.

Dysmenorrhoea refers to painful menstruations which are classified as primary or secondary dysmenorrhoeas. The former occurs in the absence of associated pelvic pathology. It is thought to be caused by a hypersecretion of certain uterine prostaglandins, since these chemicals cause painful spasms of uterine muscle. Prostaglandin antagonistics such as aspirin and ibuprofen, therefore, are sometimes used to relieve the symptoms, although oral contraceptives that inhibit uterine contractions may also be administered. Secondary dysmenorrhoea can be due to stenosis of the cervix and from various inflammatory conditions. Correction involves treating the underlying pathology.

Premenstrual syndrome

Premenstrual syndrome (PMS) is a term usually reserved for the severe physical and emotional distress which can accompany the premenstrual phase of the menstrual cycle, although sometimes it overlaps with menstruation. Its cause remains unclear, but suggested causes include:

1 an excessive level of oestrogen, with effects on fluid balance, breast development, etc.;

2 an inadequate level of progesterone;

3 an inadequate level of the neurotransmitter dopamine;

4 vitamin B_6 deficiency;

5 hypoglycaemia.

Current treatments focus on relieving the symptoms of PMS, which include oedema, breast swelling, abdominal distension, backache, constipation, fatigue, depression, or anxiety. Prostaglandin-suppressing drugs are commonly used. Diuretics and vitamin B_6 administrations have also been found to be helpful by some women.

Ovarian cysts

Ovarian cysts are benign enlargements on one or both ovaries, or within the corpus luteum. The cyst, a fluid-filled sac, develops from a follicle that fails to rupture completely, or from the corpus luteum that fails to degenerate. They rarely become dangerous and often disappear within a few months of appearance. If they remain and cause pain then surgical removal corrects the problem.

Endometriosis

The Fallopian tubes open into the peritoneal cavity of the abdomen and endometriosis, another benign condition, is the presence of functional endometrial tissue that has exited the uterus. The displaced tissue can occur in many different locations, although it is most often found in, or on pelvic and abdominal organs. The tissues develop and regress during the normal menstrual cycle and symptoms include premenstrual pain or unusual menstrual pain (dysmenorrhoea) caused by the displaced tissue being shed during menstruation.

Malignant tumours

Malignancies of the reproductive tract and related organs, especially the breast, account for the majority of cancer cases amongst women. Mammary cancers often metastasize to the ovaries, producing ovarian cancers, although ovarian cancers can occur independently. Breast cancer has one of the highest fatality rates of all cancers affecting women. It often goes undiscovered since its associated pain only becomes evident when the cancer is quite advanced. Corrective measures are dependent upon the size and type of cancer, and include lumpectomies and mastectomies. In addition, the axillary nymph nodes may be removed if metastasis is suspected.

Cervical cancer is a relatively common disorder of the female reproductive tract that begins with cervical dysplasia, that is a change in the shape, growth, and number of cervical cells. If the dysplasia is minimal, cells may regress to normal, but if severe it may progress to cancer. Depending upon the progression of the disease, cervical cancer may be detected in its early stages by a Pap smear. Treatment may consist of tissue removal by excision of lesions, by hysterectomy, and/or by radiotherapy, chemotherapy, and laser therapy to destroy discrete areas of tissue.

PSEUDOHERMAPHRODITISM

The phenotypic sex of the newborn depends upon hormonal cues received by tissues during development, and not upon the genetic sex of the individual, although the two are usually associated. Pseudohermaphroditism is a condition in which an individual's genetic and anatomical sex differ. Although such cases are relatively infrequent, the most common cause of female pseudohermaphroditism is adrenal genital syndrome (adrenal hypertrophy) in which a hypersecretion of androgens exist. This can occur in the female fetus or in the mature female, the androgens in the latter case gradually transform the female appearance into a male form. Amenorrhoea occurs, causing sterility. Other causes of female pseudohermaphroditism include androgenic drug abuse, pregnant females exposed to androgenic drug, and maternal pituitary and/or adrenal endocrine tumours.

Male pseudohermaphroditism occurs in response to a hyposecretion of androgens. A common cause is testicular feminization syndrome. This homeostatic imbalance involves a defect in the cellular receptors that respond to androgens. Consequently, embryonic and adult tissues cannot respond to the existing normal levels of these male hormones, thus the person develops and remains physically female. However, the menstrual cycle does not appear (amenorrhoea), the uterus is absent, and the vagina ends in a blind pocket. Correction involves hormonal therapy and surgery to produce a sexually functioning male or female.

HYPOSECRETION OF GONADOTROPINS

Hyposecretion of gonadotropin-releasing hormones, and gonadotropins (FSH and LH), can lead to sterility in either sex, since functional gametes will not be produced. In females, hyposecretion of oestrogens by the ovary has a similar effect. The depression of hypothalamic secretion of gonadotropin-releasing hormones may be a consequence of dietary disturbances, distress, or anaemia. In females these factors may result in an absence of the menstrual cycle (amenorrhoea). In males, fatigue, alcohol abuse, and emotional factors are more common causes of impotency. High testicular temperatures are also associated with sterility in males, by causing a depression in spermatogenesis. Pituitary, gonadal, and adrenal gland tumours may also cause infertility by secreting abnormal types and amounts of gonadotropin or sex hormones.

Summary

1 Cells are reproduced by:

(a) Mitosis – a duplication division which occurs in all body (somatic) cells and ensures that the diploid number of chromosomes is sustained, so that homeostatic functions can proceed within their normal parameters.

(b) Meiosis – a reduction division which occurs in the gonads and ensures that gametes have the haploid number of chromosomes, so that the diploid number (essential for normal embryonic/fetal development) is restored at fertilization.

2 Reproductive organs have specialized exocrine tissues adapted to produce, maintain, and transport gametes, and endocrine tissue adapted to produce steroidal hormones.

3 Primary sex organs include the male testes and the female ovaries. These organs produce spermatozoa (a process called spermatogenesis), secondary oocytes (oogenesis), and sex hormones. Accessory organs include the internal and external reproductive organs.

4 At puberty, hypothalamic gonadotropin-releasing factor/hormone stimulates the production and secretion of gonadotropins (FSH and LH) by the pituitary gland. These hormones are important in gametogenesis and in the production of the male and female sex hormones, androgens and oestrogens, and progesterone, respectively.

5 In males, mature spermatozoa are produced in the seminiferous tubules, and collect in the epididymis, where they are stored until they are catabolized and recycled or released into the vas deferens upon ejaculation. The vas continues as the urethra at the base of the bladder, and this latter part provides the exit route for both sperm and urine at the tip of the penis.

6 The seminal vesicles, prostate, and Cowper's or bulbourethral glands (and to a small extent the seminiferous tubules and the epididymis) add secretions to the sperm cells to produce the semen.

7 Testes descend via the inguinal canal into the scrotal sacs prior to birth. Cryptorchidism is an imbalance which reflects undescended testes. Inguinal hernia is a dropping of a portion of the intestines into the inguinal canal.

8 The penis is the male copulatory organ with specialized tissue (corpora cavernosa and corpus spongiosum) which becomes engorged with blood when sexually aroused, producing a rigid and erect structure necessary for the insertion into the vagina during sexual intercourse.

9 In the female, gametes are produced and matured in follicles in the ovaries at puberty, under the hormonal influence of pituitary FSH. Adequate FSH release signals the onset of menarche (the first menstrual flow).

10 The mature (or Graafian follicle) releases the secondary oocyte (and some of its surrounding follicular cells) at ovulation. These cells are taken to the uterus via the Fallopian tubes. The trigger to ovulation is an LH 'surge' from the pituitary caused by a transient positive feedback mechanism produced by oestrogen, the release of which is relatively high at this point within the menstrual cycle.

11 LH converts the follicle cells remaining in the ovary after ovulation into the corpus luteum, a body which secretes steroid hormones (progesterone and oestrogens). These hormones suppress FSH and LH release by negative feedback, in order to prevent further follicular development, and to promote further development of the endometrium.

12 The uterine cycle (average 28 days) begins with menstruation (up to the fifth day); following this steroids (from the pre-ovulatory follicles and the post-ovulatory corpus luteum) prepare the uterus for implantation of the fertilized 'ovum'. If fertilization does not occur the corpus luteum becomes the corpus albicans which then degenerates and is recycled. Consequently, steroid secretion from the ovary decreases, removing their inhibitory action over the gonadotropins; their subsequent release is associated with the next menstrual cycle.

13 The vagina is the female copulatory organ. The hymen guards its entrance in virgins. Bartholin's glandular tissue secretes a lubricant in anticipation of, and during, sexual intercourse. The external genitalia of the vulva are comprised of the mons pubis, labia majora and minora, clitoris, and vestibule.

14 During sexual arousal the engorgement of blood in the clitoris causes its erection.

15 Fertilization occurs high in the Fallopian tubes. The fusion of sperm and ovum nuclei produce the diploid zygote.

16 Contraceptive methods are designed to prevent gamete formation or prevent the sperm reaching the secondary oocyte. Methods are classified as being natural, mechanical, and chemical.

17 Homeostatic imbalances of male and female reproductive tracts are divided into anatomical and physiological abnormalities, both of which may be responsible for infertility or sterility in either sex.

Review Questions

1 List the primary sex organs of the male and female.

2 Why is it necessary that the testes descend prior to birth? Name the homeostatic imbalance in which there is a failure of this descent.

3 Describe the structure of the testes.

4 Where are sperm produced?

5 What cells are concerned with androgen production and secretion?

6 Distinguish between meiosis and mitosis.

7 Trace the path of spermatozoon and secondary oocyte exit from their respective reproductive systems.

8 List the glands associated with producing semen, and the equivalent female lubricant.

9 Describe the structure of the penis.

10 Describe the structure of the ovary.

11 Discuss the similarities and differences between the timing of oogenesis and spermatogenesis.

12 Distinguish between primary oocyte, secondary oocyte, polar bodies, ova, and zygotes.

13 Discuss the hormonal regulation of the menstrual cycle.

14 What do the abbreviations FSH and LH mean?

15 How are the gametes moved along the Fallopian tubes?

16 Draw and label the male and female reproductive tracts.

17 Describe the male and female act of sexual intercourse.

18 List five methods of contraception.

19 Describe the structure of the mammary glands.

20 List and describe the major male and female homeostatic imbalances mentioned in this chapter which may be associated with infertility and sterility.

Human development and ageing: Conception to death

Introduction: human development and homeostasis

Details of anatomical and physiological changes during the lifespan

Examples of homeostatic failure: disorders of development

Summary

Review questions

Introduction: human development and homeostasis

This book has concentrated primarily on the functions of tissues and organs evident in the adult. Some functions, however, are absent or only poorly established at birth, since growth and functional 'maturation' of certain tissues is observed during various phases of the lifespan. Anatomical and functional changes to certain systems occur during these phases and either alter homeostatic set-points, and thus promote change, or improve homeostatic control and therefore reinforce psychophysiological well-being. Some changes, such as those observed in the pregnant woman, are only transient adaptations to specific life cycle events.

Human development can therefore be envisaged as being changes in tissue growth and function during specific periods of the lifespan, appropriate to the age of the individual. On the other hand, increasing chronological age during adulthood is accompanied by declining cell and tissue functions, leading to reduced homeostatic efficiency and a resultant increase in the susceptibility to factors that promote ill-health.

Developmental events during the lifespan have a genetic basis: their sequencing is too precise for it to be otherwise. It is clear, however, that environmental factors influence the timing of events and also if they progress 'normally'. Thus, the environment of the individual may be responsible for genetic mutation, which is especially important if this involves gamete or embryo DNA, or may directly or indirectly influence gene expression, for example, by determining how substrates are metabolized, if and when hormones are secreted, and whether or not substrates are available in sufficient quantities.

Extrinsic factors may affect functional development at any stage of the lifespan, and also the rate at which physiological decline progresses during adulthood. There is only limited scope in this book to identify the factors that are known to influence human development, but some are acknowledged in the text (here and in other chapters) whilst others are highlighted in the 'Homeostatic failure' section later.

The intention of this chapter is to outline those processes which lead to the differentiation of tissues in the embryo, to fetal growth,

child development, and the advent of reproductive maturity during puberty. A discussion of human development must also include those changes observed in pregnancy, the birth process, and lactation, as all require adaptations to maternal homeostasis. Functional enhancement continues into early adulthood but thereafter systemic decline is measurable, although not necessarily apparent. Various theories have been proposed to explain the ageing process and these will be discussed in relation to recent research findings.

Details of anatomical and physiological changes during the lifespan

FERTILIZATION AND FORMATION OF THE ZYGOTE

Fertilization of the ovum normally takes place within the ampulla of a Fallopian tube and must occur within 24 hours of ovulation, since this is the period of ovum viability. Ovulation actually releases the secondary oocyte, which has already undergone the first meiotic division and so has only half the diploid number of chromosomes, from the ovarian follicle. When released it is surrounded by a glycoprotein layer called the zona pellucida, and a cloud of granulosa cells called the cumulus oophorus (the innermost cells of the cumulus form the corona radiata; Figure 19.1). Of the millions of spermatozoa ejaculated during intercourse only a few hundred will arrive in the vicinity of the oocyte, and only one will penetrate and fertilize it.

Sperm in the vicinity of the oocyte secrete the enzyme acrosin, from the acrosome at the head of the sperm, and this changes the properties of the matrix of the zona pellucida and cumulus oophorus. Once one spermatozoon has penetrated the oocyte, however, the sperm nucleus initiates further enzyme activity

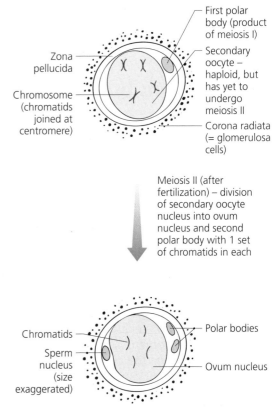

Figure 19.1 Changes in the secondary oocyte at fertilization. Only four chromosomes are shown, for clarity.

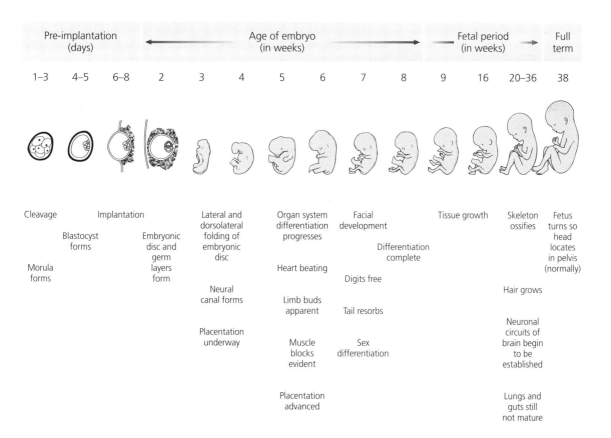

| Pre-implantation (days) | | | ← Age of embryo (in weeks) → | | | | | | | Fetal period (in weeks) → | | Full term |

| 1–3 | 4–5 | 6–8 | 2 | 3 | 4 | 5 | 6 | 7 | 8 | 9 | 16 | 20–36 | 38 |

Cleavage

Implantation

Blastocyst forms

Morula forms

Embryonic disc and germ layers form

Lateral and dorsolateral folding of embryonic disc

Neural canal forms

Placentation underway

Organ system differentiation progresses

Heart beating

Limb buds apparent

Muscle blocks evident

Placentation advanced

Facial development

Differentiation complete

Digits free

Tail resorbs

Sex differentiation

Tissue growth

Skeleton ossifies

Hair grows

Neuronal circuits of brain begin to be established

Lungs and guts still not mature

Fetus turns so head locates in pelvis (normally)

Figure 19.2 Embryo/fetal development: chronology of tissue differentiation.

in the oocyte which changes the nature of the oocytic plasma membrane and zona pellucida and so prevents the access of further sperm. The tail of the sperm separates from it during fertilization and only the head (i.e. nucleus) of the sperm will penetrate the oocyte.

For a short while the sperm and oocyte nuclei remain separate. During this period the oocyte nucleus divides to produce two daughter nuclei: the ovum nucleus and the second polar body (Figure 19.1). The polar bodies and ovum nucleus are therefore the daughter nuclei produced during gametogenesis in the female (the first polar body arises from the first meiotic division of the primary oocyte; see Chapter 18). Only the ovum nucleus remains

viable; the polar bodies have no further function and are eventually catalysed. The haploid ovum nucleus combines with the haploid sperm nucleus, thus restoring the normal (diploid) quota of chromosomes. The fertilized ovum is now called a zygote and must undergo substantial development before it can be considered an embryo.

EMBRYO AND FETAL DEVELOPMENT

Embryo development can be considered in two phases: (1) that prior to implantation in the uterine endometrium, and (2) that after implantation. The chronology of tissue differentiation is briefly described in this section, but is detailed in Figure 19.2.

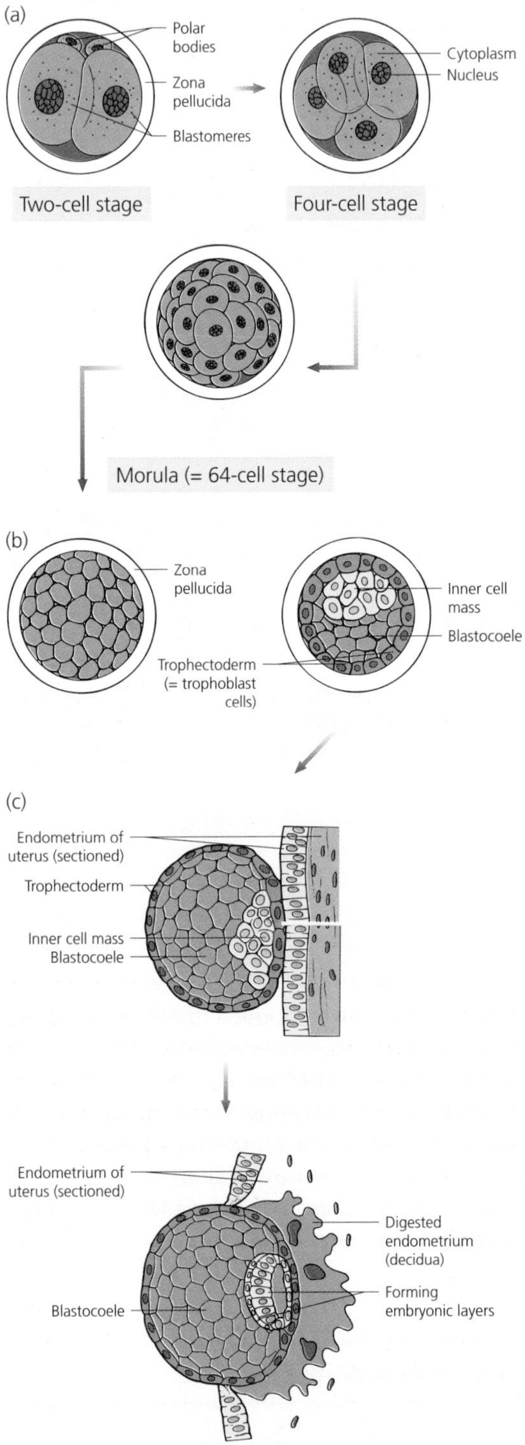

Pre-implantation development

The morula

Cell division by mitosis begins immediately after the ovum and sperm nuclei have fused. The cells divide approximately every 12 hours, eventually producing a ball of 64 cells. There is no increase in overall size, however, as the cells remain encapsulated within the zona pellucida which surrounded the oocyte at ovulation. The structure at this stage is called a morula (= 'mulberry'; Figure 19.3a). Research indicates that a cell can actually be removed during morula development without affecting future development. The cells, therefore, do not yet have a predetermined 'destiny'.

The blastocyst

Morula development occurs as the fertilized ovum is transported along the Fallopian tube. It will normally take 3 or 4 days before it arrives in the body of the uterus, by which time the morula will have been transformed. Some cells will have migrated to the outer surface, leaving a fluid-filled cavity called the blastocoele (-coele = space or compartment), whilst a small cluster of cells, called the inner cell mass, will have collected at one side or pole of the cavity. This stage of development is called a blastocyst (Figure 19.3b).

The developmental significance of the blastocyst is that cells within it have now shown a degree of specialization of role. In fact, the

Figure 19.3 Pre-implantation development. (a) Development of the morula from the zygote. (b) The blastocyst (in section). (c) Implantation.

inner cell mass is destined to become the embryo whilst cells derived from the outer surface will eventually be incorporated into the placenta. Thus the blastocyst provides the earliest evidence of functional specialization resulting from selective gene activation/deactivation.

Implantation

Two or three days after arrival within the uterus (i.e. on about the sixth day after fertilization) the blastocyst orientates itself so that the inner cell mass is adjacent to the endometrial surface. This will usually be in the upper areas of the uterus. It 'hatches' from the zona pellucida and adheres to the endometrium. Adherence is promoted by a change in the chemical and electrical properties of the surfaces of the blastocyst and endometrium.

At this point those cells forming the outer layer of the blastocyst begin to secrete enzymes which hydrolytically digest the immediate endometrial cells, and so initiate implantation (Figure 19.3c). This action explains the name given to these cells (trophoblasts; troph = nutrition) and that given to the cell layer, the trophectoderm (ecto- = outer; derm = layer). Note though that the trophectoderm bears no relation to the embryonic ectoderm mentioned later. Implantation is complete by about the eleventh day after fertilization.

Developmental changes within the implanted blastocyst now gain in momentum, but at this stage continue to be fuelled by substrates supplied by digestion of the endometrium, which by this time is rich in food deposits and blood vessels as a result of the action of progesterone secreted by the ovary of the mother.

Post-implantation development

Development after implantation can be divided for clarity into that of (1) differentiation of the inner cell mass into the embryo/fetus, (2) development of the placenta, and (3) development of the extra-embryonic membranes.

Differentiation of the inner cell mass: the embryo

The inner cell mass of the implanted blastocyst becomes organized into a flat structure called the embryonic disc. This disc of cells becomes stratified (a process called gastrulation) into three distinct layers of cells called the ectoderm, mesoderm, and endoderm (derm = layer; ecto- = outer; meso- = middle; endo- = inner). The embryo is about 14–18 days old at this stage and gastrulation represents the second phase in tissue specialization. The names of the layers refer to their final position within the developing embryo. Thus a relatively flat structure is transformed by the curling over of the ectoderm with the result that the endoderm and mesoderm form concentric tube-like layers enclosed within it (Figure 19.4).

This simple process lays down the basic body plan. If one imagines a cross-section through the adult abdomen it can be clearly envisaged how the gut and associated structures are derived from the endodermal tube, whilst the epidermis of the skin is formed from the embryonic ectoderm. Much of the structures in between, for example the skeleton, skeletal muscle layers, and blood, are derived from the mesoderm. A perforation at the 'head' and 'tail' end of the embryo eventually forms the mouth and anus.

Recent evidence indicates that chemicals produced by endometrial cells in the area influence subsequent development of the embryo. Thus, the diffusion of these chemicals into the blastocyst establishes a longitudinal concentration gradient through the inner cell mass, with its highest concentration in proximity to the endometrial surface. This gradient seems to determine which part of the embryo will form the 'head' end.

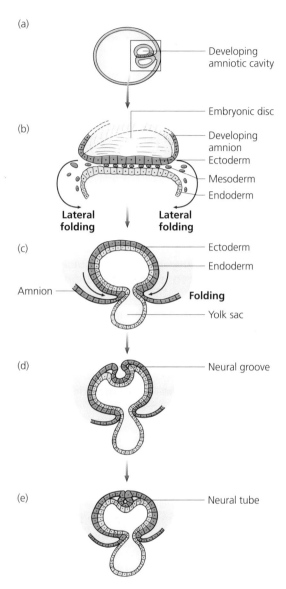

Figure 19.4 The embryonic germ layers and differentiation of the neural canal. (a) and (b) The embryonic disc. (c) Folding to internalize the endoderm. (d) Invagination of the ectoderm to form the neural groove. (e) Enclosure of the neural tube.

A more complete description of the tissues derived from the embryological layers is shown in Table 19.1 but it is worth noting here the significance of the early development of the

nervous and circulatory systems. The nervous system must begin to develop early, partly because of its ultimate complexity and partly because of its role in coordinating fetal tissue functions. Similarly, the heart and circulation must also develop early since it is this system which must ensure adequate delivery of food material to tissues to facilitate the rapid growth exhibited by the embryo.

The nervous system begins as a longitudinal groove which appears within the surface of the embryological ectoderm about 18–20 days after fertilization (Figure 19.4). The groove is eventually pinched off to form the neural tube which will develop into the spinal cord. Expansions at the head end results in the development of forebrain, midbrain, and hindbrain structures (see Chapter 13). The appearance of the neural groove is another example of genes being selectively activated. Although the embryo has undergone considerable specialization prior to this, the neural groove represents the first visible sign of the development of a specific organ.

Tissues and organs continue to differentiate during the following weeks, and the embryo becomes increasingly humanoid in shape (see Figure 19.2). Development includes the determination of the sex of the embryo, which occurs from about the seventh week.

SEX DETERMINATION

Male and female gonads develop at the same site within the fetal abdomen. Associated with this undifferentiated gonadal tissue are two sets of ducts, called the Wolffian and Müllerian ducts (Figure 19.5). Male sex determination is triggered by activation for a short period of time of genes on the Y-chromosome (if the genotype of the fetus is XY) which stimulate certain genes on the X-chromosome. These promote gonadal differentiation into testes, which begin to produce male sex steroids, (androgens) and a glycopeptide hormone called Müllerian-inhibition substance (MIS).

Androgens stimulate the differentiation of the Wolffian ducts into the vas deferens and

Table 19.1 Structures produced by the three primary germ layers

Endoderm	Mesoderm	Ectoderm
Epithelium of digestive tract (except the oral cavity and anal canal) and its associated glands	All skeletal, most smooth, and all cardiac muscle	Nervous tissue
		Epidermis of skin
Epithelium of urinary bladder, gall bladder, and liver	Cartilage, bone, and other connective tissues	Hair follicles, arrector pili muscles, nails, and epithelia of sebaceous and sudoriferous glands
Epithelium of pharynx, external auditory tube, tonsils, larynx, and airways of the lungs	Blood, bone marrow, and lymphoid tissue	
	Endothelium of blood vessels and lymphatics	Lens, cornea, and optic nerve of eye and internal eye muscles
Epithelium of thyroid, parathyroid, pancreas, and thymus glands	Dermis of skin	Inner and outer ear
	Fibrous and vascular coats of eye	Neuroepithelium of sense organs
Epithelium of prostate and bulbourethral glands, vagina, vestibule, urethra, and associated glands	Middle ear	Epithelium of oral and nasal cavities, paranasal sinuses, salivary glands, and anal canal
	Epithelium of kidneys and ureters	
	Epithelium of adrenal cortex	Epithelium of pineal gland, pituitary gland, and adrenal medulla
	Epithelium of gonads and genital ducts	

associated structures of the male reproductive tract. External genitalia develop accordingly. As its name implies, MIS causes the Mullerian ducts to degenerate. In contrast, in the absence of androgens (normally because the fetal genotype is XX) the Müllerian ducts persist and develop into the Fallopian tubes and uterus of the female tract, whilst the Wolffian ducts regress and atrophy. The gonads descend into their final positions in the body during the later stages of gestation, but the precise mechanism is unclear. The testes eventually descend into the scrotum, usually by the end of the seventh month of gestation.

Sex steroids also appear to influence brain development, and this eventually results in the mechanism by which sex steroids influence either male or female behaviours (see Chapter 13).

THE FETUS

All organs are basically defined by the end of 8 weeks of embryonic development, although their functions may be only rudimentary. The embryo is now considered to be a fetus (see Figure 19.2). Development of the fetus is primarily that of growth and functional maturation of the organs laid down during the embryonic period.

Placentation and the umbilical cord

Implantation of the blastocyst causes the endometrium to become thicker and even more vascular, as oestrogen and progesterone secretion from the corpus luteum (the remnant of the ovarian follicle which released the ovum) is stimulated by chorionic gonado-

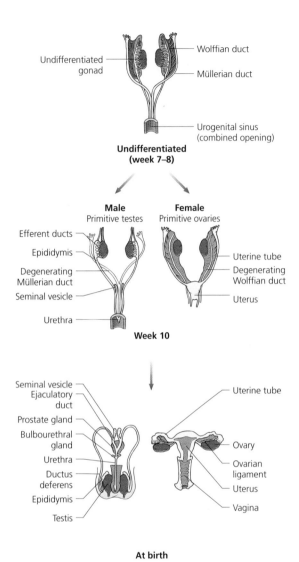

Figure 19.5 Differentiation of the sex organs.

endometrium. Placentation provides a means of direct and efficient exchange between the embryonic/fetal circulation and that of the mother, and is therefore essential for the continued development of the embryo/fetus.

THE PLACENTA

Four weeks after fertilization the implanted 'blastocyst' is about 2 cm in diameter, whilst the differentiating 'inner cell mass' – i.e. the embryo – is about 1 cm in length and already exhibits head structures, heart, and limb buds. The trophectoderm has developed finger-like projections by this time. The layer is now called the chorion and the projections are called the chorionic villi (Figure 19.6a).

The villi grow into the decidua. Some penetrate deeply and help to anchor the developing embryo, whilst others remain more superficial. Blood vessels from the embryo grow via a body stalk (formed from the allantois membrane – see below) into these latter villi, which continue to grow and branch. Maternal blood spaces within the decidua bathe the growing villi and eventually an extensive system of villi, with embryo blood vessels, 'hangs' within maternal blood spaces, providing a large surface area for the exchange of materials between mother and embryo (Figure 19.6b). The whole structure forms the placenta and the extent of its development can be gauged from its dimensions at term, when it is 18–20 cm in diameter, about 2.5 cm thick at its centre and weighs as much as 600–700 g.

The actual interface between embryo blood and maternal blood forms a delicate but effective physical barrier which prevents a mingling of the two circulations. A physical barrier is necessary because the developing embryo has a different genotype from the mother, since only half of its DNA comes from her, and embryo cells will therefore have surface antigens which will be quite different from those of the maternal tissues. Any contact between embryo cells and those of the maternal immune system will thus promote a response which could potentially kill the embryo as a 'foreign' tissue.

tropin, a hormone produced by the embryo itself. The changes in the endometrium, now called the decidua, help to maintain the nourishment of the embedded embryo.

As tissue differentiation and growth accelerates in the late embryo, the need for nutrition and excretion begins to exceed that which is provided by diffusional exchange with the

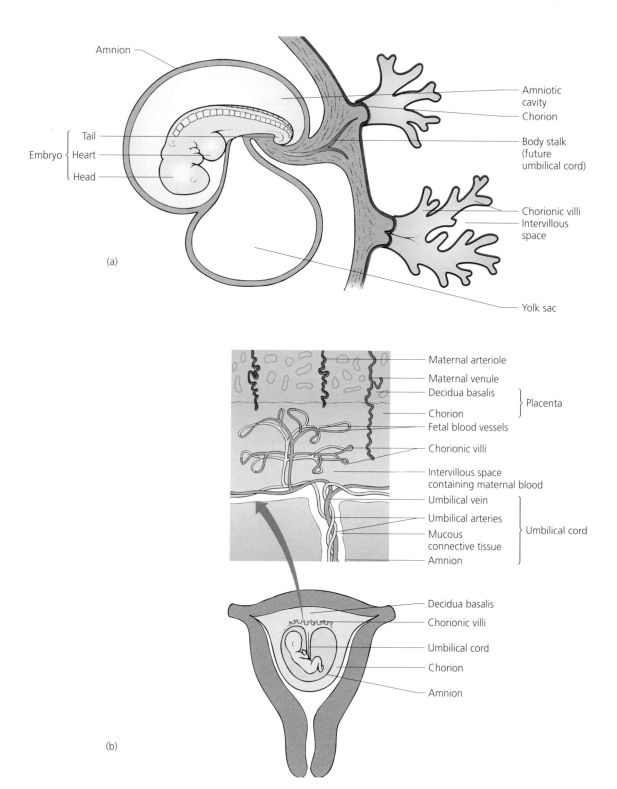

Figure 19.6 Placentation. (a) Growth of chorionic villi. (b) Development of chorionic villi to include fetal blood vessels. Note the extensive maternal blood spaces which bathe the villi.

Table 19.2 Functions of the placenta

Function	Details
Respiration	O_2, CO_2 exchange between fetal and maternal blood
Nutrition	Selective provision of nutrients from maternal blood. (Many drugs cross the placenta with ease either because they are lipid-soluble, or because they utilize membrane transport processes)
	Enzymatic catabolism of maternal proteins and complex carbohydrates
	Storage of carbohydrate for future use by the fetus
Excretion	Transfer of fetal metabolic products to the maternal blood
Protection	A physical barrier against the passage of most bacteria/viruses. Some can cross into fetal blood, however, as can some toxins
Endocrine	Oestrogens and progesterone maintain the placenta and promote changes in maternal physiology essential to support the growing fetus. Oestrogen production by the fetal adrenal gland is also important. This involvement of the fetus in influencing the maternal environment is often recognized by reference to a functional fetal–placental unit.
	Chorionic gonadotropin helps to maintain steroid production by the corpus luteum until the placenta is sufficiently developed in this respect
	Placental lactogen (also called chorionic somatomammotrophin) is involved in breast development during pregnancy. It is also a metabolic hormone and alters maternal glucose and fat metabolism. Its release increases during pregnancy and it is used clinically as an index of placental function
	Relaxin promotes cervical dilatation during birth, and relaxes the symphysis pubis joint

Essential substances will cross the placental interface either by simple diffusion or by active transport. A thin barrier with small diffusional distances, and a relatively small energy requirement for transport processes, is vital if such exchanges are to be adequate.

In addition to its nutritional role, the placenta also has important endocrine functions which help the mother to maintain her pregnancy, facilitate breast development and help to prepare the reproductive tract for the birth process. Placental functions are summarized in Table 19.2.

THE UMBILICAL CORD

Concurrent with the development of the placenta is the growth of the umbilical cord, which develops from the vascularized body stalk. The limited vasculature of the stalk, whilst adequate for the needs of the early embryo, cannot support the rapid growth observed in the fetus. The vessels of the umbilical cord provide a much more extensive circulation of blood between the fetus and placenta. The cord contains two umbilical arteries, which originate from the fetal iliac arteries, and these carry deoxygenated blood to the placenta (Figure 19.7). Following the transfer of nutrients and excretory products a single umbilical vein returns the blood to the fetus, where the vein branches to join the portal vein (which conveys blood to the liver) and the inferior vena cava (which conveys blood to the heart). The development of the placenta and umbilical cord is complete by the end of the third month of pregnancy, although nutrient exchange between maternal blood, chorionic villi, and body stalk will have commenced much earlier.

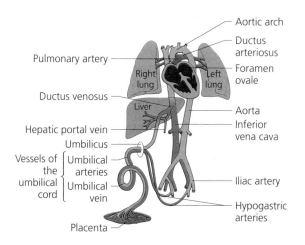

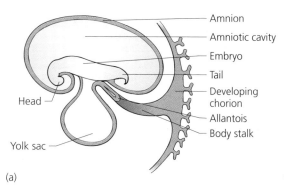

Figure 19.7 Fetal circulation.

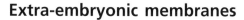

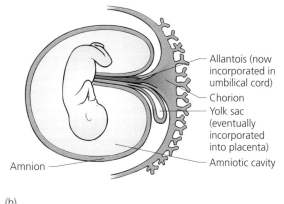

Figure 19.8 The extra-embryonic membranes.

Extra-embryonic membranes

There are four membranes – the chorion, amnion, allantois, and yolk sac. The chorion and amnion are the most extensively developed. The chorion has been mentioned previously as developing from the trophectoderm of the trophoblast stage (see Figure 19.3c). It eventually increases in size until it lines the uterine cavity. The remaining three membranes develop as outgrowths of cell layers of the actual embryo.

The amnion develops from ectoderm of the embryonic disc and distends to encompass the developing embryo (Figure 19.8). It secretes amniotic fluid (the 'waters') which provides support for the growing fetus, helps to maintain a constant temperature, and acts as a shock absorber during maternal movement. The fluid is also swallowed by the fetus, and a dilute urine excreted into it, and this facilitates the functional development of the gut and kidneys. Its volume at term is 1–1.5 litres.

The yolk sac grows from the endoderm and also incorporates migrated mesodermal cells. It projects into the cavity enclosed by the growing chorion and helps in the nutrition of the embryo (Figure 19.8). Blood vessels develop from the mesodermal cells, which are also responsible for early synthesis of red blood cells. The sac is evident only early in embryo development and it eventually becomes incorporated into the body stalk mentioned earlier, which links the growing embryo to the chorion.

The allantois is another endodermal sac and originates close to the base of the yolk sac (Figure 19.8). It also contains mesodermal cells. Blood vessels which develop from these cells help to establish the vascularization of the body stalk, and hence of the umbilical cord. The membrane is eventually incorporated into the cord although a part of it is incorporated into the growing fetal bladder.

MATERNAL PHYSIOLOGY DURING PREGNANCY

The physiology of the mother undergoes extensive changes during pregnancy and these act to support the developing embryo, and also help the mother to withstand the demands placed on her by the fetus! The changes can therefore be viewed as a shift in homeostatic set-points. For example, the growth and development of the highly vascularized placenta, which will eventually receive 500–800 ml of blood per minute, places enormous additional demands on the maternal circulatory system. Compensation is via an increased cardiac output, facilitated by an elevation of blood volume and hypertrophy of the heart (Figure 19.9). Such changes are necessary to maintain the maternal systemic blood pressure, and also ensures that placental blood flow is adequate.

Some of the major physiological changes in the mother, and their significance for embryo/fetal development, are shown in Table 19.3.

BIRTH (PARTURITION)

The total human gestation period is about 280 days from the beginning of the last menstrual period. Birth begins as a sequence of events collectively termed labour (Figure 19.10). The first stage of labour commences when the uterus begins to undergo rhythmic contractions and ends when the cervix is fully dilated. The second stage is when the fetus is expelled, and the third involves the separation and expulsion of the placenta and membranes.

What stimulates the series of rhythmic, powerful contractions of the uterus at the onset of labour is still unclear but a removal, or inhibition, of the uterus-relaxing properties of progesterone seems likely to be involved. One suggestion is that the very high concentrations of oestrogen present in the maternal circulation at term shifts the oestrogen : progesterone ratio in favour of the stimulatory actions of oestro-

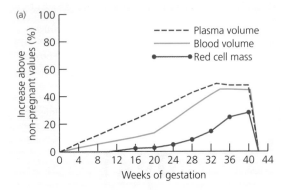

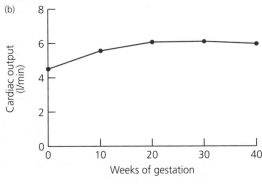

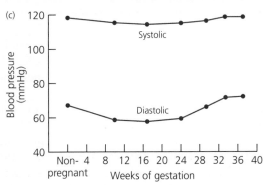

Figure 19.9 Blood volume, cardiac output, and arterial blood pressure in the pregnant woman. (a) Changes in blood volume and plasma volume. (b) Changes in cardiac output. Note that change occurs prior to the maximal increase in blood volume, reflecting cardiac growth. (c) Maternal systolic and diastolic blood pressure.

gen. Another viewpoint is that an unidentified substance is released from the placenta or fetus: some evidence has implicated fetal

Table 19.3 Changes to various homeostatic set-points in the mother during pregnancy, and their role in maintaining fetal development

Parameter	Change at 40 weeks gestation (% of pre-pregnant value)	Significance to fetus
Body water	+ 10	Supports fetal tissue growth, amniotic fluid, maternal circulation
Blood volume	+ 50	Supports placental blood flow
Cardiac output	+ 40	Supports placental blood flow, maintains maternal systemic BP
Breathing rate Tidal volume	Unchanged } +40	Increases alveolar ventilation, which facilitates gas exchange, and supports extra O_2/CO_2 demands from fetal and maternal changes
O_2 consumption	+ 250	Reflects fetal growth and increased metabolism by maternal tissues
Residual volume	−15	Results from compression of the diaphragm due to raised intra-abdominal pressure in mother. Helps accommodation of growing uterus
Glomerular filtration rate	+ 40	Facilitates excretion of nitrogenous wastes (+ others), which compensates for increased load from fetal metabolism
Endocrine secretions	Secretion of various pituitary hormones affected + fetal/placental hormones – see text	Supports changes in maternal physiology essential for maintenance of pregnancy, birth, and lactation – see text

steroid hormones from the fetal adrenal cortex as a contributory factor. Prostaglandins produced locally within the uterus also seem to be essential for the normal onset of labour but what initiates their synthesis is unknown.

Once initiated, the increased uterine tension induced by the contractions is detected by receptors within the muscle. Oxytocin is reflexly released from the posterior pituitary gland and this peptide hormone promotes further uterine contraction. This generates further tension, leading to the secretion of more oxytocin, and so on. Thus labour, once initiated, is an example of a positive feedback mechanism, that is one which is stimulated by change, and acts to promote further change.

As the interval between contractions shortens, and the contractions intensify, the uterine

cervix dilates. This process is assisted by the peptide hormone relaxin, released from the placenta. Relaxin also relaxes the symphysis pubis joint between the pelvic bones, thus providing a degree of laxity. Cervical dilatation releases any mucus and blood that has accumulated in the cervix during labour, and this is commonly referred to as the 'show'.

The separation of the placenta during the third stage of labour results from a combination of factors. The uterine contractions compress placental blood vessels and cause them to become engorged and burst, the engorged blood passing between the placenta and the deeper ('spongy') layer of the decidua. Separation of the placenta is also aided by the way in which uterine contractions pull the uterus away from the placenta, which is forced

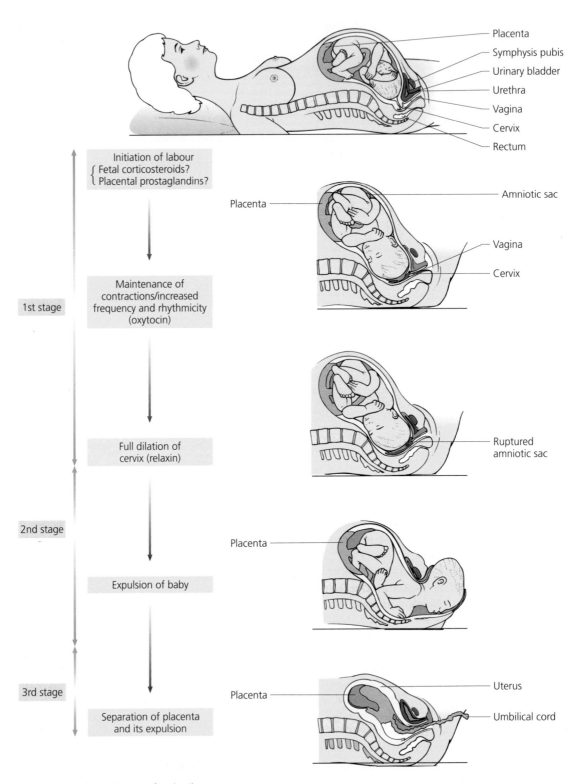

Figure 19.10 Labour. See text for details.

into the lower uterine areas and vagina. Expulsion of the placenta occurs some time after delivery via a powerful contraction of the uterus.

Blood loss during separation of the placenta from the uterus is unavoidable, and mechanisms are required to staunch that loss. The maternal vessels of the placenta follow tortuous routes between the uterine muscle fibres, and contraction of obliquely-orientated muscle fibres compresses the vessels during labour and effectively closes them. In addition, clotting is stimulated at the placental site and a fibrin mesh rapidly develops over the placenta/uterus interface.

CHANGES IN MATERNAL PHYSIOLOGY AFTER BIRTH: LACTATION

The accentuation of physiological parameters during pregnancy is inappropriate after birth. Homeostatic set-points, and hence parameters, therefore gradually return to pre-pregnancy values.

The main developmental event in the mother during the postnatal period is that of lactation, and this is hormonally controlled by the ovarian/placental steroids, and by prolactin and oxytocin from the pituitary gland.

Development of the lactiferous ducts and secretory alveoli of the breast is induced during pregnancy by oestrogens and progesterone, respectively, and is enhanced by the actions of placental lactogen (Figure 19.11a). These hormones also stimulate the hypothalamus to release prolactin-inhibitory factor, which inhibits the release of prolactin from the anterior pituitary gland. This is important because prolactin is responsible for milk secretion by the breast alveoli, and its secretion would be inappropriate during pregnancy. Declining steroid concentrations after birth removes the inhibition and prolactin release gradually increases, promoting milk secretion.

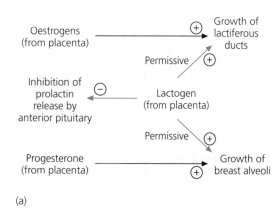

(a)

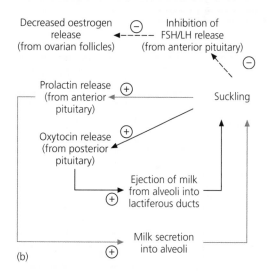

(b)

Figure 19.11 Hormonal control of (a) breast development during pregnancy and (b) lactation.

Prolactin release is maintained during breast-feeding through the actions of a neural reflex stimulated by the sucking action of the infant. Stimulation of nipple receptors also initiates the reflex release of oxytocin from the posterior pituitary. This hormone causes smooth muscle around the alveoli to contract, thus squeezing the secreted milk into the lactiferous ducts (a process called 'let-down' – Figure 19.11b). Breast-feeding also suppresses oestrogen release by inhibiting gonadotropin secretion by the pituitary gland. Ovulation can still sometimes occur, however, as the inhibition is incompletely effective.

Milk is not actually produced until a few days after birth when prolactin release is sufficiently stimulated. Colostrum is a highly proteinaceous secretion that is produced by the alveoli during late pregnancy and during this period after birth. This contains less lactose and fats than milk does, but is rich in antibodies which help to protect the infant.

PHYSIOLOGICAL CHANGES IN THE NEONATE

Physiological changes must occur in the newborn, or neonate, to equip it for life outside the body of the mother. Of the many changes observed, those to the cardiovascular system, respiratory system, and blood are of particular note.

Cardiovascular and respiratory changes

The cardiovascular system of the fetus has two important aspects which distinguish it from that of the child/adult. First, perfusion of the fetal lungs is sufficient to sustain them in their non-respiratory functional state, but must be increased if they are to function in gas exchange. Second, part of the fetal circulation includes vessels of the umbilical vasculature.

Lung perfusion and inflation

The heart and its vessels are well developed at birth but prior to birth much of the blood returning to the heart is shunted directly across to the left side, into the left atrium, via the foramen ovale, which is a perforation of the septum between the left and right atria (see Figure 19.7). Thus only a proportion of blood entering the right side of the heart actually enters the right ventricle for ejection into the pulmonary artery. Of this latter blood, much is again shunted directly from the pulmonary arterial trunk into the aorta, via a vessel called the ductus arteriosus, without passing through the lungs. Thus during fetal life, when gas exchange occurs in the placenta, the lungs receive only about 10% of the cardiac output.

At birth the fetal lungs are either collapsed or are partially filled with amniotic fluid, which is rapidly absorbed. The alveoli are inflated with air by a reflex initiation of inspiration which results from a stimulation of brainstem centres by the rising concentrations of carbon dioxide in the blood as a consequence of the loss of placental gas exchange. Oxygen uptake across the lung raises the partial pressure of oxygen in pulmonary venous blood and this stimulates closure of the ductus arteriosus. The foramen ovale also closes as a result of pressure changes in the right and left atria. These responses ensure that all blood from the right side of the heart now perfuses the lungs. Pulmonary blood flow is also facilitated by a decreased pulmonary vascular resistance. Having closed, the ductus arteriosus then atrophies into a ligament (the ligamentum arteroisum) during the following months.

Lung inflation with air requires the presence of surfactant within the alveoli to reduce surface tension (see Chapter 11). This substance is produced in adequate quantities only after about 24 weeks of development. Thus, although premature babies normally have reasonably well developed lungs, those born very early are likely to experience difficulties in inflating the alveoli; this is called infant respiratory distress syndrome. Recent developments in ventilation techniques, and the use of artificial surfactants, have improved the chances of survival of such early deliveries.

The importance of circulatory and respiratory changes are clear:

1 A persistently low partial pressure of oxygen as a consequence of inadequate gas exchange (e.g. in infant respiratory distress syndrome) prevents adequate closure of the ductus arteriosus. Blood then flows from the

aorta (in which pressure is increased at birth) into the pulmonary artery and lung, at the expense of the rest of the systemic circulation.

2 Inadequate closure of the foramen ovale (producing a 'hole in the heart') means that some blood will continue to be shunted from the right to left side of the heart, without undergoing gas exchange. If severe, this will be life-threatening, and even a small residual defect may become apparent years later when oxygen need increases in the growing child.

Nevertheless the cardiovascular changes at birth are not instantaneous or complete, and it may be weeks or months before final closure of the foramen ovale or ductus arteriosus takes place.

Umbilical vessels

The umbilical vessels consist of two arteries and a vein. The arteries originate from the iliac arteries within the fetal groin, and the vein returning blood to the fetus joins the fetal hepatic portal vein but also drains into the inferior vena cava via the ductus venosus (see Figure 19.7). Within the fetus, the two arteries are called the hypogastric arteries and these, together with the ductus venosus, rapidly close following ligation of the umbilicus at birth, and degenerate into ligaments (the lateral umbilical ligament and ligamentum venosus, respectively) during the next 2–3 months. The portal vein (which connects the gut and liver) remains patent, of course.

Blood

The neonatal blood contains a proportion of a type of haemoglobin which facilitates the uptake of oxygen from the relatively low oxygen tensions found in placental blood of the mother (see Chapter 11). This fetal-type haemoglobin (HbF) is replaced with the adult-type of pigment (HbA) within a couple of weeks but this necessitates the breakdown of

fetal erythrocytes and the pigment itself. Bile is an important route for the excretion of bilirubin produced by haemoglobin metabolism (see Chapter 7) and the immature liver of the neonate may be unable to excrete the load placed upon it. This leads to 'physiological' jaundice, which normally declines as liver function improves during succeeding days.

The blood also contains higher concentrations of white cells than is found in adult blood, and these decline during the first few days. The infant, however, is unable to produce adequate amounts of antibodies (particularly immunoglobulin G) and is dependent upon maternal sources, via breast milk. The secretion of IgG increases during the first year of life.

DEVELOPMENTAL CHANGES IN THE INFANT AND CHILD

All organs are present at birth but many are functionally immature. The first few years of life are therefore characterized by tissue growth and maturation.

Growth

Head size at birth is large relative to that of the trunk (Figure 19.12) and the brain at birth weighs about 25% of its final adult weight. The brain grows rapidly and this is facilitated by the incomplete jointing of cranial bones, which results in the presence in the infant of membrane-covered spaces called fontanelles (Figure 19.13). Most fontanelles close during the first few months but the anterior fontanelle is not fully closed for 18–24 months. The actual joints, or sutures, do not form until after 5 years of age, by which time growth of the brain and cranium has slowed considerably.

The general pattern of body growth is similar between individuals, although there is variation in the ages at which patterns change. There are slight sex differences in growth rate with girls tending to grow faster during middle childhood years, but boys exceeding

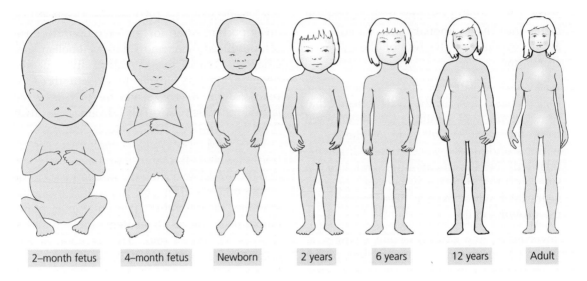

| 2–month fetus | 4–month fetus | Newborn | 2 years | 6 years | 12 years | Adult |

Figure 19.12 Fetal skull size relative to that of the trunk.

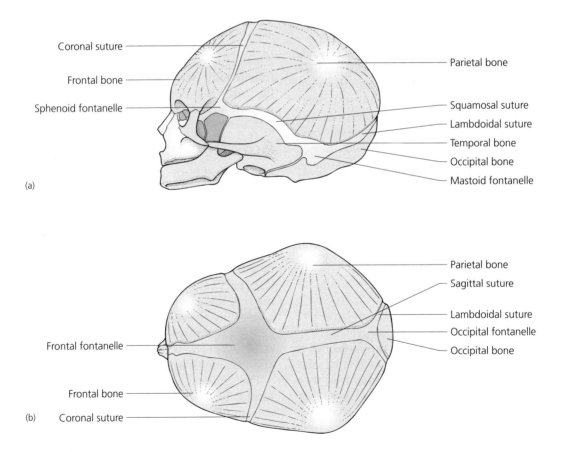

Figure 19.13 The skull of an infant: (a) side view; (b) view from above.

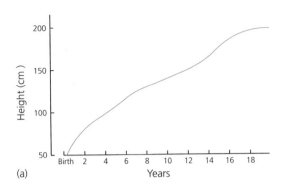

(a)

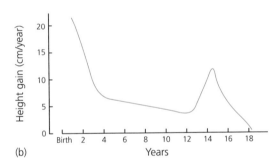

(b)

Figure 19.14 Growth during childhood and puberty. (a) Pattern of height change. (b) Growth velocity. Note the peak growth rates during infancy and puberty.

Growth is promoted by anabolic hormones, particularly growth hormone from the anterior/middle pituitary gland. Growth hormone mobilizes glucose and lipids, and enhances protein utilization by cells. It also promotes cartilage growth, which is essential if epiphyseal plates of bones are to grow (Chapter 4). Not all body growth in childhood can be ascribed to this hormone, however, and much is still unknown, although the effects of deficiency (dwarfism) and excess (gigantism) emphasize its central role. Thyroid gland activity is highest during childhood and stimulates metabolism, and thyroid hormones are also important for bone ossification and dental development. Growth in later childhood is also influenced by the increasing release of gonadal steroids.

Obesity and anorexia nervosa are relatively common in children and illustrate how the balance between nutritional needs for development and the actual intake of food can be influenced by sociopsychological factors. Likewise the environment of the child may influence the release of hormones involved in growth. Little is known, however, about how growth patterns are intrinsically organized and controlled.

Functional development

Skeletal functions

Skeletal developments in early childhood include ossification, changes in bone shape, joint strengthening, development of cervical spinal curvatures, and a 'fusion' of the pelvic girdle with the sacral vertebrae to provide strength at the body's centre of gravity. These changes are essential to support the increasing body weight and to enable the young child to assume an upright posture (see Chapter 16).

Neural integration and sensorimotor development

It is considered that most neurons which the brain will have are present at birth. Thus brain

girls during later childhood. Both sexes exhibit a pronounced increase in limb length relative to trunk length, and a broadening of the shoulders, chest, and trunk. Adipose tissue is redistributed and body shape changes accordingly.

Growth velocity is considerable during the first few years, but declines during later childhood before increasing again toward puberty (Figure 19.14). The nutritional needs to support the early rapid growth means that requirements are higher (in terms of amount per kg of body weight) in the first few years than at any time during life (Chapter 6). Increasing physical activity as the child grows places additional demands on the dietary provision of energy.

growth during childhood results from a proliferation of non-neuronal cells (the neuroglial cells) and the growth of processes from the neurons themselves. The latter establish communication links with neurons in the vicinity or at a distance. Much of the gross plan of the brain is established during fetal development, when axon growth is directed to appropriate areas by a 'scaffolding' of glial cells and by chemical attractants. Such connections are essential to the development of the circuitry of the brain, and it is their integrative functions which determine brain activities (Chapter 13). Thyroid hormones are essential for this functional development of the brain in the fetus and early childhood, particularly in relation to cognitive functions.

Motor and sensory functions mature faster than cognitive functions such as those of memory and reasoning. Early sensorimotor development is essential if the child is to be able to assume an upright posture, to walk, to acquire speech, and to gain voluntary control of urinary and anal sphincters. Autonomic efficiency will also increase, leading to better homeostatic regulation and improved physical performance. Fine motor skills therefore take time to become established.

The formation of synaptic connections between neurons is facilitated by 'reinforcement' of their activities. Accordingly physical activity, play, and other primary and secondary socialization processes promote both sensorimotor and cognitive development. This increases the complexity of activities performed, which in turn facilitate further neural development.

Digestive function and teeth

The neonatal digestive system cannot synthesize the full range of digestive enzymes necessary for a mixed diet, and gastric secretion is inadequate. The infant is therefore dependent upon milk feeds, and the tongue of babies is in a forward position to facilitate suckling. The relative position of the tongue gradually changes, and digestive enzyme secretion

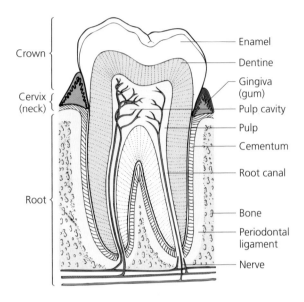

Figure 19.15 Parts of a typical tooth as seen in a section through a molar.

increases in capacity and variety, so the baby becomes able to cope with semi-solid foods.

The reliance of the infant on milk feeds necessitates the production of the gastric enzyme rennin. This coagulates milk protein and so slows its advance through the stomach giving more time for its digestion. Rennin is not to be confused with the renal enzyme renin which generates the hormone angiotensin from blood precursor.

Tooth development, essential for biting and chewing solid food, begins during fetal life but teeth do not begin to erupt until on average about 6 months after birth. These are the deciduous, or milk, teeth and one tooth on average erupts each month until all 20 are present (Chapter 7). The incisors erupt first and are chisel shaped for biting. The cuspid, or canine, teeth erupt after these and are used to tear and shred food. The molars are the last to erupt and are used to crunch and grind food.

Deciduous teeth are shed from about 6–7 years of age and are replaced with permanent teeth which are normally in place by about 12 years of age, although a further four 'wisdom' teeth may erupt during teenage or early adulthood years. Excluding the 'wisdom teeth', there are 28 permanent teeth in total, comprised of 4 incisors, 2 canines, 4 premolars and 4 molars in each jaw (Chapter 7). Since there are only 20 deciduous teeth, some permanent teeth do not have deciduous predecessors. Permanent teeth have extensive roots but are of the same basic structure as the deciduous teeth (Figure 19.15).

PUBERTY

Puberty is a period of increasing gonadal steroid secretion and so encompasses those processes which result in maturation of the reproductive system. It is also a period of rapid somatic growth.

Reproductive development

Maturation of primary sexual organs

In girls oestrogen secretion promotes maturation of the ductile system of the breast, induces fat deposition and increases nipple and areolar pigmentation. Progesterone promotes the proliferation of secretory tissue of the breast. Vaginal and uterine growth are also promoted by these steroids, and cyclical development of the endometrium and ovaries is initiated (see Chapter 18 for details).

In boys testosterone secretion induces testicular growth and elongation of the penis. Spermatogenesis begins and the prostate gland, bulbourethral glands, and seminal vesicles are stimulated to produce seminal fluid.

Secondary sexual characteristics

These are physical changes in response to gonadal steroid secretion but do not in themselves convey reproductive ability. In girls the hips broaden, fat deposition occurs,

hairs grow on the arms, legs and in the axillae. Pubic hair grows around the vaginal opening. Sweat secretion increases.

In boys there is greater muscle development, especially around the shoulders, and greater limb growth. The growth of body hair, facial hair, and pubic hair is stimulated. Laryngeal development results in a deepening of the voice. Sweat production increases.

Growth

Puberty is associated with a rapid increase in height (see Figure 19.14). Both sexes exhibit similar peak growth velocities but the growth spurt begins much later in boys, which means that they are taller at 'take-off'.

The gonadal steroids are largely responsible for this growth spurt as they promote cartilage growth and bone ossification. The steroids are also responsible, however, for the final ossification of epiphyseal cartilage toward the end of puberty and so cause bone growth eventually to cease.

The body increases its capacity for physical performance during puberty. Thus the heart doubles in weight, and blood volume, systolic blood pressure, lung volume, and muscle mass all increase.

Onset of puberty

The onset of puberty in girls is marked by the first menstrual flow (called the menarche) and this indicates that the secretion of oestrogens and progesterone is now sufficient to stimulate development of the uterine endothelium (Chapter 18). Ovulation does not normally occur in early puberty.

Onset in boys is less well defined: nocturnal emissions of semen occur only in some and thus are unreliable indicators. Spermatozoa in semen are also likely to be inviable at this time.

Puberty can only occur once the release of gonadal steroids reaches a 'threshold' point. In

Table 19.4 Selected age-related changes in homeostatic parameters and systemic functions

System	Change and/or consequence
Nervous	Loss of neurons; loss of myelin; loss of neurotransmitter; loss of synaptic receptors (e.g. memory loss, reduced reflexes, reduced postural control)
Senses	Decreased receptor density/sensitivity; decreased accommodating ability of eye lens; decreased blood flow to cochlea (e.g. loss of hearing, visual acuity, taste)
Endocrine	Decreased synthesis/release/actions of hormones (poor regulation of parameters, e.g. blood glucose)
Cardiovascular	Effects of autonomic inadequacy, atherosclerosis, and reduced peripheral circulation (e.g. hypotension, hypertension, coronary heart disease, ulceration)
Skeletal	Decreased bone density (e.g. osteoporosis); decreased vertebral column length (i.e. decreased height); fissures of joint cartilage (e.g. osteoarthrosis)
Gastrointestinal tract	Effects of autonomic inadequacy (e.g. decreased motility, decreased secretions)
Lungs	Loss of elastin (reduced vital capacity)
Kidneys	Loss of nephrons (decreased glomerular filtration rate)
Immune system	Decreased immunity; increased autoimmunity

fact hormone secretion begins during childhood and gradually increases. This early release of gonadal steroid accounts for some of the prepubertal changes in body form (the secondary sexual characteristics) but is insufficient for reproductive development. What causes their increased release toward puberty is unclear, but most evidence supports a 'maturation' either of the hypothalamic neurons responsible for the production of gonadotropin-releasing hormone, or of the portal vessels that convey this hormone from the hypothalamus to the anterior pituitary (both factors are essential if the pituitary is to secrete gonadotropins, and hence if gonadal steroids are to be secreted – see Chapter 15).

The onset of puberty may be influenced by nutritional status; obesity tends to promote early onset whilst anorexia nervosa may delay it. In addition athletic children tend to experience a late onset. The link between these factors and the release of gonadal steroids remains to be elucidated.

ADULTHOOD

Functional capacity

Developmental changes which enhance homeostasis and physiological efficiency during adulthood are difficult to define because most physiological changes during adulthood have negative connotations from the biological viewpoint. Positive functional development is observed, however, during the post-adolescent years when the 'functional capacity' of the body increases, reaching a peak during the mid–late twenties. 'Functional capacity' is a vague term that reflects increased muscle mass, cardiac growth (both of which enhance strength and maximal physical performance), and a 'fine tuning' of tissue functions, and hence homeostasis, generally. Nutritional requirements at this time are those necessary for maintenance, that is tissue repair, cell turnover, and the extra required for physical activity (see Chapter 6).

The ageing process: senescence

Peak physical performance is maintained for just a few years. Reductions in 'functional capacity' are detectable from about the age of 30 years and result in a gradual decrease in the ability to withstand physical stressors, trauma, and infection. These changes are a consequence of the ageing process and are collectively referred to as senescence, which can therefore be defined as

> a deteriorative process. . . associated with a decrease in viability and an increase in vulnerability. . . and shows itself as an increased probability of death with increasing chronological age. (Comfort, 1979)

The rate of senescent change can differ considerably between individuals and, whereas functional decline will not have a noticeable effect on the well-being of most people for many years, some are adversely affected much earlier in life.

The effects of ageing are readily observed by middle age. Visible signs include skin wrinkling as its elasticity declines, loss of hair pigmentation and, perhaps, hair loss. Internal changes are marked by a decreased homeostatic efficiency as a consequence of altered metabolic functions and loss of tissue elasticity. Such changes affect most, if not all, physiological systems (Table 19.4) By altering the constancy at which variables are homeostatically maintained, or by influencing the degree to which parameters are allowed to vary, disturbance of one system can exacerbate age-related changes in others. For example, a slowing of wound healing processes becomes apparent as a result of age-related reductions in cell division and function, but this is also influenced (particularly in the elderly) by concurrent decline in the peripheral circulation.

In women, age-related decline in physiological function is further influenced by the gradual withdrawal of gonadal steroids at the

Table 19.5 Effects of oestrogen withdrawal during and after the menopause

Early changes and symptoms
  Reproductive tract
    Cervical atrophy
    Vaginal atrophy
    Decreased cervical mucus secretion
    Uterine shrinkage
    Endometrial atrophy
  Breast
    Loss of cyclical changes to breast tissue
  Vasomotor
    Flushing
    Palpitations
    Headaches
    Night sweats

Chronic changes
  Bone
    Decreased bone density (osteoporosis)
  Blood
    Decreased high : low density lipoprotein (atheroma development)

Psychological changes
  Depression
  Insomnia

Note that vasomotor symptoms vary between individuals and may be absent. Psychological changes are not always observed and seem unlikely to relate directly to loss of oestrogens.

age of about 45–50 years. This is the menopause or climacteric.

Menopause

Ovarian steroids have widespread actions in the body, many of which are poorly understood. Thus their declining secretion during the menopause has effects in addition to causing atrophy of the reproductive system (Table 19.5), including vasomotor changes ('flushes' and sweats) associated with altered autonomic nervous system activities. Psychological effects may also be apparent, although these do not appear to result directly from the loss of the steroids. The withdrawal of ovarian steroids may facilitate expression of the actions of testosterone, which is produced in small quantities throughout life by the adrenal cortex of both sexes. This androgen can cause the growth and coarsening of facial hair, and a deepening of the voice in post-menopausal women.

In the long term the most serious consequences for physical health are reductions in the ratio of high : low density lipoproteins in blood plasma, which begins to favour the deposition of cholesterol in blood vessels (possibly resulting in heart disease and strokes), and the loss of bone matrix and mineral, leading to osteoporosis. Although such changes will be initiated in the perimenopausal period, their progress is gradual and effects are most likely to be observed many years later. Studies indicate that hormone replacement therapy during the perimenopausal and post-menopausal years prevents, or at least reduces, these changes.

The menopause has no comparable process in males. Although testosterone secretion declines with age, its metabolism also declines and so plasma concentrations are little altered. Sperm production continues well into late adulthood, although the numbers of sperm and their viability may be decreased slightly.

The effects of ageing on functional capacity, and the loss of ovarian steroids in women, cannot be regarded as 'developmental' events, although they are influential in determining the psychophysiological well-being of the individual. The increasing likelihood of ill-health or death as a consequence of the ageing process, and the ways in which extrinsic life-style factors influence ageing, are the subject of intense research. Biological ageing is still incompletely understood, however.

Theories of biological ageing

Various theories have been proposed during the last 30 years to explain physiological decline during adulthood. Most are still considered feasible today, largely based on data obtained from cells cultured *in vitro* (i.e. outside the body).

In 1961, and in subsequent studies, Hayflick and Moorhead demonstrated that cultured human cells could only undergo about 50 cell divisions before the culture declined and died, and that this was independent of such factors as nutrient supply. Findings that the maximum possible divisions (the 'Hayflick number') is considerably reduced in cultured cells from individuals with inherited forms of accelerated ageing (the syndrome called progeria), and in normally aged individuals, strongly suggest that ageing is an intracellular phenomenon. Although unrepresentative of cells which do not undergo cell division through life, the 'Hayflick number' is considered by most researchers to reflect the ageing process.

An intracellular mechanism argues against the presence of a 'central clock', or controlling tissue, which might be responsible for triggering ageing. Numerous studies have looked for such a 'clock' and the possibility still cannot be dismissed. For example, the thymus gland involutes toward the end of adolescence and then atrophies. The incidence of autoimmune disorders also increases with age and this, together with thymus changes, could implicate the immune system as an ageing 'clock'. It is also feasible, however, that autoimmune responses are a consequence and not a cause of the ageing process.

Many recent studies suggest that cumulative disturbances of enzymatic processes in cells are the cause of senescence. Generally, these metabolic disturbances can result from (1) cumulative genetic mutation, or the activation of 'ageing' genes, (2) transcription or translation errors, or (3) post-translational changes to protein structure/function (Figure 19.16).

Genetic influences

The programme theory of ageing suggests that there are specific genes which promote metabolic decline once they are activated or deactivated. These act as a genetic 'clock'. The inherited syndromes of accelerated ageing (progerias) provide strong evidence for the presence of such genes. In addition, molecular biologists have also identified genes thought to

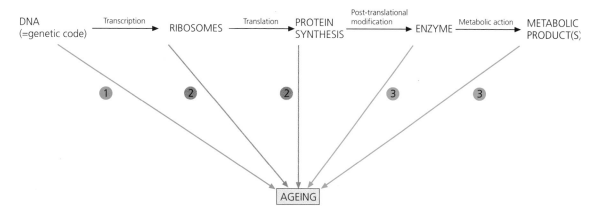

Figure 19.16 Putative effects of ageing on metabolism: 1, genetic influences; 2, effects on transcription/translation processes; 3, post-translational influences.

be activated during the normal ageing process. The role of 'ageing genes' is debatable, however, and it is considered by some researchers that such genes probably determine the maximal longevity of species and that other mechanisms promote senescence, the rate of which varies considerably between individuals.

The somatic mutation theory of ageing (review, Rao and Loeb, 1992) suggests that DNA mutations accumulate throughout life, with consequences for cell functions. There is a degree of evidence for this but the extent of nuclear DNA mutation that has been observed is debatably insufficient to account for the functional disturbances associated with ageing.

Recent studies (see Miguel, 1992) have extended this theory by showing that mitochondrial DNA and mitochondrial membranes are damaged during life. Mitochondrial DNA is extranuclear DNA which contains only a small number of genes that are particularly involved in controlling mitochondrial function. Mutation of these genes will have consequences for cellular respiratory processes and evidence indicates that oxidative metabolism does indeed decline with age.

Superoxidant chemicals, called 'free radicals', have been implicated as the cause of mitochondrial damage. These are produced by normal respiratory reactions but are so reactive that they are rapidly catabolized. Although existing only transiently, their continued production means that they are always present, albeit in small quantities, and will exert some activities. The free-radical theory (proposed by Harman, 1956) is not new, but recent advances in the study of molecular biology have only recently made it possible to investigate its implications.

Transcriptional/translational errors

The error catastrophe theory (Orgel, 1963) proposes that errors in transcribing the genetic code, or in ribosomal translation of that code, results in the loss of vital enzymes, or perhaps the production of novel ones. This theory is supported by findings that substances do indeed accumulate in cells with age, for example 'lipofucin', or age pigment. Lipofucin does not appear to be detrimental to cell function, however, although it is possible that other substances may be. The theory is 'catastrophic' as it implies that the loss of enzymes, or the production of novel substances, could disturb the activities of other enzymatic processes, which in turn causes further disruption, and so on.

Post-translational changes

Recent evidence has found that there is an accumulation of glycated proteins during ageing (e.g. Van Boeckel, 1991). Glycation is the spontaneous, but inappropriate, combination of glucose with proteins and occurs as a consequence of the continuous presence of glucose within the cell. It is distinct from the glycosylation process, in which certain proteins are metabolically combined with glucose to produce glycoproteins that are vital for cell function. Glycated enzymes will not be effective. The theory suggests that the resultant accumulation of glycated proteins, and the wider disturbances induced by loss of enzyme function, disturbs cell function.

The cross-linkage theory (Bjorksten, 1968) proposes that proteins synthesized by cells increasingly link together during life, with resultant disruption of protein structure and function. The older we are the greater will be the accumulation of glycated and cross-linked proteins. In terms of its basic proposals, the theory that post-translational changes in proteins are responsible for senescence overlaps with theories of genetic mutation and transcriptional/translational errors.

Summary

To summarize, the theories of the biological basis of ageing largely focus on the disturbances of metabolism that are observed in cell cultures, and in the whole individual. Evidence increasingly supports an accumulation of genetic disturbance and various chemicals within cells which ultimately cause cell homeostasis to decline. Such disturbances will also influence the extracellular environment. For example, the loss of intermolecular cross-linkage of collagen is largely responsible for the loss of tissue elasticity, including skin wrinkling.

With improvements in the treatment of infectious disease, and a growing understanding of the nature of many inherited disorders, senescent processes are increasingly viewed as the major challenge to health in the developed world. The brief review of ageing theories presented here illustrates that there is still debate as to which stage of protein synthesis, if one can be so pinpointed, is primarily responsible for senescence. The need for further research is clear if the actions of extrinsic factors which promote senescence in some individuals are to be understood.

When does ageing begin?

For many people biological ageing is synonymous with physiological decline during adulthood. The involution of the thymus gland in late adolescence, and the possibility that 'ageing genes' are activated at some time during the life cycle, could support the triggering of ageing as an event in early adulthood. The opposing view is that metabolic disorders accumulate throughout life, but this would mean that the ageing process is initiated much earlier in life, perhaps even before birth. The emphasis currently placed on preconceptual and antenatal care, and the possible link between maternal environment and the lifespan of progeny, would appear to support this notion (Barker, 1992).

In functional terms, however, the years between conception and adolescence mark a period of increasing physiological efficiency, and this would appear to argue against the view that cellular homeostasis declines throughout life. The two are not incompatible, however. Thus it could be that the dynamic changes induced by developmental responses, prompted by altered genetic activity and resultant hormonal changes, exceed the negative effects of the ageing process. Clearly this is a debatable area but is one which is important in the context of producing Health Promotion and Health Education programmes.

DEATH

Death occurs when the extent of functional deterioration is such that physiological disturbances are incompatible with life, and so represents the ultimate failure of homeostatic control processes. Specific disease states can frequently be pinpointed as being the cause of death, but this assumes that physiological systems can be considered as autonomous components. Rather, death is the consequence of disrupted neuronal function in the central nervous system, promoted by the disease state.

The brain is intolerant of changes to its immediate environment. It is also very active metabolically and so is susceptible to the effects of hypoxia. Loss of integrative neural function as a consequence of disease, trauma, or 'natural causes' will result in widespread systems failure largely as a consequence of inadequate functioning of the brainstem and hypothalamus. Signs of brainstem death there-fore provide confirmation of biological death: loss of the corneal touch reflex, loss of the pupillary response to light, lack of a vestibu-lar–ocular reflex in response to a sudden head turn, or to irrigation of the outer ear with cold/warm water.

Technological advances are such that now the roles of these parts of the brain can largely be replaced with artificial life-support systems, and these can potentially maintain many physiological functions for years. Under these circumstances a persistent lack of electrical activity in the brainstem would be indicative of a continuing absence of independent physio-logical control. The longer this state continues, the greater the likelihood that the damage is irreversible.

Examples of homeostatic failure: disorders of development

Development is a genetic process, modified by environmental circumstances. Disorders of development therefore arise either because there is genetic abnormality or because extrin-sic factors have modified gene expression. Genetic abnormalities are either inherited or arise because of mutation (usually in the embryo/fetus), possibly induced by extrinsic factors. Inherited disorders are discussed in the next chapter; this section focuses on additional influences.

EMBRYO/FETAL DEVELOPMENT

Development of the embryo and fetus involves the differentiation of specific tissues and organs, and tissue growth. Congenital abnor-malities (i.e. those present at birth) therefore come under two categories: (1) those arising from defective tissue differentiation and (2) lower/higher birth weights for gestational age.

Tissue differentiation

Tissue differentiation broadly depends upon two factors: the genetic complement of the embryo, and the expression of those genes.

Genetic complement

The genetic complement of an embryo is primarily determined by those genes inherited from the sperm and ovum at fertilization. Disordered development therefore arises when inherited, mutated alleles are expressed (see Chapter 20), when genes are in excess or absent because of chromosomal defects, or, alterna-tively, when genes mutate in the embryo itself either spontaneously or because of an extrinsic

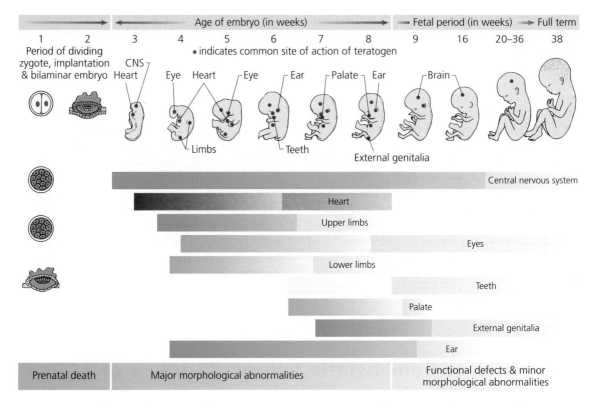

Figure 19.17 Susceptibility of the embryo/fetus to teratogens. Horizontal bars indicate period of development for those systems shown. Black shading indicates period of maximal susceptibility.

agent (e.g. radiation). Such extrinsic agents are called mutagens.

The actions of mutagens to affect embryo development are not necessarily restricted to the embryo. Thus they may also induce mutation during gametogenesis in the adult, with consequences for the subsequent embryo.

Gene expression

The actions of certain extrinsic agents to influence how genes are expressed, rather than alter gene structure itself, is of increasing concern. Numerous chemicals that are relatively harmless to the mother have been shown to influence tissue differentiation (some are shown in Table 19.6). Toxins produced by certain bacteria are also known to influence differentiation. These agents, together with

mutagenic factors, are collectively called teratogens, i.e. agents which induce physical malformities in the newborn.

Since tissue differentiation is mostly complete by the end of the eighth week, this is the period during which the embryo is particularly susceptible to teratogens (Figure 19.17). The nervous system and cardiovascular system are amongst the earliest tissues to differentiate, commencing before the woman may even be aware that she is pregnant, and these tissues are frequently the ones most affected (Table 19.6).

The importance of nutrition to embryological development also cannot be overemphasized. Apart from effects on birth weights (see below), nutrient deficiency can also influence differentiation. Recent studies, for example, have shown that the incidence of spina bifida

Table 19.6 Selected teratogenic influences on embryo/fetal development

Teratogenic influence	Possible effects on fetus or newborn
Drugs taken by mother	
Androgens	Masculinization of fetus
Anaesthetics	Depression of fetus, asphyxia
Antihistamines	Abortion, malformations
Aspirin	Persistent truncus arteriosus, abnormal heart
Diuretics	Polycystic kidney disease
Heroin and morphine	Convulsions, tremor, neonatal death
Insulin shock	Fetal death
LSD (lysergide; lysergic acid diethylamide)	Chromosomal anomalies, deformity
Nicotine (from smoking)	Stunting, accelerated heart beat, premature birth, organ congestion, fits and convulsions
Oestrogens	Malformations, hyperactivity of fetal adrenal glands
Streptomycin	Damage to auditory nerve
Thalidomide	Hearing loss, abnormal appendages, death
Maternal infection	
Chickenpox or shingles	Chickenpox or shingles, abortion, stillbirth
Syphilis	Miscarriage
Cytomegalovirus (salivary gland virus)	Small head, inflammation and hardening of brain and retina, deafness, mental retardation, enlargement of spleen and liver, anaemia, giant cells in urine from kidneys
Hepatitis	Hepatitis
Herpes simplex	Generalized herpes, inflammation of brain, cyanosis, jaundice, fever, respiratory and circulatory collapse, death
Mumps	Fetal death, endocardial fibroelastosis, anomalies
Pneumonia	Abortion in early pregnancy
Poliomyelitis	Spinal or bulbar poliomyelitis, acute poliomyelitis of newborn
Rubella (German measles)	Anomalies; haemorrhage; enlargement of spleen and liver; inflammation of brain, liver, and lungs; cataracts; small brain; deafness; various mental defects; death
Scarlet fever	Abortion in early pregnancy
Smallpox	Abortion, stillbirth, smallpox
Syphilis	Stillbirth, premature birth, syphilis
Toxoplasmosis (protozoan parasite infection)	Small eyes and head, mental retardation, cerebral oedema (encephalitis), heart damage, fetal death
Tuberculosis	Fetal death, lowered resistance to tuberculosis
Typhoid fever	Abortion in early pregnancy

can be dramatically reduced by ensuring that the maternal diet contains adequate folate, a vitamin of the B group. Spina bifida is an incomplete closure of the neural arch of one or more vertebrae. In its most severe form a fluid-filled sac (called a myelomeningocoele) protrudes through the skin, usually in the lumbar region, and this thin protection afforded to underlying spinal neurons is usually inadequate, leading to infection, damage, and resultant paralysis.

Spina bifida is detectable after about 16 weeks of gestation by monitoring the concentration in maternal blood, or amniotic fluid, of a protein called alpha-fetoprotein, which is released into the amniotic fluid as a consequence of incomplete neural tube closure.

Birth weights

Various factors such as race and gestational age affect birth weights, and there are accepted 'norms' (Figure 19.18). Excessive stimulation of fetal growth produces birth weights in excess of the norms. Thus, maternal diabetes mellitus induces increased insulin release in the fetus, with subsequent deposition of food stores.

Similarly, low birth weights reflect either inadequate placental blood flow, which restricts nutrient supply to the fetus (e.g. the effects of nicotine from smoking), or depressed metabolism (e.g. in the fetal alcohol syndrome, and possibly from carbon monoxide in cigarette smoke).

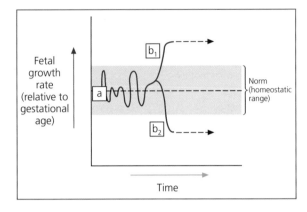

Figure 19.18 Fetal growth as a homeostatic function.
a Rate of fetal growth, appropriate to gestational age, fluctuating within normal limits.
b_1 Excessive growth rate, inappropriate for gestational age, due to maternal influence on fetal metabolism (e.g. maternal diabetes mellitus).
b_2 Deficient growth rate, inappropriate for gestational age, due to maternal influence on fetal metabolism (e.g. inadequate perfusion of the placenta; maternal alcohol intake).

INFANT AND CHILD GROWTH

Factors which influence infant and child growth, other than those arising because of congenitally malformed tissues, include a failure of circulatory and respiratory responses at birth which result in blood gas disturbances. Infant respiratory distress syndrome, as a consequence of hyaline membrane disease, arises because of a lack of surfactant. This in turn can result in a persistent ductus arteriosus (see earlier section). Septal defects of the heart may prevent normal oxygenation of blood as some of it is shunted between the heart chambers without it passing through the lungs. Blood gas disturbances induce a generalized failure to thrive, poor growth rates, and may even be fatal.

Poor growth rates may also result from a deficiency in those hormones essential for growth: growth hormone or thyroid hormone. Deficiency of the latter in infants also leads to retarded brain development (cretinism). Excessive growth hormone promotes excessive growth (gigantism). Gonadal steroids also influence growth and their deficiency can retard growth during late childhood.

ADOLESCENCE

Puberty is a time of sexual maturation, which requires the presence of the appropriate gonadal steroids. Lack of these steroids prevents normal puberty, and this commonly results from inherited disorders of the sex chromosomes (trisomy or monosomy – see Chapter 20). Infertility usually results. Impaired reproductive ability may also arise because of a congenital defect in the anatomy of the reproductive tract.

The influence of factors such as diet on the onset of puberty were mentioned earlier. In addition, growth rates during puberty also require the support of adequate nutrition, and nutritional disorders (e.g. anorexia) will have adverse effects on growth.

ADULTHOOD

The two main changes observed in adulthood – ageing and (in women) the menopause – are very much influenced by extrinsic factors. Thus symptoms of the menopause vary widely between individuals, with a minority having to obtain clinical advice and treatment. Why symptoms are more pronounced in some is unclear but could relate to the social circumstances of that person and also to the rate at which oestrogen release diminishes.

Extrinsic influences on the effects of ageing are well documented, though not entirely understood, and form the basis of current Health Promotion programmes. For example, the influence of exercise and diet on lipid composition of the blood, and the development of atheromatous deposits in blood vessels is well recognized.

References

Barker, D.J.P. (1992) *Fetal and infant origins in adult disease*. London: B.M.J.

Bjorksten, J. (1968) The cross-linkage theory of aging. *Journal of the American Geriatric Society* **16**, 408–27.

Comfort, A. (1979) *The biology of senescence*. Edinburgh: Churchill-Livingstone.

Harman, D. (1956) Aging: a theory based on free-radical and radiation chemistry. *Journal of Gerontology* **11**, 298–300.

Hayflick, L. and Moorhead, P.S. (1961) The serial subcultivation of human cell strains. *Experimental Cell Research* **25**, 585–621.

Miguel, J. (1992) An update on the mitochondrial-DNA mutation hypothesis of cell aging. *Mutation Research* **275** (3–6), 209–16.

Orgel, L.E. (1963) The maintenance of accuracy of protein synthesis and its relevance to aging. *Proceedings of the National Academy of Sciences, USA* **49**, 5117–21.

Rao, K.S. and Loeb, L.A. (1992) DNA damage and repair in brain: relationship to aging. *Mutation Research* **275** (3–6), 317–29.

Van Boeckel, M.A.M. (1991) The role of glycation in ageing and diabetes mellitus. *Molecular Biology Reports* **15** (2), 57–64.

Summary

1 Physiological development during the lifespan represents anatomical and functional changes appropriate to the life stage, and these are genetically induced, although extrinsic factors influence the process.

2 Selective gene activation is first apparent in the blastocyst phase, prior to implantation in the endometrium. Tissue differentiation continues and increases in complexity following implantation, and most tissues are basically formed by weeks 7–8 after fertilization. The embryo is now considered to be a fetus.

3 Fetal development is primarily one of growth and functional maturation. Nutrient exchange with the mother is facilitated by the development of the placenta, although this has numerous other functions also.

4 The metabolic demands of the embryo/fetus are met by changes to the maternal physiology. Such changes are hormonally mediated. Although the mechanisms are incompletely understood, some of the changes are attributable to effects of ovarian and placental oestrogens and progestins.

5 Birth also requires adaptations, both in the mother (hormonally mediated) and in the fetus.

Fetal physiology at birth must change to that compatible with air-breathing, together with adaptations to the loss of the placental circulation. Pronounced cardiovascular changes are observed, including a change to adult-type haemoglobin in erythrocytes.

6 Infant and child development is primarily one of growth and functional maturation. Perhaps the most pronounced changes are those observed in neurological function and in the digestive tract. Growth is linked to the secretion of appropriate hormones.

7 Pubertal changes involve the maturation of the reproductive tract, the development of secondary sexual characters, and growth. These changes are mediated by an increased secretion of gonadal steroids during this period.

8 Functional changes during adulthood are mainly those of declining homeostatic efficiency, with an increasing susceptibility to ill-health. Theories abound as to how the ageing process affects tissues, and most focus on interference with the synthesis of functional proteins, especially enzymes. Recent advances have pinpointed specific metabolic effects but the influence of extrinsic factors on the ageing process is still unclear.

Review Questions

1 Discuss the limitation of cell size with reference to the surface area : volume ratio.

2 Discuss the events leading to the formation of the zygote.

3 Discuss the role of the sperm in determining the sex of the offspring.

4 Distinguish between the morula and blastocyst stage of development.

5 Name the three germ layers. To what organs do the layers give rise?

6 Distinguish between the embryo and fetal stages of development.

7 List the function of the placenta.

8 What are the feedback controls involved in pregnancy?

9 Discuss the statement that the maternal homeostatic set-points are altered during pregnancy.

10 Outline the principles behind pregnancy testing (Chapter 18).

11 Describe the various stages of labour.

12 What structural changes take place in the circulatory system at birth?

13 What are the feedback controls involved in lactation?

14 Describe the role of surfactant in respiratory function.

15 Discuss the role of genes and the environment in initiation of each stage of human development.

16 Describe the hormonal changes associated with menopause.

17 How does an individual's functional capacity change in adulthood?

18 How may congenital malformation arise?

19 Discuss the homeostatic imbalances associated with mid-life and senescence mentioned in this chapter.

20 When does ageing begin?

20 Inheritance

Introduction: relation of genes to cellular homeostasis

Overview of the inheritance of characteristics

Details of the inheritance of characteristics

The inheritance of genetic disorder

Introduction to population genetics

Principles of correction/prevention

Summary

Review questions

Introduction: relation of genes to cellular homeostasis

The human body is comprised of billions of cells, each being specialized for its role within a tissue and hence in overall body function. Specialization of function largely occurs during the differentiation of cells in the embryo, and is primarily controlled by the genetic information encoded within the cell, although the expression of that information is influenced by environmental factors. Differentiation is a complex and poorly understood process but can be envisaged as resulting in the generation of cells of given structure and activity. In other words, the genes determine those processes which together are called metabolism.

Clearly the chemical reactions occurring within a cell must proceed at a rate compatible with the needs of the cell. This means speeding them up and this is achieved by the presence of catalysts: chemicals which speed up a reaction but are not themselves changed by it. The catalysts of metabolic reactions are enzymes. Cell differentiation and the maintenance of cell function require a variety of enzymes to be present at the appropriate time.

The specificity of enzyme action results from their three-dimensional shape since the reactants of a chemical reaction must combine with precise 'active' sites within the protein structure (see Chapter 3). The versatility of proteins results from variations in the number of amino acids present, the types of amino acids present, and the sequencing of those amino acids. It is the information encoded in a cell's genetic material, or DNA, that determines which protein is synthesized. The process of protein synthesis is described in Chapter 2 and the reader should familiarize himself with this process, and the nature of the genetic 'code', before continuing with this chapter.

Overview of the inheritance of characteristics

GENOTYPE AND PHENOTYPE

The genes of an individual are largely responsible for the observable or measurable characteristics, called the phenotypes of that individual. Such characteristics are normally expressed as physical ones, but, as outlined in Chapter 2, the activities of genes are observed at the biochemical level of cell activity. The term 'phenotype' could therefore be applied to characteristics ranging from a particular protein, to cell organelles, to tissue types, to organ function, to external features of the individual. The gene or genes responsible for a phenotype comprise the genotype. Collectively the entire gene composition of the DNA is called the genome.

Various factors also determine how, or if, a genotype is expressed. These include the presence or absence of gene mutations (see later), the availability of metabolic substrates, and variations in the intracellular environment, such as pH, water content, and ionic composition. In general terms:

Genotype ⟶ Phenotype
↑
Environment

Phenotypes clearly differ between individuals, even between close relatives, and (environmental influences apart) results from a 'mixing' of genes in successive generations. The variation in genotype induced by inheritance processes is considered further in the 'Details' section. In order to understand the principles of inheritance, however, it is necessary to consider first the behaviour of genetic material during cell division, particularly during the production of the sex cells or gametes.

CHROMOSOMES

During much of the time that a cell is actively performing its functional role the DNA forms an amorphous mass within the nucleus. Depending upon cell type, it might begin at some stage to prepare to divide, in order to support tissue growth, to replace cells lost by death or physical attrition, or to provide gametes for reproduction.

The DNA is packaged prior to division and this helps to reduce the hazards of attempting to divide whilst the DNA is haphazardly dispersed. The DNA actually coils around and folds in on itself and the molecule therefore becomes shorter and fatter. Eventually it can be visualized as a chromosome (chromo- = colour; soma = body).

Human cells, other than the sex cells, will normally contain 46 chromosomes; in other words there are 46 separate molecules of DNA in each cell. Two of these are called the sex chromosomes as they are involved in the development of the sexual characteristics of the fetus and eventually the adult. The remaining 44 are called autosomes (Figure 20.1). The chromosomal make-up of a cell is called its karyotype.

Each chromosome has a characteristic X-shape, though two of the arms are usually noticeably smaller than the other two. The shape arises because each chromosome actually consists of two copies of a DNA molecule joined together at one point – the centromere (Figure 20.1). Duplication of the DNA occurs as the cell prepares to divide, and each copy is called a chromatid. Cells at this stage are referred to as being diploid (diplo = double).

The principle of complementary base pairing, mentioned in Chapter 2, is essential in the success of DNA duplication. If the double helix structure of a molecule of DNA is 'unzipped' (via the actions of certain enzymes) to expose the constituent bases of the two strands, it is a relatively straightforward process for complementary bases to combine with those exposed. New deoxyribose/phosphate chains complete the process and

(a)

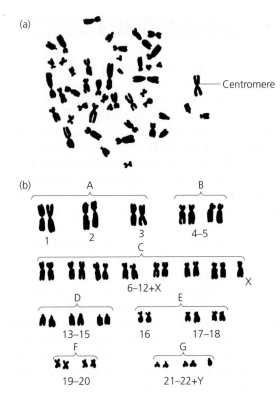

(b)

Centromere

Figure 20.1 Human karyotype. (a) Chromosomes from a normal human diploid cell (X 2000). (b) Karyotyping of chromosomes from a male.

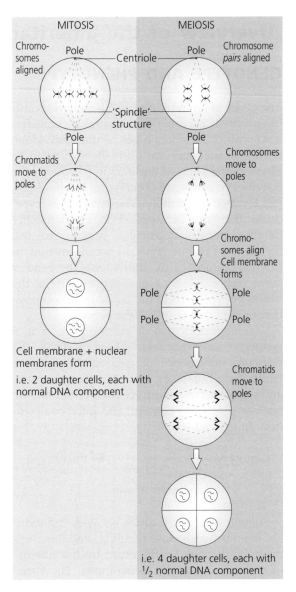

Figure 20.2 Comparison of chromosomal behaviour in mitosis and meiosis. Both processes shown at the *metaphase* stage to begin with.

two molecules of DNA, identical to the original, will have been produced. Without complementary pairing the process would be random and the new molecules, and hence the genetic code, would differ. The significance of the conservation of base sequencing can be seen during the processes of cell division called mitosis or meiosis.

CELL DIVISION

Mitosis

Mitosis is the division of cells during which the genetic make-up of a cell is conserved and passed on in its entirety into 'daughter' cells. These new cells, therefore, will have the same structure and functions of the original cells, and so mitosis is a basic process in tissue growth and in cell replacement during tissue maintenance.

The principle of cell division by mitosis is relatively simple. Thus, the molecules of DNA are duplicated, the nuclear envelope breaks down, and the chromosomes align across the centre of the cell. At this point, the chromatids separate and one from each chromosome passes to the opposite poles of the cell (Figure 20.2). Nuclear envelopes form around each cluster of chromatids and an intervening cell membrane forms. Thus two cells are produced and, providing that DNA duplication was successful, each will have DNA of identical structure to that of the original cell.

Meiosis

Meiosis is that form of cell division which occurs during gametogenesis, a process described in Chapter 18. The genetic material must be halved in the gametes to ensure that the normal amount is restored following fusion of gametes at fertilization.

The germ cells that give rise to the gametes have the usual 46 chromosomes. Through successive mitotic divisions during growth and development these are derived from the original 46 chromosomes of the zygote formed at fertilization. Thus, 23 are derived from the chromosomes of the ovum and 23 from those of the sperm cell. In other words, the 46 chromosomes are comprised of 23 pairs.

The first stage of meiosis is for the germ cell's DNA to replicate to form the characteristic X-shaped chromosomes, for the nuclear membrane to break down, and for the chromosomes to align themselves at the centre of the cell. In contrast to mitosis, the chromosomes actually align in their pairs and these now separate (this division is called meiosis I) so that members move to opposite poles of the cell. In this way the chromosome pairs are separated (Figure 20.2). The chromatids which make up the chromosomes in each 'group' immediately separate (this division is called meiosis II) and new nuclear membranes form. As a result four cells have been formed from the original cell, and each has only one set of chromosomes, or half the genetic complement of that cell; hence they are called haploid cells (haplo = single).

The separation of the pairs of chromosomes during meiosis has important implications other than just keeping the numbers correct after fertilization. The non-gamete cell contains DNA derived from that of the zygote and hence from both parents. It follows then that there must be a duplication of genes – those from the mother and those from the father. The pairs are therefore homologous (homo = same) as each member of the pair will carry a gene at the same position, or locus, for the same phenotypical characteristic (the exception is in the male as the Y-chromosome is smaller than the X and so carries fewer genes). Separation of chromosome pairs during meiosis thus separates the pairs of genes and so they are inherited independently.

Details of the inheritance of characteristics

The pairs of genes responsible for a particular phenotype may not necessarily have precisely the same genetic coding, either to each other or to those of another individual. Since the code may differ, the two forms are called allelomorphs, or alleles for short. Reference to a 'defective gene' usually means that one or both of the alleles are mutated.

ALLELE (GENE) MUTATION AND CELL FUNCTION

Differences between alleles arise through mutation, which is a change to the genetic code either as a result of deletions or substitutions of bases in the DNA, or from a rearrangement of the order of bases. Mutation can occur spontaneously or result from the actions of certain environmental agents, such as radiation, toxins, or viruses. The consequence of gene mutation is that the altered genetic code could induce the cell to synthesize novel proteins and the actions of the new protein, or alternatively the absence of the 'normal' protein, may change cell and tissue function and consequently alter the phenotype. According to evolutionary theory such changes could potentially confer a small but significant advantage to the individual. From the clinical point of view, however, some mutations change cell function to such a degree that a disease state is induced. Although mutations occur infrequently they are not unusual and it is likely that we all 'carry' some mutated genes which, if expressed, will induce a disease state.

HOMOZYGOUS AND HETEROZYGOUS GENOTYPES

If the two alleles of a particular gene have identical genetic coding then both will cause the cell to produce the same protein. Accordingly the individual is said to be homozygous for the characteristic produced. Allele mutation, however, makes it possible for the two alleles to be slightly different. In this case the individual is said to be heterozygous.

When a pair of alleles are not identical the question arises as to which will determine protein synthesis by the cell, and hence influence cell function: expression will then depend upon which allele exerts dominance.

Dominant and recessive alleles

When a pair of alleles differ, they could potentially cause the cell to produce two slightly different proteins. In practice one allele normally assumes dominance over the other one, which is then said to be recessive (or sub-dominant), and so only the dominant form determines which protein is synthesized (or at least which one predominates) and hence how the cell functions.

Mutated alleles are usually recessive in nature, though the degree to which they are suppressed by the (dominant) 'normal' allele in the heterozygous condition is variable. Some may exhibit incomplete dominance when both alleles are active, whilst some may themselves be dominant to the usual form. When expressed, the influence of mutated alleles on cell function ranges from the benign to severe (examples are given later) depending upon the consequences of either the loss of the 'normal' protein, or the activities of the 'novel' protein. The consequences to health of losing a vital enzyme is of major concern.

Polygenic phenotypes

Although phenotypical characteristics can be related to the activities of a single gene (i.e. pair of alleles), many phenotypes represent the net effect of the activities of a number of genes and therefore involve numerous alleles. The genes are not necessarily found on the same chromosome, and their net expression will depend upon how many of the alleles of the functional group are mutated – the more mutations present the greater the likelihood of an altered phenotype.

Each gene within the functional group is usually inherited independently but the expression is said to be additive. For example, skin pigmentation results from the expression of at least two genes (i.e. two pairs of alleles). If both are homozygous for the recessive alleles then skin colour is 'white'. If both are homozygous for the dominant form, which increases the amount of melanin present, then skin colour is 'black'. If one gene is heterozygous and the other homozygous, then an intermediate skin colour will be produced as expression of the homozygous genotype will not be complete. The inheritance is summarized in Figure 20.3.

Consider a pair of cofunctional autosomal alleles, A and B on homologous chromosomes

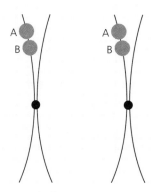

Homologous chromosomes – genotype written as AABB, i.e. homozygous A, homozygous B

If A and B determine skin colour:

Possible genotype	Phenotype (i.e. skin colour)
AABB	'Black' due to dominant A, B alleles
AaBB	'Black' due to dominant A, B alleles
AaBb	'Black' due to dominant A, B alleles
Aabb	Intermediate as only 1 dominant allele present
AAbb	Intermediate as only 1 dominant allele present
aaBB	Intermediate as only 1 dominant allele present
aaBb	Intermediate as only 1 dominant allele present
aabb	'White' as both alleles recessive

Figure 20.3 Effect of allelic variation on a phenotype determined by more than one gene.

Lethal alleles

Occasionally a mutation of an allele can occur that has such a drastic influence on tissue functions that life is impossible. Such alleles are called lethal alleles and they may be dominant or recessive in nature.

MENDELIAN PRINCIPLES OF INHERITANCE

Since most genes are comprised of two alleles, and these may be identical (homozygous) or differ slightly (heterozygous), the characteristics inherited by succeeding generations will depend upon whether dominant or recessive alleles are inherited. In order to understand how such inheritances occur, it is necessary to consider some of the general principles involved. Gregor Mendel (1822–1884) was the first person to record how 'recessive' characteristics can arise in the offspring, or progeny, even though they are not apparent in the parents, and the general principles of inheritance are frequently referred to as 'Mendelian'.

Sexual reproduction is viewed as a means of 'gene mixing' so that new generations will inherit genes that produce different, but potentially beneficial, phenotypes from those of the parental generation. There are three main processes which contribute to the mixing: (1) segregation of alleles, (2) independent assortment of alleles, and (3) crossover of alleles between chromosomes.

Segregation of alleles

In an earlier discussion it was seen how meiosis separates the homologous chromosome pairs during the formation of the gametes. By doing so the process segregates the alleles. For example, in the heterozygous state an individual may not be affected by an allele because of its recessive nature. Meiosis, however, separates it from its dominant counterpart, thus raising the possibility that it will be paired with another recessive allele in the next generation. If this is the case then homozygosity will occur and the recessive alleles will be operative.

For the segregation of alleles of a single gene it makes no difference as to which of the chromosome pair contains a mutated allele since it will pass into one or other of the gametes produced. As noted earlier, however, many phenotypical characteristics result from the expression of numerous genes located on the same homologous pair of chromosomes or on different pairs. For these alleles the inheritance of characteristics depends upon how the different chromosomes assort themselves

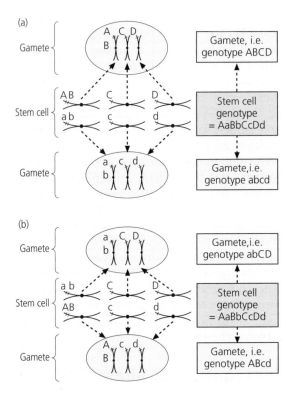

Figure 20.4 Two examples of the effects of independent assortment of just three chromosome pairs on the genotypes of gametes produced by meiosis.

during meiosis, and if alleles are exchanged between homologous chromosomes prior to their separation (see below).

Independent assortment

Figure 20.4 illustrates a possible arrangement of three pairs of homologous chromosomes during meiosis. The combination of alleles passed into the gametes will depend upon how these chromosomes are assorted before they separate. Assortment of the pairs is random and independent of the alignment of others.

Crossover or gene recombination

When a pair of homologous chromosomes align during meiosis I some of the DNA may

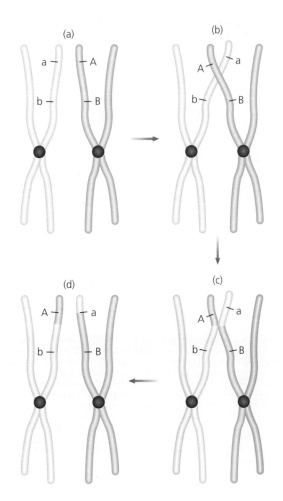

Figure 20.5 Allelic 'mixing' produced by exchange of DNA (crossover) between chromosomal pairs during meiosis. (a) Chromosome pair aligns at metaphase stage of meiosis. (b) Arms of the two chromosomes interact. (c) Crossover of DNA from one chromosome to another complete. (d) Chromosome pair ready to separate during the next stage of meiosis. Note the different allelic pairing on each chromosome, compared with (a).

be exchanged between the chromosomes, taking with it the constituent alleles (Figure 20.5). If the alleles on each chromosome were identical then this would be of no consequence. If different, then crossing over causes a mixing of alleles. This has the effect of varying the alleles that are inherited on a particular chromosome.

The inheritance of genetic disorder

Inborn errors of embryological development can arise for a number of reasons:

1 because a mutated gene has been inherited from the parents or a gene has mutated at a critical stage during intrauterine development;

2 because the number of chromosomes inherited from the parents is more or less than 46. Similarly additional chromosome fragments might be inherited, or a chromosome may not be complete; and

3 because the expression of genes has been disrupted by environmental agents, either in terms of transcription, ribosomal translation of the genetic code, or perhaps in the actions of the products of metabolism.

Point (3) provides the basis for the actions of teratogenic substances and is discussed in Chapter 19. This section is concerned with describing the consequences of inheritance *per se*.

The familial occurrence of certain disorders has long been recognized. Mendelian principles help to explain the frequency of such inherited conditions, and why some disorders can 'skip' generations.

INHERITANCE OF GENE MUTATIONS

The likelihood of progeny inheriting mutated alleles that will influence cell function depends upon whether the alleles are recessive or dominant, or if they are found on the autosomes or sex chromosomes.

Autosomal recessive inheritance

When meiosis separates homologous chromosomes it also separates the gene alleles and, if the individual is heterozygous, then half of the gametes will contain the dominant allele and half the recessive form. Should his/her partner also be heterozygous it can be seen that there is a 1 in 4 statistical chance that a zygote formed will be homozygous for the recessive allele (Figure 20.6).

In contrast, there is no possibility of a recessive homozygous offspring when one parent is heterozygous and the other homozygous for the 'normal' (i.e. dominant) alleles. There is, however, a 1 in 2 chance that the child will be heterozygous (Figure 20.6). In this case any disorder associated with the recessive allele will 'skip' that generation but there remains the possibility that the homozygous form will appear in the following one. The heterozygous individual is referred to as a carrier of the recessive allele.

There are many examples of recessive disorder that result from a single gene defect. The genes responsible for some of the commoner disorders have now been identified, and the defective cell process studied. The commoner disorders include the following.

CYSTIC FIBROSIS
This is a condition that is characterized by the secretion of viscous mucus, particularly in the lungs and alimentary tract. The disorder actually arises because of a defect in chloride transport, and hence water movement, across the cell membranes of mucosal cells as a consequence of a failure of the recessive gene to cause the synthesis of the appropriate enzyme.

PHENYLKETONURIA (PKU)
This condition is characterized by an accumulation of the essential amino acid phenylalanine in tissues. The amino acid is obtained from dietary protein and some is converted in the liver to tyrosine which is used by the body to synthesize proteins, melanin and catecholamine hormones. Tyrosine synthesis is catalysed by the enzyme phenylalanine hydroxylase and it is the absence of this enzyme which promotes the disorder. Young

Consider autosomal gene A, possible genotypes: AA Homozygous for dominant alleles
Aa Heterozygous
aa Homozygous for recessive alleles

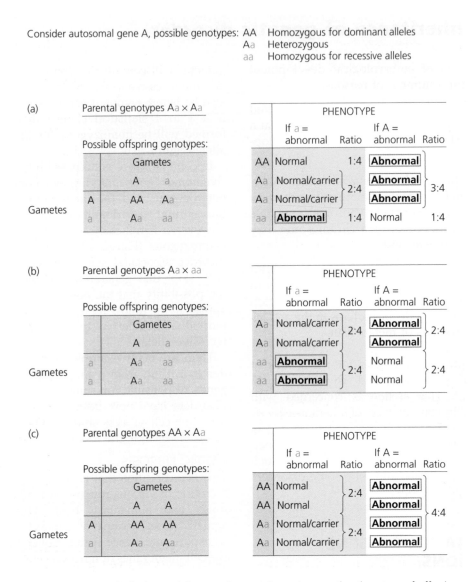

Figure 20.6 Autosomal inheritance: influence of parental genotype on the phenotype of offspring.

children in particular are at risk of the consequences of this problem (phenylalanine accumulation retards brain development) but the condition is controllable by reducing the dietary intake as compensation for the decreased utilization. Analysis of a blood sample (the Guthrie test) will clearly show if excessive phenylalanine is present.

FAMILIAL HYPERLIPIDAEMIA

In this condition there is an excessively high lipid concentration in the blood which promotes the development of atheromatous deposits in vessels. The elevated lipid results from a defect in the uptake mechanism in liver cells.

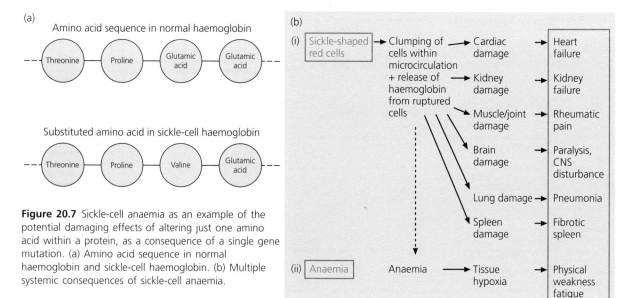

Figure 20.7 Sickle-cell anaemia as an example of the potential damaging effects of altering just one amino acid within a protein, as a consequence of a single gene mutation. (a) Amino acid sequence in normal haemoglobin and sickle-cell haemoglobin. (b) Multiple systemic consequences of sickle-cell anaemia.

INCOMPLETE DOMINANCE

An example of incomplete dominance, in which the mutated allele is neither recessive nor completely dominant to the normal allele, is that shown by the allele responsible for sickle-cell anaemia. This condition arises because one of the polypeptide chains in the haemoglobin molecule contains a single amino acid substitution when compared with 'normal' haemoglobin. This small change alters the properties of the pigment, causing it to distort after releasing oxygen and so produce the sickling of the erythrocyte. The cell membrane is more fragile in the sickled state, resulting in haemolysis, and hence the anaemia. Various tissues are affected as a consequence (Figure 20.7 and Chapter 8).

Although the disorder is seen in the homozygous condition, blood samples from heterozygous individuals will also show numbers of sickled erythrocytes, in addition to normal ones, as both alleles are expressed. The degree of sickling may not be sufficient to produce severe symptoms of the condition, and the heterozygous state is actually advantageous in certain countries because the sickled cells convey resistance to infection by malarial parasites.

Autosomal dominant inheritance

It was mentioned earlier that a mutated allele will occasionally behave in a dominant fashion. This means that the influences of that allele will be observed even in the heterozygous condition. Thus, with two heterozygous parents, there is a 75% chance that the offspring will have the phenotype associated with the allele because of a 2 in 4 chance that the progeny will be heterozygous, and a 1 in 4 chance that a child will be homozygous for the dominant allele (see Figure 20.6).

If only one parent is heterozygous, and the other is homozygous for the 'normal' (now recessive) allele, then there is still a 50% chance that the dominant phenotype will be inherited (Figure 20.6). Clearly if a parent is homozygous for that gene then all children will inherit the phenotype.

An example of a dominant mutation that is detrimental to health is that which produces the neurological disorder Huntington's chorea, but the expression of this disorder typically does not occur until well into adulthood. The condition is characterized by a deficiency of

Consider gene A present on the X-chromosome but absent on the Y:

Possible genotypes

Female (XX)	AA	Homozygous for dominant alleles
	Aa	Heterozygous
Male (XY)	AO	where O indicates lack of homologous
	aO	allele on Y-chromosome

Figure 20.8 Sex-linked inheritance.

Parental genotypes Aa × AO

i.e. the female is a carrier (heterozygous) for the recessive allele, the male has the normal allele

Possible offspring genotypes:

		♂ Gametes	
		A	O
♀ Gametes	A	AA	AO
	a	Aa	aO
		female	male

	PHENOTYPES	
AA	Normal ♀	1:2 females will be carriers
Aa	Normal/carrier ♀	
AO	Normal ♂	1:2 males will be affected
aO	**Abnormal** ♂	

Note that there cannot be a 'carrier' male

the neurotransmitter gamma aminobutyric acid (GABA) from neurological areas involved in the control of movement. Why there should be a delay in expression of the disorder is unclear. Some childhood cancers also appear to result from the expression of dominant alleles.

Sex-linked recessive inheritance

The discrepancy between the sizes of the X- and Y-chromosomes has important implications for conditions arising from gene mutations on the X-chromosome (the Y-chromosome appears generally to be functionally 'quiet' after birth). This is because there are some 200–300 alleles on the X-chromosome but only a handful on the Y-chromosome. Thus alleles on the X will not have homologous alleles on the Y. In the female, the expression of recessive, mutated alleles on the X-chromosome will only be observed if both chromosomes have a copy of the allele, but in the male a recessive allele on the X-chromosome will be expressed as there can be no dominant 'normal' allele on the Y-chromosome.

The means of inheritance is illustrated in Figure 20.8. In this example, the inheritance of Duchenne's muscular dystrophy results from the passing down into the next generation of the recessive allele on the X-chromosome. Duchenne's muscular dystrophy is characterized by loss of the skeletal muscle protein dystrophin, which has a role in the maintenance of the sarcolemma. Loss of the protein results in chronic wastage of muscle.

The example given in Figure 20.8 assumes a 'normal' father and a heterozygous 'carrier' mother and is the most likely pattern of inheritance for this condition. The alternatives of a father with the dystrophy allele on his X-chromosome (i.e. a sufferer of the condition) or a mother who is homozygous for the condition (i.e. a sufferer who must have inherited one of the alleles from her dystrophied father) are unlikely. This is because it is a fatal condition which progresses during childhood, and so it is unlikely that anyone with the condition will have children. Girls receive one of their X-chromosomes from their father and so are unlikely to be homozygous, although a handful of cases are known world-wide. Heterozygous girls will have inherited the recessive allele from their mothers.

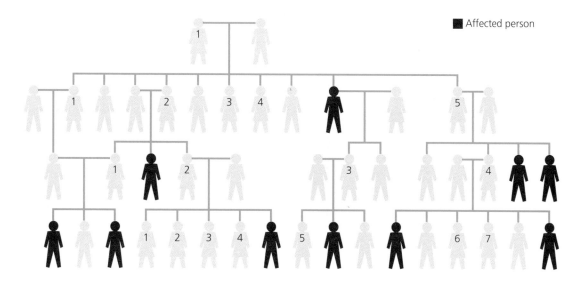

Figure 20.9 An example of a pedigree analysis. Female carriers are identified by numbers.

Other known X-linked conditions do not place reproductive restrictions on the inherited genotype. For example, haemophilia A has been known for many years to be primarily a condition of boys (see Figure 20.9), although a few incidences in girls have been documented. The condition results from a loss of the liver enzyme necessary for the synthesis of clotting factor VIII.

In this case sex linkage arises because of the low frequency of the mutated allele within the population. Thus, the female progeny of a male haemophiliac will inherit the recessive allele but, unless another copy is obtained from the mother (who would either have to have both alleles or at least be heterozygous) then the female child will be heterozygous and not develop the condition. The frequency of female carriers in the population is low and it is estimated that, whilst 1 in 10 000 males may inherit the condition, the chances of a homozygous female arising are as low as 1 in 100 million.

Polygenic inheritance

With an increased number of alleles involved, it is not surprising that the frequency of congenital disturbances arising from mutations is small. Pronounced changes in cell function will arise only if a 'vital' gene within the sequence is mutated, or if a number of the genes within the group are mutated.

It has been proposed, however, that the inheritance of homozygous recessive and heterozygous genotypes within the functional 'group' provides a predisposition to a condition which may arise later in life should further mutation of the remaining genes (especially those which are heterozygous in which only one dominant normal allele would have to be altered) occur due to environmental influences. This influence of life-style on genetic expression is increasingly being recognized. From the inheritance viewpoint it could explain why, for some individuals at least, many diseases of adulthood seem to have a weak familial linkage (e.g. colonic cancer, heart disease, Alzheimer's disease, insulin-independent diabetes mellitus).

CHROMOSOMAL DEFECTS

In addition to the presence or absence of gene mutations, the development of the embryo and the resultant health of the neonate (and adult)

(a)

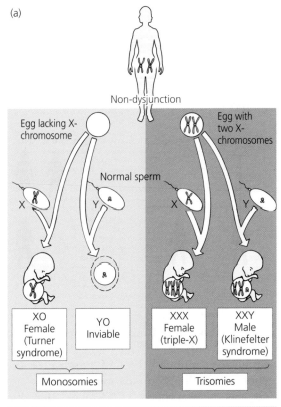

(b)

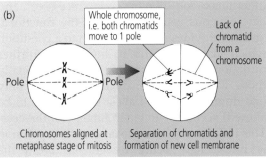

Figure 20.10 Non-dysjunction of (a) sex chromosomes during meiosis and (b) chromatids during mitosis (or second meiotic division).

is also influenced by the loss or gain of chromosomes, or parts of chromosomes. The disorders associated with such changes are distinct from those induced by single gene mutations because they involve the loss or gain of large numbers of genes. Accordingly their symptoms are frequently severe and the survival rates are low.

Chromosome number

Cells other than the gametes normally contain two copies of each autosome and two sex chromosomes. Trisomy (literally three chromosomes of one type) usually arises because either the chromosome pair involved failed to separate at meiosis when the gametes were formed or the chromatids of a chromosome in the second stage of meiosis failed to separate (Figure 20.10).

The failure of chromosomes or chromatids to separate is called non-dysjunction. Whether it occurs in the first or second phase of meiosis it will result in a gamete which contains two of the same chromosome (similarly there must also be a gamete which is lacking it). Fertilization will therefore produce a zygote with either three of the chromosome (two from one partner, one from the other), or just one copy (from just one partner; this is called monosomy).

Trisomy of the sex cells is not unusual. Klinefelter's syndrome is a relatively common occurrence in males, in whom there is an extra X-chromosome (i.e. these individuals are XXY). The consequence is that the testes are small and androgen secretion is low. Sperm may be absent, though some people with the syndrome have fathered children (note that the presence of the Y-chromosome makes these people male). Intelligence is usually normal or at most only slightly affected.

Trisomy of the X-chromosome is called triple X syndrome and is also frequently found within a population, but individuals usually do not have distinctive phenotypic characteristics. Although some of these females have menstrual difficulties, many are fertile.

Non-dysjunction during meiosis may also lead to the inheritance of multiple sex chromosomes. Even the pentasomy XXXXX has been observed, though the consequences are more severe than for trisomy and it is associated with learning disabilities.

A relatively common monosomy is that which leads to Turner's syndrome, in which individuals are XO; 98% of such fetuses spontaneously abort. The 2% born are female as no Y-chromosome is present. Intelligence is largely unaffected but development of the gonads, and growth, are retarded.

Trisomy of chromosome 21 is the only viable autosomal trisomy. Others are known (e.g. 3×18 and 3×13) but are usually fatal in the first year or abort during pregnancy. Trisomy 21 (Down's syndrome) usually arises because of non-dysjunction during the formation of the 'ova' (though some are 'mosaics' – see below). Its incidence increases as maternal age increases, presumably because of ageing of the primary oocytes in the ovary.

Mosaicism

As the name implies, mosaicism means that a proportion of cells within the individual have chromosomal defects whilst the rest are normal. Within the embryo such an occurrence could not be explained by the inheritance of a defect from the parents as all cells would be expected to have the same genotype as the zygote. The condition arises because of incomplete separation of chromatids during mitotic division of cells in the embryo itself, especially in the early embryo or in the early stages of tissue differentiation. Thus, new cells formed by mitosis may contain two chromatids of a chromosome (i.e. the whole chromosome from the original cell) whilst others will now be lacking that particular DNA molecule. Subsequent cell divisions will then increase the numbers of trisomic and monosomic cells in a tissue.

Mosaicism is frequently encountered in Down's syndrome, i.e. many cells are trisomic for chromosome 21 whilst others have only one copy. Yet other cells, derived from embryonic cells which divided normally, will have the usual two copies. Clearly the consequences for development will depend upon the extent of the mosaicism, and this relates to the period of embryo/fetal development when the non-dysjunction occurred.

Chromosomal fragmentation

The inheritance of extra DNA, or of a chromosome deficient in DNA, can occur if there is an error in crossover, or translocation, during meiosis. Thus a chromosome could receive DNA from its homologous partner but does not 'release' its own DNA. The chromosome with the additional fragment will therefore contain some duplicated alleles, and these will therefore be present in triplicate in the zygote after fertilization. Sometimes the fragment translocates and attaches to a different chromosome altogether. The effects on health will depend upon how many additional alleles have been inherited, or how many have been lost if the deficient chromosome is inherited.

Fragile X syndrome results from fragmentation of the X-chromosome. In this case the error is due to a 'fragile' section of DNA which tends to break during meiosis. As a consequence any resultant zygote will be deficient in the alleles found on the lost fragment. The lack of homologous alleles on the Y-chromosome means that the effects will be particularly pronounced in males. The condition is a frequent cause of learning disability.

Introduction to population genetics

The above section considered the likelihood of a gene mutation carried by the parents being inherited in the offspring. By extrapolation, the incidence of genetic disorder within a population as a whole will therefore depend upon the frequency of the alleles within the genes of the population (called the gene pool). This is determined by various factors.

INBREEDING

Inbreeding within a family increases the likelihood that a defective gene present in members of a family will be inherited. This, for example, is why the incidence of haemophilia A in the royal line traced back to Queen Victoria is much greater than that of the population as a whole (Figure 20.10). The effect is not just confined to inbreeding between close relatives, however. If a population is small and stable with little immigration or emigration, then the likelihood of people being related, perhaps from several generations earlier, increases. The incidence of an inherited condition will increase accordingly within that population. This is a cause of clusters of inherited conditions being found in some districts, when compared with national figures.

MUTATION

Mutations arise when the genetic code of a section of DNA is altered. Such alterations can occur spontaneously and, although DNA can self-repair, some mutations may persist and therefore be inherited. This means that inherited conditions are unlikely to be eradicated from a population as new mutations will continuously occur within the gene pool.

Mutations can also arise through the actions of environmental agents and there is no doubt that this is the cause of disorders in some adults. Changing the DNA of gametes, or of gamete stem cells raises the possibility that the mutated gene(s) will be passed on to the next generation. Environmentally induced mutation is another cause for local clusters of disorders, for example the leukaemias induced by radon gas emission from granite rocks.

SELECTION

If the advantage of 'gene mixing' is to produce offspring with genotypes that may prove beneficial when compared with the population as a whole, then the success of such offspring should, over many generations, increase the incidence of the advantageous alleles within the population. Similarly, any gene which is detrimental to life should tend to reduce in frequency in the gene pool. This is the basis of the proposals forwarded by Charles Darwin in the nineteenth century in his theory of evolution. Darwin called the process natural selection.

Selection might be expected to reduce the incidence of severe genetic disorders, and this is a factor in the rarity of conditions. For some conditions, however, there is a reasonable chance that a child will survive into adulthood and have children of his/her own. Medical advances in recent years have also increased the survival rate and, to some degree, negated selection processes.

POPULATION DRIFT

Immigration or emigration of individuals into or out of a population will respectively add to or remove genes from that population. The process can alter the incidence of a particular gene mutation within a gene pool and may even result in the introduction of novel mutations.

Principles of correction/prevention

Genetic disorders have proved extremely resistant to curative methods. Therapies have generally been directed at the maintenance of health for as long as possible, rather than cure. Recent advances in molecular biology, however, have furthered knowledge and understanding of genetic disease and advances in the treatment of such disorders are on the horizon.

The identification of fetuses at risk is not new. Techniques such as amniocentesis and chorionic villus sampling have for a long time enabled clinicians to obtain samples of fetal cells for chromosomal analysis. In this way, the sex of the fetus is readily identified, and chromosomal defects determined. Also now available are techniques which can identify the presence of certain mutated genes in fetal cells, although this might only be looked for if there is a known risk. Such techniques allow the prospective parents to be aware prior to birth of the likelihood of certain neonatal abnormalities.

PEDIGREE ANALYSIS

The risk of genetic disorder in offspring is established by pedigree analysis. Thus familial incidences of a disorder, going back through a number of generations, can identify the presence of a mutated allele within the family line (Figure 20.9). Such analyses can only highlight the possibility that an individual is a carrier of the allele, and likewise if his/her partner might also be a carrier. Frequently a couple become aware that they are carriers of a recessive allele only after the birth of an affected (homozygous recessive) offspring. Counselling may then be initiated should the parents plan further pregnancies.

Pedigree analysis cannot on its own prevent a child from being affected, and amniocentesis techniques only yield information regarding an already formed fetus. Recent scientific advances are beginning to increase the options for couples of known risk. For some disorders it is now possible to have unaffected embryos selected *in vitro* for implantation.

EMBRYO SELECTION

The screening of *in vitro* early embryos is possible because cells can be removed from the morula stage without affecting later development. Chromosomal and gene analysis (for a few disorders only at present) of the extracted cell can identify which embryos will be affected. Unaffected embryos might then be chosen for implantation. Such techniques might be considered a form of Darwinian 'natural' selection! Recent methodological advances have also opened up the possibility of manipulating the genome through genetic engineering.

GENETIC ENGINEERING AND GENE THERAPIES

Genetic engineering, or recombinant DNA technology, developed during the 1970s and 1980s as a means of producing large quantities of a particular gene or gene product. The methodology involves either (1) the incorporation of a fragment of DNA into that of a host cell (usually a bacterium) which, by multiple cell division, produces multiple copies, or clones, of the DNA fragment and its genes; or (2) utilizing the enzyme DNA polymerase to produce multiple copies of DNA fragments from an original small sample. Such techniques enable production of quantities of (pure) genes or gene products sufficient for further study. More recently, techniques have been developed as a means of incorporating a normal gene into defective host cells within the body.

Gene transplantation (called transgenics) involves incorporating a piece of DNA containing the required allele into a vector (usually a modified virus) and allowing the vector to penetrate the target cells. By nature of the life cycle of the virus, the DNA will be incorporated into the genome of the recipient cell. If the transplanted allele is a dominant form, then this will influence cell function.

Transplantation of genes into embryos has been confined to animal studies to date, and understandably raises concern regarding the legal and ethical position of embryo manipulation, and regarding the prevention of abuse of these techniques to enable parents to select 'desirable' characteristics for their offspring. Transgenics, however, is an exciting development which could aid the prevention of recessive disorders.

Genetic engineering has also opened up the possibility of treating individuals with genetic disorder. Gene therapies may provide a definitive means of curing, or at least preventing deterioration of, sufferers of many conditions. To be effective, a normal allele must be transplanted into the majority of the affected cells in extensive, already differentiated, tissues. One way is to transplant the gene into stem, or germinative, cells from which new tissue cells will be derived; another is to use a method which provides access to large areas of tissue, using either specific viruses or small lipid droplets called 'liposomes' as vectors.

A spin-off from gene research is that drugs can be 'designed' to target inappropriately functioning genes, or the actions of those genes. Some areas of cancer research are currently investigating this approach by, for example, using antibody–drug complexes to target abnormal antigens on tumour cells.

GENETIC FINGERPRINTING

With the advent of technology to determine genetic coding, it has become possible genetically to 'type' individuals. Although the human genome is vast, it contains within it sequences which mutate little and which will be almost constant between closely related individuals. The family link can also be assessed by comparing mitochondrial DNA (i.e. extranuclear DNA found within the cell mitochondria). This DNA is only inherited through the female line as the mitochondria of sperm are jettisoned with the tail at fertilization.

Sequencing can be performed on minute amounts of tissue, but only after the DNA has been replicated many times in the laboratory. The method has been of value in forensic science, legal (paternity) cases, in identifying related species of plant or animal (both extant and extinct!) and in the debate as to the evolutionary links of human cultures.

Summary

1 Genes are sections of DNA and a sequence of constituent bases which contains the information necessary for a cell to synthesize a specific polypeptide.

2 The four different bases present in DNA are 'complementary' pairs. That is, within DNA adenosine will only pair (i.e. bond) with thymine, guanine with cytosine. This pairing is vital because it is the basis for conserving the genetic code during DNA duplication prior to somatic cell division (so that succeeding generations of cells will function identically).

3 The DNA of a cell is packaged prior to cell division as chromosomes. There are 23 pairs of chromosomes in each somatic cell, i.e. 23 chromosomes inherited from each parent. There is thus a duplication of genes (except on the sex chromosomes of males where the Y-chromosome is considerably smaller than the X-chromosome). Each member of a pair of genes is called an allele. The pairs of alleles separate in meiosis during the formation of the gametes, however, and the alleles on either chromosome can potentially be inherited by offspring.

4 Mutation, or alteration, of the genetic code in one of a pair of alleles is possible, in which case the person is said to be heterozygous. Such a mutation may be of no consequence if the mutated allele is recessive to the normal dominant one on the homologous chromosome, since the normal protein associated with the gene will be synthesized. If the mutation is dominant, however, then the cell will synthesize the protein determined by that allele, with possible damaging effects.

5 Although recessive alleles may remain 'hidden' in heterozygous individuals, there is always a possibility that a child may inherit copies of the allele from each (heterozygous) parent. With no dominant counterpart to suppress it, the mutated allele will now contribute to protein synthesis and cell function. The poten-

tial effects of losing a normal protein, or of producing the novel protein, can be devastating and is the basis of most recognized genetic diseases.

6 Mutated alleles on the X-chromosome are unlikely to have corresponding alleles on the smaller Y-chromosome. Thus male offspring will always be affected even if the mutation is recessive to the normal form. This means that males cannot be 'carriers' of a recessive allele in the usual sense and some disorders typically are observed more frequently in boys than girls.

7 Characteristics produced by the net effects of multiple genes are less sensitive to the effects of mutation of an individual allele within the group, but the more mutations that are inherited the greater the likelihood will be that mutation of the remainder of the 'group' will occur during life. Thus a propensity to a disorder can be inherited with consequences later in life.

8 Pedigree analysis can identify people at risk of genetic disorder and so pregnancies can be avoided (depriving a couple of children) or couples prepared for the outcome. Traditional therapies for inherited disorder have been aimed at maintaining as high a standard of life as possible – cures have not been possible. Alternatively, affected fetuses may be aborted.

9 The development of *in vitro* fertilization techniques, coupled with recent advances in the identification of mutated genes, has meant that the implantation of embryos known to be lacking certain mutations is possible, and will result in an unaffected child.

10 Advances in genetic engineering are beginning to make the treatment of certain genetic disorders appear possible, and such genetic therapies would represent a major breakthrough in medicine.

Review Questions

1 Explain the nature of intracellular homeostatic principles with reference to gene expression and list all the ways that you can think of by which the amount of gene product in the cell can be altered.

2 Explain why it is desirable that organisms are able to regulate the expression of genes.

3 Define the following:
(a) mutation, (b) mutagen, (c) recombination, (d) phenotype, (e) genotype, (f) teratogen, (g) selection, (h) population drift.

4 Distinguish between the following terms:
(a) point mutation, (b) substitution, (c) chromosomal mutation.

5 Why are some mutations lethal?

6 Define the following terms:
(a) alleles, (b) lethal alleles, (c) gamete, (d) dominant, (e) recessive, (f) co-dominant, (g) homozygous, (h) heterozygous.

7 Explain what is meant by incomplete dominance and co-dominance.

8 What are multiple alleles?

9 What would be the offspring genotype and phenotypes with the following genetic crosses of parental ABO blood groupings:
(a) AO × BO; (b) AA × OB; (c) AB × AB.

10 Define the following:
(a) chromosome, (b) autosome, (c) sex chromosome, (d) linkage group, (e) zygote, (f) sex-linked inheritance, (g) independent assortment.

11 What is crossover?

12 Outline the principles of the operon theory as a model for gene expression (Chapter 2).

13 Describe the processes that can lead to maternal and paternal trisomies and monosomies, giving appropriate examples.

14 Discuss the principles behind genetic engineering.

Pain

21

Introduction

Neurophysiology of pain

The subjectivity of pain and pain therapies

Assessment of pain

The clinical measurement of pain

Summary

Review questions

Introduction

Most people think they know what pain is and yet, from a scientific point of view, it is a state about which relatively little is known! It is difficult for researchers to agree upon a definition and further difficulties arise in developing a suitable theory to account for all the different observations that have been made (Melzack and Wall, 1990). An individual's personality, culture, anxiety level, their perception of the painful situation, mood, and social influence, have all been suggested to affect the perception and expression of pain. Although pain perception can be considered to be a 'sense', to understand how pain can be subjective necessitates more discussion than was possible when the senses were described in Chapter 14. The aim of this chapter is to consider some of the determinants of pain, and also to examine the statement by Fordham (1986) that:

> The experience of pain is dependent upon the integrated function of the nervous system. Therefore, to say pain is either body or mind is meaningless.

This statement will be investigated from a sociopsychophysiological perspective, using Melzack and Wall's (1965) gate control theory of pain as a basis. This involves linking and integrating the sociopsychology with the neurophysiology associated with pain perception. The chapter begins with a definition of pain, and then investigates the functions of pain and the types of pain a person may perceive. In addition, various assessment tools will be reviewed, and those factors which must be taken into consideration during objective assessment of pain will be discussed. Finally, the basis of analgesic methods employed by the health care professional will be briefly mentioned.

DEFINITION OF PAIN

The word pain is derived from the Greek word 'poine' for 'penalty' and thus suggests the concept of punishment and retribution. Despite the importance of pain control in medicine, nursing, and allied health care professions, it is astonishing to discover that pain has never been defined satisfactorily. Any credible definition must include the subjective nature of pain, as emphasized by McCaffery's (1983) definition that:

> Pain is whatever the experiencing person says it is, existing whenever he says it does.

PAIN THRESHOLDS AND PAIN TOLERANCE

Pain threshold refers to the level of stimulation at which the subject just begins to perceive pain. There is considerable debate over the existence of an absolute pain threshold for each individual, since the threshold is affected by sociopsychological and 'physical' factors, such as anxiety, hospitalization, and the pain relief technique administered. Thus, individual thresholds are dynamic as well as subjective. Some of the factors that account for this subjectivity are highlighted later in the chapter. Thresholds can be divided into that of pain perception, when the perception of stimuli, for example temperature change, and pressure, reaches a level when the subject begins to feel pain for the first time, and that of severe pain, i.e. the point when the pain becomes unbearable if stimulus strength is increased further.

There is little difference between the values obtained for pain perception thresholds across different social and ethnic groups (Melzack and Wall, 1990). However, values for the severe pain threshold differ markedly, and this may be explained by cultural and psychophysiological variations.

FUNCTIONS OF PAIN

Pain has survival and protective values. For instance, the pain sensation that occurs before serious injury, such as when picking up a hot plate, produces immediate withdrawal in order to prevent further damage. Subsequently, through conditioned learning and socialization, one avoids future injurious objects.

Pain associated with injuries may be considered a homeostatic imbalance, since damaged cells are involved in hyperproduction and/or hypersecretion of pain-producing substances. Injuries set limits on activity by enforcing inactivity and rest, which itself aids a faster recovery. In this sense, rest and inactivity could be considered as crude homeostatic adaptive mechanisms. Injury pain, therefore, serves useful purposes (Melzack, 1992). However, on occasions pain seems to have no useful value; for example, some amputees suffer excruciating phantom limb pain for years.

VARIETIES OF PAIN

Classifying the type of pain aids the selection of appropriate assessment tools and therapies to suit the individualistic needs of the patient. Clinically, pain is classified as being either acute or chronic.

Acute pain

Acute pain is usually adequately dealt with, and is relatively short-lived; a beginning and an end are often identifiable. It is viewed positively as a warning signal which draws attention to injury or illness and is experienced by everyone at some stage in their lives. It can range from a relatively minor acute pain, such as toothache, to a relatively major pain such as post-operative pain. The characteristics of acute pain are usually those associated with tissue damage, and anxiety-led features exhibited in the psychophysiological 'fight and flight' reactions (Chapter 22). Accompanying these reactions is a preoccupation with the cause of the pain and its consequences.

Chronic (intractable) pain

In contrast to acute pain, chronic pain has no biological value (Morris, 1986); it is disabling, easily recognizable, but poorly understood. The pain overwhelms the patient and is often associated with anxiety, depression, and insomnia. Saunders *et al.* (1981) reported a qualitative difference between acute and chronic pain since it affects the whole person differently, whether psychologically, physiologically, emotionally, or spiritually. Twycross and Lack (1983) referred to chronic pain as a situation and not an event, in which it is impossible to predict when it will end, it often gets worse rather than better, it is also poorly controlled, and therapies are generally ineffective. Examples include arthritic and cancer pains. In fact, chronic pain can be so terrible and detrimental to one's life that some people would sooner die than continue living with it.

Neurophysiology of pain

In order to perceive pain there is usually cellular damage, for example in a myocardial infarction, but this is not always the case, for example in angina pectoris. In these examples pain results from insufficient coronary blood flow, called cardiac ischaemia, and the presence or absence of cellular damage should be a consideration in the practitioner's pain assessment, since this is the foundation of planning appropriate analgesic care. Thus assessment of the patient's pain and accompanying symptoms, together with biochemical and X-ray analysis, determine the different care regimens for angina and myocardial infarction patients.

Cellular damage results in the release of pain-producing substances, such as histamine, bradykinin, and potassium ions. Prostaglandins are also released and potentiate the effects of these pain-producing substances (Tempest, 1990). The substances combine with receptor sites on nociceptors (receptors which respond to harmful stimuli) and are therefore the initiators of the neural transmission associated with the perception of pain following cell damage. In order to evoke a neural impulse, the interaction between pain-producing substances and nociceptors must reach threshold level, i.e. the minimal level of noxious stimulus required to initiate neural transmission. Depolarization (activation) of the nociceptor membrane then occurs and a wave of depolarization passes along the associated neurons in the form of action potentials (see Chapter 13).

Pain neurons are small diameter, myelinated fibres (classified as Aδ fibres) and smaller unmyelinated (or C) fibres. These are classified as the 'fast' and 'slow' pain fibres respectively, since faster transmission is associated with thicker fibres and the presence of a myelin sheath. If the pain is identified as being sharp, localized, and distinct, this informs the practitioner that the pain fibres involved are mainly of the Aδ type. If the assessment indicates that the pain is characteristically a dull, burning, poorly localized, visceral and persistent pain, then the pain fibres involved are of the C variety (Puntillo, 1988).

The 'gate' control theory

Melzack and Wall (1965) proposed a gating mechanism within the dorsal horn of grey matter of the spinal cord, in the layer called the substantia gelatinosa, through which sensory information has to pass before it is relayed to, and perceived in, the 'pain centre(s)' of the brain. It is now generally accepted that there are gating mechanisms at each level of the spinal cord and also at several sites within the

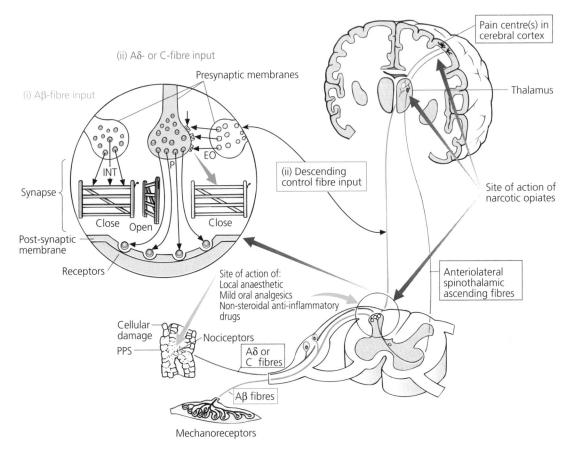

Figure 21.1 The gate control theory of pain perception and pain management. (i)–(iii) Presynaptic fibres. P, substance P; EO, endogenous opiates; INT, inhibitory neurotransmitters; PPS, pain-producing substance. See text for details.

brain (the thalamus, reticular formation, and areas of the limbic system). The gates are symbolic of synapses between afferent neurons and various ascending and descending tract neurons. The gate control theory suggests that information can only pass through when the gate is 'open' and not when the gate is 'closed' (Figure 21.1). The opening of the gate is by the release at the synapse of excitatory neurotransmitter chemicals. The closing of the gate is brought about by the release of other chemicals, which are inhibitory neurotransmitters and neuromodulators. Clinically, the closing of the gate forms the basis of pain relief.

The gating mechanism depends upon two modifying factors:

1 The balance of activity of afferent neurons.

2 The control provided by descending fibres from the brain's higher centres.

Balance of activity of afferent neurons

The afferent neurons which provide input to the gate are:

1 the Aδ- and C-pain fibres from nociceptors which release substance P, an excitatory neurotransmitter, at synapses within the central nervous system; and

2 the faster-transmitting Aβ neurons from mechanoreceptors, that release inhibitory neurotransmitters.

If the dominant input to the gate is via the faster-transmitting Aβ fibres, then the gate will close due to the release and action of the inhibitory neurotransmitters. This modifying influence is thought to be the mechanism that relieves pain when the painful area is gently rubbed, massaged or touched since the mechanoreceptors are stimulated and the Aβ fibre input to the gate (or gates) dominates (Tempest, 1990). According to Melzack and Wall (1988) the application of transcutaneous nerve stimulation (TNS), and acupuncture, also operate via this method.

There are many possible modes of action of these inhibitory neurotransmitters (Clancy and McVicar, 1992). These are as follows.

Presynaptic inhibition

Upon release the inhibitory transmitters from the Aβ fibres may interact with the pain neurons and either:

1 repress the gene activity necessary for substance P synthesis;

2 Block enzyme action by competitive binding (lock and key) when it is necesary to produce substance P;

3 destroy vacuolated substance P in the pre-synaptic fibres;

4 prevent substance P release by decreasing the presynaptic membrane permeability, or by inducing its hyperpolarization (Chapter 13).

Synaptic inhibition

Substance P may be destroyed within the synapse (although this seems unlikely).

Post-synaptic inhibition

There may be competitive inhibition of the binding of substance P to post-synaptic membrane receptor sites.

In contrast, if the dominant input to the gate is from the Aδ and/or C pain fibres, the gate may be open, owing to the release of the excitatory neurotransmitter substance P, and the patient then perceives pain. Pain perception will still only occur, however, if there is no interference from descending fibres from higher centres within the central nervous system.

Descending control from higher centres

The gate theory proposes that, even if pain fibre input into the central nervous system dominates, the gate may still close since higher brain centres such as the raphe nuclei, trigeminal nuclei, and vestibular nuclei of the brainstem, various nuclei of the hypothalamus, and the cerebral cortex, can modify the gating process via descending neural mechanisms. These neurons release a variety of opiate chemicals (enkephalins, endorphins, and dynorphins) which are the body's own natural 'pain killers'. When released, these neuromodulators act at the presynaptic membrane and may close the gate by inhibiting substance P release (Figure 21.1).

The descending route of pain control forms the psychophysiological basis of distraction and diversion therapies, counselling, and placebo (Melzack and Wall, 1988), and according to Whipple (1990) TNS also causes the release of these endogenous opiates. The communication skills used by nurses and allied health care professionals, in admission procedures, pre- and post-operative counselling, and in the daily ward routine, all help to reduce a patient's anxiety levels, which is generally reported to decrease pain perception.

INTERIM SUMMARY

If the combined effect of pain modifiers (i.e. inhibitory neurotransmitters and endogenous neuromodulators) does not exceed the pain fibre input to the gate, the gate is opened, and afferent neurons transmit activity mainly to the anterolateral spinothalamic tracts and hence to the thalamus (Figure 21.1). Within the thalamus they synapse with other neurons which transmit the impulses to the cortical pain centre(s). Melzack and Wall (1988) stated that the cerebral cortex may not contain specific pain centres, and it may just process the information it receives before transmitting it deeper into the brain tissue. Thus, specific pain centre(s) have not yet been located and,

> the dream of some researchers of finding one pain centre which, if removed, would obliterate pain, has been abandoned. (Fordham, 1986)

The subjectivity of pain and pain therapies

Pain is a subjective experience since each individual has a unique range of anatomical, physiological, social, and psychological identities. These identities can be applied to the gate control theory to help to explain the subjective nature of pain perception. The concept of individualized pain relief is based upon a knowledge of the patient's background, the progress of his illness, its associated pain and his personal interpretation of his current situation, since all are relevant to successful pain management.

ANATOMICAL SUBJECTIVITY

A tremendous variation in human body shapes and sizes exists and it is not surprising, therefore, that the distribution of nociceptors varies between individuals. This could be expected to produce regional variations of anatomical subjectivity, in sensitivity to stimuli.

BIOCHEMICAL AND PHYSIOLOGICAL SUBJECTIVITY

Individuals have different production capacities of the biochemicals involved in the transmission of pain (Figure 21.1). The person's genome is responsible for the production of physiologically active enzymes necessary for the biochemical synthesis of pain-producing substances, substance P, inhibitory endogenous opiates, and inhibitory neurotransmitters. If the genes responsible for the synthesis of pain-producing substances or substance P were mutated or repressed, or the nociceptors become desensitized to them, then it would be possible to experience tissue injury without perceiving pain. Alternatively, people may not report pain, despite tissue damage, if the genes necessary for the production of the endogenous opiates or inhibitory neurotransmitters are repeatedly expressed, since their high levels would close the gate. Conversely, high levels of pain-producing substances, and consequently substance P or low levels of endogenous opiates and/or inhibitory neurotransmitters as a consequence of gene activity or inactivity respectively would lead to pain hypersensitivity. Congenital disorders of pain perception do exist and thus some people are born insensitive to pain, whilst others feel pain without any detectable injury (Melzack and Wall, 1988).

SOCIOPSYCHOLOGICAL SUBJECTIVITY

Sociopsychological factors affect physiological processes and may be indirectly responsible for either opening or closing the gate. Social factors influence the development of the brain and these higher cortical centres may conceivably influence the physiological, neuronal, and synaptic activity of the gate by influencing the descending control.

Anxiety is a state that may be genetically determined and/or environmentally socialized. Elevated anxiety levels are associated with an increased pain perception (Seers, 1987). The gate control theory would attribute this to depressed endogenous opiate levels, or to an increased substance P level; the former is most likely according to descending control theory. Whichever the case, Sofaer (1983) argued that nursing care should aim to reduce the patient's anxiety levels before attempting to quantify the pain that the patient is perceiving. Perhaps, then, an appropriate nursing action might be just to empathize, sit and support the patient in pain since this physical assurance can have analgesic qualities.

Cultural differences in the perception of pain are also observed, according to Melzack and Wall (1988), and therefore need to be taken into consideration when assessing pain. This could suggest that past socializing experiences and individual conditioning have important influences on the subjective elements of pain. Socialization determines psychological behaviour, which could conceivably affect the output of endogenous opiates. Thus practitioners should be concerned with management of a particular type of pain by using constant patient monitoring, rather than have different treatment regimens according to the patient's perception of their pain. The health care professional should be familiar with cultural differences when reducing the patient's anxiety prior to assessing the appropriate care to be implemented.

The importance or meaning of a situation can affect one's perception of pain. For example, prior to entering hospital (particularly with emergency) pre-admission pain can seem almost unbearable, whereas post-admission interviews indicate that the pain may have lessened or even disappeared. Perhaps the fear of a serious diagnosis results in a surge of endogenous opiate gene activity, resulting in high levels of these pain killers! If this is the case, then it demonstrates how environmental factors, such as the clinical setting, presence of doctors and nurses, and unfamiliar and possibly high-technology equipment, may influence gene activity and subsequent opiate release, thus reducing or abolishing the pain.

PAIN CONTROL AND THERAPEUTIC SUBJECTIVITY

The different characteristics associated with acute, chronic benign, chronic malignant, phantom, bone and muscle pains, necessitates different therapeutic approaches emphasizing the subjectivity of pain perception and consequently of pain management. Nurses adopt a psychological approach in assisting the patient to understand and to cope with their pain, whilst doctors are more concerned with the physiological role of diagnosing pain and instigating treatment (Caunt, 1992). However, a considerable degree of overlap exists depending upon the philosophy of the ward staff, a factor itself which demonstrates subjectivity. On the whole, it could be argued that the nurse should be fully aware of the sociopsychophysiological aspects of pain in order to manage the patient's pain successfully since she is the practitioner who has most frequent contact with the patient.

Pain is treated either pharmacologically or non-pharmacologically. The analgesic qualities of these methods are briefly reviewed in the next section, and the reader is directed to numerous other texts for further detail. Prior to the discussion, however, it must be stressed that a good rapport and verbal communication with the patient (if conscious) are essential aspects of caring, so that the patient feels confident in the practitioner's ability to reduce or abolish their pain. According to Richardson (1991) this operates via a placebo effect.

PHARMACOLOGICAL THERAPEUTIC SUBJECTIVITY

Analgesic drug administration can be via a variety of routes: oral, sublingual, rectal, inhalation, intramuscular, intravenous, subcutaneous, transdermal, spinal, and epidural. In addition, the infiltration of an area with local anaesthetics may be used to provide nerve blocks. However, these methods are only of pharmacological benefit if the nurse/practitioner is familiar with, and safe in her management of, these treatments (Caunt, 1992). There is, therefore, potential subjectivity in the administration routes and management of pain according to the expertise of the nurse/practitioner. Furthermore, the choice of drug depends upon the type of pain experienced, its location, its severity, its mode of action, its side-effects; this further emphasizes therapeutic subjectivity (Table 21.1).

For example:

1 Simple analgesics are administered for mild to moderate pain.

2 Non-steroidal anti-inflammatory drugs are used for painful generalized or local inflammation.

3 Weak opioids are administered for moderate to severe visceral pain.

4 Stronger opioids are used for severe visceral pain.

If the pain is poorly controlled then an analgesic 'staircase' is used in an attempt to manage the pain (Figure 21.2). Smith (1985) used the anatomical pathways associated with the gate theory in order to explain the site of pharmacological actions (Figure 21.1).

The operation of this gating mechanism may explain other therapeutic regimens that are used to control the patient's pain. Although the effectiveness of pain management techniques, such as diversion, distraction, placebo, and transcutaneous nerve stimulation, is dependent upon the application skills of the practitioner, the patient also needs to believe that pain relief will be successful. For example, placebos are effective

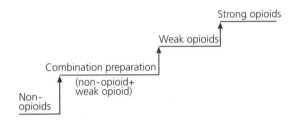

Figure 21.2 The analgesic staircase. The analgesic pathway may be used in order to reduce or abolish a patient's pain. That is, if the pain is not removed using non–opioids (e.g. paracetamol), then a combined preparation may be given (e.g. paracetamol + codeine phosphate). If the pain is still not removed, then weak opioids are given and if pain still persists, then a strong opioid is given.

because individuals are socialized to accept that pain killers abolish pain. Whether these pain killers mimic traditional forms, such as aspirin, morphine, or are 'magic potions' administered by a 'witch doctor' is irrelevant; the recipient needs to believe that the analgesic (placebo) is going to be effective. Therefore the nurse's reliability in the eyes of the patient, and the trust a patient places in his practitioner, becomes an essential element in analgesic success. However, the lack of placebo effectiveness in others demonstrates the subjective nature of placebo pain control. Other factors that affect analgesic success are briefly discussed later.

According to Puntillo (1988) the appropriate choice of therapeutic intervention also depends upon the setting where treatment occurs. For example, therapies appropriate to the critical care patient include opioid analgesia, transcutaneous nerve stimulation, relaxation techniques, distraction, and control of the patient environment. The analgesic qualities of these therapies are now discussed.

OPIOID THERAPY

Intravenous opioid therapy is the most frequently used method of pain relief for patients who are in chronic pain. Patient's

Table 21.1 Which analgesic?

Analgesic used	Examples	Type of pain	Other actions	Site and mode of action	Side-effects
Non-opioids					
Non-steroidal anti-inflammatory drugs (NSAIDs)	Aspirin Ibuprofen Indomethacin Diclofenac	Mild to moderate	Anti-inflammatory Anti-pyretic	Incompletely understood Peripheral and central acting – inhibit prostaglandin synthetase (cyclo-oxygenase)	Gastrointestinal irritation Asymptomatic bleeding Increased bleeding time Ulceration Bronchospasm Skin reactions
	Paracetamol	Mild to moderate	Anti-pyretic	Incompletely understood Weak peripheral action (thus no inflammatory action?) Central action on nervous and hypothalamic tissue; in both cases inhibits prostaglandin synthetase	Rare side-effects include skin reactions, blood disorders, acute pancreatitis Overdosage leads to liver failure, kidney failure
Opioids		All used with pain associated with visceral origin			
Weak (mild) opioids	Codeine* Dextropropoxyphene* Dihydrocodeine*	Mild to moderate Moderate to severe	Constipating Cough suppressant	Centrally acting via opioid receptors on pain fibre presynaptic membrane (Figure 21.1) Action raises pain threshold and pain tolerance	Nausea, vomiting, constipation, drowsiness Large dosages: respiratory depression and hypotension (less marked side-effects with codeine and dextropropoxyphene)
Strong opioids	Morphine Diamorphine Pethidine	Severe pain	As above	As above	As above but side-effects more marked

The type of analgesic used depends upon the type of pain: its location, the other actions and side-effects of the analgesic. This reflects subjectivity in pharmacological pain management.
*Mild opioids in combination with aspirin or paracetamol.

anxieties are also modulated by this form of medication. Administration routes also include epidural or spinal routes. The advantages of epidural administration are that lower dosages are needed, the effects are longer-lasting, mobilization is improved, the effects are limited to the immediate area, and respiratory depression resulting from the effects of the analgesics on the brainstem is minimized.

A disadvantage of opioid therapy is the associated risk of vasodilatation and subsequent hypotension near the site of the epidural injection. This can be particularly profound if the patient is elderly, and so is another consideration in pain management. Other potential problems include infection, spinal cord damage, and injury caused by improper techniques.

NON-PHARMACOLOGICAL TECHNIQUES

Non-pharmacological techniques are frequently more within the direct control of the health care practitioner, and they may be used in isolation or combination with medically prescribed analgesics (Caunt, 1992).

Neurosurgery

Neurosurgery is used as a short-term analgesic control and, according to Melzack and Wall (1988), is regarded as being fully justified to improve the quality of life of patients who have a limited time to live, as in the later stages of terminal cancer. Long-term analgesia is rarely achieved and this method may be associated with additional unpleasant sensations. For example, surgical section of peripheral nerves permanently disturbs 'normal' input patterning, but may also produce 'abnormal' inputs from scar tissue. Neurosurgeons are minimizing the use of such techniques (which include rhizotomies, cordotomies, etc. – Figure 21.3) in favour of non-destructive methods, such as devices which electrically stimulate nerves, spinal cord, and discrete but accessible areas of the brain.

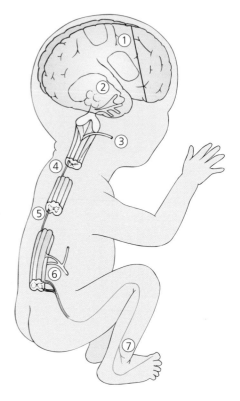

Figure 21.3 A schematic diagram illustrating various neurosurgical procedures designed to alleviate pain: 1, prefrontal lobotomy; 2, thalamotomy; 3, fifth nerve rhizotomy; 4, cervical cordotomy; 5, thoracic cordotomy; 6, posterior rhizotomy; 7, neurectomy.

Transcutaneous electrical nerve stimulation

Transcutaneous electrical nerve stimulation (TNS) involves the electrical stimulation of the nervous system using a pulse generator, an amplifier and a system of electrodes (Figure 21.4). Although the mode of action of TNS is controversial, the technique requires very little training and its effectiveness increases when combined with pharmacological techniques. Latham (1987) stated that TNS can be used to treat any localized pain associated with:

1 acute trauma (such as sports injuries);

2 major trauma (such as multiple injuries);

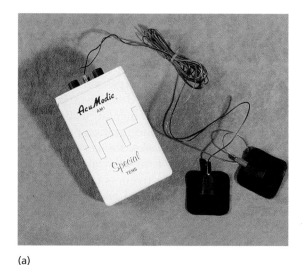

(a)

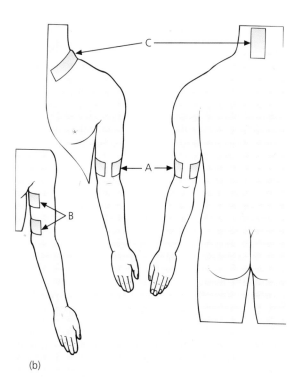

(b)

Figure 21.4 (a) TENS machine with electrodes attached. Photo kindly supplied by the Acumedic Centre, London. (b) Electrode placement for brachial plexus lesion: A, complete anaesthesia below the elbow and pain in the whole hand; B, complete anaesthesia below the elbow and pain in the little and ring fingers; C, complete anaesthesia below the shoulder.

3 the first stages of labour;

4 chronic pain situations, such as phantom limb pain, back pain, arthritic joint pains, and nerve compressions.

The advantages for its use post-operatively are that it provides continuous pain relief, and reduces the need for narcotics.

Puntillo (1988) stated that, although TNS has led to excellent pain relief after surgery, it is only effective with certain types of pain, thus emphasizing the therapeutic subjectivity of this technique.

Distraction touch and imagery

Anxiety, muscle spasms, and increased sympathetic activity are all associated with pain. Anxiety has already been mentioned. Regarding spasms and sympathetic activity, the former increases pain via the release of pain-producing substances and through compromising blood flow to tissues, causing ischaemia, whereas the latter can lead to pulmonary problems, increased cardiovascular work, altered muscle metabolism, increased oxygen consumption, and even death. Herlitz *et al.* (1989) stated that relaxation therapy is designed to increase comfort levels, decrease pain medication usage, and decrease pain distress. The Royal College of Surgeons and the College of Anaesthetists Commission (1990) acknowledged the value of such a therapy in reducing post-operative pain, a factor which results in shorter post-operative hospital stays.

Distraction draws attention away from the pain, refocusing it to a pleasant sensory stimulus. Music, as demonstrated by Munro and Mount (1976), lowers the pain response and the use of pain medication following abdominal surgery. It could be argued that the music must be pleasing to the patient to be beneficial, otherwise it may be a source of irritation, which raises one's anxiety and perception of pain. Also, according to Munro and Mount (1976), music therapy is used as a form of palliative care for patients with advanced malignant disease and has the following advantages:

1 Physically, it assists muscle relaxation therefore relieves anxiety/depression and perception of pain.

2 Socially, it enhances a sense of bonding between the therapist, patient, and family members.

3 Psychologically, it provides a non-verbal means of expressing conscious and unconscious feelings.

4 Spiritually, it acts as an avenue of expressing doubts, questions, etc. on the 'meaning of life'.

Touch includes massage, aromatherapy, acupressure, or reflexology. It may even simply involve holding a patient's hand, or lightly stroking the patient's forehead or forearm. Caunt (1992) argued that touch promotes hypothalamic stimulation of the parasympathetic nervous system. One must be careful with this therapy, however, as the practitioner may invade the patient's 'personal space', and this may elevate anxiety levels, again emphasizing therapeutic subjectivity.

Imagery involves the patient focusing on a situation which is completely incompatible with pain. It may include one or a combination of all senses, incorporating a pleasurable sensation. This ranges from a simple sensation, such as getting the patient to describe a favourite pastime, to a complex mental visualization which involves deep concentration on detailed tasks, such as work tasks. Imagery promotes relaxation which in turn alleviates or eliminates anxiety. The effectiveness of this therapy depends on the image used and the ability of the individual patient concerned.

INTERIM SUMMARY

Many pain therapies exist, and numerous texts are available for further detail. However, it is hoped that the reader will be aware that any pain therapy is only effective if it is adapted to the patient's subjective needs and individualized environment. In our opinion the criteria which should be part of any pain relief plan are based upon establishing a good patient–practitioner relationship and in teaching the patient about the appropriate health education regarding his/her 'condition'.

Assessment of pain

Pain and nursing are inextricably linked because assessment and management of the pain process is one of the commoner roles of the nurse. The measurement of pain, however, is a contentious and controversial issue with debate from two schools of thought.

One school of thought believes that pain measurement is necessary and feasible. McCaffery (1983) argued that communication is an essential step towards measurement and pain relief. Therefore problems in communication and poor understanding of the complexity of pain can result in its poor management. However, it must be stated that the success of

communication is influenced by the ward environment. For example, critical care patients are often vulnerable to communication barriers, such as the presence of highly technical equipment and the sight of other critically ill patients. Technical equipment may increase or decrease anxiety levels since its presence may or may not aid the knowledgeable patient's understanding of his condition and alleviate the fear of the 'unknown'. The presence of other critically ill patients also may or may not increase anxiety, according to individual experience.

A second school of thought believes that pain experiences can never be measured because of its subjective nature. Puntillo (1988) argued that no objective test exists to diagnose pain. In support of this Hunt *et al.* (1981) acknowledged several pain assessment studies which demonstrated that nurses tend to underestimate the patient's pain, and if assessment of pain is judged simply on a patient's behaviour (such as restlessness, groaning, or grimacing) it can be misleading. In addition, classical signs such as an increased heart rate and lowered blood pressure may also be absent in some patients experiencing pain, thus exposing the dangers of using generalizations.

Both schools of thought emphasize that there is no easy way of understanding what a patient is suffering, or of conveying information from one person to another, though doctors, nurses, and other health care practitioners need to do so.

In short, many factors affect pain assessment and these are often interrelated. They all stem from the complex nature of pain and one cannot expect a certain stimulus to produce a predictable outcome, as other factors may intervene. This is supported by Willets (1989) who stated that pain cannot be measured directly, so one cannot be sure how much pain someone is suffering. It could also be argued, however, that accurate pain assessment and measurement are essential if the sufferer is to obtain appropriate and successful pain relief; perhaps before one can assess pain successfully, one must be aware of its sociopsychophysiological subjectivity.

Clinicians treating patients need to know how the pain changes throughout the day, the descriptive quality of pain, and if there are any aggravating or relieving factors. Such information, according to Tempest (1991), will make clinical diagnosis more accurate and allow easier evaluation of treatments.

An individualized approach to the assessment and control of pain is the obvious solution. This is easier said than done, as Seers (1987) acknowledged, because in order to assess pain, one must take into account individuality with respect to those who have the pain (patients/clients) and those who are trying to assess it (practitioners).

Patient factors

Patient factors affect the patient's expression of pain, rather than the amount of pain perceived, and consequently assessment must also be affected. This is complicated further by the 'fact' that patients have difficulty in describing the pain and in expressing its location. The Royal College of Surgeons and College of Anaesthetists Working Party (1990) acknowledged that the more the patient feels in control of their own pain management, the lower the requirement for analgesia is, hence the advocacy of patient-controlled analgesia (PCA).

Cultural backgrounds

Previously it was stated that different cultures have different socialization attitudes and behaviours and thus the cultural background of the patient may be responsible for some aspects of inadequate pain assessment and management. It is important to recognize how cultural bias can influence patient care.

Personality typing

Bond and Pearson (1969) reported that introverts had more intense pain, but complain less than extroverts. Chapman and Cox (1977) suggested that anxiety levels also lead to an increased perception of pain and a worrying feature noted by Hollinworth (1994) is that anxiety is heightened by hospitalization and surgery and therefore exacerbates the individual's interpretation of pain. Personality and anxiety can be interrelated and this is supported by Friedman and Rosenmann (1974) who correlated personality types 'A', 'B', and 'C' with the incidence of anxiety-provoked myocardial infarctions (Chapter 22).

Social class

Social class, according to Mienhart and McCaffery (1983), is an instrumental factor in pain assessment and if the nurse's and patient's social class are comparable, the more sympathy and better management of pain ensues. Also, higher social class patients are usually more effective in expressing their pain and thus are more likely to receive better pain management. Language, therefore, is another significant factor (Seers, 1987) and an impairment of communication (for example, impaired hearing, sight, or foreign languages) makes pain assessment, and hence management, more difficult.

Past experiences

The patient's past experiences are significant since attitudes to pain and suffering are, in part, socially learned responses (Davitz and Davitz, 1985) and hence affect one's judgement of pain and what the pain means to the patient. For example, upon the lay person's first visit for an electrocardiogram they may be horrified, and suffer psychosomatic pain, if it is not clarified by the practitioner that the electrodes do not produce painful electric currents when they are applied to the chest and limbs. However, on subsequent visits, when the client has had time to reflect on the method, socially learned responses result in the patient not experiencing psychosomatic pain.

Location of the pain

The location of the pain is important since some areas of the body are more acceptable discussion topics than others. For example, a rectal pain may be an unacceptable topic and needs to be assessed differently from pain associated with a sore finger.

Gender differences

Gender differences need to be taken into consideration when assessing a patient's pain, since in westernized societies males tend to be socialized into being courageous, females to express their emotions. However, the practitioner must not sexually stereotype since Seers (1988), in reviewing the literature, showed that an effect of a person's sex on pain and its expression is inconclusive. More recently, McCaffery and Ferrel (1992) demonstrated that generally there are differences in how a nurse thinks men and women respond to pain. They observed that, of 362 nurses, approximately one-third argued that there were gender differences in pain expression. Regarding the patient's pain tolerance, approximately 50% of the nurses thought that females tolerated pain better than males, whilst only 15% thought men had a better tolerance. Pain and distress trends seemed to be reversed, that is, 41% believed men showed greater distress when in pain, whilst only 18% believed women exhibited more distress. Fifty-three per cent, compared with 27%, believed that men rather than women were likely to under-report their pain.

Practitioner factors

The individual factors that affect the patient's experience and interpretation of pain are equally likely to affect that of the practitioner. In addition, a number of other factors are important, and, regarding the nursing profession, Lockstone (1982) argued that training placed the responsibility of pain control with the doctors and consequently nurses were unaware of their importance in pain control. Nurse training affects attitudes to pain killers and misplaced concerns, such as opioid analgesic addiction and dependency, may cause the nurse to give less than the prescribed analgesia, both in terms of frequency and amount (Hollinworth, 1994). Therefore a more realistic training in pharmacology would help reduce such fears and would benefit patient care.

According to Willets (1989) the practitioner has to infer the amount of pain and suffering a patient is experiencing since it cannot be directly assessed. Although complex, a knowledge of the sociopsychophysiological subjective nature of pain is therefore essential to improve the practitioner's assessment and management of pain. The nurse's own beliefs and values might influence her/his assessment of pain (Seers, 1987) and she/he must be aware of this in order to be objective.

Pain relief may be further affected by busy

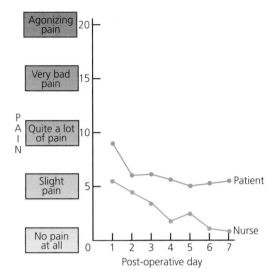

Figure 21.5 Nurses' and patients' mean daily ratings of patients' pain (*n* = 221 nurse/patient pairs). (Reproduced by kind permission, from Seers, K. (1988) Factors affecting pain assessment. *The Professional Nurse* **3**, 201–206, Austen Cornish Publishers Ltd.)

ward routines, staff shortages, and by frequent staff changes, all of which increase the difficulties in establishing a good practitioner–patient relationship. Frequent patient change-over in a ward also affects patient–patient relationships and this can affect the expression of pain by the patient. Thus, ward policy may influence assessment, and hence pain management. Current cost-cutting changes to the skill mix in nursing may well compound the problem (Hollinworth, 1994).

It will always be difficult to assess adequately an individual's perception of pain because of the complexity in understanding subjectivity. The concept of holistic care attempts to close this gap and minimize the differences between practitioner and patient assessments which still exist. For example, Seers (1987) found that nurses constantly rated the patient's pain as being less than the patient's own appraisal

(Figure 21.5). Superficially, pain assessment seems easy and nurses may underestimate the difficulties associated with pain perception/ assessment, etc. In addition, communication skills need time and training to develop, and may cause inaccuracies in assessment, because some patients assume that the practitioner knows when they are in pain. Sometimes nurses assume patients will report their pain. It is not surprising that the pain then goes unchecked and is inadequately controlled. Thus, there needs to be a good working relationship between the patient and the practitioner in which both parties must have mutual trust in one another.

INTERIM SUMMARY

The experience of pain is so complex, being influenced by so many variables (subjective to the patient and practitioner), that the practitioner may or may not be able to predict them. It must be stressed, however, that at all times it is important not to stereotype the factors mentioned above. For example, when caring for patients from different cultures, the practitioner must not only be aware that cultural difference exist in pain expression, but also that individual differences occur within each culture. That is, if the practitioner expects a Caucasian patient to be stoic and he is not, then there may be a danger that he could be labelled as attention seeking or even malingering! Thus it is still the patient who is the only one who knows how much pain he/she has. The patient must be involved, whenever possible, in any assessment of pain. Thus, an individualized approach in assessing and controlling pain is the obvious solution. To conclude, nurses who operate on the basis of stereotyping (for cultural, gender, social class, etc.) are in danger of ignoring the individuality of pain perception, and consequently pain assessment and

The clinical measurement of pain

management becomes unsatisfactory.

An accurate assessment of pain is essential for adequate therapy. The subjective nature of pain, both in the sufferer and in the observations made by the health practitioner, makes assessment difficult. This section highlights the strengths and shortcomings of frequently used clinical assessment methods.

Measurements of pain involve informal and formal observations. The former observations are made when the patient is unaware that he is being assessed, since this is when the most natural reactions occur. These involve monitoring facial expression, difficulties in performing physical movement, and mood.

Formal observations encourage a more accurate assessment and are important in providing continuity of care. They stress the objective measurements performed by doctors and nurses and are based on the patient's experiences and comments, and the observer's own experience of pain and/or traditional/cultural beliefs about pain and the level to be expressed in a given illness, etc. Verbal report is of obvious significance since:

> pain occurs when the patient says it does. (McCaffery, 1983)

A 'word' scale could be used in the clinical measurement of pain, but these are open to distortion and observer bias. This is why more attention is currently being paid to pain involving the patient's own estimate of pain as a basis for treatment.

Such measures include the following scales and charts.

SIMPLE VERBAL RATING SCALES (DESCRIPTIVE SCALE)

For example:

| No | Mild | Moderate | Severe | Unbearable |

pain   pain   pain   pain   pain

Verbal rating scales are crude and give only a rough approximation of the pain experienced. In addition, individuals cannot be readily compared. Thompson (1989) acknowledged further problems and stated that, although these scales are easy to use, they can have a limited usefulness in that there may be misinterpretation of words by the patient/practitioner, a limit to the number of words one uses, and different assumptions made by the practitioner or patient that the intervals between the words are of equal value. Thompson (1989) also stated that descriptive scales are too complicated for use in acute pain.

VISUAL ANALOGUE SCALE (VAS)

Visual analogue scales are also known as graphic rating scales and have been used in an attempt to overcome the problem of expressing 'pain language'. The analogue scale might consist of a line 100 cm long.

No pain ——————————— Worst possible pain
100 cm

The patient marks the line, and this represents the level of pain at that moment. The distance of the mark from the left end is measured and is called the 'pain score'. This may be repeated several times each day to form the basis of a pain profile for that patient. This type of scale avoids the use of gradation, reduces the misinterpretation of language, is user friendly and may be modified to assess pain relief, by having 'no pain relief' and 'complete pain relief' at opposite ends of the scale.

Shortcomings of the scale are that it is an abstract concept which can be difficult to understand, most answers cluster around the extremes of the scale with little use of the midpoints (Bond, 1984), and the relevance to patients experiencing acute pain is questionable. Both the verbal and visual scales view pain unidimensionally, since they do not take into account other variables which may have an impact on the amount of pain experienced.

NUMERICAL SCALES

Numerical scales use a continuum comprising a numerical rating scale of either 1–10 or 1–100, 0 signifying no pain and 10 or 100 signifying unbearable pain. For example:

| 1 | 2 | 3 | 4 | 5 | 6 | 7 | 8 | 9 | 10 |

These scales allow for greater sensitivity and avoid misinterpretation of the meaning of words. Such scales are commonly used in assessing pain associated with acute myocardial infarction patients, relating pain scores with morphine requirements.

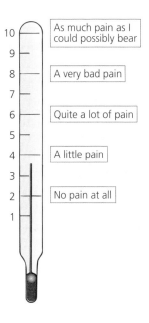

Figure 21.6 Pain thermometer.

PAIN THERMOMETER ('PAINMETER')

The pain thermometer (designed by the Burford Nursing Development Unit at Oxford – Figure 21.6) acts as a visual aid for the patient to describe his/her pain experience. It has been used extensively in the care of the elderly, where patients find it easy to understand. The practitioner and the patient decide how often the painmeter is used and the analgesia can be administered accordingly. Although limited in range, it is helpful in assisting the nurse to improve the control of pain relief (Cooperman, 1987).

THE LONDON HOSPITAL PAIN OBSERVATION CHART

The London Hospital pain chart is illustrated in Figure 21.7. It improves communication

between the practitioner and the patient by making the recording of pain more systematic, makes readily available in one place the information that is useful when making decisions about the management of pain, focuses attention on the mechanisms of different pains by recording each site of pain separately, and is a means of communication to be used *with* the patient and not *on* the patient. Occasionally, it is a good idea to have two separate charts, one kept by the patient and the other by the staff.

MCGILL–MELZACK PAIN QUESTIONNAIRE

Rather than viewing pain as a specific sensory experience, this questionnaire attempts to measure pain on a broader level by categorizing it into dimensions of pain experience: the sensory, affective, and evaluative levels

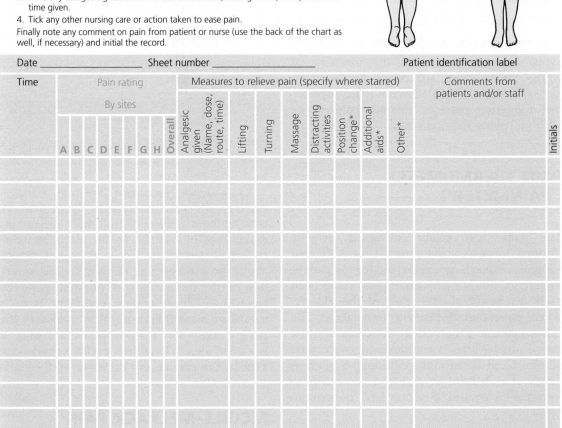

The London Hospital
Pain Observation Chart

This chart records where a patient's pain is and how bad it is, by the nurse asking the patient at regular intervals. If analgesics are being given regularly, make an observation with each dose and another half-way between each dose. If analgesics are given only 'as required', observe two-hourly. When the observations are stable and the patient is comfortable, any regular time interval between observations may be chosen.

To use this chart, ask the patient to mark all his or her pains on the body diagram below. Label each site of pain with a letter (i.e. A, B, C, etc).

Then at each observation time ask the patient to assess:

1. The pain in each separate site since the last observation. Use the scale above the body diagram, and enter the number or letter in the appropriate column.
2. The pain overall since the last observation. Use the same scale and enter in column marked overall.

Next, record what has been done to relieve pain. In particular:

3. Note any analgesic given since the last observation, stating name, dose, route and time given.
4. Tick any other nursing care or action taken to ease pain.

Finally note any comment on pain from patient or nurse (use the back of the chart as well, if necessary) and initial the record.

| Date _____ | Sheet number _____ | | Patient identification label |

Time	Pain rating By sites								Overall	Measures to relieve pain (specify where starred)								Comments from patients and/or staff	Initials
	A	B	C	D	E	F	G	H		Analgesic given (Name, dose, route, time)	Lifting	Turning	Massage	Distracting activities	Position change*	Additional aids*	Other*		

Figure 21.7 The London Hospital pain observation chart. (Reproduced, with permission, from Latham, J. (1989) *Pain control*. Austen Cornish, p. 33.)

1	8	16
Flickering	Tingling	Annoying
Quivering	Itchy	Troublesome
Pulsing	Smarting	Miserable
Throbbing	Stinging	Intense
Beating	9	Unbearable
Pounding	Dull	17
2	Sore	Spreading
Jumping	Hurting	Radiating
Flashing	Aching	Penetrating
Shooting	Heavy	Piercing
3	10	18
Pricking	Tender	Tight
Boring	Taut	Numb
Drilling	Rasping	Drawing
Stabbing	Splitting	Squeezing
Lancinating	11	Tearing
4	Tiring	19
Sharp	Exhausting	Cool
Cutting	12	Cold
Lacerating	Sickening	Freezing
5	Suffocating	20
Pinching	13	Nagging
Pressing	Fearful	Nauseating
Gnawing	Frightful	Agonizing
Cramping	Terrifying	Dreadful
Crushing	14	Torturing
6	Punishing	PPI
Tugging	Gruelling	0 No pain
Pulling	Cruel	1 Mild
Wrenching	Vicious	2 Discomforting
7	Killing	3 Distressing
Hot	15	4 Horrible
Burning	Wretched	5 Excruciating
Scalding	Binding	
Searing		Constant
		Periodic
		Brief

This questionnaire enables researchers to compare to some extent people's level of pain. Each descriptive word carries its own score – the lower down in its group, the higher its value. The sum of the scores gives what is termed a person's "pain rating index" – in other words, their overall pain intensity. The final "present pain intensity" (PPI) section gives an idea of the pain level at the moment the questionnaire is completed.

Figure 21.8 The McGill–Melzack pain questionnaire.

(Thompson, 1989) (Figure 21.8).

From the list presented, the patient selects those words which best describes his pain and from these measurements the pain is quantifiably and quantitatively assessed (i.e. the higher the total scores are, the greater the pain).

Tempest (1991) acknowledged the questionnaire's value for the assessment of chronic pain. It is frequently used in clinical practice, mainly for work in pain clinics with chronic pain sufferers. However, difficulties arise in the interpretation of the words into the dimension of pain experienced, and it appears diffi-

cult to adapt its bulky format to the acute pain setting. Possibly the questionnaire benefits from being used with other assessment tools, and is in need of some refinement before it can become widely applicable.

HOME DIARY

Home diaries are useful in combining measurements with the patient's description of the pain (Figure 21.9). These include how the pain changes with respect to time, the precipitating factors of pain, and the success of the analgesic method used to alleviate the pain.

INDIRECT CLINICAL MEASURES OF PAIN

Such techniques depend upon the effect that pain has on bodily functions, or on the amount of analgesia required to bring pain relief. Specific ones have been developed for use in specific clinical environments. For example, Thompson (1989) acknowledged the use of the following questions in the coronary care setting:

1 How do you feel? Describe the sensation.

2 Where does it hurt?

3 Does the sensation travel anywhere?

4 Did anything trigger it off?

5 How long did it last?

6 Has anything made it worse or better?

7 Are there any other relevant signs or symptoms?

This has the advantage of being a quick procedure with the questions overlapping with each other in the scope of the answers and allowing a place for physical signs and symptoms which may be relevant.

The disadvantages of the method is that the replies cannot be standardized, and the assessment is still subjected to the practitioner's

	NOTES of any different pain, symptom or problem, and any unusual activity or exercise during each day	ANY OTHER COMMENTS
Day 1		
Day 2		
Day 3		
Day 4		
Day 5		
Day 6		
Day 7		

HOME DIARY

NAME.............................
DATE STARTED ....

HOW TO FILL IN THE HOME DIARY

1 *Sleep:* In this column, fill in hours slept, then ring word which best describes how much your pain disturbed your rest.

2 *Pain:* In the column for each part of the day, write the number of doses of pain killer (tablets, spoonfuls) taken. Then choose the best word to describe your pain for that part of the day. Put in the chart the *pain number* next to the word you chose.

3 On the back of the diary, make a note of any different pains, symptoms, or problems and note any unusual activities or exercise that day.

4 Add any other comments of your own.

Excruciating	5
Very severe	4
Severe	3
Moderate	2
Just noticeable	1
No pain at all	0

	SLEEP	MORNING (to 12 noon)	AFTERNOON (noon to 4pm)	EARLY EVENING (4 – 8 pm)	LATE EVENING (from 8 pm)
Day 1	Hours of sleep / Pain disturbed sleep / never/a bit/often/a lot	No. of pain killers / Pain number	No. of pain killers / Pain number	No. of pain killers / Pain number	No. of pain killers / Pain number
Day 2	Hours of sleep / Pain disturbed sleep / never/a bit/often/a lot	No. of pain killers / Pain number	No. of pain killers / Pain number	No. of pain killers / Pain number	No. of pain killers / Pain number
Day 3	Hours of sleep / Pain disturbed sleep / never/a bit/often/a lot	No. of pain killers / Pain number	No. of pain killers / Pain number	No. of pain killers / Pain number	No. of pain killers / Pain number
Day 4	Hours of sleep / Pain disturbed sleep / never/a bit/often/a lot	No. of pain killers / Pain number	No. of pain killers / Pain number	No. of pain killers / Pain number	No. of pain killers / Pain number
Day 5	Hours of sleep / Pain disturbed sleep / never/a bit/often/a lot	No. of pain killers / Pain number	No. of pain killers / Pain number	No. of pain killers / Pain number	No. of pain killers / Pain number
Day 6	Hours of sleep / Pain disturbed sleep / never/a bit/often/a lot	No. of pain killers / Pain number	No. of pain killers / Pain number	No. of pain killers / Pain number	No. of pain killers / Pain number
Day 7	Hours of sleep / Pain disturbed sleep / never/a bit/often/a lot	No. of pain killers / Pain number	No. of pain killers / Pain number	No. of pain killers / Pain number	No. of pain killers / Pain number

Figure 21.9 Home diary.

interpretation of the patient's reply.

INTERIM SUMMARY

The use of pain assessment tools has been shown to improve pain control and aid care. The tools, however, are still not in common practice (Berker and Hughes, 1990). Introducing a pain system of measurement would improve the practitioner's awareness of pain, which would inevitably result in improved patient care. However, which tool is chosen is dependent on the type of pain, the clinical setting, the client group, etc. Measurement tools are essential to avoid possible difficulties in practitioner–patient communication and to avoid unnecessary patient suffering. However, it could be argued that the assessment of pain barely considers the patient's sociopsychophysiological factors, all of which must be considered if assessment is to be accurate. The development of appropriate assessment tools specific to certain clinical

References

settings must be considered of vital importance in the practitioner's bid to improve the quality of patient care.

Bond, M.R. (1984) *Pain: its nature, analysis and treatment*. Edinburgh: Churchill Livingstone.

Bond, M.R. and Pearson, I.B. (1969) Psychological aspects of pain in women with advanced cancer of the cervix. *Journal of Psychosomatic Research* **13**, 13–19.

Caunt, H. (1992) Reducing the psychological impact of postoperative pain. *British Journal of Nursing* **1**(1), 13–19.

Chapman, C.R. and Cox, G.B. (1977) Anxiety, pain and depression surrounding elective surgery: a multivariate comparison of abdominal surgery patients with kidney donors and recipients. *Journal of Psychosomatic Research* **21**, 7–15.

Clancy, J. and McVicar, A.J. (1992) The subjectivity of pain. *British Journal of Nursing* **1**(1), 8–12.

Cooperman, H. (1987) Symptom relief. How can you help? *Nursing Standard* Sept. 23, pp. 28–9.

Davitz, L.L, and Davitz, J.R. (1985) Cultures and nurses' inferences of suffering. *Nursing Times* **73**(15), 521–3.

Fordham, M. (1986) Neurophysiological pain theories. *Nursing* **10**, 360–4.

Friedman, H. and Rosenmann, R.H. (1974) *Type A behaviour and your heart*. London: Wildwood House.

Hoerlitz, J., Hjalmarson, A. and Wagstein, F. (1989) Treatment of pain in myocardial infarction. *British Heart Journal* **61**, 9–13.

Hollinworth, H. (1994) No gain? *Nursing Times*. **90**(1), 24–7.

Hunt, J.M., Stolar, T.D., Littlejohns, D.W., Twycross, R.G. and Vere, D.W. (1981) Patients with protracted pain: a survey conducted at the London Hospital. *Journal of Medical Ethics* **3**, 61–73.

Latham, J. (1987) Transcutaneous nerve stimulation. *The Professional Nurse* **8**, 133–5.

Lockstone, C. (1982) Pain – it's what the patient says it is. *Nursing Mirror* **154**(7), ii–xii.

McCaffery, M. (1983) *Nursing the patient in pain*. London: Harper Row.

McCaffery, M. and Ferrell, B.R. (1992) Does the gender gap affect your pain control? *Nursing* **22**(8), 48–51.

Melzack, R. (1992) The tragedy of needless pain. *Scientific American* **262**(2), 19–25.

Melzack, R. and Wall, P.D. (1965) Cited in Melzack, R. and Wall, P.D. (1988) *The challenge of pain*. Harmondsworth: Penguin.

Melzack, R. and Wall, P.D. (1988) *The challenge of pain* Hamondsworth: Penguin.

Melzack, R. and Wall, P.D. (1990) *Textbook of pain*. Edinburgh: Churchill Livingstone.

Mienhart, N.T. and McCaffery, M. (1983) *Neurophysiological aspects in pain. A nursing approach to assessment and analysis*. Newark, CT: Appleton–Century–Crofts.

Morris, R. (1986) A personal account: life goes on with chronic pain. *Nursing* **10**, 375–376.

Munro, J. and Mount, D. (1976) Cited in Autton, N. (1988) *Pain. An exploration*. London: Darton.

Puntillo, K.A. (1988) The phenomenon of pain and critical care nursing. *Heart and Lung* **17**(3), 262–73.

Richardson, F. (1991) Pain and its placebo effects. *Front Pain* **2**, 1–2.

Royal College of Surgeons and College of Anaesthetists Working Party (1990) *Report of the working party on pain after surgery*. Sept. London: Royal College of Surgeons.

Royal College of Surgeons and the College of Anaesthetists Commission (1990) *The provision of surgical services*. London: Royal College of Surgeons.

Saunders, Dame C., Summers, H. and Teller, N. (1981) *Hospice, the living idea*. London: Edward Arnold

Seers, K. (1987) Perceptions of pain. *Nursing Times* **83**, 37–9.

Seers, K. (1988) Factors affecting pain assessment. *The Professional Nurse* **Mar.**, 201–4.

Smith, S. (1985) Drugs and pain. *Nursing Times* **81**(5), 36–7.

Soafer, B. (1983) Pain relief – the core of nursing practice. *Nursing Times* **Nov**, 38–42.

Tempest, S. (1990) Pain and pain control. 1. Sensory perception. *Current practice in pharmacy and therapeutics*. Vol. 3, No. 6. London: Medical Tribune UK.

Tempest, S. (1991) Pain and pain control. 3. Treatment considerations. *Current practice in pharmacy and therapeutics*. Vol. 3, No. 8. London: Medical Tribune UK.

Thompson, C. (1989) The nursing assessment of the patient with cardiac pain on the coronary care unit. *Intensive Care Nursing* **5**, 147–54.

Twycross, R.S. and Lack, S.A. (1983) Symptom control in far advanced cancer. *Pain relief*. London: Pitman.

Whipple, B. (1990) Neurophysiology of pain. *Orthopaedic Nursing* **9**(4), 21–32.

Willets, K. (1989) Assessing cardiac pain. *Nursing Times* **85**(47), 52–4.

Summary

1 Pain is a subjective experience dependent upon the sociopsychophysiological characteristics of the individual.

2 Melzack and Wall's gate control theory of pain perception is a credible model which explains pain perception and control.

3 Pain perception is dependent upon:
(a) the balance of afferent neuron input to the gating mechanisms, and,
(b) the descending neuron input to the gating mechanism.

If the afferent pain fibre input dominates, the gate is 'open' and one perceives pain. If the mechanoreceptor afferent input and/or the descending neuron input dominates, the gate is 'closed' and pain is not perceived.

4 The subjectivity of pain is determined by the individual's unique blend of genes and his/her unique environmental experiences.

5 The subjective nature of pain has wide implications for assessing, evaluating, planning, and monitoring the care of people who are in pain. Thus, the complexity of pain states demands a multifaceted and multidisciplinary approach if the patient/client is to achieve effective pain relief.

6 Assessment of pain is multifactorial. It is affected by factors attributed to the patient, the practitioner, ward policy, and hospital environments, and it must be questioned if it can really be assessed adequately.

7 Pain assessment tools, it could be argued, are of limited use in measuring pain. Their usefulness is largely in monitoring the effectiveness/appropriateness of the analgesic method used.

8 A prerequisite to good patient care is that the practitioner actually believes the patient. Unless this happens one cannot get much further with pain assessment, and consequently its management. We suggest that a good understanding of the individualistic nature of the patient's pain is essential before practitioners attempt to plan and rationalize a patient's care.

9 Biomedical and physiological research have provided great understanding of some dimensions associated with pain, and psychological research has increased knowledge of the relationships between stress, anxiety, and pain. Psychometric studies have generated various methods of measuring pain. However, because of the complexity of the sociopsychophysiological phenomenon we label pain, there are many unanswered questions and continued research into the interrelations of these disciplines is the only way forward to unfold some of these mysteries.

Review Questions

1 Distinguish between the following:
(a) pain perception threshold;
(b) severe pain threshold;
(c) pain tolerance.

2 Distinguish between acute and chronic pains.

3 List the pain-producing substances released from cells following injury and the body's endogenous opiates which attempt to counteract their actions.

4 Differentiate between the following:
(a) nociceptor and polymodal nociceptor;
(b) Aδ and C-pain fibres, and Aβ fibres;
(c) inhibitory neurotransmitters, excitatory neurotransmitters, and neuromodulators.

5 Outline the principles behind the 'gate control theory' of pain perception, using the following terms:
pain-producing substances; inhibitory neurotransmitters; excitatory neurotransmitters; neuromodulators; nociceptor; endogenous opiates; Aδ pain fibres; C-pain fibres; Aβ fibres; threshold; afferent input; descending fibres; pain centre; higher cortical centres, kinins, prostaglandins, endorphins, enkephalins.

6 Suggest:
(a) how it is possible to perceive pain in the absence of cellular damage; and
(b) how it is possible not to perceive pain in the presence of cellular damage.

7 What do you understand by the following statement: 'pain is a subjective experience depending upon an individual's sociopsychophysiological characteristics'.

8 What factors should be taken into consideration when assessing pain?

9 List the clinical tools used to assess pain and comment on the usefulness and drawbacks of such tools.

10 Pain is an homeostatic imbalance. Discuss.

Stress

22

Introduction

The subjectivity of stress

Coping mechanisms and features of failure

Summary

Review questions

Introduction

Stress is a phenomenon that is observable as both psychological and physiological responses. Responses to particular situations are highly individualistic, however, and there is a strong subjective element. The multi-definitional aspects of stress will be briefly explored in this chapter and the authors will suggest that stress is a psychophysiological response caused by environmental (social) stressors, thus emphasizing that stress is a sociopsychophysiological phenomenon. The concept of individualism will be the main focus and the subjective nature of stressors, the stress response, coping methods, and stress-related illnesses will be discussed with this in mind. The stress models used in reviewing this subjectivity are those of: Cox and Mckay (transactional), Selye's physiological theory (the general adaptation syndrome or GAS) and the Selye–Lazarus psychophysiological model.

DEFINITIONS OF STRESS

Various attempts have been made to find a suitable definition of stress, and it can be concluded that stress has different connotations for different people.

Stimulus-based definition

Cox (1978) stated that a lay-person views stress as an environmental phenomenon (stimulus) which causes strain within the body in the form of fatigue and/or distress (Figure 22.1a). These environmental stresses, for example, could be a situation or conditions at work, the divorce process, low income support for a single parent family, the highly technical equipment used in the intensive care setting, or life-style problems created after being diagnosed HIV positive.

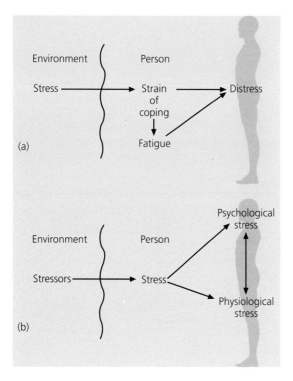

Figure 22.1 (a) Layperson's model of stress. (b) Response-based model of stress.

Such stimulus-based definitions are incomplete, since any situation may or may not be stressful, depending upon the individual and the meaning of the situation for him/her.

Response-based definition

Although there is no generally accepted definition of 'a state of stress' in biological or social systems, Hinkle (1987) acknowledged that biologists and behavioural scientists continue to use the term. Biologists and medical scientists tend to be concerned with the sources of stress that are concrete and observable and can otherwise be considered as 'causes' of illness and injury. The response-based definition views stress as bodily psychophysiological responses to environmental stressors. What is not explained satisfactorily is the uniqueness of these stressors to individuals, and the individ-ualistic responses, presumably because the complexity of humans always makes it impossible to comprehend fully the interrelationships of psychophysiological processes which arise due to environmental influences. Thus, the layperson's environmental stresses are recognized as stressors to the biomedical scientist, and it is the accumulation of these which produce stress within the body. This can be identified as physiological stress or psychological stress (Cox, 1978). However, these two disciplines are inseparable from one another (Figure 22.1b) and from the environment. For example, in a state of anxiety one may become consciously aware of a faster and more powerful heart beat (a 'physiological' stress indicator), which in turn may increase the individual's perception of his/her anxiety state (a 'psychological' stress indicator). Which indicator is the starting trigger, we will never know! Thus, in reality, anxiety is better described as a psychophysiological bodily state induced by environmental stressors.

According to Hinkle (1987), social and behavioural scientists tend to be concerned with sources of stress that represent information arising from outside the person, and responses are mediated by higher centres of the central nervous system. It is clear that such 'psychological stresses' can lead to alterations of internal functions even at the biochemical level, and that these are potential 'causes' of disease. Equally so, psychological responses are a consequence of biochemical (enzymatic) changes. These are not, however, independent of other mechanisms, including environmental stressors which ultimately are of a sociocultural origin. In other words the sources of stress are environmental/social stressors outside (exogenous) and/or inside (endogenous) the body that may produce a psychophysiological stress response.

Selye (1956) defined stress as:

> the non-specific response of the body and that freedom from stress is death.

This definition views stress as being the non-specific (i.e. common) result of any mental or

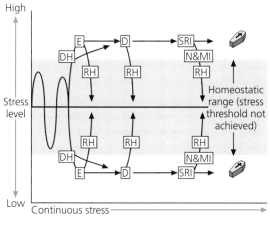

KEY:

DH	– Disturbed homeostasis (stress threshold reached or superseded)
E	– Eustress
RH	– Re-established homeostasis
D	– Distress
SRI	– Stress-related illness
N&MI	– Nursing and medical intervention
⚰	– Death

Figure 22.2 Stress, a disturbed homeostasis (Clancy and McVicar, 1993).

somatic demand placed upon the body. That is, stress is the response to a 'threat' (a change in the environment), and its integrity is based on evaluating the information received. However, we regard it as being common or stereotypical only within the effector mechanism's homeostatic ranges; it is actually subjective since a limited number of these effectors exist and there is a limited extent to which they can be targeted on a given threat.

We view stress as being a disturbed homeostasis which manifests itself by many psychophysiological indicators (Table 22.1). Thus, although stress is viewed in terms of physiological, psychological, and sociological phenomena (Monat and Lazarus, 1985), the authors feel that theorists need to integrate the scientific disciplines in order to appreciate the subjective nature of stress, or what the nursing/medical professions term phenomenological holism.

Milkhail (1985) defined stress as:

> a state which arises from an actual or perceived demand–capability imbalance in the organism's vital adjustment actions which is partially manifested by a nonspecific response.

This definition emphasizes the continuity between physiological and psychological theory. However, we feel the need for a wider definition in order to integrate the three disciplines, and view stress as being a psychophysiological homeostatic imbalance which arises when there is an actual or perceived demand–capability mismatch between the individual and his/her environment.

Figure 22.2 illustrates homeostasis as a dynamic concept, with parameters always fluctuating around the mean, either within (stress threshold not achieved) or outside (threshold reached or superseded) the homeostatic range, the latter producing psychophysiological imbalances as indicated in Table 22.1. This imbalance depends upon the cumulative effects of the stressors. These include everyday and long-term stressors.

Everyday stressors ('eustressors')

Eustressors are beneficial stressors which trigger homeostatic controls to remove, adapt or cope with the initiating stressor(s) and so restore homeostasis. This stress is eustress, which promotes the 'healthy' stress response.

Extreme, long-lasting, or unusual stressors ('distressors')

Distressors produce distress, that is, the negative or 'unhealthy' stress response. If homeostasis is restored, it is at a cost to the body (i.e. the individual's resistance to stress is reduced). If, however, homeostatic mechanisms are not re-established, then a stress-related illness, or even death, may occur.

Table 22.1 Some psychophysiological indicators of the stress response

'Physical' indicators	'Behavioural' indicators	'Emotional' indicators
▲ High blood pressure	● Poor work performance	● Emotional outbursts/crying
● Increased heart rate	● Accidents at work and home	● Irritability with people
● Increased respiratory rate	● Overindulgence in smoking,	▲ Depression
▲ Increased muscle tension	alcohol, and drugs	● Tendency to blame others
▲ Increased restlessness	● Loss of interest	● Hostile and insulting behaviour
▲ Upset stomach	● Daydreaming	● Tiredness
● Sweaty palms	● Diminished attention to detail	● Anxiety
● Loss of appetite	● Forgetfulness	
▲ Indigestion or heartburn	● Mental blocking	
● Change in sleep patterns	▲ Social isolation	
▲ Tension headaches	▲ Marital and family breakdowns	
▲ Cold hands and feet		
▲ Nausea		
▲ Nail biting		
▲ Constipation or diarrhoea		
▲ Backaches		

● Usually short-term effects.   ▲ Usually long-term effects.

Note: The above are termed psychophysiological indicators because physical, behavioural and emotional indicators are inseparable, being both cause and effect, i.e.

Physical ⟷ Behavioural
Emotional

Figure 22.2 also illustrates that eustress is time-dependent. When homeostasis is not restored within a certain time (which is individually subjective, depending on the causes of the imbalance and the homeostatic control efficiency), then eustress becomes distress. As a result a different psychological perception of the stressors occurs producing the disturbed homeostasis. Accompanying eustress is a sense of 'psychological' well-being, whereas distress is associated with many negative feelings such as those emotional and behavioural indicators illustrated by Table 22.2.

An example of the transition of eustress into distress can be found in competitive sports, such as boxing. At the commencement of a fight, a boxer usually believes he is going to beat his opponent, and so experiences eustress-

Table 22.2 'Psychological' classification of the stress response

Eustress	Distress
Increased mental acuity	Diminished attention to detail, forgetfulness, poor work performance
Pleasure, happiness Euphoria	Emotional outbursts, sadness Lethargy, apathy

ful responses on the first bell. The perception extends until the boxer gets tired or is hurt and then he doubts winning; eustress is then transformed into distress.

The subjectivity of stress

Stress is the psychophysiological response of the body to environmental (exogenous and endogenous) stimuli we call stressors (eustressors or distressors). The perceptions of stressors differ, quantitatively and qualitatively, between individuals, as do the stress thresholds, i.e. the minimum cumulative stressor value necessary to evoke a stress response. Psychophysiological responses to stressors are also subjective, since individuals experience either eustress or distress depending upon their perception of the stressors. In addition, Table 22.1 demonstrates the range of physical, emotional, and behavioural indicators that occur when people are stressed (the main emphasis is on indicators when one is distressed) and it is unlikely that two people will display the same indicators. The psychophysiological response is also time-dependent. For example, as mentioned previously, eustress may be converted to distress, and perceptions of the response varies daily and even within the same day, since humans are social beings who display circadian rhythmicity (Chapter 23).

The individualistic nature of the psychophysiological stress response can be explained using arguments based in the nature–nurture debate, i.e.

$$\text{Genotype} \xrightarrow{\hspace{3cm}} \text{Phenotype}$$
$$\uparrow$$
$$\text{Environment}$$

The 'unique' blend of genes or genotype that one possesses partly determines the measurable psychophysiological indicators, or phenotypes, of the stress response. Genes are expressed or repressed when the necessary environmental factors (stressors) prevail. For example, everyone has a genetic potential for intelligence, but the necessary environmental factors must be present for that potential to be achieved: primary, secondary, and tertiary

socialization. These are associated with the necessary environmental 'triggers' such as books, intellectual peers, etc. Hence the environment modifies the expression of the genotype.

As a further example, crying (a phenotype) is a common indicator of the psychophysiological stress response. This act is labelled an emotion and as such is usually dealt with in the realms of psychological teaching. However, crying is a result of excessive tear production and secretion. Tears are chemicals and thus are the end product of enzymatically controlled chemical reactions and enzymes themselves are produced as a result of gene expression, which is influenced by the dominant environmental stressor within the cumulative stressors one is perceiving at that point in time. Crying can be a distressful or eustressful response depending upon how the individual perceives the major contributory stressor (or stressors), that is as joyful or unhappy events. It must be remembered, however, that psychological perception of environmental stressors is a consequence of physiological processes called nerve impulses.

THE SOCIOPSYCHOPHYSIOLOGICAL SUBJECTIVITY OF STRESS

Livingston-Booth (1985) argued that we react to stress in different ways because of the differing societies we live in, the way we live our lives within that society, the type and dynamic fluctuations of societal stressors, and genetic variation.

Individualism, therefore, is a combination of our own unique blend of genes and how we react to the individualized environment in which we live. Even identical twins differ in their biochemistry, due to their genetic uniqueness (genetic mutations will occur during uterine development and with age) and in their family experiences. Although parents think they treat their children the same, the 'fact' is they do not! Different experiences occur even in the womb, depending upon how the mother is living her life in different gestatory periods, and the position and the degree of placentation influences development, even with identical twins.

Before we become aware of the bodily stress response, the cumulative stressors one perceives at that point must have reached or superseded the stress threshold. These stressors, and the threshold, are dynamic and subjective, fluctuating with circadian rhythms in the individual and between individuals.

THE SUBJECTIVITY OF STRESSORS

People are constantly exposed to stressors, and are either consciously or unconsciously aware of their existence. Thompson (1982) classified stressors as being (1) social, (2) physical, (3) psychological, (4) environmental, and (5) developmental.

SOCIAL STRESSORS

Holmes and Rahe (1967) argued that there is an increase in incidences of stress-related illnesses following stressful life events because of the extent of coping activities such 'adaptive' changes require. 'Negative' and 'positive' perceived events, such as divorce and marriage respectively, are stressful since they necessitate adjustments by the individual to a new life-style. Using their 'social readjustment rating scale' (Table 22.3), the person reports any change in life-style and each change is assigned a life change unit (LCU) score and a total LCU score is calculated. Rahe and Holmes ranked people as experiencing mild, moderate or severe stress, i.e.

Table 22.3 The Rahe and Holmes social readjustment rating scale

Events	Life crisis score (points)
Death of spouse	100
Divorce	73
Marital separation	65
Personal injury or illness	53
Marriage	50
Pregnancy	40
Sexual problems	39
Change in responsibilities at work	29
Outstanding personal achievement	28
Trouble with the boss	23
Change in working hours or conditions	20
Change in social activity	18
Vacation	13
Christmas	12

Magnitude of life crisis	LCU score
Mild	150–199
Moderate	200–299
Severe	300+

In support of such scales Thompson (1982) traced these numerically documented life events retrospectively over a 10-year period in one of his coronary patients, a condition frequently mentioned as a stress related illness. Figure 22.3 highlights the most dominant (with regard to the LCU score) stressor the patient perceived during that period.

Maes *et al.* (1987) viewed life events operating as stressors to the extent that they tax or exceed the adaptive resources of the person. They divided events into major and minor; the former includes events such as divorce, unemployment, serious illness, or death of a loved one, whereas the latter includes daily stressors such as noise, crime, job dissatisfaction, or enjoyment.

The stressor scales are useful in:

1 Identifying potential distressors, so that the individual can avoid them or learn how to cope with them.

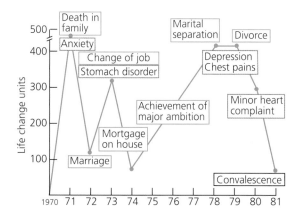

Figure 22.3 How stress affects your health. Life change units used from Rahe and Holmes SRRS (see Table 22.3).

2 Emphasizing the cumulative effects of multiple stressors in a person's life, which cause the resultant signs of distress.

3 In researching stress. For example, Rowland (1977) found an increased incidence of mortality in widowers and widows within the first few months following the death of their spouse.

However, there are theoretical and methodological weaknesses associated with such scales. Some individuals undergo considerable life event changes without experiencing illness of any kind (Monat and Lazarus, 1985). Even Holmes and Rahe (1967) stated that 20% of scores bordering severe stress levels (LCU = 300), are not associated with a stress-related illness. Attempts to quantify stressors in numerical order are also crude and unscientific, since individuals rank life events differently according to their own perceptions. Thus one cannot quantify subjective experiences. For example, when caring for a spouse during the terminal stage of cancer, death may not be the highest ranked distressor in that person's life (at that particular moment in time). It may bring 'relief' to some and even be a eustressful experience, as it does not prolong the agony associated with seeing a loved one 'waste'

away. Finally the scales focus only on distressful events, and omit eustressful experiences.

This variation demonstrates that subjectivity exists even in the measurement of stress and we would argue that this is due to differences in the adaptability of individuals to cope with stressors.

Cultural parity was acknowledged by Lepore *et al.* (1991) when considering common daily hassles of an urban centre of India with economically advantaged westernized countries. Conversely, cultural disparity was observed with the same population groups when considering 'hassle' frequency and mental health problems. Lepore *et al.* also found that chronic stressors, for example substandard housing, inadequate access to water, etc. were associated with greater levels of psychosomatic symptoms. Furthermore, the correlation between chronic stressors and psychosomatic symptoms increased when the effects of income were statistically controlled, suggesting that income attenuates these effects.

Pearlin (1983) suggested that adult emotional distress relied upon personality characteristics formed early in life, but indicated that primary, secondary, and tertiary socialization must also be taken into account. These included current experiences which take place with continuing changes (stressors) in one's life. Values, beliefs, ideologies, interactional patterns, interests and activities, indeed the entire range of dispositions and behaviours, are subject to modification as one proceeds through the lifespan.

Whilst exposure to stressful situations varies with the social circumstances of people, it is also true that identical circumstances have different effects on individuals within the group depending upon the social contexts. For example, retirement may be eustressful to a person who had an unstimulating job, or in a culture, such as Japan, that values its elders. Alternatively, retirement may lead to chronic distress and consequently depression in the person who thoroughly enjoyed his work and now has not enough to occupy his mind, or in a culture, such as Britain, that views the elderly negatively.

Societies influence individual change and adaptation. They are sources of hardship and challenges and, by providing contexts that give meaning to the consequences of these hardships, help people fend off the harmful emotional distress that may otherwise result.

The strains amongst people of different ages is especially relevant to developmental concerns. They can be simply summarized because of their uniqueness to particular individuals, whether it be work-related, or the strains associated with being single, married, or divorced. Temperamentally, however, everyone is different. Thus, how we respond to stressors is subjective. Personality, it could be argued, is largely socially determined, since the family is important in providing mental stability or instability in developing our attitudes to pain (Chapter 21), distress, etc. The ways in which we face a crisis or disaster is learned from those around us in our youth.

Physical stressors

Physical stressors involve over-exertion as well as bodily change which may affect one's mood. They result from malnutrition, hormonal–biochemical imbalances, illnesses, injuries caused, for example, by too much activity and strain on the skeletomuscular system, or from drug and alcohol abuse.

Psychological stressors

Psychological stressors include innate and socialized 'fears' and 'fantasies' that, if provoked, will produce either distressed (anxiety) or eustressed responses.

Environmental stressors

Environmental distressors include:

1 Societal pressures (distressors) such as overcrowding, antisocial behaviour, conforming to societal norms and values, parental wishes.

2 Work distressors associated with imposed conditions, such as levels of noise, glare, or restricted movement, or 'work overload' in terms of too much work (quantitative overload) or too difficult work (qualitative overload) and, conversely, quantitative and qualitative 'underload'. Conditions of employment, such as low pay, low status, shiftwork, staff shortages, lack of resources, etc. are also included. Relationships at work are also important, and poor communication channels within these may be a source of distress. A lack of understanding of social support, and accountability levels, and other aspects, including career and promotion prospects may all result in frustrations and distress which may be associated with high absenteeism, work-related illnesses and can result in the individual leaving that employment.

3 Organizational stressors such as work policy and procedures could be restrictive for the individual. No positive feedback on performance, or acceptance of new ideas, etc. could all be perceived as a source of frustration and distress.

4 The individual's organizational role; this could be a source of irritation, for example there may be a lack of defined authority, or no definite role specification. Interdepartmental conflicts with superiors, or with colleagues/staff may occur. A difficulty in delegation, a lack of involvement in decision making, a lack of training for management, etc. are also perceived as sources of distress.

5 Work–home interactions. According to Cooper and Marshall (1980) there are two broad categories of stress for the person in work: occupational and private (domestic/personal). They argued that the greatest source of stress occurs when there is conflict between the two, most obviously between the family, fame, and fortune. Stress, whether eustress or distress, in one part of life tends to spill over into other areas. Home and work conflicts may also arise

with women's 'double-shifts'. Their domestic labour, child care, caring for dependants, etc. result in a lack of time for their choice of employment. This may be related to the lack of recognition of work by colleagues or spouse.

Developmental stressors

In an attempt to make sense of the 'meaning of life', science has always tried to classify objects, living matter, etc. Human development is no exception: various stages of development have been attributed a label, so one can distinguish one developmental stage from another in order to aid advances in specialist knowledge in these areas. Thus, we have the 'beginnings of life' stage known as the zygote: this stage progresses into the morula; the blastocyst; the embryo; the fetus; the neonate; the infant; the child; the pubertal adolescent; the adult; the stage we equate to the elderly, retirement and beyond; and finally the terminal stage of 'death', which according to Selye is when we are free from stress!

Each stage is considered by the authors to be a macrophenotype, identifiable from one another by differential psychophysiological responses. For example, the emotional and physical characteristics of the adolescent and adult are obviously different from one another. Each psychophysiological characteristic is also regarded as a phenotype which arises through enzymatically-controlled reactions that are ultimately controlled by gene expression. This expression is influenced by environmental factors (stressors), and the timing of exposure to such factors, and these are responsible for the range of onset of developmental stages. For example, the onset of puberty is between 10 and 12 years for girls and 12 and 14 years for boys, and results from the production of adequate quantities of the male and female steroid hormones which promote the development of the secondary sexual characteristics. Genes must be expressed to produce the enzymes necessary for hormone synthesis. Most people have the genetic potential for pubertal onset and the age range above demonstrates subjectivity. Perhaps premature or delayed pubertal onset may be a result of premature or delayed exposure to those environmental factors necessary for gene expression.

Therefore psychophysiological subjectivity exists across the lifespan. Society also has positive and negative effects on development, for example technological advancement is usually centred around the young who are more adaptable to changes, and this, according to Seligman (1975), can lead to the elderly feeling depersonalized and helpless.

INTERIM SUMMARY: THE SUBJECTIVITY OF STRESSOR PERCEPTION

So far this discussion has focused on the subjectivity of how people perceive stressors. The cumulative effect on an individual of such stressors (social, developmental, physical, environmental, and psychological) also demonstrates subjectivity. Thus, stressors may or may not be consciously perceived as such by different individuals because no two people are alike. It is also unlikely that any two people will experience identical stressors. Furthermore, the perceived stressors must reach or supersede the stress threshold of the individual. Stress thresholds are dynamic and are not fixed entities. They are subjective to individuals, according to the individual's resistance to stressors, their available 'adaptation energy', and to the stress-related conditions they have experienced throughout their lives.

Subjectivity is based upon at least five factors:

1 An individual's genotype.

2 An individual's upbringing.

3 An individual's environment.

4 An individual's personality (this depends on 1 and 2).

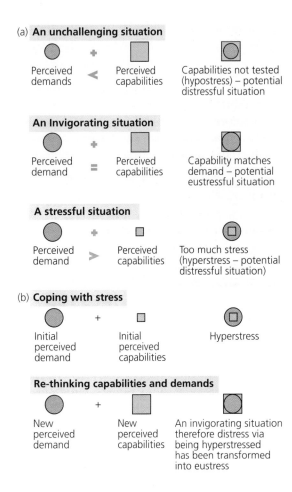

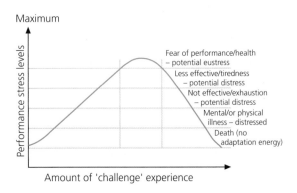

Figure 22.5 Yerkes–Dodson's law on human performance and stress.

Figure 22.4 (a) Cox and McKay transactional model of stress. (b) Coping with stress.

5 Circadian rhythm fluctuations, as I'm sure we are all aware of 'moody' people first thing in the morning!

Once the cumulative effect of the stressors have reached or superseded the stress threshold, then individuality of the psychophysiological bodily response is observed and the individual experiences either distress or eustress depending upon the cognitive interpretation of the stressors. Using Cox and McKay's (1976) transactional model of stress,

one can describe this stress response as occurring when there is a mismatch between the perceived environmental demands and the individual's perceived capabilities (Figure 22.4a). An important aspect of their model is that it is the individual's perception (not actual demands and capabilities) of demands placed upon him/her that may produce the stress response. That is, if the individual's perception of demands exceeds his/her perceived capabilities to cope with them, then too much stress (or hyperstress) becomes apparent. Conversely, if perceived capabilities of coping exceed the perceived demands, then too little stress (or hypostress) is evident. When capabilities and demands are matched then, the authors would argue, the individual experiences eustress. Thus coping or adapting to hyperstress or hypostress situations involves changing one's perceptions of demands according to one's capabilities and vice versa respectively (Figure 22.4b). Yerkes-Dodson's (1982) 'law' stated that optimum stress provides maximum performance and from this one may then potentially experience eustress. Stress levels below or above this optimum results in deteriorating performance and can be a potential source of distress (Figure 22.5).

The subjectivity of the stress response

THE GENERAL ADAPTATION SYNDROME (GAS)

The demand–capability model could be linked with earlier work of Selye who in 1956 described the general adaptation syndrome (GAS), which attempted to explain the physiological responses to stress. He labelled this a non-specific (stereotypic) response, 'the sick syndrome', as he realized that patients with a variety of diseases had similar signs and symptoms including weight loss, appetite loss, decreased muscular strength, and no ambition. His animal studies demonstrated that three changes occurred during exposure to continued or extreme stress:

1 The adrenal cortex hypertrophied and was hypersecretive.

2 The thymus, spleen, and lymph nodes atrophied.

3 Bleeding ulcers appeared in the gastro-intestinal tract.

He argued that a variety of dissimilar situations, such as arousal, grief, pain, fear, unexpected success, or loss of blood, are all capable of producing similar physiological stress responses. Thus, although people may face quite different stressors, in some respects their bodies respond in a stereotypical pattern. According to Selye this involved identical biochemical changes which enabled them to cope with any type of increased demand on the body. Thus, he believed that stress was the non-specific adaptive response of the body to any demand placed upon it. Later, he argued that stress, whether pleasurable (eustress) or threatening (distress), produces physiological changes to restore the body's homeostasis, which has been disrupted by the stressors. Selye suggested that continued exposure to stressors results in a triphasic response of alarm, resistance (adaptation), and exhaustion.

Alarm stage

Alarm is predominantly initiated and controlled by the sympathetic nervous system and affects visceral effector organs such as the brain, heart, and skeletal muscles (Figure 22.6). These initial sympathetic effects are prolonged by the simultaneous release of the adrenal medullary catecholamines (adrenaline and noradrenaline) which function at the sympathetic neuromuscular and neurosecretory effector sites. The alarm stage, therefore, is equivalent to Cannon's (1935) famous 'fight and flight' statement when describing the adrenomedullary effects of adrenaline and noradrenaline. The effects of this stage can be viewed as short-term homeostatic controls operating, hopefully, to enable us to cope with, or adapt to, the dominant stressor(s) which contributed to the individual reaching the stress threshold. If these controls are successful, or the dominant stressor is perceived to have fallen below threshold level, then visceral organ functions return to their 'normal' baselines (i.e. within their homeostatic ranges). However, if the stressors remain at or above threshold level, and/or additional stressors occur, then Selye argued that the individual goes into the second stage of resistance.

Resistance or adaptation stage

Resistance is predominantly endocrine controlled and is mediated by the hypothalamus. Such events are analogous to intermediate and long-term homeostatic controls which act to re-establish homeostasis. The majority of hormones released are hyperglycaemic agents

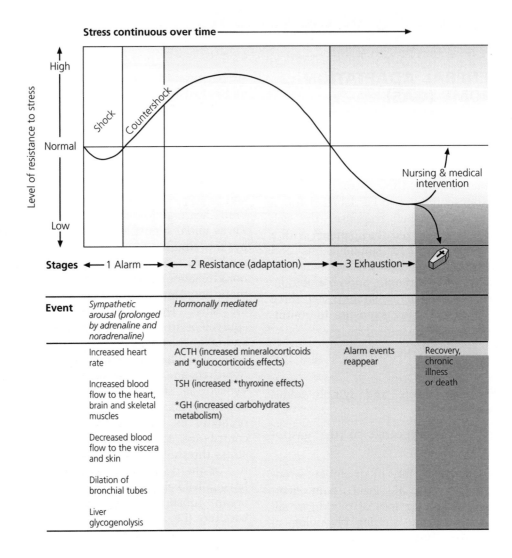

Figure 22.6 Selye's general adaptation syndrome (GAS). ACTH, adrenocorticotrophic hormone; TSH, thyroid-stimulating hormone; GH, growth hormone; *increased glucose availability for catabolism (possibly provides a source of adaptation energy).

(i.e. chemicals which raise the blood sugar levels) to provide cells with energy to cope with the effects of the stressors. Selye (1956) called this 'adaptation energy'.

The amount of adaptation energy might be compared to our inherited bank account, determined by our individualistic genotype, from which we can make withdrawals, but into which we apparently cannot make deposits. Every stressor causes wear and tear, leaving some irreversible scars which accumulate and contribute to the signs of ageing (see Chapter 19). If ageing is defined as a disturbance of homeostatic control systems, then it could be argued that age-related conditions are in reality stress-related conditions. In other words there is functional decline owing to wear and tear, due to overexposure to environmental/ social demands (stressors). If this is the case adaptability should be used wisely rather than squandered. It is still not understood what is lost, except that it is unlikely to be simply calorific energy. If there is no adaptation (or resistance), or if attempts to reduce the cumulative effects of the stressors below threshold level are unsuccessful, then, Selye argued, we would go into the final stage of exhaustion.

Exhaustion

In exhaustion the signs of the alarm stage reappear, and this is an indication that the body's homeostatic control systems have failed. Consequently stress-related illnesses appear; Selye called these 'diseases of adaptation'. In the context of this book, this is when clinical intervention is required to restore the patient's homeostatic processes. First there is a need to identify the major stressors associated with this illness, then these must be removed or treated. For example, bacteria or social problems would be treated with antibiotics, or controlled by teaching stress management techniques, respectively. We would argue that serious conditions, that are not commonly recognized as being stress-related, such as terminal cancers, and acquired immune deficiency syndrome (AIDS) are in fact just that, and the agents (i.e. carcinogens and HIV) that instigate these conditions are stressors. These conditions are fatal as the individual cannot adapt. Could this be due to depleted adaptation energy? Arguably depleted adaptation energy as a consequence of ageing reduces our capacity to cope with disease.

Only the most severe stress leads rapidly to the exhaustion stage and maybe death. Most physical and/or psychological exertions, infections, and other stressors act upon us for a limited period of time and produce changes corresponding only to the first and second stages. At first the stressors of the alarm stage

upset us, that is if we are distressed, but then we adapt, either consciously because alarm signs cause us to employ stress management techniques, or unconsciously in the resistance stage via our hormonally-mediated homeostatic controls. Thus throughout life we go through these first two stages many times, in order to adapt to all the demands within our environment.

The triphasic nature of the GAS indicates that the body's adaptation energy is finite, since continuous distress eventually produces exhaustion, and individuals succumb to a stress-related condition. The type and severity of these conditions reflect yet again subjectivity elements. Selye (1976) classified GAS responses as synotoxic and catatoxic reactions of the body's defence against potential internal and/or external aggressors (stressors). The former helps us put up with the aggressor, the latter helps us to destroy it. Synotoxic stimuli act as tissue tranquillizers permitting a peaceful coexistence with the aggressors, whereas catatoxic agents mainly involve the induction of destructive enzymes, which generate an attack on the pathogen, usually by accelerating its metabolic degradation.

Corticoids are amongst the most effective synotoxic hormones. This hormonal group inhibits inflammation and promotes other defence mechanisms, such as transplant rejection. The main purpose of inflammation is to prevent irritants from entering the circulation by localizing them. However, once the foreign agent is rendered innocuous and causes disorders only as a consequence of an exaggerated defence reaction, the suppression of inflammation becomes advantageous. Clinically, anti-inflammatory corticoids are given in such cases and have proven to be effective in treating diseases in which the major complaint is inflammation of the eyes, joints or respiratory passageways.

Alternatively, when the aggressor is dangerous the defence reaction should be increased above the normal level. This is achieved by catatoxic substances such as antibodies, lysozymes, and pain-producing substances, which carry messages to fight the 'invaders' (stressors) even more actively than normal.

The major physiological response of the body to excessive stress is vascular collapse. The body may overcome this by neural/endocrine changes which re-establish vascular homeostasis. This response is potentially life-saving in acute situations, but if stressors are prolonged, or intense, it can lead to organ system failure, resulting in, for example, cardiovascular and gastrointestinal disease. The interdependency of organ systems and their component parts means that if one system is affected, then others will also be affected. A good example of this is in maturity-onset diabetes mellitus, which demonstrates that a failure at cellular level results in multiple organ system failure. This condition is exacerbated by the prolonged effects of carbohydrate-rich (distressor) diets which promote the hyperglycaemia (= excessively high glucose concentration in blood) as the insulin target receptor sites become 'desensitized' to the hormone insulin. The hyperglycaemia (now a distressor) must be corrected. Glycosuria occurs which helps to moderate the hyperglycaemia but there are no endogenous agents, other than insulin, which will reverse it. In addition, diabetes is also associated with fat breakdown and this produces hyperlipidaemia (another distressor) with an atherosclerotic effect. Atherosclerosis is another distressor in diabetes, and diminishes the functions of the blood vessels of multiple organs, and partly explains why the diabetic's eyes, heart, blood pressure, and kidneys may be affected. Although diabetic individuals exhibit the same biochemical and response mechanisms, the degree of change is individualistic, and so which organs are affected, and how much they are affected, varies. Perhaps this variation is also explained by the host of factors which form the basis of sociopsychophysiological subjectivity.

A severely stressed individual also presents a clinical picture which is the result of the cumulative effects of various stress hormones. For example, hypertension could be due to the vasoconstrictory actions of adrenaline, nor-adrenaline, and angiotensin II, or to the circulatory volume-expanding effects of aldosterone and antidiuretic hormone, or to increased cardiac output caused by adrenaline and noradrenaline. The latter hormones may also cause a tachycardia, hyperventilation, bowel dysfunction, and other fight and flight response (alarm reactions). Again, however, there is individual variability.

AN ANALYSIS OF THE GAS

Although on the whole the authors agree with Selye's ideas, looking at Table 22.1 one could argue that stressed individuals do not have consistent physiological, behavioural, and emotional response indicators. In addition, when stressed, individuality is again observed in the way a person perceives the stress response either as distress or eustress, and also whether the individual is consciously aware of this stress response.

Mason (1971) demonstrated that the pituitary–adrenocortical activity in response to stress was not as broad and consistent as Selye suggested. He found that some physically harmful stressors, such as fasting, did not increase 17-hydroxycorticosteroid (17-OHCS) levels when the stressors were weak. However, when fasting was strengthened by psychological factors, the non-specific response occurred. Thus, it is only demands which tax the individual's capabilities that are stressful, i.e. those which reach or exceed the individual's stress threshold. The extent of the stress response depends upon the individual's evaluation of the consequences of unfulfilled demands. The stress response is not stereotypical and stress is not manifested as a single syndrome such as the GAS. Multiple factors governed by situational and individualistic variables are involved (Clancy and McVicar, 1993).

Monat and Lazarus (1985) argued that the disadvantages of Selye's GAS are that it fails to clarify what conditions cause stress or what constitutes a demanding stressor capable of initiating it, and it does not take into account situational and individualistic variables involved in the activation of this stress response. Consequently, it really describes a theory of adaptation to stress rather than a stress theory.

Selye's work, however, can be easily defended using the stress threshold concept. If stressor strength is below threshold level ('mild' stress) then the reactions of the GAS do not appear and it is only when the threshold is met or superseded that the reactions of the GAS come into operation.

The influence of Lazarus in 1966 marked a change in the stress research field which previously had been dominated by Selye. Lazarus identified three important aspects of stress:

1 Individuals differ in their reactivity to stress.

2 Stress is determined by the perception of a stressful situation rather than by the situation itself.

3 The extent of stress depends partly on the capabilities of the individual to cope.

Therefore, according to Lazarus (1966),

stress occurs when there are demands on the person which tax or exceed his adaptive resources.

This definition views stress as involving a cognitive appraisal of a demand–capability imbalance (Lazarus, 1966; Cox, 1978). Factors important in the perception of environmental stressors involve:

1 Perception of control. If one is not in control then distress is more likely.

2 Predictability of the outcome. If one cannot predict the outcome then distress is more likely.

3 Past experiences. If one has no past experience with potential distressors then one is more likely to experience distress until a coping strategy can be developed.

In contrast to Selye's biological theory, the emphasis of 'psychological' stress is on the

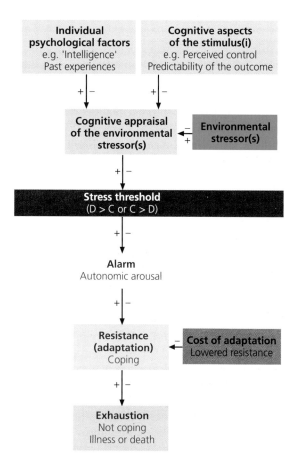

Figure 22.7 'Psychophysiological' model of stress. D, demands; C, capabilities; +, continue; –, removal; >, greater than; <, less than.

input side, in particular on the kind of situation and the individual interaction that evokes a stress state. Both approaches are complementary. Lazarus's psychological theory outlines the conditions which determine the evocation of stress, while Selye's physiological theory describes its form (Figure 22.7). This integrated approach provides Selye's formulations with the breadth needed to encompass the stress of living.

The psychological effects of stress are subjective and multiple. They may result in depression, lack of personal accomplishment, avoidance of decisions, depersonalization or a feeling of emotional emptiness. Spencer (1986) stated that the effects of these stressors can result in a shift from a positive to a negative view, which can lead to an uncaring disposition. Absenteeism, guilt, error and helplessness can follow.

Scientific breakthroughs include the use of tranquillizers in combating 'mental' illnesses, and the use of anti-ulcer drugs. Most of these agents are not actually directed against stress,

but rather against some of its manifestations. Increasing attention is being given to psychological and behavioural techniques that anyone can use to avoid producing the stress response. Relaxation techniques, such as transcendental meditation, must be given the respect they deserve as they work on some of those who try them. People tend to mock such stress relievers but only because medical science cannot explain them!

Coping mechanisms and features of failure

Stress management attempts to reduce or prevent distress and its harmful effects. There are three classes of management: to change one's environment and/or life-style, to change one's personality and/or one's perceptions, or to change the biological response to stress.

These three classes of management equate with the sociopsychophysiological coping mechanisms since stress is an integration of these influences. In general, the term 'coping' is usually reserved for behavioural (psychological) responses and 'adaptation' is applied to the physiological responses. Thus as stress is viewed by the authors as a psychophysiological bodily response then we prefer the usage of 'adaptive-coping' as stress management techniques are employed to alleviate the negative consequences of the whole-body stress response. It is obviously outside the scope of this chapter to describe stress management techniques in any detail; however some methods are illustrated in Table 22.4. The important point to note is that the usefulness of each technique is subjective to an individual's beliefs and that these beliefs are time-dependent and dynamic.

COPING

This section is concerned with how people generally cope with stress using cognitive appraisal of distressors, and does not discuss individual coping strategies.

It is hoped that this book has demonstrated that stressors are necessary to perform the 'characteristics of life'; and that it is how the individual copes or fails to adapt to distressors which is important in determining whether the individual succumbs to stress-related conditions, or progresses through developmental stages of the lifespan.

Cognitive coping

A cognitive approach to coping involves transferring distress into eustress, or removing distressors to below the individual's stress threshold level by reducing perceived or actual stresses (Clancy and McVicar, 1993). According to Maes *et al.* (1987) the success of coping methods is subjective, since individuals differ in respect of their cognitive and behavioural efforts to manage, reduce, or tolerate the internal and external demands of the person–environment transactions, and it is time-dependent, since individuals have circadian rhythm fluctuations (Chapter 23), which influence cognitive and behavioural appraisals and responses.

A mismatch between perceived demands and capabilities produces a source of distress

Table 22.4 Some stress management techniques

Environmental/life-style	Personality/perception	Biological response
Time management	Assertiveness training	Progressive relaxation
Proper nutrition	Thought stopping	Relaxation response
Exercise	Refuting irrational ideas	Meditation
Finding alternatives to frustrated goals, i.e. stopping smoking, drinking, etc.	Stress inoculation modifying type A behaviour	Breathing exercise, biofeedback autogenics

(Cox and McKay, 1976), and so it is important that the individual copes or adapts to these distressors in order to prevent the occurrence of stress-related illness. This can be achieved by rethinking our capabilities and demands (Figure 22.4b) by cognitively reassessing the demands (stressors) according to our capabilities (Figure 22.7). For example, rather than trying to understand all of this book, you can only do your best and understand what is within your capabilities.

Another method of cognitive coping could involve 'moulding' one's personality into a less distressed or even a eustressful personality. For example, personality type A (Friedman and Rosenmann, 1974), is often described as being hard-driving, hasty, hostile, hurried, agitated, impatient, irritable, frequently poor listeners, rushed, overcompetitive and overambitious. People who have few of these characteristics are referred to as personality type B, being calm, content, controlled, easy-going personality, good-listeners, not easily irritated, patient, and unhurried. Type A often state that 'they thrive on stress' (perhaps they are addicted to adrenaline and noradrenaline which are released in the stress response alarm and exhaustion stages). Excessive, frequent and prolonged release of these catecholamines is thought to increase one's susceptibility to stress-related conditions, such as heart disease, hypertension, migraines, and ulcers. However, not all type A personalities succumb to the ill-effects of stress. Freidman and Rosenmann (1974) suggested that if someone of type A consciously recognizes what is happening to

him/herself, they can actually become more resistant to stress, that is they become type C (sometimes referred to as type H or hardy personality personalities). These people now look upon situations as challenges rather than threats, and convert the distressful life events of type A into opportunities or possibilities (eustressful life events) for personal growth and benefit. According to the Cox and McKay transactional model they have rethought their demands and capabilities.

In order to be 'stress-wise' it is important, therefore, to identify type A behaviour in ourselves by recognizing attitudes and expectations that engage us in a constant struggle to gain control over our environment. For example, when a type A personality perceives emotional threats or challenges, the stress response is automatically triggered, even when there is no real danger, as when waiting in a traffic jam, queuing in banks, etc. As a result, much unnecessary 'stress' (and loss of adaptation energy) is created which keeps the individual frequently outside the normal range of the stress balance and in the distressed area. The difficulty is in appraising our behaviour and altering our responses to stressors. Lazarus (1966) put forward a stress appraisal model based on coping with mental illnesses. According to Lazarus primary appraisal of the initiating situation involved three possibilities:

1 A stressor is considered irrelevant.

2 A stressor is seen as being positive with respect to well-being, having positive and pleasant emotions.

3 The stressors are regarded as damaging and threatening, with negative emotions such as anxiety.

These three possibilities can therefore be equated to being unconsciously aware of the psychophysiological indicators of the stress response, eustress and distress.

The outcome of these possibilities determines the emotions experienced (Lazarus, 1976). This experience promotes the necessary action to be taken and results in a secondary appraisal which involves planning and evaluating possible coping methods: to change the stressors or situation, to modify the meaning of the situation, or to regulate the experienced emotions.

In other words distress may be transferred into eustress or the situation fled, one's perceptions of demands and capabilities may be altered, or distressful emotions may be minimized.

Coping, like stress, has acquired many meanings. It may refer to efforts to master conditions of harm, or threat, of challenge, when a routine or automatic response is not readily available. Here environmental demands must be met with new behavioural solutions or old ones must be adapted to meet the current stress. Folkman and Lazarus (1984) suggested two sources of coping: problem- and emotion-focused coping.

Problem-focused coping

Problem-focused coping involves efforts to change distressors (i.e. problems) in order to cope with the troubled person–environment relationship. The answer according to Hawkins (1980) lies in direct action involving an ergonomics approach. He argued it is first necessary to identify the potential distressors, such as a quantitative work overload as experienced with time pressures and staff shortages. Although an ergonomic approach to stress management might reduce workload, it cannot increase staff numbers. It operates on the principle of optimizing efficiency levels and so reduces the time spent on specific tasks. This can be achieved by keeping abreast of professional developments, perhaps with the aid of advanced technology. For example, centralizing information can reduce the time spent in unnecessary meetings and the 'freed' time can be used in other ways, including to ease the burden of time-pressurizing tasks. If the problem or distress is caused by a lack of involvement in decision making, then restructuring gives more emphasis to a team approach. If the distress is a result of desynchronizing circadian rhythms by the removal of the natural light and dark cues, as occurs with night work or during periods of hospitalization (Chapter 23), the ergonomic approach of coping could involve the use of solar spectrum artificial lighting, as an aid to the shift worker and the hospitalized patient in order to reduce the extent of the desynchronization.

Emotion-focused coping

Emotion-focused coping is a palliative process, since these methods do not actually alter the damaging conditions, but are used to make the person feel better. Traditionally, emotion-focused coping can become pathological or maladaptive (Lazarus, 1966). For example, denial defence mechanisms may be used to deny that a suspicious lump may be cancerous. Such coping strategies can become dangerous when they prevent essential direct action, but are considered beneficial in providing the individual with a sense of 'psychological' well-being.

Voluntary behaviour habits such as the use of alcohol, cigarettes, tranquillizers, sedatives, and excessive caffeine, act as distressors themselves, and have long-term pathological consequences and thus may be detrimental to one's health. In addition, there are involuntary reactions in the stressed individual, such as decreased appetite, and disturbed sleeping patterns. (Chapter 23), which are also potential distressors and thus can affect one's resistance to disease.

Individuals usually employ a combination of these coping mechanisms either consciously or unconsciously in an attempt to counteract stress. Some coping methods are more successful than others, not only from an individual's point of view but also within one of the three domains of physiology, psychology, or sociology (Folkman and Lazarus, 1984). However, coping affects all three domains since they are inseparable entities.

COPING FAILURE: PSEUDO-ORGANIC AND ORGANIC DISEASE

Pseudo-organic disease

Some people with coping failure present symptoms that suggest the presence of an organic disease, for example pseudo-angina, which upon consultation and examination show no evidence of the actual disorder. Frequently, such patients are treated with mild analgesics and if these prove ineffective, then more powerful analgesics may be administered. The patients may be very anxious and complain that it is the pain which is the stressor and that this is causing a lack of sleep. Consequently they may be prescribed antidepressants and, after taking a few months to recover, rarely complain of the 'angina' again. It may be speculated that the reason for an increased pain perception is that there is a decrease in arousal levels in the depressed state. That is, the depression is a failure of adaptation, and is a sign that may be attributed to the exhaustion stage of the GAS when the level of endogenous pain killers such as endorphins might be expected to be low. Guillemin was awarded the Nobel Prize in 1977 for discovering endorphins which have anti-stress effects by acting as pain killers. They may be amongst the first mediators in the alarm stress response.

Organic disease

According to Maes *et al.* (1987) there are two pathways whereby stress is related to the onset of disease. First, stress may have direct psychophysiological effects which affect one's health via disturbed homeostatic controls within cells influenced by the neuroendocrine responses to stress. Second, stress may lead to health-impairing habits and altered behaviours, such as smoking and biting one's nails, respectively. These are referred to as palliative coping methods.

These two pathways explain the relationship between stress and the onset of disease. For example, hormonal changes and immune system decline are thought to reduce the host's resistance, thereby increasing the risk of disease. Once an illness occurs then one may be subjected to illness behaviour, which influences the course of the disease, and so would form a third pathway. For example, in the case of bereavement, Rowland (1977) demonstrated a clear link between the increased incidence of mortality and an increased likelihood of an illness amongst widows and widowers who suffered a recent bereavement of their spouses. One may argue that the evidence is suggestive, but not conclusive. However, what is important is that the dominant stressor (death of the spouse) demonstrates individuality with respect to the differing illnesses acquired, and even death in those who seem unable to cope with the bereavement. As far as cardiovascular diseases are concerned, there are a number of well designed retrospective studies (Thompson, 1982; Figure 22.3; and Freidman and Rosenmann, 1974) that provide evidence in favour of the hypothesis that factors such as personality type may be important in the aetiology of disease.

Hinkle (1987) questioned whether ischaemic heart disease was a disease of stress. In a 'biological' sense it is, however, since 90% of myocardial infarctions are due to atherosclerosis (Meltzner, 1987), and a contributory factor (stressor) to this process is a constant and heavy intake of saturated fat as a source of 'stress' for the affected person. In this instance the liver responds to the hyperlipidaemia by synthesizing large amounts of cholesterol from circulatory fats. As time passes more and more cholesterol is deposited in blood vessels, including the coronary arteries, and this may be sufficient to restrict blood flow to the organs they supply. At first, this may be transient or partial (e.g. at times of high oxygen demand angina pectoris may be induced) and, later, total and permanent (e.g. in myocardial infarctions). The stress response observed will vary according to the sociopsychophysiological subjectivity associated with the resultant ischaemic pain (Chapter 21). According to Brundy (1988) myocardial oxygen demands are not within the affected individual's capabilities, but the degree of angina or the extent of the myocardial infarction emphasizes the subjectivity of this process. Following the classic formulation of Selye, individuals with ischaemic heart disease either adapt partially – angina – or do not adapt at all – myocardial infarction.

In our opinion, diseases are not solely due to one predisposing factor (stressor), but due to the cumulative affects of multiple stressors. Using the above example, the stressors include all the risk factors associated with cardiovascular disease. These can generally be classified as being:

1 Within the body, for example, a genetic predisposition (endogenous stressor) to hypercholesterolaemia. A gene was identified in 1992 which predisposes the individual to a myocardial infarction.

2 Outside the body, for example, cigarette smoking, high dietary fat, distressful life events (exogenous stressors), all of which are hypercholesterolaemic agents. This again demonstrates stressor subjectivity with relation to an individual's exposure to such a diverse range of stressors.

It is the cumulative effect of all coronary risk factors which is responsible for the resultant cardiac problem. The common view of stress is that it results from difficulties associated with life-style and professional or personal relationships. We believe, however, that every illness can be viewed ultimately as a stress-related illness (a disturbed homeostasis), whereby the individual's homeostatic controls have failed or 'adaptation energy' has been depleted. This applies whether it be:

1 A commonly referred to stress-related condition, such as coronary heart disease or an infection. Then all the risk factors could be referred to as stressors which may be linked to environmental influences on gene expression.

2 Serious conditions not commonly labelled as being stress related, for example, AIDS. The stressors associated with AIDS are HIV and the pathogenic stressors of the opportunistic infections which have led to the individual being diagnosed as having AIDS. This idea stems from the work of Hinkle (1987) who stated that disease can be regarded as a phenomenon that occurs when an agent or condition threatens to destroy the dynamic state (i.e. homeostatic mechanisms), upon which the integrity of the organism depends, and the manifestations of disease appear to be, in large measure, manifestations of the organism's efforts to adapt to and contain threats to its integrity. In this sense, all diseases are to some extent disorders of adaptation, as Selye suggested in 1956.

References

Brundy, C. (1988) Stress and coronary disease. *Nursing Times* **84**(44), 18–21.

Cannon, W.B. (1935) Stressses and strains of homeostasis. *American Journal of Medical Sciences* **189**, 1.

Clancy, J. and McVicar, A.J. (1993) Subjectivity of stress. *British Journal of Nursing* **2**(8), 410–17.

Copper, C. and Marshall, J. (1980) *White collar and professional stress*. Chichester: John Wiley & Sons.

Cox, T. (1978) Stress. London: Macmillan.

Cox. T. and McKay, C.J. (1976) Psychological model of occupational stress. A paper presented to the Medical Research Council Meeting – *Mental Health in Industry*, London.

Folkman, S. and Lazarus, R.S. (1984) *Stress appraisal and coping*. New York: Springer.

Friedman, H. and Rosenmann, R.H. (1974) *Type A behaviour and your heart*. London: Wildwood House.

Hawkins, L. (1980) Circadian rhythms and shift working. *Journal of Occupational Health* **33**(2), 86–90.

Hinkle, L.E. (1987) Stress and disease: the concept after fifty years. *Social Science and Medicine* **25**(6), 561–6.

Holmes, T.H. and Rahe, R.H. (1967) The social readjustment rating scale. *Journal of Psychosomatic Research* **11**(2), 213–18.

Lazarus, R.S. (1966) *Psychological stress and coping process*. New York: McGraw-Hill.

Lepore, J.S., Palsane, M.N. and Evans, G.W. (1991) Daily hassels and chronic strains: a hierarchy of stressors. *Social Science and Medicine* **33**(9), 1029–36.

Livingston-Booth, A. (1985) *Stressmanship*. Wallington, Surrey: Severn House.

Maes, S., Vingerhoets, A., Van Heck, G.H. and Evans, G. (1987) The study of stress and disease. Some developments and requirements. *Social Science and Medicine* **25**(6), 567–78.

Mason, J.W. (1971) A historical view of the stress-field. *Journal of Human Sleep* **1**, 65–8.

Meltzner, L.E. (1987) *Intensive coronary care – A manual for nurses*. Hemel Hempstead: Brady Company.

Milkhail, A.(1985) Stress: a psychophysiological conception. Cited in Monat, A. and Lazarus, R.S. *Stress and coping*. Columbia, OH: Columbia University Press.

Monat, A. and Lazarus, R.S. (1985) *Stress and coping*. Columbia, OH: Columbia University Press.

Pearlin, L.I. (1983) Role strains and personal stress. Cited in Kaplan, H.B. (1983) *Trends in theory and research*. New York: Academic Press, 3–32.

Rowlands, K.F. (1977) Environmental events predicting death for the elderly. *Psychological Bulletin* **84**, 349–72.

Seligman, W.M.P. (1975) *Helplessness*. Oxford: Freeman and Company.

Selye, H. (1956) The general adaptation syndrome and diseases of adaptation. *Journal of Clinical Endocrinology* **6**, 117–18.

Selye, H. (1976) *The stress of life*. New York: McGraw-Hill.

Spencer, D. (1986) Concern for the carers. *Holistic Medicine* **1**, 225–31.

Thompson, R. (1982) *A pocket guide to stress*. London: Arlington Books.

Yerkes-Dodson, P. (1982) Cited in Dodson, C.R. (1982) *Stress. The hidden adversary*. Lancaster: MTP Press, 29–30.

Summary

1 Stress is a disturbed homeostasis which manifests itself via certain psychophysiological bodily responses (imbalances).

2 Stress occurs only when the cumulative effects of stressors reach or supersede the stress threshold, which varies between individuals and within the individual with time, since it may be influenced by circadian fluctuations.

3 The stress experienced is either eustress or distress. The former is regarded as a healthy bodily response, the latter an unhealthy response.

4 The person's perception of stressors, stress thresholds, their resistance or adaptation to stress, their coping strategies, the stress-related illnesses people experience in their lives, and their eventual outcome are all subjective.

5 The basis of subjectivity is dependent upon an individual's genotype and the unique environmental perceptions they are exposed to throughout their lives.

6 Integration of sociology, psychology, and physiology is required to investigate stress as a sociopsychophysiological phenomenon. This would involve focusing attention on the multiple cumulative stressors, which are responsible for each stress-related condition, since it is our opinion that all diseases are a result of cumulative stressors (including physical, psychological, environmental, social, developmental, etc.). Some disorders are easily identifiable, whilst others are difficult to pinpoint.

7 Since stress is a sociopsychophysiological phenomenon, then it follows that stress management must involve a multidimensional approach. Organizations and individuals must work together for their mutual self-interests, It is important for everyone to become educated in this area of research, in order to identify distress in oneself and then to take appropriate action via individualized coping methods so as to transfer distress into eustress, or to remove or adapt to distressors. It may be a matter of 'life and death' – YOURS!

Review Questions

1 'Freedom from stress is death' (Selye, 1956). Discuss.

2 Define the concept of stress threshold.

3 Distinguish between the following terms:
(a) Eustress and distress.
(b) Exogenous and endogenous stressors.
(c) Perceived demand and perceived capability.

4 Describe the events associated with the triphasic stages of the GAS syndrome.

5 Stress is said to be a psychophysiological bodily response arising through environmental stressors. What do you understand by this statement?

6 Stress is a perception. Discuss this statement using the principles of Cox and McKay's transactional model of stress.

7 Stress is a subjective phenomenon. Discuss this in relation to the individualistic nature of the following:
(a) stressors, (b) stress threshold, (c) stress response, (d) stress-related illnesses.

8 Suggest why it is difficult to measure or assess subjective experiences such as stress.

9 Coping is a cognitive act. Discuss.

10 What do you understand by the statement that all illnesses are stress-related?

Circadian rhythms

Introduction: relation of rhythms to humans

Circadian rhythm patterns

Role of circadian rhythms in homeostasis

Circadian rhythm desynchronization: a homeostatic imbalance

Summary

Review questions

Introduction: relation of rhythms to humans

The term 'circadian' was introduced by Halberg in 1959 and stems from the Latin word 'circa' meaning 'about' and 'dies' meaning 'one day' (Burgener, 1985). A rhythm refers to a sequence of events that repeat themselves through time in the same order and at the same interval (Palmer, 1977). Thus human circadian rhythms refer to the events that are repeated in the body every 24 hours. Armstrong-Esther and Hawkins (1982) described circadian rhythms as

a periodicity or rhythmicity of a number of physiological, biochemical, behavioural functions.

Halberg (1959) and Aschoff (1966) argued that rhythms are associated with all forms of life, and, because organisms are a part of the physical environment they live in, they are responsive to natural rhythmical changes within that environment.

Humans are not obviously a rhythmic or cyclical species as they have no breeding season, migration, hibernation, etc. Some human rhythms are persistent and not circadian, but are of shorter duration frequencies, for example, heart rate, with approximately 70 beats/min. Luce (1977) reported that it was Ogle in 1866 who first identified human circadian rhythm (of body temperature) and it was Simpson and Galbraith in 1906 who established that the monkey's temperature rhythm was synchronized according to the light and dark cycle. Most human studies came much later and in 1959 Halberg stated that physical, psychological, and biochemical oscillators are intrinsic to individuals with a day and night periodicity of 20–30 hours.

Circannual rhythms are of a yearly periodicity and are very important in plant and animal species as they control breeding and hibernation. It is debatable whether these rhythms are present in humans, although they may be responsible for mood swings at certain times of the year and a link with suicides has been suggested by Luce (1977). That is, some people feel good and are at their happiest during the spring and summer months and this may partly explain why suicide rates are at their lowest at this time of the year. In contrast, some people feel low and depressed in winter months (this corresponds with a seasonal affected disorder, or SAD, syndrome) and this may be linked to the higher suicide rates during this time of the year. The mood swings may be related to the amount of natural daylight since light is arguably one of the most important environmental stimuli which controls human rhythms.

CIRCADIAN RHYTHM PATTERNS

It is obviously outside the scope of this book to credibly discuss Armstrong-Esther and Hawkin's (1982) broad definition of circadian rhythms; thus, 'psychological' rhythms will be omitted owing to the nature of this textbook and biochemical rhythms will be limited to just a few common examples associated with physiological rhythms. The reader should be aware, however, that these three parameters of bodily function are inseparable and are inter-dependent entities. Although physiological rhythms such as body temperature will be described, the reader should bear in mind that heat is produced as a consequence of metabolic reactions and these are dependent upon cellular biochemistry. In addition, physiological parameters can be influenced by one's psychological functions (or vice versa), for example most 'psychological' performance peaks are associated with peaks in body temperature. The purpose of this chapter is to emphasize that if one were to 'look inside our body', then one would see a number of repetitive psychophysiological patterns. Some cells would be more active in the morning, when the body is in an awake state, whilst others will be more pronounced at night when one is asleep. These 'normal' patterns become disturbed in illness or when we change our natural timing of sleep–wake patterns, such as in shift work, travelling across different time zones, admission to hospitals or staying up late at weekends.

Technical advances now mean that non-invasive assessment of physiological variables can be performed, or that measurements can be made on very small samples of fluids, including plasma and urine. Thus, sequential measurements can be carried out during the circadian period.

Body temperature, heart, respiratory, and metabolic rates

Body temperature is one of the most stable rhythms in humans (Samples *et al.*, 1985), and thus is one of the most reliable indicators of 'time inside the body'. It is convenient to measure body temperature and, according to Minors and Waterhouse (1985), the rhythm does not markedly differ in 'normal' healthy people.

Body temperature, heart, respiratory, and metabolic rates all follow the same pattern. This is not surprising because of their interdependency: for example, body temperature is an indicator of the level of one's metabolism and, according to Luce (1977), may reflect activity in the central nervous system. That is, an increased body temperature is associated with a high rate of metabolism, and this necessitates quicker heart and respiratory rates in order to deliver more nutrients and oxygen to the active cells. A high rate of metabolism requires more energy (ATP, another 'key chemical of life') to drive the metabolic reactions. Consequently, the metabolic pathways of cellular respiration are faster, with the result that more heat energy is produced, thus increasing one's body temperature.

Figure 23.1 illustrates the expected rhythmicity of oral temperature and its interdependent circadian rhythms. The pattern of change is:

1 A steep rise in the morning, becoming maximimal during late morning (or early afternoon in some).

2 A slight decline from the maximum followed by a return to the maximum or a value close to it later in the afternoon; this is called the post-lunch dip.

3 A decline in the afternoon or early evening, continuing through the night.

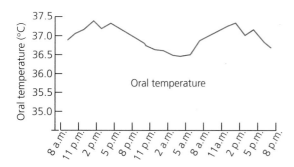

Figure 23.1 Oral temperature over 36 hours.

4 The minimum value (nadir) occurs in the early hours of the morning.

One would expect such rhythmicity since the increase which begins just before awakening prepares the body for the waking process and subsequent events. The rise continues during the morning and early afternoon, which are the times when we require a higher rate of metabolism to deal with the daily activities. The fall-off during late afternoon and the declining levels in the evening are a consequence of our activities slowing down and getting ready for sleep. Upon sleeping such parameters are at their lowest (body temperature falls at night by about 0.5 degrees Centigrade and this represents a considerable change in metabolic activity), as we replenish energy levels in preparation for the following daily activities. Only people who are very sick, for example, with cancer, fevers (pyrexias), or encephalitis, show distortions of this rhythm.

Body temperature is actually more closely related to changes in skin temperature than it is to metabolism; constriction of cutaneous blood vessels reduces heat loss and so promotes a rise in body temperature. The change in skin temperature occurs before the body temperature is elevated and so body core temperature changes seem also to be a consequence of rhythmic vasomotor changes in the skin vessels, in addition to a change in metabolic rate.

Blake (1967) and Klietman (1967) both demonstrated that the diurnal rhythm of performance paralleled that of body temperature and stated that, generally, there is a positive correlation between temperature, performance and arousal levels. The most consistent improvement in efficiency occurred during the first 3 hours when the temperature rise was most noticeable. On a general note, peak performance corresponds to the peak temperature and arousal levels, occurring between 12 noon and 6 p.m., and this was also the period of quickest reaction times and best psychomotor coordination. The poorest performance coincides with the intervals of lowest temperature and arousal; this is between 3 a.m. and 6 p.m. (this is generally referred to as the 'dead spot'). This is not surprising since, between 2 a.m. and 7 a.m., there is a natural urge to sleep. The timing or duration of maximum temperature and 'post-lunch dips' (PLDs) may vary depending on the individual but the rhythmicity tends to be consistent in the same individual. 'Morning people' (who tend to be introverts), in whom temperature shows a faster rise and peaks earlier in the morning (in Figure 23.1 the peak would move to the left), claim that they perform better in the morning compared with evening people, who tend to be extroverts, in whom in the day temperature rises more slowly and peaks later (the peak moves to the right). The steepness of rise, the timing and duration of the peaks of temperatures (morning and evening people), PLD variations, the steepness of the decline, dead spot times, etc. all demonstrate that there is subjectivity of circadian rhythmicity.

The PLD phenomenon has not been satisfactorily explained as it occurs irrespective of whether we have lunch or not. The PLD does not affect one's performance during this period simply because an increased proportion of the cardiac output is diverted to the gastrointestinal tract, since there are no post-breakfast or post-dinner dips. However, if one becomes consciously aware of the slight 'lull' in performance, one may arrange to perform automatic tasks in this period! According to

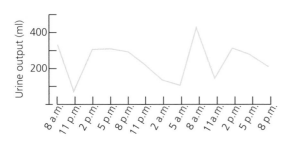

Figure 23.2 Urine output over 36 hours.

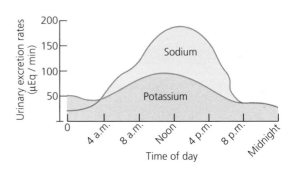

Figure 23.3 Urinary excretion of potassium (K+) and sodium (Na+).

Lanuza (1976) the small rhythmical change in body temperature is also not so large that motivation cannot compensate for it. Therefore, performance is not greatly affected in the highly motivated shift worker.

Other functions of the body have a reverse or an intermediate rhythmicity to that of temperature. For example, growth hormone release and the concentrations of some electrolytes in body fluids tend to have their maximal value nocturnally (Campbell *et al.*, 1986).

Urination

Figure 23.2 demonstrates a rhythm in urinary excretion which involves the production of a large volume of urine in the morning and mid-day, and lower volumes at night. The urinary circadian rhythm may result from the influence of bodily rhythms in such parameters as glomerular filtration rate (GFR), tubular reabsorption, antidiuretic hormone (ADH) secretion, or from fluid intake. The rise in urine flow is dependent on the switch-over from dark to light. A decreased recognition of light and dark cues in the elderly and the blind, therefore, may result in abnormal rhythms. For example, the elderly produce more urine at night in comparison with during the day. According to Armstrong-Esther and Hawkins (1982) this can lead to social problems, such as insomnia, nocturia, and nocturnal wandering

and thus could be labelled as confusional behaviour.

Urinary excretory products, for example that of sodium (Na+), and potassium (K+), demonstrate separate activities as illustrated by Figure 23.3. Potassium excretion changes are pronounced and, generally, for one who went to bed at 11 p.m. and arose at 7 a.m., most potassium excretion would be between 10:30 p.m. and 2:30 a.m. Variations in these are explained by individualistic differences in diets and routines.

Blood components

Wesson (1964) demonstrated circadian rhythms in the concentrations of certain plasma components. Figure 23.4 illustrates individuality with reference to the timing of their peaks, nadirs, and the duration of troughs and plateaux. The rhythms of iron, phosphate, and hydrocorticosteroids demonstrate considerable consistency, and, thus, can be of practical importance. For example, hydrocorticosteroids are released from the adrenal gland in a series of discrete episodes which include an increase in release early in the morning, and a declining frequency as the day proceeds, though throughout this broad pattern there is a series of small sharp peaks. Figure 23.5 illustrates a typical circadian pattern in a 'normal' healthy subject. A steep rise from low nocturnal values to a maximum about 1 hour before waking is observed and the

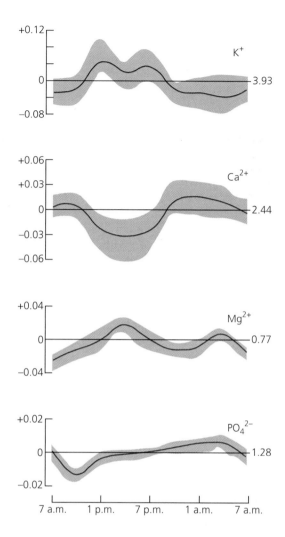

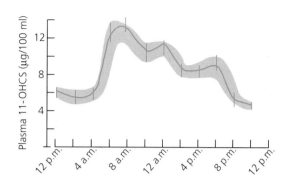

Figure 23.5 Circadian rhythm of plasma 11–hydrocorticosteroid concentrations. Shaded area represents subjectivity in population studied.

Figure 23.4 Mean diurnal cycles of plasma concentrations of potassium (K^+), calcium (Ca^{2+}), magnesium (Mg^{2+}), and phosphate (PO_4^{2-}). Shaded area indicates subjectivity of individual circadian parameters.

peak is just before the end of the dark phase at a time when we are usually awakening. According to Harker (1964) this may promote central nervous system arousal which causes waking up. Many of us may be aware of this, since it is reflected by us awakening to switch the alarm off before it has been activated!

A knowledge of circadian parameters is of clinical importance. However, pathology reports only indicate the upper and lower normal values which are associated with 'health' and the homeostatic ranges which have been frequently referred to throughout this book. We would argue that the sampling of blood, urine, etc. should ideally coincide with the patient's mean values and daily comparative sampling is of greater value if it is performed at the same time of the day. For example, the neural outputs from the respiration and cardiac control centres of the brainstem are at their lowest in the middle of the night, and the subsequent higher blood carbon dioxide and lower oxygen means the person may become quite hypoxic. Consequently, the individual's life functions are at their lowest and therefore it is not surprising that most deaths occur in this 'critical period'.

Sleep–wake cycle

At rest the basic innate rhythm is generally longer than 24 hours and the observed circadian (24-hour) periodicity is dependent upon:

1 Environmental cues such as the night–day cues (Norton, 1991). The removal of these in underground cave studies by Aschoff in 1966 produced a free-running sleep–wake cycle with a periodicity range of 16–50

hours, demonstrating subjectivity of the individual's control over the sleep–wake 'activity' cycles.

2 Levels of circulating compounds which influence the sleep–wake cycle. For example, as previously mentioned, waking may be associated with the stimulatory effects of corticosteroids on the brainstem, including the respiratory and cardiac areas.

Body temperature curves strongly suggest that poor sleepers might be out of synchrony with the 24-hour day. Their temperature declined less when compared with good sleepers and was still declining when they arose in the morning. A poor sleeper, according to Luce (1977), may wish that he could go to bed later and rise later than is socially convenient, for the body time actually may lag behind the clock time (showing a longer period than 24 hours). These free-running periods are common in response to distress and may help to explain the insomnia which accompanies many illnesses, particularly in the mentally ill patient. Thus, during this free-running period, the individual is performing his waking tasks with a 'sleeping' body and subsequently may develop psychosomatic and emotional symptoms as a result of this desynchronization.

When all the rhythms are following their expected patterns then the body is said to be in a state of internal synchronization. It is now considered unusual to find a 'physiological' variable without a rhythm. Moore-Ede and Richardson (1982) argued that we should not consider circadian timing systems as being distinct from the functioning of physiological systems. They argued that there is a need for a counterbalance between rhythms. We support this, and believe that this counterbalance can only be achieved by integrating psychophysiological rhythms and observing how the environment affects each rhythm. In this way sociopsychophysiological subjectivity can be identified in circadian rhythms, or what the nursing and medical professions prefer to call

phenomenological holism. An understanding of such integration would enhance the understanding of illnesses and how, for example, hospitalization affects patients.

CONTROL OF CIRCADIAN RHYTHMS

Although Brown (1972) suggested that circadian rhythms are passive to environmental cues, this is not now generally accepted. Aschoff (1966) suggested a genetic (endogenous) basis of control, with environmental (exogenous) modification of the rhythms. Takahashi (1994) has confirmed the endogenous component in mice by identifying the so called 'clock' gene on chromosome 5 (see Mestel, 1994). He and his colleagues are now working to narrow the location, and once this is achieved scientists will be able to clone the gene and test whether clocks in humans are similar. Consequently, they may identify the link between the clock(s) and seasonal affective disorders; furthermore an understanding of the clock's molecular working might suggest therapies for these conditions, as well as means of alleviating the problems associated with jet lag and shift work.

Endogenous rhythms are 'free-running' (that is, longer than 24 hours), being exogenously modified to give a 24-hour rhythmicity; this is the process of entrainment or synchronization. Aschoff (1966) called these modifying exogenous cues 'zeitgebers', whilst Halberg (1959) referred to them as 'synchronisers'. Examples of exogenous cues are clocks, radio, television, and a regular life-style involving work, leisure, and mealtimes (Armstrong-Esther and Hawkins, 1982). However, Reinberg and Smolensky (1983) argued that mealtimes in humans have not been shown to be an important zeitgeber, in so far as they do not seem to influence the timing of the internal clock. We would argue that it is a combination of exogenous cues and endogenous components which determine mealtimes and, in the majority of instances, this is dominated by exogenous cues, such as socially acceptable times of the day to which an individual is conditioned. Rhythms vary in the relative influence of their endogenous and exogenous components. For example, body temperature has a large endogenous component, whilst cardiovascular and respiratory rhythms have large exogenous components.

Light and dark cues are generally considered to be the most important exogenous cues to which species synchronize their bodily rhythms (Wurtman, 1975). In man the importance of light as an exogenous zietgeber is supported by isolation studies, studies involving the blind and in studies in Eskimos.

Isolation studies

Mills (1973) studied a young man who wore a wrist-watch throughout a 3-month stay in a cave. Although the subject resolved to sustain a 24-hour routine, Mills demonstrated that the subject got out of bed later, slept when tired and generally lived on an activity–rest cycle which was longer than 24 hours. In other words free-running rhythms were exhibited because of the removal of exogenous cues. Most other studies have demonstrated sleep–wake (endogenous) rhythms to be of a greater periodicity than 24 hours, although the range documented for this cycle has been between 16– and 50-hourly rhythms. The difference in the free-running periods demonstrates subjectivity of the control of sleep–wake cycle. Subjectivity is not surprising as each individual is comprised of their own unique blend of genes and their unique environmental perceptions. Although the environment is controlled to a certain extent in isolating studies by the removal of exogenous cues, we would argue that what cannot be controlled is the individual's perceptions of that removal.

In contrast to the sleep–wake cycle, rhythms such as body temperature are more genetically controlled and less dependent upon environmental modification, as they exhibit a 25-hour

rhythmicity in isolation studies (Burgener, 1985). Aschoff (1966) proposed that there were two classes of circadian oscillations:

1 A poorly entrained and easily modified sleep–wake cycle.

2 Strongly sustained rhythms which include body temperature, hormone secretion, enzyme production, urine excretion, etc.

Studies involving the blind and elderly

The endogenous control and exogenous modification of circadian rhythms is evident in studies involving congenitally blind people. These people still exhibit rhythmicity, although the rhythms are a little disorganized (low in amplitude; these are referred to by Armstrong-Esther and Hawkins in 1982 as 'flattened' rhythms). However, they still show some degree of periodicity that approximates to about 25 hours. These researchers argued that this rhythmicity is brought about by blind people putting a greater emphasis (compared with sighted people) on exogenous cues such as television and clocks, in order to entrain their rhythmicity. This has also been demonstrated in the elderly who have a decreased sensitivity to light and this will be discussed later.

Eskimo studies

The Eskimo year includes 6 months of continuous light and 6 months of continuous dark (twilight). They are therefore devoid of night/day circadian rhythms, and their rhythms are free-running. There seems to be no adverse effects, although this is difficult to quantify because of the apparent lack of longitudinal studies, and so it could be questioned as to why we have circadian rhythms.

Whether or not light is the most important zeitgeber in humans remains unresolved. Luce (1977) stated that, although light has profound physiological effects, man's most powerful synchronizers are social. What is certain is that human circadian rhythms are a result of the cumulative zeitgebers, such as choice of mealtimes, sleep times, time to be sociable, etc. that enable us to cooperate as a social group. Thus, cultural difference, and differences within the same culture, produce individual variation. Dobree (1993) recognized this when she stated that:

> for humans the most powerful zeitgebers are socio-economic and lifestyle.

LOCATION OF CIRCADIAN CONTROL

Early suggestions of a 'biological clock' within the hypothalamus was put forward as the 'inherited clock theory'. That is, a group of hypothalamic cells were suggested to be responsible for the inherent 24-hour rhythmicity, and these control the activity of the rest of the body, probably through pituitary endocrine activity, and so the rhythm may be 'born not made'.

There is almost certainly more than one clock, however, and Harker (1964) claimed that there are a number of clocks all operating at once. These may, however, be controlled or synchronized by a 'master' clock. The clocks may be the homeostatic control centres of the brain, such as the medullary, cardiac, respiratory, and vasomotor centres, which in turn would be responsible for free-running periodicities. Considerable research has tried to establish the clock(s) location(s) and the neuroendocrine communicating channels between them. The hypothalamic suprachiasmatic nucleus (SCN) was strongly advocated as being the link between the clocks, and hence could be the master clock (Moore-Ede *et al.*, 1982). This is a plausible theory since the hypothalamus is the centre of many activities, for example, satiety, hunger, temperature control. Furthermore, Tureck (1981) identified

a direct retino-hypothalamic link which terminates in the SCN, and this may explain why light is an important exogenous cue.

If the hypothalamus is the master clock then damage to it will result in damage to other circadian functions. Evidence suggests that damage to the hypothalamic temperature control area (as occurs when one is subjected to recurrent fever), results in other bodily rhythms being affected, for example, those of heart rate and respiratory rates. Which circadian rhythms become desynchronized presumably depends upon which area of hypothalamus is damaged.

Wurtman (1975) believed that the pineal gland is the 'master' clock since it is the gland which responds to light and dark, and it is an important link between light and dark reception and CNS function. Wurtman identified an anatomical pathway which linked the gland with the eye:

Retina
↓
Nucleus of Bochenek (cerebral peduncles)
↓
Medulla (brainstem)
↓
Superior cervical ganglia
(a pair of sympathetic ganglia)
↓
Pineal gland

In this way light incident on the retina will stimulate the pineal gland. Noradrenaline is secreted at the neuropineal synapses, thereby acting as an inhibitory neurotransmitter for the release of a pineal hormone called melatonin. Thus, light suppresses melatonin secretion, and Figure 23.6 indicates that melatonin secretion is 20 times higher in the dark compared with during the light phase. The functions of melatonin seem to be to induce sleep, increase endocrine secretion from the pituitary, gonads, and the adrenal glands, and to increase the secretion of the neurotransmitter serotonin (a vasoconstrictor).

Melatonin release in the elderly is elevated during daylight because they have a reduced sensitivity to light–dark as a result of:

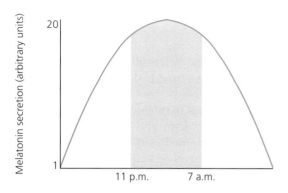

Figure 23.6 Melatonin secretion during the night.

1 The eye becoming opaque, for example in glaucoma, which therefore limits the amount of light penetrating the eye.

2 Retina–pineal gland neural pathways losing their function or certainly having a diminished function in the elderly.

3 Calcification of the pineal gland, which affects 60% of the population over 65 years of age (Armstrong-Esther and Hawkins, 1982).

If the pineal is the 'master' clock, the elderly potentially have disturbed endogenous circadian rhythms and so have to rely more on exogenous (social) synchronizers, for example the arrival of the milkman, radio programmes, etc., to give them 24-hour rhythmicity. If these synchronizers are disturbed, for example upon hospital admission, then circadian rhythm desynchronization may occur.

The 'fact' is that we still don't know where the clock is, or even if there are many clocks controlled by a 'master' clock and, although the inherited clock theory receives most support, other theories do exist. For example, the basis of the 'imprint theory' is that initially an animal is arrhythmic (without rhythms), and it then learns from environmental conditions and parental behaviour what is 24 hours. This theory does not receive much support and is contradicted by Pittendrigh (1974) who demonstrated that rhythms are not a learnt phenomenon, as some rhythms such as that of heart rate appear in uterine development. It cannot be demonstrated, however, that these rhythms are inherent in the fetus or result from changes in the mother, but it is likely that the fetus does respond to maternal rhythms, and that we are born with some form of rhythmicity. Neonatal rhythms are low in amplitude (flattened). As the body adapts to the light–dark activity, the rhythm becomes more mature, and eventually full maturity is developed in a light and dark environment. The rate of maturation varies with respect to the different rhythms. For example, the heart rate rhythm takes a few days to mature, whereas the sleep–wake cycle must develop before there is a capability to entrain to light–dark cues (Klietman and Engelman, 1963). At approximately 20 weeks of age some infants begin to synchronize with parents, but in others it takes longer (up to a few years), before synchronization is fully mature. Bladder control can take up to 10–11 years; this late control is thought to be a result of a lack of light and dark cue modification of endogenous control of urine volume early on in the developmental processes. Further support comes from studies of children in nurseries, in which artificial light predominates and is thought to delay control in some children. Other evidence includes studies involving the jaundiced newborn. These babies are put into high-intensity light to reduce the jaundice but the light prolongs the time for maturation.

Pittendrigh (1974) put forward a theory that those cellular mechanisms which underpin circadian oscillators may be the products of divergent evolution and so differ between species. Alternatively, an ancient mechanism may have been preserved and diversely applied.

Role of circadian rhythms in homeostasis

Cells are the 'basic units of life' and therefore must ultimately control each circadian rhythm, and hence homeostatic function, via:

Genotype
(controller of the ⟶ Phenotype
endogenous rhythms) (circadian
parameters)

↑

Environment
(exogenous modulators)

Phenotypes include all the measurable psychophysiological parameters, for example, temperature; levels of biochemicals, such as neurotransmitters (acetylcholine, adrenaline, etc.); hormones (growth hormone, insulin); chemicals such as glucose, amino acids, electrolytes; and others such as pain-producing substances (kinins, prostaglandins, etc.), and pain-relieving substances (endorphins, enkephalins). Thus, psychophysiological func-

tions normally referred to as 'behavioural' factors, such as mood, sleep, IQs, will also be affected.

All circadian parameters are influenced by cellular metabolism and thus, ultimately, are enzymatically mediated. The production of these enzymes is genetically (endogenously) determined and environmentally (exogenously) influenced by social modulators. For example, noise disturbances (exogenous modulator) may lead to less sleep, which affects the psychophysiological activity–rest (wake–sleep) cycle which in turn can alter neural metabolism and affect one's mood. Therefore, is it the genetic, biochemical, physiological, and psychological homeostatic disturbances which affect circadian rhythmicity, or is it circadian rhythm disturbances that lead to psychophysiological disturbances? Your guess is as good as ours!

Circadian rhythm desynchronization: a homeostatic imbalance

Health is a state of complete physical, mental, social well-being and not merely the absence of disease or infirmity. (World Health Organization 1947)

Alternatively, we would argue that health only occurs when the body has normal synchronized psychophysiological circadian rhythms. Once these rhythms are acquired, then their disturbance or desynchronization must be due to unnatural or 'abnormal' exogenous cues, such as shift work, travelling across time zones, illness, and hospitalization. These cues can modify the expression of one's genotype to produce psychophysiological

imbalances by changing the body's pronounced daily rhythms of eating, sleeping, body temperature, performance, etc. This requires the body to resynchronize, or re-establish homeostasis; otherwise, if desynchronization is chronically imposed, it can be detrimental to one's health. Such disturbances are referred to as 'phase shifts' because rhythms persist but the peaks and nadirs occur at times out of phase with periods of activity and inactivity (Figure 23.7).

The following sections discuss the consequences of such phase shifts as experienced by shift workers, and by patients through their illness and hospital admission.

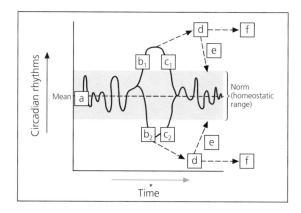

Figure 23.7 Circadian rhythms, a homeostatic function.
a Homeostasis = synchronized psychophysiological circadian rhythmicity = health. Range is dynamic, reflecting subjectivity of parameter rhythmicity within the population based upon the individual's unique genotype and perceptions of environmental cues.
b_1/b_2 Disturbed homeostasis = desynchronized psychophysiological 'circadian' rhythms = phase shifts due to: (i) extreme, unusual, or abnormal exogenous cues (stressors, zeitgebers, etc.), e.g. shift work, travelling across time zones, potential pathogens, and hospitalization; (ii) a deviation in genotypes, e.g. congenital malformations, cancers, etc.
c_1/c_2 Homeostatic control systems re-establishing the balance = circadian rhythm resynchronization as occurs following the removal of extreme, unusual, or abnormal exogenous cues, e.g. shift working patterns, cease chronic travelling across time zones, body's successful defence against potential pathogens, and community care.
d Homeostatic imbalances as a result of control failure = free-running psychophysiological rhythms = ill-health/illness.
e Clinical intervention, e.g. health education, community care, etc.
f Untreatable clinical imbalances, e.g. institutionalized patients, terminal illnesses, etc.

SHIFT WORK

Health consequences of shift work

According to Kostreva and Genevier (1989), 15–25% of the working population of industrialized countries are shift workers. Continuous shift work is necessary for a variety of reasons:

1 Economic gain. Shift work is a high priority for the country's gross national profit.

2 Technological reasons. Some industries, for example petroleum and steel, need to operate on a 24-hour basis.

3 Human services. The population requires public services throughout 24 hours for security reasons (police, military, etc.) and for health reasons (health care workers).

4 Job security. Workers may have to choose between shift work or redundancy.

5 Economic necessity for the workers. Shift work brings financial bonuses that may be needed in order to maintain standards of living.

Various shift patterns exist, but studies are few and controversial. Shifts are classified according to the number of hours worked; generally, 8 hours constitutes a shift and shifts are split into mornings (earlies), afternoons (lates), or nights. Twelve-hourly shifts may also be used and this usually involves a reduced number of working 'days' from 5 down to 4 or 3.

Shifts in health care, especially nursing, are dependent upon regional and hospital policies; there are either two shifts, being early–lates and permanent night, or three shifts of mornings (e.g. 7 a.m.–3 p.m.), afternoons (e.g. 2 p.m.–10 p.m.), and nights (e.g. 9.30 p.m.–7.30 a.m.). The latter pattern is described as rotational as workers rotate their shifts between afternoons, nights, and earlies. According to Rutenfranz (1982) shifts produce a chronic alteration in environmental time (or exogenous cues). This is supported by Figure 23.8. As a result of this alteration

> shiftwork has important implications for both the personal well being of the workers and the safety of the general public both in and out of the work place. (Fossey, 1990)

There are many sociopsychophysiological implications for the unsynchronized

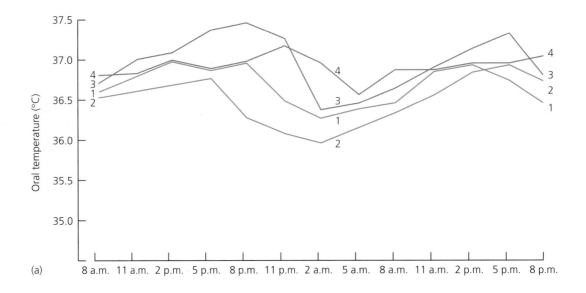

(a)

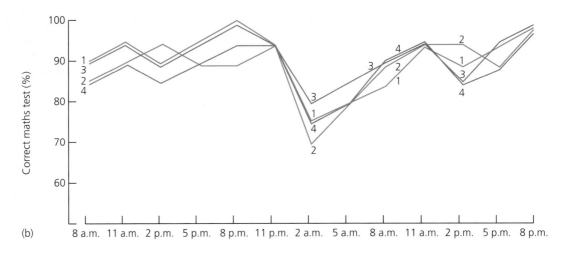

(b)

Figure 23.8 (a) Relationship between oral temperature and time over 36 hours. (b) Relationship between mathematical testing efficiency (%) and time over 36 hours. (c) Graph representing the time of the peak temperature values in non–shift workers and shift workers over a 7–day period. (d) Graph representing the time of the peak performance levels in mathematical testing between non–shift workers and shift workers over a 7–day period. 1 and 2, Control subjects (non–shift workers); 3 and 4, experimental subjects (shift workers prior to commencing the shift) (Clancy and Miller, 1989).

(unadapted) shift worker. 'Social' problems may exist as a result of a lack of qualitative and quantitative time spent with the family, and no regular leisure time with family and friends as documented by Taffa (1984). According to Luce (1977) this may partly explain the high divorce rate amongst shift workers. These social stressors can lead to a sense of isolation and helplessness in the shift worker (Samples *et al.*, 1985), resulting in psychophysiological imbalances including:

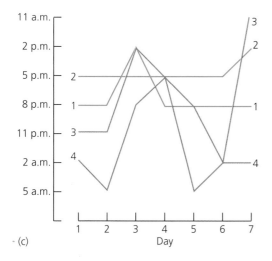

(c)

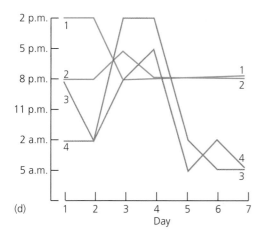

(d)

1 'Psychiatrically' labelled mood conditions associated with:
- neurosis (Luce, 1977);
- depression (Taub, 1974) – according to Fossey (1990) depression is more common in night workers and men;

- some cases of schizophrenia (Wehr and Goodwin, 1983).

2 'Physiologically' labelled conditions associated with:
- disorganized and poor eating patterns: this leads to significantly higher incidence (10–12%) of gastrointestinal tract disorders (Luce, 1977; Taffa, 1984). Common complaints are peptic and duodenal ulcers, and shift workers are eight times more likely to get stomach disease and ulcers (Rutenfranz, 1982). An increased incidence of gastroduodenitis and other gastro-intestinal-associated problems like anorexia and constipation, were noted by Fossey (1990). Rutenfranz (1982) also claimed that shifts seem to promote more 'junk' food being eaten, and increased caffeine and smoking consumption, and they argued that it is these which are responsible for, or contribute to, the gut disorders.
- disorganized sleep patterns. Some workers have difficulty falling asleep, because their sleep–wake pattern is affected. According to Fossey (1990):

In night workers the cycle of sleep and wakefulness is completely reversed and is initially at odds with other rhythms?

Sleep disturbances are more common in the evening shift, whilst fatigue is associated with the night shift because day sleep is shorter. According to Minors and Waterhouse (1985) the shift worker on average gets 1.5 hours less sleep than a day worker (i.e. 6 hours versus 7.5). The quality of sleep is reduced even when daily noises are absent. That is, rapid eye movement (REM) sleep which is important in relaxation, is of a low amplitude. There is also less REM sleep and sleep is of shorter periods.

Changing sleep patterns can have dramatic effects, since sleep is one of the most important circadian rhythms and its desynchronization has multiple effects on other circadian rhythms (Klietman, 1967).

Sleep disturbance is reported to be a contributory factor as to why there is a higher consumption of alcohol, cigarettes, sleeping pills and tranquillizers in the shift worker (Fossey, 1990). The interdependency of rhythm desynchronization in shift workers was recognized by Oswald (1980) who stated that:

> low levels of corticosteroids and adrenalin at night when night-workers must function at their best cause them to be less efficient.

Performance is affected because the night worker is working when bodily rhythms are geared up to sleep, and they sleep when the rhythms are geared for activity. It is not, therefore, surprising that sleep is of a poor quality and quantity.

- Cardiovascular problems (Taffa, 1984). According to Knuttson *et al.* (1986) shift work is associated with an increased risk of myocardial infarctions (MIs) when the shift pattern lasted between 11 and 15 years, although the incidence appears to decrease if the shift is continued for more than 20 years. Alfredsson *et al.* (1989) supported these findings when they demonstrated greater incidences of hyper-cholesterolaemia amongst shift workers, the link being that 90% of MIs are a result of atheroscelerosis (Meltzner, 1987). Conversely, Rutenfranz (1982) concluded that mortality due to cardiovascular problems is not associated with shift work.
- Nervousness, tension and fatigue are particular problems for the shift worker (Taub, 1974; Lanuza, 1976).

Shifts and work performance

The above psychophysiological imbalances (distressors) are likely to affect an individual's work performance. General accidents in factories and cars are greater at 1 a.m., whilst most industrial accidents occur between 2 a.m. and 4 a.m., and doctors and nurses are less efficient at night (Luce, 1977). Sweden's meter readers also recorded most errors at night, followed by afternoon, then the morning and telephone operators identified 3 a.m.–4 a.m. as their 'dead spot' since greater number of errors were recorded. In addition, impaired retention, decreased factual recall, poorer manual dexterity, slow information processing, slow problem solving, increased anxiety, hyper-irritability, less social affection, depersonalization, and divorce problems are also frequently quoted as a consequence of shift work. These stressors may cause stress-related conditions such as ulcers, hypertension, cardiac complaints, depression, neurosis, and even an increase in suicidal tendencies.

Night shifts, in particular, are associated with a high rate of absenteeism because of reported 'stress-related' conditions. The question is whether these conditions are due to the night work itself or are a consequence of the individual's daily activities. Whichever is the case, we can safely say that night work is less efficient from the employers' and employees' points of view.

Afternoon (late) shifts are the most popular amongst shift workers, followed by morning (early) shifts and nights. Factors contributing to the popularity of late shifts are the lesser effects on social life, less susceptibility to gut disorders, and less fatigue.

Of those aware of problems associated with shift work, a study by Minors (1988) demonstrated that 20–30% dislike shift work so much that they would abandon it. This was supported by Kostreva and Genevier (1989) who demonstrated that the scheduling of nursing shifts was cited most often as a reason for resignation. Thus, one can only assume the financial gain, job security, and in the case of nurses, devotion to patients, are a few reasons why they remained.

ADAPTATION TO SHIFT WORK

Difficulties in rhythm resynchronization

Evidence that adaptation is a problem comes from several studies. For example:

It takes several days to completely readjust to just a 1 hour shift. (Monk and Folkard, 1976)

night work patterns have to be continuous, and a period of 2 days of night sleeping is sufficient to revert back to normal daily circadian rhythm. (Bunning, 1984).

Luce (1977) stated that when a person works on night shift, his entire body enters a state of transition for many days. Although the individual responds to 'resetting' or synchronizing sleep and activity cycles, the problem is that our numerous psychophysiological rhythms do not reset at once. Indeed certain cardiac rhythms take up to 3 or 4 days to resynchronize, whereas others may take up to 2 weeks to reset to a new schedule of sleep and rest.

Monk and Folkard (1976) stated that there is a significant increase in road traffic accidents in the week after a change of shift, and suggests that this may be caused by the rhythms being desynchronized (maladapted). The positive correlation between shift workers and disorders also indicates maladaptation. But the 'adaptability' of some individuals suggests that some people are more able to do shift work than others. This is difficult to analyse because shift workers tend to be self-selected groups. The nature of this transitional vulnerability arising through phase shifting, perhaps arising from a desynchronization of internal rhythms, remains one of the interesting questions of work–rest scheduling (Luce, 1977).

Although longitudinal studies which investigate the desynchronizing effects on the human lifespan are not forthcoming, we would argue that the cumulative effects of shift-induced psychophysiological imbalances (stressors), would result in squandering one's adaptation energy levels (resistance to stress) at a greater rate in shift workers, and that a removal of shift work may actually decrease or diminish the stressors associated with the shift worker's situation.

We believe that shifts affect individuals differently, because there is sociopsychophysi-ological subjectivity of circadian rhythms, i.e. an individual's psychophysiological tolerance varies, as this is dependent upon the individual's genotype and their perceived environmental (socializing) experiences. In addition, the rate and direction of shift change varies as a result of social, societal, organizational, and public requirements, and this is very important in one's perception of adaptation. The problem is that the individual may think that he is in control and adapted, but most people are unaware of the damaging effects of shift work on their bodies and their relationships. This was supported by the Rhone Valley survey of 1000 industrial workers, 45% of whom could not adjust to a 7-day shift rotation, and 34% could not adjust to a 2-day rotation. Thus, 55% and 66% respectively thought they were adapted; interestingly body temperature did not adapt in either group. Moore-Ede and Richardson (1982) introduced the term 'shift maladaptation syndrome' to describe a condition befalling individuals who cannot adapt to shifts. They argued that this was characterized by a higher incidence of sleep–wake problems, and gastrointestinal and cardiovascular pathology.

Body temperature is often used as an index of adaptation, and in shift work which involves consecutive night work for periods of 1–3 weeks, a phase shifting of the minimal body temperature was observed (Luce, 1977). The temperature shifted to a point within the new sleeping period after 7+ days of night shift, i.e. adaptation had occurred. However, in shift systems with a single night shift, the natural circadian rhythm of body temperature was not significantly altered; linking this with performance, then less errors would be recorded. Perhaps this is why certain health authorities employ a rapid rotation shift system for their nursing staff. Felton (1976) demonstrated that blood pressure took 2 days to adapt, but body temperature took more than 5 days, in response to a 1-hour time change in shifts amongst student nurses.

Plasma potassium (K^+) concentration has also been used as it is a good indicator of how quickly a person is adjusting to phase shifts and living to non-circadian schedules. For a reversal of the patterns, the shift worker must work 14 nights to achieve adaptation, i.e. 14 consecutive nights before the K^+ concentrations have been inverted from their daily pattern of change.

Most night shifts are approximately of 5 nights' duration and therefore some rhythmic patterns will be adapted, whilst others will not. For example, body temperature takes a week to adapt, but then reverts back to normal during subsequent rest days. Because of the body's attempt to resynchronize during rest days there can be no shift pattern with totally synchronized circadian rhythms, with the exception of the 'normal' (socialized) synchronized daily shift, that is between 8 a.m.–6 p.m.

Hypothetically, an ideal shift pattern would be one which takes into account the adaptation of all the rhythms. Thus, since 14 nights are necessary for adaptations of some rhythms, such as K^+, then one would have to be constantly at work, as days off would result in the individual trying to resynchronize to the 'normal' circadian pattern. Even constant working (without time off) would not help, however, since the worker would become easily fatigued, exhausted, and consequently enhance the likelihood of illness and absenteeism. During absence from work, the individual would revert back to the 'innate' rhythms associated with a daily work routine! Thus, the reasoning of shift work in nursing, for example, is that:

1 Slow rotation results in slow adaptation, and so efficiency of work declines for up to 1 week. Thus, upon a month of shifts there will be 3 efficient weeks and 1 inefficient week. However, improved safety measures for the nurse and the patient are needed at lower efficiency levels, and, as mentioned above, the nurses' body clocks are tending to revert back to their normal circadian patterns during the days off. In our opinion 3 efficient weeks is a misconception.

2 Rapid rotation (the majority of nurse shifts) produce very little adaptation of circadian rhythms, and workers just feel tired and fatigued (Fossey 1990). It is generally considered that rapidly rotating shifts do not affect efficiency but substantive data to support this is required; not only short-term data but also long-term data which looks at the cumulative effects of rapidly rotating shifts on the well-being of the nurse, and on efficiency levels, which are going to affect the well-being of the patients.

Three major strategies have been used to address the problem of adaptation to shifts. The first is to schedule workers on straight shifts without rotation. The problem would be staffing the night shift. The second is to use a rapid rotation of shifts in order to escape the consequences of partial adaptation. The problem is that the circadian rhythms may be affected even upon rapid rotation, or else why should one feel tired and fatigued if the rest–activity cycle was within its homeostatic parameters? The third is to select individuals who seem to have the best tolerance to shift work or have abnormal sleeping rhythms, i.e. those with rhythms of low amplitude.

Recently, Wild (1992) replaced her 'normally' revised 2-week rota with a repeating rota shift system in nursing. This new system involved a work pattern of 5 days off and 9 days on over a fortnightly period. It also incorporated the following elements: days off prior to night duty, early shifts before days off, late shifts following time on the ward, as far as possible no single days off, alternate weekends off, and a 'scallywag' system. These staff would vary their shifts according to the needs of the ward, i.e. cover for sickness, double up during 'busy times, etc. The benefits of such a system after a 3-monthly trial noted by her staff were:

1 Being able to predict shifts in advance meant that staff could plan their social life better.

2 Individual request for time off was accommodated by swapping shifts.

3 Alternate weekends off were seen as an advantage even to staff who worked weekends as it provided time to do other things.

4 From a managerial point of view it was much easier to organize.

In summary, shift work will always be a necessity because of its importance to the country's economy. This will become more of a problem to health as more and more of the world becomes industrialized and trends to run continuous around-the-clock operations increase. Since it is our view that no shift can provide totally synchronized circadian rhythms (except 'normal' day work), then one must seek compensatory behaviours to reduce the desynchronizing effect of shift work. Such interventions were suggested by Fossey (1990). These included napping and exercise.

Napping

Napping can be used as a sleep supplement and many Japanese companies offer their workers rest rooms for this 'activity' during their shift. They believe that this results in decreased fatigue and reinstated arousal which increases the performance of their workforce. However, to the individual 'napper', this can reduce the quality and quantitative nature of the subsequent night's sleep and Akerstedt *et al.* (1989) believed that naps need to be controlled with reference to the individual's shift pattern if the individual is to benefit. For example, if the next main sleep is on the following night, it is better not to take a nap in order to ensure that the sleep is of good restorable quality. However, if the following night is a working night, an afternoon nap is advisable to reduce the inevitable fatigue that accompanies night work.

Exercise

Regular, moderate exercise increases one's fitness and, as a result, decreases skeletomuscular signs of fatigue. There is also an increased alertness, resulting in an increase in the efficiency of memory-loaded tasks. Fossey (1990) claimed that exercise can increase resynchronization efficiency, resulting in quicker adaptation rates.

Interim summary

Further research is needed in this area in an attempt to minimize the effects of shift work. This is recognized in North America where there are chronobiological departments which study circadian rhythms in an attempt to improve schedules. Chronobiologists believe that the best shift is the one which takes account of the natural circadian patterns. They also believe that night workers are able to accommodate their sleep disruption more satisfactorily if they go to sleep as soon as they finish their night shift, rather than staying up until around mid-day and going to sleep before normal sleep time. Chronobiologists have demonstrated that improved shift change patterns are those which rotate clockwise; that is mornings to afternoons to evening and back to morning. In most shifts, this is usually at a frequency of 1 or 2 days, but if this period is extended then it also improves circadian effects. Rotational shift patterns are a source of debate as rhythms are constantly being disrupted and adaptation depends upon the speed of rotation. The time interval between each shift in a slow rotation is generally only long enough for the rhythms partially to adapt and this partial resynchronization is potentially harmful to rhythms which do not fully adapt. Rapid rotation avoids problems of continued partial resynchronization and so is considered more satisfactory. The major problems associated with rapid rotation are the greater disruptions they cause to domestic and social life, and this is why many prefer slow rotation. With regard to rapid rotation it is not known what cumulative psychophysiological effects will result over a long period of time. German companies provide optional medical check-ups for their employees and provide special hospital admission arrangements for them to normalize their desynchronized rhythms in an attempt to avoid long-term problems for their employees.

TRAVELLING ACROSS TIME ZONES

Upon crossing time zones the individual becomes desynchronized as the body time is not in phase with the external cues. Body temperature adjustment times vary from 5 to 21 days according to different studies, demonstrating subjectivity. This is hardly surprising when one considers that if one flies west, from Britain to the USA, there is a time difference of between 5 and 8 hours (east and west coasts respectively). Simpson (1965) demonstrated equally pronounced rhythms in both Europeans and Americans; however, the phases of Americans are approximately 5 hours behind, and consequently their peaks and troughs occur earlier than those of Europeans (Figure 23.9). Individuals find it hard to adjust and every traveller is aware of the fatigue associated with 'jet lag'. Furthermore, continued exposure to this causes the 'jet syndrome', with symptoms of general malaise, sleep disruptions, feelings of disorientation, headaches, burning or unfocused eyes, gastrointestinal tract problems, sweating, and shortness of breath. According to Winget *et al.* (1984) these are very similar problems to those experienced by shift workers. Life expectancy of persistent flyers is reduced by 10%; however, this is not irreversible, the symptoms disappearing with time when persistent flyers cease flying. According to Campbell *et al.* (1986) hallucinations are reported by some around-the-world travellers. What is not known, however, is the extent to which cumulative sleep loss is responsible for this.

The components responsible for travel fatigue are:

1 External desynchronization. The weak time cues on arrival lead to slow adjustment.

2 Internal desynchronization, leading to a decrease in psychomotor skills (Winget *et al.*, 1984).

When we invert our sleep pattern by east–west travel (or stay up late at parties), we

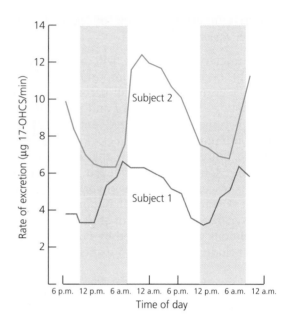

Figure 23.9 Excretion rates of 17–hydroxycorticosteroids in adults at different times of the day: Subject 1, Americans; Subject 2, Europeans.

expose our bodies to viruses and infection during the very phase when production of antibodies, or gammaglobulins is at its lowest, and this may account for the high incidences of colds and infections that many travellers, students studying for exams and people doing shift work experience (Luce, 1977). Petrie *et al.* (1989) demonstrated a decreased incidence of jet lag, and a quicker recovery in sufferers, following melatonin administration. This supports the evidence that the light and dark cycle is one of the most important circadian rhythms and that the pineal and other light and dark centres may be the master synchronizer(s) of other circadian rhythms.

ILLNESS

Some illnesses produce changes in normal circadian rhythms. For example, Alberti *et al.*

(1975) demonstrated variations and desynchronized patterns of blood glucose in his diabetic patients. Bartoli (1967) found that peripheral circulation in the arms and legs reached a low point between midnight and 4 a.m. Tissues receive less oxygen during this period, and therefore it is not surprising that some people with peripheral arterial disease are awakened with acute pain from their sleep at this time. Menzel (1968) used 'time charts' with his patients and he observed that sickness is associated with disordered rhythms in body temperature and urinary components. He reported that a child with a lymphatic disease displayed a 12-hourly body temperature rhythm, and liver-diseased patients had urination and temperature peaks at night instead of in the morning. Night studies have also shown that abnormal gastric secretions occur when the stomach is empty, at times when increasing levels of corticosteroids are observed in sleeping people (Luce, 1977). Menzel suspected that desynchronization of circadian rhythms could eventually explain recurrent symptoms. Perhaps all illnesses need to be studied for disturbed circadian rhythms so as to contribute to the understanding of the associated signs and symptoms. Constant exposure to distressors (in this case desynchronized rhythms) leads to a deterioration of one's adaptive system and consequently one succumbs to an illness (stress-related illness). It is possible, perhaps, that this deterioration may even be caused by one or more circadian rhythm(s) moving out of phase.

Observations of circadian patterns have demonstrated that there are times in the day–night cycle which correlate with specific illnesses. For example, Reinberg and Smolensky (1983) found that the peak frequency for the onset of myocardial infarctions occurs between 8 a.m. and 10 a.m. Evidence also suggests that some psychiatric conditions are influenced by circadian rhythm disturbances, and Taub (1974) suggested that phase shifts lead to emotional disruption.

There also appears to be a peak time for births and deaths. Most labours begin around midnight, and the births are more frequent in the early hours of the morning. Induced births, however, are opposite to natural labour, since from an economic point of view more staff are available during the day. Interestingly, the number of stillbirths follow the induced curves, and it is tempting to speculate, therefore, that the timing of the induction may be a contributory factor to the number of stillbirths, since it is not the natural time for delivery. Deaths are more likely to occur at night, but this is not surprising, since metabolism is at its lowest and so we are more at risk!

Illnesses are all associated with desynchronized circadian rhythms. Which rhythms are most disturbed depends upon the illness. For example, feverish illnesses produce pronounced desynchronized body temperature rhythms (and associated rhythms i.e. heart, respiratory, and metabolic rates, etc.). Campbell *et al.* (1986) argued that illness affects the patient's internal clock. However, this chapter has already provided evidence that alterations in exogenous cues as experienced by shift work produce illness, and these cues are markedly altered by hospitalization.

HOSPITALIZATION

Effect on exogenous cues

As previously mentioned, illnesses induce desynchronized circadian rhythms. These, and other unaffected rhythms, may be further disturbed upon hospitalization, since exogenous synchronizers are partly replaced by those cues determined by the ward policy and new environment. In addition, admission to hospital can potentially produce a greater desynchronization in those individuals (for example, the blind and the elderly) who are more dependent upon set exogenous cues for their circadian rhythmicity (Armstrong-Esther and Hawkins, 1982). In support of this Norton (1991) argued that adaptability decreases with age. Thus, not only are the elderly desynchronized to a greater

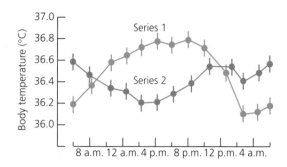

Figure 23.10 Normal circadian rhythm of body temperature in control subjects (series 1) and experimental group (series 2) (n = 15 in each group; • mean and standard deviation). Reproduced by kind permission of Nursing Times where these figures first appeared with the article 'Day For Night – Circadian Rhythms in the Elderly' on July 28th, 1982.

extent following hospital admission, but they find it more difficult to adapt to the imposed hospital zeitgebers. Armstrong-Esther and Hawkins (1982) observed an inverted body temperature in psychogeriatric patients who had been hospitalized for several months (Figure 23.10); i.e. the temperature peaked when they are expected to sleep, and was at its lowest during the day. Consequently an increased metabolism and urine production was more likely at night. As a result, psychogeriatric patients may be reported as having a disturbed urinary output which exhibits itself as incontinence and nocturia, confusion, and sleep disturbances which may lead to nocturnal wandering (Figure 23.11).

All patients upon admission lose some of their exogenous synchronizers. Some wards still awaken their 'geriatric' patients during the night to commode, and this further disrupts sleep–wake and associated rhythms; the nurse may report this as confusion. However, we would argue that any person may appear temporarily confused and distressed when awakened at these times, especially if they were awakened when in stage IV (deep) sleep. When labelled confused, the patient may be sedated, thus disrupting sleep–wake and

associated circadian rhythms further, and unfortunately this may lead to permanent sedation. Awakening policies are not restricted to care of the elderly wards. For example, Walker (1972) reported that patients were disrupted during sleep as much as 14 times in 1 hour, and for as long as 50 minutes, during 3 days after a heart operation.

The hospitalized patient, whether elderly or not, has many additional routines or zeitgebers. For example, the last drug round is at about 10 p.m. with lights out soon after this. The patient is awakened at 6:30 a.m.–7 a.m. and there are specific meal times (i.e. breakfast 8:30 a.m.; lunch 12 noon; dinner 5:30 p.m.). Complicated and unfamiliar machinery is also present to which they must adapt. During this period of adaptation the patient may appear to be confused. Increasing social interaction may be the way to reduce or remove this confusion. For example, Burgener (1985) highlighted the importance of face-to-face therapy at the patient's level of understanding, since this researcher argued:

> the greatest disturbance to patients comes from communication between nurses and staff.

The removal of wall-to-wall seating, which still occurs in many hospital rest rooms, may improve social contact and so help remove confusion in patients and abolish unnecessary sedation. Perhaps it may also decrease the amplitude of circadian rhythm disturbances and reduce the adaptation period, thus improving the quality of care.

Armstrong-Esther and Hawkins (1982) argued that the study of circadian rhythms may aid the assessment of the individual needs of elderly patients, and that compressing the elderly into a rigidly conforming pattern of care is only going to make them worse, more confused and disorientated or incontinent, and therefore increase the level of dependency on the nurse. Conversely, Wessler et al. (1976) argued that rhythmicity can be promoted by adopting a highly regularized living routine even if different from the one previously

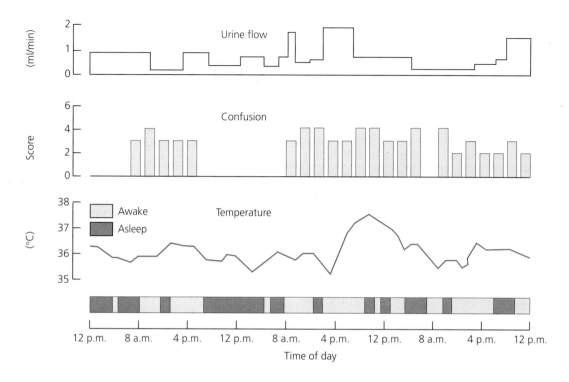

Figure 23.11 Comparison of renal activity, confusion rating, body temperature, sleep, and activity level in a subject showing nocturnal confusion and incontinence. Reproduced by kind permission of Nursing Times where these figures first appeared with the article 'Day For Night – Circadian Rhythms in the Elderly' on July 28th, 1982.

followed. Thus it remains controversial whether the well-being of the older adult is better fostered by imposing environmental rhythms which do not coincide with his/her own internal rhythms.

Circadian rhythms and vulnerability to drugs

Chronopharmacology and chronopharmacokinetics are comparatively 'new' areas of research, hence little is known. However, there is much evidence to suggest that a lower pharmacological tolerance exists at night-time, and thus if the same dosages are given at night they have greater pharmacological effects. For example, digitalis is 40 times more effective at night than during the day (Luce, 1977). It is common ward practice to administer digitalis in the morning. This is 'normal' practice with drugs that are administered once daily, and depressed tolerance levels are not, on the whole, taken into account for drugs which are needed two, three or four times per day, as the same dosage is given at night as during the day.

Tolerance depends upon the absorption rates of drugs, their distribution rates, their metabolism by the liver, and their excretory rates. All are depressed at night. Drug tolerance variation is even more pronounced in the elderly. Bleathman (1985) stated that absorption rates are much slower in the elderly. Conversely, Draper (1983) argued that absorption is not significantly slower, but the main problem is that the elderly are more likely to be affected by drug combinations, since many of the elderly are on multiple drugs. Both Draper and Bleathman demonstrated that there is an increased drug distribution, resulting in a longer half-life of the drugs. This arises because the elderly have lower plasma albumin (which binds to certain drugs) concentrations, leaving more 'free' drug, and, therefore, increased pharmacological activity occurs.

Draper and Bleathman also both found decreased activities of drug-metabolizing enzymes in the liver of the elderly. Bleathman suggested that depressed drug metabolism in the elderly was also due to a decrease in hepatic blood flow, and therefore reduced dosages are required, and dosage intervals need to be less frequent, in this section of the population. Kidney clearance of drugs by the elderly is also reduced (Simpkins and Williams, 1987), and this also supports the need for decreased dosages and for less frequent intervals.

A misunderstanding of drug dosages and drug intervals could conceivably lead to further desynchronization of circadian rhythms and, as a result, hospitalization. This is supported by Williamson and Chopin (1980) who found that 10% of 2000 admissions were solely or partly due to adverse drug reactions, and 6.6% were as a consequence of two drug groups: first, cardiovascular drugs, and second, central nervous system acting drugs. In support of the above Bliss (1981) argued that adverse drug reactions in the elderly stems from

1 Multi pharmacology: 75% of 75+-year-olds have some drug medication, whilst 66% have one to three drugs administered and 33% have four or more drugs administered.

2 Repeat prescriptions given without regular medical 'check-ups'.

3 Self-medication: evident in the elderly, because they self-administered certain drugs prior to the introduction of the National Health Service. As a result, the elderly may exhibit drug-induced diseases. For example, an overindulgence in laxatives (drugs to counteract constipation) has been demonstrated to have a strong link with the incidence of colonic cancers. Bleathman (1985) documented that adverse drug reactions are equally a problem in the United States of America and apparently are also increased with age.

Campbell *et al.* (1986) claimed that drugs given by continuous infusion, or intramuscularly at precise regular intervals, throughout the 24 hours prevent an improvement in this perception of an environmental 24-hour rhythmicity. Sedatives and opiates also alter that patient's perception and ability to respond to environmental cues.

Implication for care

There is a need for the health care professions to study patients' circadian rhythms, and their disturbances, as rhythm desynchronizations are important diagnostic tools (Halberg *et al.*, 1973). For example, a continued increase in plasma calcium ion concentration could represent a gradual decalcification of bone, which is known to accompany continuous recumbency, and a fall in blood nitrogen is typical of the effects of starvation (Mills, 1973). Deviation in patterns can be indicative of disturbed homeostatic functions. For example, in Addison's disease and Cushing's syndrome, the normal variation in cortisol release is largely or entirely absent. In the former disease, cortisol concentrations are lower, but may not be any lower than is observed in normal subjects at night. Conversely, with Cushing's syndrome, elevated cortisol levels may be no higher than those shown in a healthy subject when rising in the morning. Diagnosis is thus best aided by taking a morning and evening sample. If only single samples are permitted by hospital policy, then a morning sample would more clearly detect Addison's, an evening sample would be better to detect Cushing's. The timing of samples, however, is complicated if the patient is a shift worker, as there is no guarantee of their 'adapted' rhythmicity. In addition, an individual's nationality may have to be taken into consideration. For example, an unadapted (resynchronizing) American visitor would have rhythms at 5–8 hours (depending upon which coast the visitor came from) ahead of Europeans (Figure 23.9). All these variations yet again demonstrate the importance of individualized care for patients.

Where possible circadian rhythms should be routinely applied to all aspects of care. The following should become a matter of routine in order to improve the quality of care administered:

1 Clinical staff could investigate optimal times (i.e. increased responsiveness) for chemotherapeutic administration, especially for medications that commonly cause allergic responses (Burgener, 1985). Allergy testing should be investigated in the evening, when allergic responses are at their highest.

2 Clinical staff could investigate optimal times for laboratory specimens. Since variations in the peaks of leucocyte counts, electrolyte concentration, haematocrit, blood gas composition, temperature, urinary output, etc. all exist, it makes the common practice for collection of samples questionable. The 'typical' sample should be collected closest to the mean for that person rather than the time when it would be at its highest or lowest values. In addition, daily comparative sampling will be of maximal value only if it is performed at the same time of the day to take into account circadian fluctuations. Presently, samples are usually drawn at 6 a.m. in order that they be ready for when the physician arrives at the unit, a time when some of the rhythmic values are at their minimum. If regular samples (for example, every 4 hours), were taken, a circadian pattern for the patient could be plotted after a few days (a process called 'circadian mapping'). Once established, circadian patterns can be used to avoid:
  • Reactionary responses. For example, decreased urinary output at night should not be diuretically controlled.

  • Increased stressors or exercise at the patient's lowest resource point. For example, the lowest pain response is between midnight and 4 a.m. (Luce, 1977); intravenous catheterization and other painful procedures could be started early in the rest cycle in order to minimize the pain response. The optimal time for treatment and surgery scheduling is thought to be in the early morning hours when the patient's metabolism is low, despite the practitioner's metabolism also being low and consequently risking error and accident. Also, care may be improved by monitoring patients closely at more susceptible times. For example, exaggerated broncho-constrictory rhythm occurs in asthmatics at approximately 6 a.m., and special alertness is required at this time (Bleathman, 1985).

3 A knowledge of circadian patterns can be of value from a health education point of view, since the body temperature peak is associated with a better performance in relation to both teaching (practitioner) and learning (patient). We would argue that the most important teaching time ideally will coincide with the patient's peak temperatures times, in order for them to gain maximum benefit from the teaching. However, body temperature cannot always be used as a reliable indicator of the person's performance since illness and hospital admission may be associated with rhythm desynchronization in the patient.

4 Research needs to investigate the circadian timing of 'stress-related' events, in order to avoid 'stressors', which can potentially affect the circadian rhythms of the patient.

5 One could minimize circadian problems for patients by maintaining the patient's natural social synchronizers, for example emphasizing community care, particularly for the elderly. Night admission wards could be introduced to cater for insomniacs, those who are nocturnally disturbed, or for those

who are frightened of being alone at night. In addition to providing an extra element of care, this would also remove the 'burden' from families who obviously have their sleep patterns disturbed by the nocturnal activities within their homes.

According to Myco (1981) the patient is in a period of resynchronization or entrainment because of the illness itself, the admission process, and the stressors associated with being a patient. Therefore care should support previous circadian rhythms where possible and not be associated with ward conformity. For example, sleep is usually influenced by social and occupational pressure, and removal of these pressures, as with retirement, or hospital admission, may result in a 'polycyclic' sleep pattern, i.e. 'cat naps' during the day. Napping reduces the quality and quantity of night-time sleeping and if the person in the community or the patient on the ward (particularly the elderly) complains of sleep disturbances, this may result in narcotic prescription. Thus, we would argue that the best treatment would be to detect the stressor (e.g. boredom) which cause the naps, and remove the stressor (e.g. by increased social interaction) or replace it (e.g. with face-to-face therapy). The need for narcotics may be diminished, or better still abolished, thus benefiting the patient by removing the effects of the drugs, and also giving a sense of time.

If on the wards polycyclic sleep is evident, then one must question whether it is imposed or if it is a normal routine for the patient. The nurse must try to remove it only if it is not the patient's normal routine, since a disturbed rest–activity cycle can lead to desynchronization of other rhythms. It can be prevented by providing a stimulating environment specific to each patient. If polycyclic sleep is a normal occurrence for the patient, we would argue

that this should be encouraged in hospitals. Myco (1981) argued that the patient was usually overloaded with many additional stressors, and that nurses should minimize these potential desynchronizers by various means. Interviews should be conducted as a series of short interviews rather than a long-winded interview, in order to develop a care plan. This should be by the same nurse, whenever possible. The interviews should coincide with the patient's most receptive time, borne out by the body temperature peak. The patient should be involved in the decision-making process. Also, subsequent to discussions with the nurse, the patient should be allowed to 'sleep on it' before coming to a final decision. The patient should also be involved in rehabilitation since increasing sensory input can transform distress into eustress. Finally, the patient's individuality should be considered. For example, the nurse could investigate whether the patient is a 'morning' or an 'evening' person, a shift worker, or an unacclimatized overseas person, as this could influence assessment, planning, implementing and evaluation of care.

Care of the unconscious or comatose patient necessitates clinical intervention to maintain physiological equilibrium, so that the endogenous rhythm approximates to its innate time minus the zeitgebers. The nurse has to assume, therefore, that the rhythms are free-running. If the patient is unconscious for a long period of time, or if there is brain injury, then desynchronization must be assumed. In such cases it is essential that the nurse supports the previous circadian rhythms; in order to do this she/he must maintain the patient's physiological equilibrium. Second, the patient must be helped to reorient the brain to previous temporal and life experiences. This sometimes involves the playing of favourite audio tapes or a relative talking about the past, etc.

References

Akerstedt, T., Torstall, L. and Gilberg, M. (1989) *Sleep and alertness – chronological, behavioural and medical aspects of napping*. New York: Raven Press.

Alberti, K.G.M.M., Dornhorst, A. and Rowe, A.S. (1975) Metabolic rhythms in old age. *Biochemical Society Transactions* **3**, 132–3.

Alfredsson, L., Karasek, R. and Theorell, T. (1989) Myocardial infarction risk and psychosocial work environment: an analysis of male Swedish working force. *Social Sciences Medicine* **16**, 463–7.

Armstrong-Esther, C.A. and Hawkins, L.H. (1982) Day for night. Circadian rhythms in the elderly. *Nursing Times* **78**, 1263–5.

Aschoff, J. (1966) Adaptive cycles. *International Journal of Biometeorology* **10**, 305–24.

Bartoli, C. (1967) Cited in Luce, G.G. (1977) *Body time*. St Albans: Palidin.

Blake, M.J.F. (1967) Relationship between circadian rhythms of body temperature and introversion and extroversion. *Nature* **215**, 304–9.

Bleathman, C. (1985) Pharmacology. Effects of drugs on older people. *Nursing* **2**(41), 1213–17.

Bliss, M.R. (1981) Prescribing drugs for the elderly. *British Medical Journal* **283**, 203–5.

Brown, F.A. (1972) *Interrelations between biological rhythms and clocks. Aging and biological rhythms*. New York: Plenum Press.

Bunning, E. (1984) *The physiological clock*. New York: Springer-Verlag.

Burgener, S. (1985) Circadian rhythms: implications for evaluation of the critically ill patient. *Critical Care Nurse* **5**(5), 43–7.

Campbell, I.T., Minors, D.S. and Waterhouse, J.M. (1986) Are circadian rhythms important in intensive care? *Intensive Care Nursing* **1**(3), 170–5.

Clancy, J. and Miller, C. (1989) (unpublished data). Cited in Clancy, J. and McVicar, A.J. (1994) Circadian rhythms 2: shift work and health. *British Journal of Nursing* **3**(14), 712–17.

Clancy, J. and McVicar, A.J. (1994) Circadian Rhythms 1. Physiology. *British Journal of Nursing* **3**(13), 657–61.

Dobree, L. (1993) How do we keep time? *Professional Nurse* **8**, 444–9.

Draper, B. (1983) Keep taking the tablets. *Nursing Mirror* **156**(13), 26–9.

Felton, G. (1976) Body rhythm effects on rotating work shifts. *Nursing Digest* **4**, 45–77.

Fossey, E. (1990) Shiftwork can seriously damage your health. *Professional Nurse* **5**, 476–80.

Halberg, F. (1959) Chronobiology. *Annual Review of Physiology* **31**, 675-725.

Halberg, F., Johnson, E.A., Nelson, W., Runge, W.

and Sothern, K. (1973) Autorhythmicity procedures for physiologic self-monitoring and their analysis. *The Physiology Teacher* **1**(4), 1–11.

Harker, J.E. (1964) *The physiology of diurnal rhythms*. Cambridge: Cambridge University Press.

Klietman, N. (1967) *Sleep and wakefulness*. Chicago: University of Chicago Press.

Klietman, N. and Engelman, R.G. (1963). Sleep characteristics of infants. *Journal of Applied Physiology* **6**, 269–82.

Knuttson, A., Akerstedt, T., Jonsson, B. and Orth-Gomer, K. (1986) Increased risk of ischaemic heart disease in shift workers. *Lancet*, **ii**, 89–91.

Kostreva, M. M. and Genevier, P. (1989) Nurse preference vs. circadian rhythms in scheduling. *Nursing Management* **20**(7), 50–62.

Lanuza, D.M. (1976) Circadian rhythms of mental efficiency and performance. *Nursing Clinics of North America* **11**, 585–94.

Luce, G.G. (1977) *Body time*. St Albans: Paldin.

Meltner, L.E. (1977) *Intensive coronary care – a manual for nurses*. Hemel Hempstead: Brady Company.

Menzel, J.W. (1968) Biological cycles and psychiatry. Cited in Luce, G.G. (1977) *Body time*. St Albans: Palidin, 205–21.

Mestel, R. (1994) Mouse gene could help master rhythm. *New Scientist* **7**, 15.

Mills, J.N. (1973) *Biological aspects of circadian rhythms*. New York: Plenum Press.

Minors, D.S. (1988) *Practical applications of circadian rhythms to shiftwork. The biological clock – current approaches*. Southampton: Inprint (litho) Limited.

Minors, D.S. and Waterhouse, J.M. (1985) Circadian rhythms in deep body temperature, urinary excretion and alertness in nurses on night work. *Ergonomics* **28**(11), 523–30.

Monk, T. H. and Folkard, S. (1976) *Hours of work*. Chichester: John Wiley & Sons.

Moore-Ede, M.C. and Richardson, G.S. (1982) Medical implications of shift work. *Annual Reviews of Medicine* **36**, 607–17.

Moore-Ede, M.C., Sulzman, F.M. and Fuller, C.A. (1982) *The clocks that time us*. Cambridge, MA: Harvard University Press.

Myco, F. (1981) Clocking in. *Nursing Mirror* **152**(18), 32–4.

Norton, D. (1991) Investigating the sundown syndrome. *Nursing Standard* **14**(47), 26–9.

Oswald, L. (1980) Sleep as a restorative process: human cues. *Progress in Brain Research* **53**, 279–88.

Palmer, S. (1977) *Biological rhythms and living clocks*. Chapel Hill, North Carolina, USA: Scientific Publications.

Petrie, K., Conagelen, J.V., Thompson, L. and Chamberlain, K. (1989) Effects of melatonin on jet lag after long haul flights. *British Medical Journal* **298**, 705–7.

Pittendrigh, C.S. (1974) *Circadian oscillations in cells and circadian organization of multicellular systems. The neurosciences third study program.* Cambridge, MA: MIT Press.

Reinberg, A. and Smolensky, M.H. (1983) *Biological rhythms and medicine. Cellular, metabolic, physiopathologic and pharmocologic aspects.* New York: Springer-Verlag, 265–300.

Rutenfranz, E. (1982) Occupational health measures for night and day shift workers. *Journal of Human Ergology* **11**, Suppl. 17.

Samples, J.F., Van Cott, M.L., Long, C., King, I.M. and Kersenbrock, A. (1985) Circadian rhythms: basis for screening for fever. *Nursing Research* **34**(6), 377–9.

Simpkins, J. and Williams, J.I. (1987) *Advanced human biology.* London: Harper-Collins.

Simpson, H.W. (1965) Transatlantic differences in circadian rhythms. *Journal of Endocrinology* **32**, 179–81.

Taffa, P. (1984) Shift work and nurses. *The Lamp (Sydney)* **41**, 22–30.

Taub, J.M. (1974) Acute shifts in sleep-wakefulness: effects on performance and moods. *Psychosomatic Medicine* **36**, 164–73.

Tureck, F.W. (1981) Are the suprachiasmic nuclei the location of the biological clock in mammals? *Nature* **229**, 289–99.

Walker, B.B. (1972) The post-surgical heart patient: amount of uninterrupted time for sleep and rest during the first, second and third post-operative days in a teaching hospital. *Nursing Research* **21**, 19–24.

Wehr, T.A. and Goodwin, F.K. (1983) *Circadian rhythms in psychiatry.* California: Boxwood Press.

Wessler, S., Ferrans, S. and Powers, J. (1976) Quality of life index – cancer version. Cited in Fuller, S. and Swenson, C.H. (1992) Martial quality and quality of life among cancer patients and their spouses. *Journal of Psychosocial Oncology* **10**(3), 41–56.

Wesson, L.G. (1964) Circadian rhythms of serum electrolytes. *Medicine* **43**, 547–8.

Wild, W. (1992) Changing times. *Nursing Times* **88**(29), 34–5.

Williamson, J. and Chopin, J.M. (1980) Adverse reactions to prescribed drugs in the elderly. *Age and Ageing* **9**, 273–80.

Winget, C.M., De Roshia, C.W., Markley, C.L. and Holley, D.C. (1984) A review of the human physiological and psychological changes associated with the desynchronization of biological rhythms. *Aviation Space and Environmental Medicine* **55**, 1085–96.

World Health Organization (1947) Cited in Dixon, J.K., Dixon J.P. and Hickey, M. (1993) Energy as a central factor in self-assessment. *Advances in Nursing Science* **15**(4), 1–12.

Wurtman, R.J. (1975) The effects of light on man and other mammals. *Annual Review of Physiology* **37**, 467–83.

Summary

1 Human circadian rhythms are psychophysiological bodily processes which are repeated every 24 hours.

2 The genetic (endogenous) component of such rhythms (demonstrated by studies of isolation, the elderly, the congenitally blind, and of Eskimos) is responsible for producing innate rhythms which are free-running, that is, outside the 24-hour periodicity.

3 The free-running rhythms are synchronized (or entrained) by environmental cues (zeitgebers or synchronizers) to give the 24 hour (circadian) periodicity. Therefore circadian rhythms are a sociopsychophysiological phenomenon.

4 Most circadian patterns (e.g. body temperature) show a rise and plateau during the waking hours, and a fall and nadir during the sleeping hours, although some (e.g. the release of growth hormone) display a reversal of this pattern.

5 Subjectivity of circadian parameters occurs with relation to the timing of peaks, and troughs, the degree of inclines and declines, and the timing of post-lunch dips and dead spots, according to an individual's genotype and their perception of environmental cues.

6 The hypothalamus appears to be the master clock synchronizing the free-running rhythms of the homeostatic control centres. There may also be a link with the pineal gland, since this is responsive to light/dark cues which are very important zeitgebers.

7 Health is associated with internal synchronization, i.e. all the circadian rhythms being within their homeostatic ranges.

8 Desynchronization occurs when the circadian rhythms are outside their homeostatic range; such a disturbance is known as a phase shift.

9 Phase shifts have been demonstrated in shift workers, people who travel across different time zones, during illnesses, and upon hospitalization.

10 Chronobiologists suggest compensatory changes are necessary to minimize the circadian disturbances. For example, with regard to:

(a) Shift work: shifts must be changed clockwise (i.e. morning to afternoon to evening, etc.). Longer intervals between changes must be introduced so that individuals have time to 'normalize' their patterns.

(b) The health care setting: chronopharmacology removes some adverse drug interactions and decreases the need for hospitalization, and consequently the person's exogenous cues are maintained. This involves dosages and timing of dosages being calculated using the circadian changes that are associated with the illness and the process of hospitalization. Finally, if the nurse is hoping to meet the total needs of the patient, she/he must take into account the effects of circadian rhythmicity on temporal, physiological, and psychological coordination when planning, assessing, implementing and evaluating care, and use this knowledge to aid a more speedy recovery.

Review Questions

1 Distinguish between circadian and circannual rhythms.

2 Distinguish between the following terms: synchronization, desynchronization, and resynchronization.

3 Describe the 'normal' circadian pattern of body temperature.

4 Discuss what is meant by circadian pattern subjectivity.

5 Circadian rhythms are said to be endogenously controlled and exogenously modified. What do you understand by this statement?

6 Discuss the suggested role of the hypothalamus in circadian rhythms.

7 Describe why shift work, travelling across different time zones, illness, and hospitalization are said to cause circadian rhythm desynchronization.

8 Suggest what interventionary schemes may be used to compensate for desynchronized rhythms associated with shift work.

9 Suggest why the elderly are more reliant upon exogenous time-givers for circadian rhythmicity.

10 What is the possible link between community care and circadian rhythm resynchronization?

Appendix

Units of measurement

INTERNATIONAL SYSTEM OF UNITS

The International System of Units (Système Internationale, or SI units) is a system of standard units used by the scientific, medical, and technical fraternity throughout most of the world. Most units used in this country are now SI units (e.g. grams, litres) but some imperial units (e.g. pounds, stones, pints, and gallons) are still in everyday usage.

The following are SI units for various parameters. Note that the basic SI unit for temperature is the Kelvin but the use of a Celsius scale is more practical for most measurements, since 0 Kelvin is –273°C!

Measurement	SI unit and symbol
Mass	gram (g)
Length	metre (m)
Volume	litre (l)
Temperature	degrees Kelvin (K) (or Celsius, °C)
Time	second (s)
Amount of substance	mole (mol)
Pressure	pascal (Pa)
Frequency	hertz (Hz)
Energy/heat	joule (J)
Radioactivity	becquerel (Bq)
Force	newton (N)
Electrical potential	volt (V)
Electric current	ampere (A)
Power	watt (W)

The following are some useful conversions from Imperial into SI units.

Lengths

Length	Metric equivalent
1 yard (yd)	0.9144 metre (m)
1 foot (ft)	0.31 metre (m)
1 inch (in)	2.54 centimetres (cm)
	25.4 millimetres (mm)

Metric length	Equivalent
1 metre (m)	100 centimetres (cm)
	1000 millimetres (mm)
	39.37 inches (in)
1 centimetre (cm)	10 millimetres (mm)
	0.39 inches (in)
1 millimetre (mm)	0.1 centimetre (cm)
	1000 micrometres (μm)
1 micrometre (μm)	1000 nanometres (nm)

Weights

Weights	Metric equivalent
1 pound (lb)	373 grams (g)
	373 000 milligrams (mg)
1 ounce (oz)	31.1 grams (g)
	31 000 milligrams (mg)

Metric weight	Equivalent
1 kilogram (kg)	1000 grams (g)
	1000 000 milligrams (mg)
	1000 000 000 micrograms (μg)
	32 ounces (oz)
	2.7 pounds (lb)
1 gram (g)	1000 milligrams (mg)
	1000 000 micrograms (μg)
1 milligram (mg)	1000 micrograms (μg)

Volumes

Volume	Metric equivalent
1 fluid ounce (fl oz)	29.6 millilitres (ml)
	29.6 cubic centimetres (cm³)
1 pint (pt)	473 millilitres (ml)
	473 cubic centimetres (cm³)

Metric volume	Equivalent
1 litre (l)	1000 millilitres (ml)
	1000 cubic centimetres (cm³)
	2.1 pints (pt)
1 millilitre (ml)	1 cubic centimetre (cm³)

FACTORS, PREFIXES AND SYMBOLS FOR DECIMAL MULTIPLES

Factor	Prefix	Symbol
10^6	mega	M
10^3	kilo	k
10^2	hecto	h
10^1	deca	da
10^{-1}	deci	d
10^{-2}	centi	c
10^{-3}	milli	m
10^{-6}	micro	µ
10^{-9}	nano	n
10^{-12}	pico	p

UNITS OF CONCENTRATION, PRESSURE AND OSMOTIC PRESSURE

Substance concentration, the pressure of a gas or fluid, and the osmotic pressure of a fluid, are important measurements in physiology and it is worthwhile considering the units used in more detail.

Units of concentration

The concentrations of substances in body fluids and urine may be expressed as grams or milligrams per unit volume, for example grams per litre (written as g/1). Although widely used, such units are of limited use in considering chemical activities because they give no indication of the concentration of atoms or molecules present. Atoms of different elements are of different size and mass and so the number of atoms in, say, a milligram will vary between substances. The SI unit of concentration is called the mole, and 1 mole of an element will contain 6.02×10^{23} atoms (called Avogadro's number); if the substance consists of molecules then a mole of the substance will contain that number of molecules. A mole of atoms or molecules is also equal to the atomic, or molecular, weight of the substance.

Consider glucose (chemical formula $C_6H_{12}O_6$):

$$\begin{array}{ccc} 1 \text{ mole} & & 180 \text{ g} \\ \text{of} & = & \text{of} \qquad (= \text{its molecular weight}) \\ \text{glucose} & & \text{glucose} \end{array}$$

made up of 6 moles of carbon atoms

$6 \times$ atomic weight of carbon = $(6 \times 12 = 72 \text{ g})$
12 moles of hydrogen atoms $\quad (12 \times 1 = 12 \text{ g})$
and 6 moles of oxygen atoms $\quad (6 \times 16 = 96 \text{ g})$

$$\overline{\qquad 180 \text{ g}}$$

(Note that hydrogen is the atomic 'standard', i.e. 1 mole weighs 1 g.)

A molar solution of a substance contains 1 mole of it per litre of solution (usually dissolved in water). A molar solution of glucose, therefore, will contain 180 g of glucose per litre. This is actually a very high concentration, far higher than is found in body fluids. The concentrations of substances in physiological fluids are usually given in millimoles (1 mmol = 1 mole $\times 10^{-3}$) or micromole (1 µmol = 1 mole $\times 10^{-6}$). Some biochemicals are of even lower concentrations and are measured in nanomoles (1 nmol = 1 mole $\times 10^{-9}$) or even picomoles (1 pmol = 1 mole $\times 10^{-12}$).

Sometimes the concentration of a hormone or an enzyme is recorded in Units or milliUnits per millilitre. In this case, the unit relates to the biological activity of the substance, with 1 milliUnit producing a known, quantified physiological response.

Units of pressure

Fluids are non-compressible. Gases, however, can be compressed into a smaller volume or expanded into a larger one. Such compressions and expansions alter the concentration of gas molecules as the same number of molecules are now contained in different volumes. Pressure is a measure of the interactions made between gas molecules and the surface of its container or chamber – the greater the concentration of a gas, the more interactions there will be per unit time. Traditionally, pressure was measured by observing how high mercury would rise up a thin tube as a consequence of collisions between gas molecules and the surface of the pool of mercury in which the tube stood. At sea level, standard air pressure is 760 mm of mercury (written as 760 mmHg; the symbol for mercury is Hg).

The SI unit for pressure is the pascal (Pa) although mmHg (or even mmH_2O for low pressure; water has a lower density than mercury) is still used for many parameters, such as blood pressure (note that pressure also applies to fluids within enclosed chambers, such as blood vessels). The pressures of respiratory gases are usually given in kilopascals (kPa) and 1 kPa approximates to 7.6 mmHg. For example, the pressure of oxygen in the alveoli after inspiration is 13.3 kPa (equivalent to about 100 mmHg).

Units of osmotic pressure (osmolarity)

The direct measurement of osmotic pressure of a solution is difficult when dealing with small samples of body fluid. However, osmotic pressure is directly related to the concentration of solute in the solution. A convenient means of measuring the total concentration of solute, and therefore its osmotic potential, is to measure how much the freezing point of the solvent (i.e. water) has been depressed by the solute. Body fluids contain a variety of substances and the unit of concentration of solute used is the osmole, to distinguish it from the mole unit for the concentrations of individual substances present. Physiological fluids are normally in the milliosmole range, for example plasma has an osmolarity of about 285 mosmol per litre. The higher the osmolar concentration, the greater the osmotic potential of the fluid.

B # Appendix

Blood, plasma, or serum values

Test	Normal values*	Significance of change
Bicarbonate	22–26 mmol/l	↑in metabolic alkalosis ↑in respiratory alkalosis ↓in metabolic acidosis
Blood urea nitrogen (BUN)	5–25 mg/dl	↑with increased protein intake ↓in kidney failure
Blood volume	*Women*: 65 ml/kg body weight *Men*: 69 ml/kg body weight	↓during a haemorrhage
Calcium	8.4–10.5 mg/dl	↑in hypervitaminosis D ↑in hyperparathyroidism ↑in bone cancer and other bone diseases ↓in severe diarrhoea ↓in hypoparathyroidism ↓in avitaminosis D (rickets and osteomalacia)
Chloride	96–107 mmol/l	↑in hyperventilation ↑in kidney disease ↑in Cushing's syndrome ↓in diabetic acidosis ↓in severe diarrhoea ↓in severe burns ↓in Addison's disease
Clotting time	5–10 minutes	↓in haemophilia ↓(occasionally) in other clotting disorders
Creatine phosphokinase (CPK)	*Women*: 0–14 IU/l *Men*: 0–20 IU/l	↑in Duchenne muscular dystrophy ↑during myocardial infarction ↑in muscle trauma
Glucose	70–110 mg/dl (fasting) (4–6 mmol/l approx.)	↑in diabetes mellitus ↑in liver disease ↑during pregnancy ↑in hyperthyroidism ↓in hypothyroidism ↓in Addison's disease ↓in hyperinsulinism
Haematocrit (packed cell volume)	*Women*: 38–47% *Men*: 40–54%	↑in polycythaemia ↑in severe dehydration ↓in anaemia ↓in leukaemia ↓in hyperthyroidism ↓in cirrhosis of liver

Haemoglobin	Women: 12–16 g/dl Men: 13–18 g/dl Newborn: 14–20 g/dl	↑in polycythaemia ↑in chronic obstructive pulmonary disease ↑in congestive heart failure ↓in anaemia ↓in hyperthyroidism ↓in cirrhosis of liver
Iron	50–150 μg/dl (can be higher in male)	↑in liver disease ↑in anaemia (some forms) ↓in iron-deficiency anaemia
Lactate dehydrogenase isoenzymes (LDH$_{1-5}$)	60–120 u/ml	↑during myocardial infarction ↑in anaemia (several forms) ↑in liver disease ↑in acute leukaemia and other cancers

Lipids – total
  Cholesterol – total
    High-density
      lipoprotein (HDL)
    Low-density
      lipoprotein (LDL)
	450–1000 mg/dl
	120–220 mg/dl
	
	>40 mg/dl
	
	<180 mg/dl
		↑(total) in diabetes mellitus
		↑(total) in kidney disease
		↑(total) in hypothyroidism
		↓(total) in hyperthyroidism
		↑in inherited hypercholesterolaemia
		↑(cholesterol) in chronic hepatitis
		↓(cholesterol) in acute hepatitis
		↑(HDL) with regular exercise

Mean corpuscular volume	82–98 μl	↑or↓in various forms of anaemia
Osmolality	285–295 mosmol/l	↑or↓in fluid and electrolyte imbalances
PCO$_2$	35–43 mmHg (4.6–5.7 kPa)	↑in severe vomiting ↑in respiratory disorders ↑in obstruction of intestines ↓in acidosis ↓in severe diarrhoea ↓in kidney disease
pH	7.35–7.45	↑during hyperventilation ↑in Cushing's syndrome ↓during hypoventilation ↓in acidosis ↓in Addison's disease
Plasma volume	Women: 40 ml/kg body weight Men: 39 ml/kg body weight	↑or↓in fluid and electrolyte imbalances ↓during haemorrhage
Platelet count	150 000–400 000/mm³	↑in heart disease ↑in cancer ↑in cirrhosis of liver ↑after trauma ↓in anaemia (some forms) ↓during chemotherapy ↓in some allergies
PO$_2$	75–100 mmHg (breathing standard air) (10–13.3 kPa)	↑in polycythaemia ↓in anaemia ↓in chronic obstructive pulmonary disease
Potassium	3.8–5.1 mmol/l	↑in hypoaldosteronism ↑in acute kidney failure ↓in vomiting or diarrhoea ↓in starvation
Protein – total Albumin	6–8.4 g/dl 3.5–5 g/dl	↑(total) in severe dehydration ↓(total) during haemorrhage

Globulin	2.3–3.5 g/dl	↓(total) in starvation
Red blood cell count	*Women*: 4.2–5.4 million/mm³ *Men*: 4.5–6.2 million/mm³	↑in polycythaemia ↑in dehydration ↓in anaemia (several forms) ↓in Addison's disease ↓in systemic lupus erythematosus
Reticulocyte count	25 000–75 000/mm³ (0.5–1.5% of RBC count)	↑in haemolytic anaemia ↑in leukaemia and metastatic carcinoma ↓in pernicious anaemia ↓in iron-deficiency anaemia ↓during radiation therapy
Sodium	136–145 mmol/l	↑in dehydration ↑in trauma or disease of the central nervous system ↑or↓in kidney disorders ↓in excessive sweating, vomiting, diarrhoea ↓in burns (sodium shift into cells)
Transaminase	10–40 u/ml	↑during myocardial infarction ↑in liver disease
Viscosity	1.4–1.8 times the viscosity of water	↑in polycythaemia ↑in dehydration

White blood cell count
  Total
  Neutrophils
  Eosinophils
  Basophils
  Lymphocytes
  Monocytes
	
	4500–11 000/mm³
	60–70% of total
	2–4% of total
	0.5–1% of total
	20–25% of total
	3–8% of total
		↑(total) in acute infections
		↑(total) in trauma
		↑(total) some cancers
		↓(total) in anaemia (some forms)
		↓(total) during chemotherapy
		↑(neutrophils) in acute infection
		↑(eosinophils) in allergies
		↓(basophil) in severe allergies
		↑(lymphocyte) during antibody reactions
		↑(monocyte) in chronic infections

*Values vary with the analysis method used and between individuals.
1 dl = 100 ml.

Urine components

Test	Normal values*	Significance of change
Routine urinalysis		
Acetone and acetoacetate	None	↑during fasting ↑in diabetic acidosis
Albumin	None to trace	↑in hypertension ↑in kidney disease ↑after strenuous exercise (temporary)
Calcium	<150 mg/day	↑in hyperparathyroidism ↓in hypoparathyroidism
Colour	Transparent yellow, straw-coloured, or amber	Abnormal colour or cloudiness may indicate: blood in urine, bile, bacteria, drugs, food pigments, or high solute concentration
Odour	Characteristics slight odour	Acetone odour in diabetes mellitus (diabetic ketosis)
Osmolality	500–800 mosmol/l	↑in dehydration ↑in heart failure ↓in diabetes insipidus ↓in aldosteronism
pH	4.6–8.0	↑in alkalosis ↑during urinary infections ↓in dehydration ↓in emphysema
Potassium	25–100 mmol/l	↑dehydration ↑in chronic kidney failure ↓in diarrhoea or vomiting ↓in adrenal insufficiency
Sodium	75–200 mg/day	↑in starvation ↑in dehydration ↓acute kidney failure ↓in Cushing's syndrome
Creatinine clearance	100–140 ml/min	↑in kidney disease
Glucose	0	↑in diabetes mellitus ↑in hyperthyroidism ↑in hypersecretion of adrenal cortex
Urea clearance Urea	>40 ml blood cleared per min 25–35 g/day	↑in some kidney diseases ↑in some liver diseases ↑in haemolytic anaemia ↓during obstruction of bile ducts ↓in severe diarrhoea
Microscopic examination		
Bacteria	<10 000/ml	↑during urinary infections
Blood cells (RBC)	0–trace	↑in pyelonephritis ↑from damage by calculi ↑in infection ↑in cancer
Blood cells (WBC)	0–trace	↑in infections

Appendix

WORD PARTS COMMONLY USED AS PREFIXES

Word part	Meaning	Example	Meaning of example
a-	Without, not	Apnoea	Cessation of breathing
af-	Toward	Afferent	Carrying toward
an-	Without, not	Anuria	Absence of urination
ante-	Before	Antenatal	Before birth
anti-	Against, resisting	Antibody	Unit that resists foreign substances
auto-	Self	Autoimmunity	Self-immunity
bi-	Two; double	Bicuspid	Two-pointed
circum-	Around	Circumcision	Cutting around
co-, con-	With; together	Congenital	Born with
contra-	Against	Contraceptive	Against conception
de-	Down from, undoing	Defibrillation	Stop fibrillation
dia-	Across, through	Diarrhoea	Flow through (intestine)
dipl-	Twofold, double	Diploid	Two sets of chromosomes
dys-	Bad; disordered; difficult	Dysplasia	Disordered growth
ectop-	Displaced	Ectopic pregnancy	Displaced pregnancy
ef-	Away from	Efferent	Carrying away from
endo-	Within	Endocarditis	Inflammation of heart lining
epi-	Upon	Epimysium	Covering of a muscle
ex-, exo-	Out of, out from	Exophthalmos	Protruding eyes
extra-	Outside of	Extraperitoneal	Outside of peritoneum
eu-	Good	Eupnoea	Good (normal) breathing
hapl-	Single	Haploid	Single set of chromosomes
Haem-, haemat-	Blood	Haematuria	Bloody urine
hemi-	Half	Hemiplegia	Paralysis in half the body
Hom(e)o-	Same; equal	Homeostasis	Standing the same
hyper-	Over; above	Hyperplasia	Excessive growth
hypo-	Under; below	Hypodermic	Below the skin
infra-	Below, beneath	Infraorbital	Below the (eye) orbit
inter-	Between	Intervertebral	between vertebrae
intra-	Within	Intracranial	Within the skull
iso-	Same, equal	Isometric	Same length
macro-	Large	Macrophage	Large eater (phagocyte)
mes-	Middle	Mesentery	Middle of intestine
micro-	Small; millionth	Microcytic	Small-celled
milli-	Thousandth	Millilitre	Thousandth of a litre
mono-	One (single)	Monosomy	Single chromosome
non-	Not	Non-dysjunction	Not disjoined
para-	By the side of; near	Parathyroid	Near the thyroid
per-	Through	Permeable	Able to go through
peri-	Around; surrounding	Pericardium	Covering of the heart
poly-	Many	Polycythaemia	Condition of many blood cells
post-	After	Postmortem	After death
pre-	Before	Premenstrual	Before menstruation

pro-	First; promoting	Progesterone	Hormone that promotes pregnancy
quadr-	Four	Quadriplegia	Paralysis in four limbs
re-	Back again	Reflux	Backflow
retro-	Behind	Retroperitoneal	Behind the peritoneum
semi-	Half	Semilunar	Half-moon
sub-	Under	Subcutaneous	Under the skin
super-, supra-	Over, above, excessive	Superior	Above
trans-	Across; through	Transcutaneous	Through the skin
tri-	Three; triple	Triplegia	Paralysis of three limbs

WORD PARTS COMMONLY USED AS SUFFIXES

Word part	Meaning	Example	Meaning of example
-aemia	Refers to blood condition	Hypercholesterolaemia	High blood cholesterol level
-al, -ac	Pertaining to	Intestinal	Pertaining to the intestines
-algia	Pain	Neuralgia	Nerve pain
-aps, -apt	Fit; fasten	Synapse	Fasten together
-arche	Beginning; origin	Menarche	First menstruation
-ase	Signifies an enzyme	Lipase	Enzyme that acts on lipids
-blast	Sprout; make	Osteoblast	Bone maker
-centesis	A piercing	Amniocentesis	Piercing the amniotic sac
-cide	To kill	Fungicide	Fungus killer
-clast	Break; destroy	Osteoclast	Bone breaker
-crine	Release; secrete	Endocrine	Secrete within
-ectomy	A cutting out	Appendectomy	Removal of the appendix
-emesis	Vomiting	Haematemesis	Vomiting blood
-gen	Creates; forms	Lactogen	Milk producer
-genesis	Creation, production	Oogenesis	Egg production
-graph(y)	To write, draw	Electrocardiograph	Apparatus that records heart's electrical activity
-hydrate	Containing H_2O (water)	Dehydration	Loss of water
-ia, -sia	Condition; process	Arthralgia	Condition of joint pain
-iasis	Abnormal condition	Giardiasis	*Giardia* infestation
-ic, -ac	Pertaining to	Cardiac	Pertaining to the heart
-in	Signifies a protein	Renin	Kidney protein
-ism	Signifies 'condition of'	Gigantism	Condition of gigantic size
-itis	Signifies 'inflammation of'	Gastritis	Stomach inflammation
-lepsy	Seizure	Epilepsy	Seizure upon seizure
-logy	Study of	Cardiology	Study of the heart
-lunar	Moon; moon-like	Semilunar	Half-moon
-malacia	Softening	Osteomalacia	Bone softening
-megaly	Enlargement	Splenomegaly	Spleen enlargement
-metric, -metry	Measurement, length	Isometric	Same length
-oma	Tumour	Lipoma	Fatty tumour
-opia	Vision, vision condition	Myopia	Nearsightedness
-ose	Signifies a carbohydrate (especially sugar)	Lactose	Milk sugar
-osis	Condition, process	Dermatosis	Skin condition
-oscopy	Viewing	Laparoscopy	Viewing the abdominal cavity
-ostomy	Formation of an opening	Tracheostomy	Forming an opening in the trachea
-otomy	Cut	Lobotomy	Cut of a lobe
-philic	Loving	Hydrophilic	Water-loving
-penia	Lack	Leucopenia	Lack of white (cells)
-phobic	Fearing	Hydrophobic	Water-fearing
-plasia	Growth, formation	Hyperplasia	Excessive growth

-plasm	Substance, matter	Neoplasm	New matter
-plegia	Paralysis	Triplegia	Paralysis in three limbs
-pnoea	Breath, breathing	Apnoea	Cessation of breathing
-(r)rhage, -(r)rhagia	Breaking out, discharge	Haemorrhage	Blood discharge
-(r)rhoea	Flow	Diarrhoea	Flow through (intestines)
-some	Body	Chromosome	Stained body
-tensin, -tension	Pressure	Hypertension	High pressure
-tonic	Pressure, tension	Isotonic	Same pressure
-uria	Refers to urine condition	Proteinuria	Protein in the urine

WORD PARTS COMMONLY USED AS ROOTS

Word part	Meaning	Example	Meaning of example
acro-	Extremity	Acromegaly	Enlargement of extremities
aden-	Gland	Adenoma	Tumour of glandular tissue
aesthe-	Sensation	Anaesthesia	Condition of no sensation
alveol-	Small, hollow, cavity	Alveolus	Small air sac in the lung
angi-	Vessel	Angioplasty	Reshaping a vessel
arthr-	Joint	Arthritis	Joint inflammation
bar-	Pressure	Baroreceptor	Pressure receptor
bili-	Bile	Bilirubin	Orange-yellow bile pigment
brachi-	Arm	Brachial	Pertaining to the arm
brady-	Slow	Bradycardia	Slow heart rate
bronch-	Air passage	Bronchitis	Inflammation of pulmonary passages (bronchi)
calc-	Calcium; limestone	Hypocalcaemia	Low blood calcium level
carcin-	Cancer	Carcinogen	Cancer-producer
card-	Heart	Cardiology	Study of the heart
cephal-	Head, brain	Encephalitis	Brain inflammation
cerv-	Neck	Cervicitis	Inflammation of (uterine) cervix
chem-	Chemical	Chemotherapy	Chemical treatment
chol-	Bile	Cholecystectomy	Removal of bile (gall) bladder
chondr-	Cartilage	Chondroma	Tumour of cartilage tissue
chrom-	Colour	Chromosome	Stained body
corp-	Body	Corpus luteum	Yellow body
cortico-	Pertaining to cortex	Corticosteroid	Steroid secreted by (adrenal) cortex
crani-	Skull	Intracranial	Within the skull
crypt-	Hidden	Cryptorchidism	Undescended testis
cusp-	Point	Tricuspid	Three-pointed
cut(an)-	Skin	Transcutaneous	Through the skin
cyan-	Blue	Cyanosis	Condition of blueness
cyst-	Bladder	Cystitis	Bladder inflammation
cyt-	Cell	Cytotoxin	Cell poison
dactyl-	Fingers, toes (digits)	Syndactyly	Joined digits
dendr-	Tree; branched	Oligodendrocyte	Branched nervous tissue cell
derm-	Skin	Dermatitis	Skin inflammation
diastol-	Relax; stand apart	Diastole	Relaxation phase of heart beat
ejacul-	To throw out	Ejaculation	Expulsion (of semen)
electr-	Electrical	Electrocardiogram	Record of electrical activity of heart
enter-	Intestine	Enteritis	Intestinal inflammation
eryth(r)-	Red	Erythrocyte	Red (blood) cell
gastr-	Stomach	Gastritis	Stomach inflammation
gest-	To bear, carry	Gestation	Pregnancy
gingiv-	Gums	Gingivitis	Gum inflammation
glomer-	Wound into a ball	Glomerulus	Rounded tuft of vessels

gloss-	Tongue	Hypoglossal	Under the tongue
gluc-	Glucose, sugar	Glucosuria	Glucose in urine
glyc-	Sugar (carbohydrate); glucose	Glycolipid	Carbohydrate–lipid combination
hepat-	Liver	Hepatitis	Liver inflammation
hist-	Tissue	Histology	Study of tissues
hydro-	Water	Hydrocephalus	Water on the brain
hyster-	Uterus	Hysterectomy	Removal of the uterus
kal-	Potassium	Hyperkalaemia	Elevated blood potassium level
kary-	Nucleus	Karyotype	Array of chromosomes from nucleus
lact-	Milk; milk production	Lactose	Milk sugar
leuc-	White	Leucorrhoea	White flow (discharge)
lig-	To tie, bind	Ligament	Tissue that binds bones
lip-	Lipid (fat)	Lipoma	Fatty tumour
lys-	Break apart	Haemolysis	Breaking of blood cells
mal-	Bad	Malabsorption	Improper absorption
melan-	Black	Melanin	Black protein
men-, mens-, (menstru-)	Month (monthly)	Amenorrhoea	Absence of monthly flow
metr-	Uterus	Endometrium	Uterine lining
muta-	Change	Mutagen	Change-maker
my-, myo-	Muscle	Myopathy	Muscle disease
myel-	Marrow	Myeloma	(Bone) marrow tumour
myx-	Mucus	Myxoedema	Mucous oedema
nat-	Birth	Neonatal	Pertaining to newborns (infants)
natr-	Sodium	Natriuresis	Elevated sodium in urine
nephr-	Nephron, kidney	Nephritis	Kidney inflammation
neur-	Nerve	Neuralgia	Nerve pain
noct-, nyct-	Night	Nocturia	Urination at night
ocul-	Eye	Binocular	Two-eyed
odont-	Tooth	Periodonitis	Inflammation (of tissue) around the teeth
onco-	Cancer	Oncogene	Cancer gene
ophthalm-	Eye	Ophthalmology	Study of the eye
osteo-	Bone	Osteoma	Bone tumour
oto-	Ear	Otosclerosis	Hardening of ear tissue
ov-, oo-	Egg	Oogenesis	Egg production
oxy-	Oxygen	Oxyhaemoglobin	Oxygen–haemoglobin combination
path-	Disease	Neuropathy	Nerve disease
phag-	Eat	Phagocytosis	cell eating
pharm-	drug	Pharmacology	Study of drugs
photo-	Light	Photopigment	Light-sensitive pigment
physio-	Nature (function) of	Physiology	Study of biological function
pino-	Drink	Pinocytosis	Cell drinking
plex-	Twisted; woven	Nerve plexus	Complex of interwoven nerve fibres
pneumo-	Air, breath	Pneumothorax	Air in the thorax
pneumon-	Lung	Pneumonia	Lung condition
pod-	Foot	Podocyte	Cell with feet
poie-	Make; produce	Haemopoiesis	Blood cell production
presby-	Old	Presbyopia	Old vision
proct-	Rectum	Proctoscope	Instrument for viewing the rectum
pseud-	False	Pseudopodia	False feet
psych-	Mind	Psychiatry	Treatment of the mind
pyel-	Pelvis	Pyelogram	Image of the kidney pelvis
pyro-	Heat; fever	Pyrogen	Fever producer
ren-	Kidney	Renocortical	Referring to the cortex of the kidney
sarco-	Flesh; muscle	Sarcolemma	Muscle fibre membrane
semen-, semin-	Seed; sperm	Seminiferous tubule	Sperm-bearing tubule

sept-	Contamination	Septicaemia	Contamination of the blood
sigm-	Greek Σ or Roman S	Sigmoid colon	S-shaped colon
son-	Sound	Sonography	Imaging using sound
spiro-, -spire	Breathe	Spirometry	Measurement of breathing
stat-, stas-	A standing, stopping	Homeostasis	Staying the same
syn-	Together	Syndrome	Sings appearing together
systol-	Contract; stand together	Systole	Contraction phase of the heart beat
tachy-	Fast	Tachycardia	Rapid heart rate
therm-	Heat	Thermoreceptor	Heat receptor
thromb-	Clot	Thrombosis	Condition of abnormal blood clotting
tox-	Poison	Cytotoxin	Cell poison
troph-	Grow; nourish	Hypertrophy	Excessive growth
tympan-	Drum	Tympanum	Eardrum
varic-	Enlarged vessel	Varicose vein	Enlarged vein
vas-	Vessel, duct	Vasoconstriction	Vessel narrowing
vol-	Volume	Hypovolaemic	Characterized by low volume

* Tables in Appendix C are reproduced, with permission from Thibeaudeau, G.A. and Patton, K.T. (1992). *The human body in health and disease*. St Louis: Mosby.

* A term ending in -*graph* refers to apparatus that results in a visual and/or recorded representation of biological phenomena, whereas a term ending in -*graphy* is the technique or process of using the apparatus. A term ending in -*gram* is the record itself. Example: In electrocardio*graphy*, an electrocardio*graph* is used in producing an electrocardio*gram*.

Appendix

Symbols and abbreviations

Many medical terms are commonly expressed in abbreviated form. The following list is designed to familiarize you with some of these abbreviations. Most of the terms have been used in the book however some are included because they are frequently used.

SYMBOLS

♀, O	female
♂,	male
∞	infinity
α	alpha
β	beta
γ	gamma

ABBREVIATIONS

Ab	antibody; abortion
ACTH	adrenocorticotropic hormone
ADH	antidiuretic hormone
Ag	antigen
AIDS	acquired immune deficiency syndrome
ANS	autonomic nervous system
ARD	acute respiratory system
ARF	acute renal failure
ATP	adenosine triphosphate
AV	atrioventricular
BBB	blood–brain barrier; bundle branch block
BBT	basal body temperature
BMR	basal metabolic rate
BP	blood pressure
BPM	beats per minute
BS	blood sugar
C	Celsius
CABG	coronary artery bypass grafting
CAD	coronary artery disease
CCU	cardiac care unit; coronary care unit
CF	cystic fibrosis; cardiac failure
CH	cholesterol
CHF	congestive heart failure
CNS	central nervous system
CO	cardiac output; carbon monoxide
COAD	chronic obstructive airways disease

CSF	cerebrospinal fluid
CVA	cerebrovascular accident
CVD	cardiovascular disease
CVS	chorionic villus sampling
DBP	diastolic blood pressure
DNA	deoxyribonucleic acid
DVT	deep venous thrombosis
ECF	extracellular fluid
ECG	electrocardiogram
EEG	electroencephalogram
EM	electron micrograph
EMG	electromyogram
EPSP	excitatory post-synaptic potential
ER	endoplasmic reticulum
ESR	erythrocyte sedimentation rate
ESV	end-systolic volume
F	Fahrenheit
FAS	fetal alcohol syndrome
FSH	follicle-stimulating hormone
GAS	general adaptation syndrome
GFR	glomerular filtration rate
GI	gastrointestinal
GIFT	gamete intrafallopian transfer
Hb	haemoglobin
hCG	human chorionic gonadotropin
Hct	haematocrit

HDL	high-density lipoprotein	PMS	premenstrual syndrome
HDN	haemolytic disease of newborn	PNS	peripheral nervous system
HF	heart failure	PRL	prolactin
hGH	human growth hormone	PROG	progesterone
HR	heart rate	PTH	parathyroid hormone
HSV	herpes simplex virus	RBC	red blood cell; red blood count
ICF	intracellular fluid	RDS	respiratory distress syndrome
Ig	immunoglobin	REM	rapid eye movement
IPSP	inhibitory post-synaptic potential	Rh	rhesus
IUD	intrauterine device	RNA	ribonucleic acid
i.v.	intravenous	RR	respiratory rate
IVC	inferior vena cava	RRR	regular rate and rhythm (heart)
IVF	*in vitro* fertilization	SA	sinoatrial
KS	Kaposi's sarcoma	SBP	systolic blood pressure
kPa	kilopascal	SCA	sickle cell anaemia
LDL	low-density lipoprotein	SCD	sudden cardiac death
LH	luteinizing hormone	SCID	severe combined immunodeficiency syndrome
mEq/l	milliequivalents per litre	SIDS	sudden infant death syndrome
MI	myocardial infarction	SNS	somatic nervous system
mm³	cubic millimetre	STD	sexually transmitted disease
mmHg	millimetres of mercury	SV	stroke volume
MS	multiple sclerosis	SVC	superior vena cava
MSH	melanocyte-stimulating hormone	T	temperature
NSAID	non-steroidal anti-inflammatory drug	TB	tuberculosis
NTP	normal temperature and pressure	TIA	transient ischaemic attack
OD	overdose	TPR	temperature, pulse, and respiration
OT	oxytocin	TSH	thyroid-stimulating hormone
P	pressure	URI	upper respiratory infection
PCP	*Pneumocystis carinii* pneumonia	UTI	urinary tract infection
PCV	packed cell volume	UV	ultraviolet
PG	prostaglandin	VF	ventricular fibrillation
pH	hydrogen ion concentration	VS	vital signs
PKU	phenylketonuria	WBC	white blood cell; white blood count

Index

abbreviations 699–700
abducens nerve 378
Aβ fibres 617
abortion 553
ABO system 186–187, 199
    see also haemolytic disease of the
        newborn
abscesses 83
absorption
    nutrients 122
        intestine 145–149
        large intestine 150
    vs reabsorption 327
accessory muscles of respiration
    298, 299
accessory nerve 378
accessory optic nuclei 413–414
accessory organs, alimentary tract
    124
accessory sex glands
    female 536
    male 529–530
accidents, shift work 672, 673
accommodation (pupil) 411
    disorders 423
ACD, for blood samples 195
acetabulum 467
acetone, urine 693
acetylcholine 227, 367, 391
    memory 382
    myasthenia gravis 395
    neuromuscular junctions 501
acetylcholinesterase inhibitors 395
achilles tendon 471
acid-base regulation 342–343
acidosis, metabolic 158, 159
acid phosphatase, plasma levels
    172
acids 87–89
acinar cells, pancreas 139–140
acinar glands 69
acne 520–521
acoustic nerve 378, 419
acquired immunity 282–283

acquired immunodeficiency
    syndrome, *see* AIDS
acrosin 563
acrosomal caps, spermatozoa 541
actin 26, 77, 475, 476
action potentials 362–364, 394–395
    cardiac conduction system 212
active immunity
    artificial 283–284
    natural 282–283
active transport 17, 20–21
    intestinal absorption 149
acupuncture 617
adaptation
    vs coping in stress 652
    receptors 401–402
    shift work 672–673
    smell 422
    visual 412
adaptation energy (Selye) 648
adaptation stage, general
        adaptation syndrome 647–649
adaptive responses, immune 279
Addison's disease 249
    circadian rhythms 680
Aδ fibres 615, 616
adenohypophysis, *see* anterior
    pituitary gland
adenosine diphosphate 20, 56
adenosine triphosphate 20, 56–57
    intracellular hypoxia 34
    skeletal muscle contraction 476
adherence, phagocytes 268–269
adhesion, bacteria, prevention 274
adipocytes 28
adipose tissue 73, 515
admission to hospital, *see* hospital
    admission
adolescence, *see* puberty
adrenal genital syndrome 558
adrenal glands 444–446
    autonomic innervation 390
    cortex 433, 444–445
        hypertension 248

hydrocorticosteroids, circadian
    rhythms 662–663
medulla 433, 445–446
adrenaline 238, 391, 437, 445–446
    addiction 653
    glucose release 61, 435
    heart rate 227–228
    for hypersensitivity reactions
        289
    hypertension 650
adrenergic neurons 366
adrenocorticotropic hormone 432,
    444
    hypertension 248
    stress 281
adulthood 582–586
adult respiratory distress syndrome
    318
adverse drug reactions, elderly
    patients 680
aerobic metabolism, fatty acids and
    amino acids 59–60
aerobic respiration 9, 24
afferent neurons 76, 351
    autonomic nervous system 387
    gate control theory 616–617
agammaglobulinaemia 196
age
    and cancer 39
    cardiac function 228
    core temperature 518
ageing 33, 40, 582, 583–586, 648–649
    circadian rhythms 665, 677–678
        drugs 679–680
    melatonin release 666–667
    nocturia 662, 678
    nutrition 117
    onset 586
age pigment (lipofucin) 585
agglutination 274
agglutinins 274
    ABO system 185
    see also haemolytic disease of the
        newborn

agglutinogens 173
  blood groups 185
aggressive behaviours 383
agonists, muscle action 486
agranular endoplasmic reticulum
  23
agranulocytes 172, 174, 179,
  180–181
agranulopoiesis 181
AIDS 286–287, 553
  as adaptation disorder 656
AIDS-related complex 287
air, partial pressures of gases 305
air pressure, middle ear 416
airways 295–297
  ciliated epithelia 66
  resistance 298, 299, 317
alanine aminotransferase, plasma
  levels 172
alarm stage, general adaptation
  syndrome 647
albinism 508
albumins
  deficiency 196
  plasma 170, 171
  plasma levels 691
  urine 693
alcohol
  absorption 146–147
  birth weights 590
  cardiomyopathies 247
  cirrhosis 162
  haemophilia 196
aldosterone 239, 248, 339–340, 341,
  445
alimentary tract, see gastrointestinal
  tract
alkaline phosphatase, plasma levels
  172
alkaline solutions 88
alkalosis, metabolic 158
allantois 571–572
allergens 271, 287
allergy
  testing, circadian rhythms 681
  see also hypersensitivity reactions
allografts 290
alpha-adrenergic receptors 391
alpha-cells 139
alpha-fetoprotein, amniotic fluid
  590
alphaglobulins 170
altitude hypoxia 315
  polycythaemia 189, 191
  2,3-diphosphoglycerate 309
alveolar-capillary membranes 303
alveolar ducts 297
alveolar gases, analysis 303
alveolar ventilation 301
alveoli (breasts) 538
alveoli (lungs) 297, 299–300
amenorrhoea 556, 558
amino acids 55, 104–105
  absorption 147

and fatty acids, aerobic
  metabolism 59–60
genetic codes 30, 32
from haemoglobin breakdown
  178
and hunger 122
metabolism 153
milk feeding 116
size 12
aminoexopeptidases 132
aminopeptidases, alimentary 142
ammonia 154
amniocentesis 608
amnion 571
amniotic fluid 571
  alpha-fetoprotein 590
amphetamine abuse 381
amplification, second messenger
  systems 435
amplifier T-cells 277
ampulla (Fallopian tube) 534
ampulla (vestibular apparatus) 404,
  488
amygdala 372, 381
amylase
  pancreas 142, 143
  plasma levels 172
  saliva 131, 142
anabolism 48, 49
anaemia 118, 189–190
  haemolytic disease of the
    newborn 198
  renal failure 344
  tongue 156
  see also pernicious anaemia
anaemic hypoxia 316
anaerobic metabolism, glucose 60
anaerobic respiration, erythrocytes
  176
anaesthetic agents, on fetus 589
anal canal 150, 151
analgesics 620–622
anamnestic responses 279, 280
anaphylaxis 250, 287–288, 289
anastomoses
  arterial, arteriovenous 218, 516
anatomical dead space 300–301
androgen-binding protein 527–529,
  543
androgens 433
  adrenal 445
  on fetus 589
  testicular 446
aneurysms, atherosclerotic 252
angina pectoris 252–253, 615, 656
  glyceryl trinitrate 146
angiotensin-converting enzyme 239
angiotensinogen 155, 239, 445
angiotensins 239, 247, 445
anions 15, 16, 47, 87
ankle joint 482
ankylosing spondylitis 500
anorexia nervosa 119, 579
  puberty 581

antagonists, muscle action 486
anterior cerebral artery 359
  CVA 394
anterior corticospinal tract 498
anterior pituitary gland 440–441
  hormones 432
  portal system 221
anterior spinothalamic tracts 407
antibiotics
  antigenicity 272
  on colonic bacteria 150
antibodies 170, 270, 272–274,
  278–279
  fetus 280
  IgE 180
  maternal 257–258, 280, 282, 577
  monoclonal 282
antibody-antigen complexes 289
anticoagulants 195
anticodons 33
anti-D agglutinins 187, 198
antidiuretic hormone 239, 338–339,
  432, 437, 441
  hypertension 248
antigenic determinant sites 272
antigen-presenting cells 274–275
antigens 267, 271–272
  blood groups 185
  erythrocytes 173
  lymph nodes 260–261
antihaemophilic factor (factor VIII)
  184, 188
antihistamines, on fetus 589
anti-hypertensive therapy 248
anti-sera 284
  tetanus 170
antitoxins 273
anus, see anal canal
anxiety 638
  pain 619, 625
aorta 208, 221
aortic pressure, coronary blood
  flow 210
aortic valve 206, 224
apex, cardiac 203
apical membranes, epithelia 147
apneustic centre 312, 377
apocrine glands 69, 511
aponeuroses 471
appendicular skeleton 464–468
appendix 149
  histology 126
appetite 117
  for salt 117, 420
appositional growth, cartilage
  73–74
aqueduct, cerebral 373
aqueous humour 408
  glaucoma 425
arachidonic acid 105
arachnoid mater 379–380
arachnoid villi 380
ARC (AIDS-related complex) 287
arches, foot 484

arcuate fasciculus 382
areola 538
areolar connective tissue 72
argentaffine cells, gastric glands
    138
argon atom 45
arm, bones 465
arousal, brain activity 381
arousal (sexual), see sexual act;
    sexual stimulation
arrector muscles 509, 514
arrhythmias 212, 213
arterial anastomoses 218
arterial baroreceptors 237
arterial disease, peripheral,
    circadian rhythms 677
arterial pressure, systemic, see
    blood pressure
arterial thrombosis 195
arterial-venous anastomoses, skin
    218, 516
arteries 214–216
    layout (fig.) 222
arterioles 216, 232
arteriosclerosis 216, 250–252
arthroplasty 500
Arthus reactions 289
artificial immunity
    active 283–284
    passive 284
ascending neurons (tracts), spinal
    cord 354, 384, 407
ascites 99
ascorbic acid, see vitamin C
aspartate aminotransferase, plasma
    levels 172
aspirin 621
    capillary fragility 194
    enteric coated 157
    fetus 589
    stomach 156–157
assimilation 122, 153–154
asthma 317
    circadian rhythms 681
astigmatism 423
astrocytes 355
atherosclerosis 250–252
    diabetes mellitus 650
    shift work 672
athletes, cardiac function 228, 245
athletic build, puberty 581
atlas 460–463
atomic mass 44–45
atomic number 44
atoms 44–47
    size 12
ATP, see adenosine triphosphate
atria 205, 208
    atrophy, ECG 213
    baroreceptors 237
    systole 226
atrial natriuretic factor 239, 339,
    340, 449
atrial reflex 227

atrioventricular bundle 210, 211
atrioventricular node 211, 225
    autorhythmicity 212
atrioventricular valves 205–206
    see also mitral valve
audiograms 418–419
auditory meatus 416
auditory nerve 378, 419
auditory pathways 382
auditory tube (Eustachian tube) 416
Auerbach's plexus 126
autocrine secretions 430
autografts 290
autoimmune diseases 271, 289–290
    hormone hypersecretion 450
    rheumatoid disease 290, 500
autolysis 24, 269
autonomic nerves 350
    vs somatic nerves 392
autonomic nervous system 386–391
    heart 213, 227
autoregulation
    arterioles 216
    kidneys 328
autorhythmicity 212
autosomal inheritance
    dominant 603
    recessive 601–603
autosomes 595
AV block (heart block) 212
Avogadro's number 688
AV shunts, see arterial-venous
    anastomoses
awakening policies, hospital wards
    678
axial skeleton 457–464
axis 463
axons 353
    conduction velocity 364
axoplasm 365

bacteria
    adhesion, prevention 274
    colon 150, 194
    infections, skin damage 265
    size 12
    toxins, neutralization 273
    urine 693
Bainbridge reflex 227
balance, sense 404–405, 488
ball and socket joints 470
baroreceptors 237, 441
barrier methods, birth control 552
Bartholin's glands (vestibular
    glands) 536
basal bodies, flagella 26
basal ganglia 372, 497
basal metabolic rate 106
basement membranes 64
base pairs, DNA 30
bases 87–89
basilar artery 359
basilar membrane 405, 418

basolateral membrane, see lamina
    propria
basophils 174, 180, 267
    counts 192, 692
beans 105
beef, fats 106
beetroot, urine 324
behaviours 383
benign tumours 38
bereavement 643, 655
Bernard, Claude 2–3
beta-adrenergic receptors 391
beta-blockers 248
beta-cells 139
beta-galactosidase, E. coli 36, 37
betaglobulins 170
bicarbonate 88, 95
    blood 91
    erythrocytes 309–310
    fluid compartments 90
    intracellular 92
    plasma levels 172, 690
    reabsorption 343
bicuspid valve, see mitral valve
bile 140–141
    flow 152
    ionic composition 91
bile pigments 141
bile salts 141, 154
bile sinusoids 151–152
biliary colic 162
bilirubin 141, 178
    bacterial conversion 150
    plasma levels 172
    protein binding 170
biliverdin 141
biochemistry 43–62
biological activity, units 689
biorhythms, see circadian
    rhythms
biotin 108
bipolar cells, retina 413
birth 572–575
    time of night 677
birth control 551–553
birth weights 590
bladder, see urinary bladder
blastocoele 565
blastocyst 38, 535, 565, 568
bleeding (therapy) 191
blindness, congenital, and circadian
    rhythms 665
blind spot 408
blood 3, 75, 165–200
    clotting 7, 183, 185
    components 690–692
        circadian rhythms 662–663
    loss, third stage of labour 575
    neonate 577
    pH 91, 691
    production, see haemopoiesis
    spleen 263
    see also plasma; serum
blood–brain barrier 313, 358

blood flow 230–231, 241
  see also specific organs and
    tissues
blood groupings 185–187
  homeostatic failures 196–198
blood islands, yolk sac 168
blood pressure 231
  autonomic effects 390
  on blood flow 230–231
  measurement 232–233
  pregnancy 572
  regulation 235–240
  set-points 7
  units 689
  see also hypertension
blood reservoirs (capacitance
  vessels) 219–220
blood sinusoids, liver 151–152
blood urea nitrogen, serum levels
  690
blood vessels 214–223
  autonomic innervation 390
  nomenclature 221
  resistance 231–232
blood volume 167
  distribution 220
  pregnancy 572, 573
  regulation 235–236, 339–340
  values 690
blurred vision 423
B-lymphocytes 180, 260, 270,
  278–279
body fluids 3, 86–100
  compartments 89–94
  and nutrition 102
  regulation 97–98, 335–343
  role in homeostasis 98
body region, stomach 136
body stalk 568, 570
body surface area, *see* surface
  area
Bohr shift 308
bolus 132
bonds, covalent 47
bone 74, 455–457
  calcium 74, 341–342, 499
  disorders 498–499
  relationship to muscle 485
  remodelling 480
  repair 82
bone conduction, sound 419
bone marrow 74, 169
  biopsy 188
  transplantation 193
    SCID 287
booster doses, immunization 279
bottle feeding 115–116
boutons (end-bulbs of synapses)
  365
Bowman's capsules 325, 328–329,
  331
Boyle's law 298
brachial pulse 233
bradycardia 245, 246

brain 355–356
  blood supply 358–360
  growth 577, 579–580
  see also central nervous system
brainstem death 587
breast feeding 112–116, 441,
  575–576, 580
breasts 537–539
  cancer 557
  development 581
  pregnancy 575
breathing
  initiation at birth 576
  neural control 350–351
  rate 294
    circadian rhythms 660
    pregnancy 573
  see also respiration
Broca's area 382
bronchi 295–297
bronchioles 297
bronchoconstriction,
    hypersensitivity 288
brown fat 515
Brunner's glands 139
buffers 88–89, 343
  carbon dioxide carriage 310
  intracellular 92
  plasma proteins as 170
bulbourethral glands 530, 531
bulimia 118
bulk flow 92
bundle of His (atrioventricular
    bundle) 210, 211
burns 265, 520
  shock 249
bursae 470

cachexia, *see* wasting
caecum 149
calcaneus 468, 482
calcitonin 342, 432, 443
calcium 57, 109
  action potentials, imbalances 394
  balance 443–444
  bone 74, 341–342, 499
  coagulation of blood 7, 184, 194
  dietary 110
  estimated average requirements
    114
  fluid compartments 90–91
  intestinal absorption 149
  intracellular 92, 95
  kidney fluids 325
  on myocardium 228
  plasma levels 172, 690
    hospital patients 680
  protein binding 170, 341
  regulation 98, 341–342
  renal failure 344
  skeletal muscle contraction
    476–477, 501
  urine 693

calcium-binding compounds, for
    blood samples 195
calculi
  renal 345
  see also gallstones
callus 82
calories 106
camphor 421–422
canaliculi, bone 75, 455
canal of Schlemm 408
cancellous tissue (spongy bone) 74,
    455
cancers 38–40
  colon 680
    risk 107
  female reproductive system
    557–558
  and immunology 281–282
  prostate 556
  testes 556
  see also leukaemias; tumours
canine teeth 131, 580
capabilities, *vs* demands 646, 651
capacitance vessels 219, 220
capillaries 214–218
  blood flow 243
  fluid and solute exchange 92–94
  fragility 194
  glucocorticoids on 281
  permeability 90
  pressure 234
    hydrostatic, oedema 99
  pulmonary 303–304
capillary buds, skin healing 81
capsules, synovial joints 469
carbaminohaemoglobin 309
carbohydrates 51–53, 102–104
  cell membrane 15
  chyme 141
  energy 106
  vs lipids 54
  excess in diet 650
  see also fibre (diet)
carbon (atom) 48
carbon, isotopic 45
carbon dioxide 87–88, 322
  blood carriage 309–310
  on brain tissue 242
  excretion 294
  movement 16
  partial pressures
    alveoli 303
    blood 691
    respiratory gases 305
    tissues 311
  regulation 343
  transport 166, 169
carbonic acid 87, 88, 310
carbonic anhydrase 310
carboxyexopeptidases 132
carboxypeptidases, alimentary 142
carcinogens 23, 39
carcinoma 39
  see also named organs

cardiac cycle 224–226
cardiac failure, *see* heart failure
cardiac glycosides 247
cardiac muscle, *see* myocardium
cardiac output 226–227
  abnormal 245, 246–247
  assessment 230
  effect of reduction 236–237
  pregnancy 572, 573
  regulation 235
cardiac reserve 226
cardiac sphincter 134–135, 136
cardiac veins 209
cardiodynamics 226–230
cardiogenic shock 250
cardiomyopathies 247
cardiovascular system 165–255
  ageing 581
  autonomic innervation 390
  disorders
    personality types 655
    shift work 672
  fetus 576
  heart 202–213
  skin healing 81
carotid body 313–314
carpals 465
carrier molecules 18
cartilage 70, 73–74
  repair 81–82
cartilaginous joints 468, 469
cascades
  blood clotting 7, 183, 185
  hormone action 435
casein 116
Castle's factor, *see* intrinsic factor of
  Castle
catabolism 48
catalysts 49, 594
cataract 423
catatoxic reactions 649
catching balls, muscle action 493
catecholamines 431–432, 433
  addiction 653
  hypertension 650
  see also adrenaline; noradrenaline
cations 15, 16, 47, 87
cauda equina 383
cave studies, sleep-wake cycle
  663–664, 665
cell-mediated hypersensitivity 289
cell membranes 11, 12–15, 94
  electrical potentials 95
cells 2, 9–40, 101
  death (autolysis) 24, 269
  differentiation, *see* tissue
    differentiation
  division 26, 33–34, 539, 596–597
    disorder 38–40
    loss of capacity 63–64
    see also meiosis
  form 11–15
  optimum size 33
  specialization 63–64

cells of Leydig 543
cellular immunity 269–270, 275–278
  development 280
cellular respiration 58–60
cellulose 103
Celsius scale 687
central clock, ageing 584
central nervous system 354–360
  AIDS 287
  arousal 381
    circadian rhythms 663
  disorders, on movements
    501–502
  haemodynamic control 238
  ischaemic response 216, 231
  temperature effects 519
  see also brain; spinal cord
central sulcus, cerebrum 370
central veins, liver 152
centre of gravity 481–482
centrioles 26
centromeres 595
centrosomes 26
cephalic stage, gastric function 138
cerebellar arteries 360
cerebellar peduncles 375
cerebellum 375
cerebrospinal fluid 357–358
  chemoreceptors 313
  ionic composition 91
cerebrovascular accidents 394
  constipation 161
cerebrum 355–356, 369–372
  aqueduct 373
  blood flow 242
  cortex 356, 370–371
    motor association area 497
    primary somatosensory cortex
      370, 495–496
  functional integration 380–383
  ischaemia, *see* central nervous
    system, ischaemic response
  nuclei 497
cerumen (wax) 425
ceruminous glands 68, 511
cervicolumbar system, *see*
  sympathetic nervous system
cervix 535
  cancer 557–558
  dilatation 573
C fibres (slow fibres) 484, 615, 616
chalk mixtures 159
chambers, heart 205
chancre 554
channels, cell membranes 15
  neurons 362, 367, 394
charge, molecular 15
chemical digestion 127
chemistry 43–62
chemoreceptors 237–238, 312–314,
  403–404, 423
chemotaxis 268
chewing 131
chickenpox, on fetus 589

chief cells, gastric glands 137
chloride 45, 94, 95
  dietary 110
  fluid compartments 90
  kidney fluids 325
  neurons 361, 367
  plasma levels 172, 690
  reabsorption 330
chloride shift 310
chlorine, atom 46
cholecystokinin-pancreozymin
  (CCK-PZ) 138, 144, 433, 446,
  448
choleglobin 178
cholesterol 54–55, 105
  cell membranes 13
  coronary arteries 656
  gallstones 161–162
  serum levels 105, 691
  see also hypercholesterolaemia
cholinergic receptors 391
cholinergic synapses 366
chondrocytes 73
chordae tendineae 206
chorion 568, 571
chorionic gonadotropin 546, 549,
  568, 570
chorionic somatomammotrophin
  (lactogen) 570, 575
chorionic villi 568
  sampling 608
choroid, eye 408
choroid plexus 358
Christmas disease 196
Christmas factor 184
chromatids 34, 595
chromatin 29
chromium, dietary 110
chromosome number 605–606
chromosomes 11–12, 29, 34, 595–596
  ABO system 187
  defects 605–607
  fragmentation 607
chronic lymphatic leukaemia, white
  cell counts 192
chronopharmacology 679–680
chronotropic drugs 228
chylomicrons 147
chyme 141–143
chymotrypsin 143
chymotrypsinogen 142
cilia 26–27, 265
ciliary body 408
ciliated epithelia 66–67
  respiratory tract 295, 297
cingulate gyrus 372
circadian mapping 681
circadian rhythms 449, 660–686
  control 664–667
  core temperature 517–518
  disturbance, coping 654
  sleep 381
  stress 652
  stress response 641

circannual rhythms 660–661
circle of Willis 360
circulation 201–202, 214, 220–221, 230–240
  collateral 218
  coronary 208–210
  disorders 248–253
  fetus 570, 576, 577
  hepatic 152, 221
  see also cardiovascular system
circulatory pressure 231
circumflex branch, coronary artery 209
cirrhosis 162
cisternae 22
cistrons 29
class, social, pain assessment 625–626
clavicle 465
clearance, renal 334–335
climacteric 550, 583–584
clitoris 536
'clock' gene, circadian rhythms 664
clocks (biological) 666–667
  ageing 584
coagulation of blood 7, 183–185
  clotting time 690
  factors
    imbalances 194
    inflammation 267
coal dust 269
cobalt, erythropoiesis 177
coccyx 460
cochlea 418–419
cochlear nuclei 419–420
codeine 621
codons 30, 32
coeliac disease 158
coeliac ganglion 389
coenzymes 57
cofactors 50
cognitive coping 652–653
cognitive disorders 393
coitus, see sexual act
coitus interruptus 551
cold sores 521
collagen fibres 71
collateral circulation 218
collecting ducts 331
collecting tubules 330
colliculi
  inferior and superior 373
  superior 414, 496
collisions, postural reflexes 493
colloid osmotic pressure, see oncotic pressure
colon 149–150
  absorption 147
  bacteria 150, 194
  cancers 680
    risk 107
  histology 126
  see also large intestine
colostrum 576

colour vision 412–413
columnar epithelia 66–67
  stratified 67
columns, spinal cord 384
coma, care 682
combination pill, oral contraceptive 552
comfort zone 515
common carotid arteries 358
community care, night admission wards 681–682
compact bone 74, 455
compartments, body fluids 12, 89–94
  fluid movements 92–94, 243
compensated heart failure 247
competitive binding 50–51
competitive sports, stress 640
complementary proteins 105
complement system 267, 269, 274
  cytotoxic reactions 288
complete antigens 271–272
compliance, lungs 298–299
compound epithelia, see stratified epithelia
compounds (chemical) 47–48
concentrated red cells (infusion) 190
concentration, units 688
conchae 295
condensation reactions 53
conditional learning 381
conditioned reflexes 129–130
condoms 552, 553–554
conduction
  heat 513
  neurons 363–365
    velocity 364, 395
  sound, bone 419
conductive tissue, cardiac muscle 77, 210–212
condyles 457
  femur 467
  humerus 465
cones 410, 411–413
confusion, hospital patients 678
congenital abnormalities 587–590
  heart defects 246
conjugated bilirubin 178
conjunctiva 408
conjunctivitis 425
connective tissues 70–75
Conn's syndrome 248
constant regions, antibodies 272–273
constipation 159, 161
contact inhibition 79
continuous capillaries 217
contraception 551–553
control mechanisms 5–7
convection, heat loss 513
coping 652–656
copper
  assimilation 154

dietary 110
  estimated average requirements 114
  role in erythropoiesis 177
copulation, see sexual act
core temperature 517–518
cornea 410
coronary care, pain measurement 631
coronary circulation 208–210
  atherosclerosis 252
  blood flow 209–210
  cholesterol 656
  thrombosis, see myocardial infarction
coronary sinus 208, 209
corpora cavernosa 531
corpus albicans 532
corpus callosum 369–370
corpus luteum 532, 549
corpus spongiosum 531
cortex, see adrenal gland; cerebrum; lymph nodes
corticobulbar tracts 498
corticospinal tracts 498
corticosteroids, see steroids
corticosterone 444
cortisol 61, 438, 444
  hypersecretion 450
  hypertension 248
coughing 265, 314
countercurrent flow, heat regulation 515
countercurrent multipliers 337
covalent bonds 47
covering epithelia 65–67
Cowper's glands (bulbourethral glands) 530, 531
cow's milk, vs human milk 115, 116
cranial nerves 351, 377–379
craniosacral system, see parasympathetic nervous system
cranium 457
  sutures 460, 469, 577
creatine 322
creatine kinase, plasma levels 172
creatine phosphate 476
creatine phosphokinase, serum levels 690
creatinine 322, 334, 476
  clearance 693
  excretion 327, 329
  plasma levels 172
crenation, erythrocytes 19
crests, bones 457
cretinism 590
crista 488
  vestibular apparatus 404
critical care, pain assessment 624
cross-linkage theory 586
crossover (recombination) 600
cruciate ligaments 482
crying 641

cryoprecipitate, for infusion 188
cryptorchidism 556
crypts of Lieberkühn 139
cuboidal epithelia 65–66
   stratified 67
cultural parity, and stress 643
culture, pain expression 627
cumulus oophorus 562
cuneate fasciculi 375
cupula 488
   vestibular apparatus 404
curare-like drugs 501
Cushing's syndrome 450
   circadian rhythms 680
cuspid teeth, see canine teeth
cutaneous receptors 403
cyanide poisoning 59
cyanocobalamin 108
cyanosis 246
cysteine 57
cystic duct 141, 152
cystic fibrosis 158, 601
cystitis 346
cysts
   from abscesses 83
   ovaries 557
cytochromes 59
cytology 11
cytomegalovirus, on fetus 589
cytoplasm 11, 14
   inclusions 12, 28
cytoplasmic membranes, see cell
   membranes
cytoplasmic streaming 92
cytoskeleton 25–26
cytotoxic cells (killer T-cells)
   275–276
cytotoxic drugs,
   immunosuppressant therapy
   291
cytotoxic reactions 288

Dalton's law 303
Darwin, Charles 608
DDT 154
dead space 297, 300–301
deafness 425
deamination 37, 153
death 586–587, 645
   and stress 643
   time of night 663, 677
decibel (unit) 416
decidua 568
deciduous teeth 131, 580, 581
decompensated heart failure 247
decubitus ulcers 520
decussation 375, 498
deep fascia 471
deep venous thrombosis 195
defecation 122, 151
defence mechanisms 264–291
   blood 167
   digestive system 122
   skin 264, 265, 512

   see also immune system;
      lymphatic system
defensive behaviours 383
defibrillation 213
deglutition 133–134
   Eustachian tubes 416
   regulation 135
dehydration 97, 99, 129, 336, 338
   diarrhoea 159
   polycythaemia 190
   prevention by skin 512
dehydrogenases 49
delayed hypersensitivity 289
   T-cells 277
delta-cells 140
deltoid muscle 473
demands, vs capabilities 646, 651
demineralization 109
demyelinating diseases 394, 395,
   501
denaturing, enzymes 505
dendrites 353
dendritic cells, immune response
   274–275
dendrons 353
denial 654
dens (odontoid process) 463
dentition 131
   development 580–581
deoxycholate 107
deoxyribonucleases, alimentary 144
dependency 454
depolarization 362
depressive illness 396, 655
dermis 510
descending neurons, spinal cord
   354
descending tracts, spinal cord 384
desensitization 288
desmosomes, cardiac muscle 210
detoxification 154
development
   disorders 587–591
   gene expression 37–38
   human 561–582
developmental stressors 645
dextropropoxyphene 621
diabetes insipidus 451
diabetes mellitus 6, 61, 290,
   451–452
   birth weights 590
   circadian rhythms 677
   maturity-onset 650
diamorphine 621
diapedesis 268
diaphragm (contraceptive) 552
diaphragm (muscle) 295, 298
diaries, pain 631
diarrhoea 159
   faecal incontinence 161
   shock 249
diastole 224, 226
diastolic pressure 231
diclofenac 621

dicoumarol 195
dicrotic notch 226
diencephalon 356, 372–373
diet, nutrition 101–120
dietary reference values 111
differential white cell counts 174,
   179, 191, 692
diffusion 16–18, 169
   gas exchange 303–304
DiGeorge's syndrome 286
digestion 121, 122, 127–145
   development 580–581
   leucocytosis 192
   see also gastrointestinal tract;
      intracellular digestion
digestive bodies, see lysosomes
digitalis 247
   circadian rhythms 679–680
diglycerides 105
dihydrocodeine 621
diluting segment, nephron 330
dipeptidases, alimentary 144
dipeptides 55, 143
   absorption 147
2,3-diphosphoglycerate 309, 315
diploid number 34, 539
disaccharidases, alimentary 142,
   144
disaccharides 52–53, 102–104
discontinuous capillaries 217
discrimination, sensory 401
discs, intervertebral 463
diseases of adaptation (Selye) 281,
   649
dissolving bodies, see lysosomes
distal nephron 330
distraction, for pain 623
distress
   vs eustress 652
   and immunity 281
distressors 639, 640
distributing arteries (muscular
   arteries) 216
diuretics 246, 330
   on fetus 589
   for hypertension 248
diurnal rhythms, see circadian
   rhythms
diverticulosis, -itis 160
DNA 28–29, 29–31, 595–596
doctors, factors in pain assessment
   626–627
dominance, incomplete 598, 603
dominant inheritance 598, 603
dopamine 367, 391
   memory 382
   release deficiency 395, 396
dorsal column nuclei, medulla
   oblongata 495
dorsal columns, spinal cord 384,
   407
dorsal horn 385
dorsal nerve root ganglia 353, 383
dorsal nerve roots 383, 407

dorsal nucleus of vagus 379
Down's syndrome 606, 607
dreaming 380
drug rounds, hospital wards 678
drugs
 circadian rhythms 679–680
 on fetus 589
Duchenne's muscular dystrophy
 500, 604
ductless glands, *see* endocrine
 glands, system
ductus arteriosus 576–577
ductus deferens 529
ductus efferentia, testis 529
ductus venosus 577
duodenum 139
 histology 126
 hormones 433
 ulcers 157
duplication division (mitosis)
 33–34, 539, 596–597
dural sinuses 360, 379
dura mater 379
dynorphin 367
dysmenorroea 556–557
dystrophin 500

ear 416–420
 disorders 425
 wax 425
 see also vestibular apparatus
eardrum 416
eccrine glands 511
ECG, *see* electrocardiogram
ectoderm 565, 567
ectopic beats 227
EDTA, *see* ethylene ditetraacetic
 acid
efferent arterioles, kidneys 328
efferent neurons 76, 351
efferent renal nerves 324
efficiency, biorhythms 661
ejaculation 531
elastic arteries 214–216
elastic tissue 72
elastin fibres 71, 72
elasto-cartilage 74
elderly patients, *see* ageing
electrical burns 520
electrical potentials, cell
 membranes 95
electrocardiogram 212–213
 psychosomatic pain 626
electrochemistry, neurons 361–369
electroencephalography, sleep 380
electrolytes 45–47, 87–89
 balance 96–97
 intestinal absorption 149
 loss, diarrhoea 159
 on myocardium 228
 neurons 361
 obligatory excretion 322
 reabsorption 337
 receptor excitation 400

electrons 44, 46
electron transport chain 59
eleidin 507
elements (chemical) 44
ellipsoidal joints 470
emboli 195
embryo
 blood production 168
 development 564, 565–567
embryonic disc 565
embryo selection 609
emetics 158
emotional behaviours 383
emotional factors, breathing 314
emotional shock, autonomic effects
 390–391
emotion-focused coping 654
emphysema 317
emulsification 141
end-bulbs, synapses 365
end diastolic volume 228–229
endocarditis 246
endocardium 205
endocrine cells, pancreas 139–140
endocrine glands, system 70, 430
 ageing 582
 heart rate control 227–228
 metabolism 61
 see also hormones
endocytosis 17, 20–21
 receptor-mediated 17, 21
endoderm 565, 567
endogenous growth, *see* interstitial
 growth
endogenous rhythms 664
endogenous stressors 638
endolymph 404, 418
 excess 425
endometriosis 557
endometrium 535, 545
 embryonic development 566
 implantation 565
endomysium 473
endoneurium 349
endopeptidases 132, 137
 pancreatic 143
endoplasmic reticulum 14, 22–23
endorphins 367, 617
endoscopy 155
endosomes 21
endothelium, blood vessels 214
endothelium-derived relaxing
 factor 449
endotoxins, haemolysis 288
end systolic volume 226, 228–229
energy 2, 20
 adenosine triphosphate 56–57
 estimated average requirements
 112
 kidneys, usage 331
 lipids *vs* carbohydrates 54
 nutrition 106
 pregnancy 117
 production 293–294

energy levels, atoms 46
enkephalins 367
enterokinase 142, 143
enteroreceptors 403–404
entrainment, biorhythms 664
environmental stresses 637
environmental stressors
 644–645
 perception 651, 652–653
enzymes 29, 49–51
 denaturing 505
 digestive 132
 intracellular 34
 lysosomes 23–24
 pH 95
 production control 35–37
 tissue differentiation 594
eosinophils 174, 180, 267
 allergy 288
 counts 192, 692
ependyma 355
epicardium 203
epidermal growth factor 507
epidermis 67, 265, 506–510
epididymis 529
epidural opioids 622
epiglottis 295
epimysium 471
epinephrine, *see* adrenaline
epineurium 349
epiphyseal plates 74
epiphyses 74, 469
episiotomy 537
epithelia 64–70
 blood-brain barrier 313
 cell size 12
 ileum 145
 olfactory, nasal cavity 421
epithelial membranes 77–78
 see also mucous membranes
equilibrium, *see* balance
erectile tissue, penis 531
erect posture 480–481
error catastrophe theory 585
error detectors, *see* sensory
 receptors
erythroblastosis fetalis 198–199
erythroblasts 175
erythrocytes 11, 28, 167, 172–178
 counts 692
 osmotic effects 19–20
 population imbalances
 189–190
 size 12
 urine 693
erythrocyte sedimentation rate
 196
erythrogenin 177, 449
erythropoiesis 176–177
erythropoietin 177, 449
 secretion 239
erythropoietinogen 449
Escherichia coli, enzyme
 production control 35–36

Eskimos, circadian rhythms 665–666
essential amino acids 104–105
  infant feeding 116
essential hypertension 249
estimated average requirements, nutrition 111–117
ethylene ditetraacetic acid 335
  for blood samples 195
Eustachian tube 416
eustress
  vs distress 652
  and immunity 281
eustressors 639, 640
evaporation, heat loss 513
exchange vessels 217
excitability, neurons 363
excitatory neurotransmitters 229, 366–367
  imbalances with inhibitory neurotransmitters 395–396
excitatory post-synaptic potentials (EPSP) 366–367
excretion 1, 2, 321–347
  biliary 141
  skin 323, 512
  water and electrolytes 97
exercise 315
  blood flow 241, 243–245
  blood vessels 220
  cardiac function 228, 229
  metabolism 60
  oxygen requirements 294, 315
  shift work 675
  sympathetic nervous system 244, 389–390
exhaustion, general adaptation syndrome 649–650
exocrine cells, pancreas 139
exocrine glands 68–69, 430
exocytosis 20–21, 22
exogenous growth, *see* appositional growth
exogenous stressors 638
exopeptidases 143
expiration 298–300
expiratory rate 299
expiratory reserve volume 301
expression, genes 37–38
external anal sphincter 151
external auditory canal 416
external carotid arteries 358
external jugular veins 360
exteroreceptors 403
extracellular compartment 12
  interchanges with intracellular compartment 94
extracellular fluid 89–90, 100
  volume 339–340
extrafusal muscle spindles 490
extrapyramidal pathway 498
extrinsic muscles, eyes 408
extrinsic pathway, blood coagulation 184–185

extrinsic sugars 104, 116
eyes 408–415
  autonomic innervation 390
  disorders 423–425
  movements 351
    control 415
    head movements 496

Fab parts, antibodies 273
facial bones 457–460
facial nerve 378, 406, 421
facilitated diffusion 17, 18
factors VIII, IX, concentrates for infusion 188
faecal incontinence 161
faeces 150, 322
  constipation 161
fainting 249
  see also vasovagal attacks; syncope
fallen arches 484
Fallopian tubes 534–535
  ciliated epithelia 66–67
  infection 555
  ligation 551
Fallot, tetralogy of 246
false ribs 464
falx cerebri 360
familial hyperlipidaemia 602–603
family trees (pedigree analysis) 609
fascia, deep 471
fascicles 473
fast fibres (Aδ fibres) 615, 616
fast twitch muscle fibres 484, 485
fatigue resistance, muscles 484–485
fats, *see* adipose tissue; lipids
fat-soluble vitamins 57, 107
  assimilation 154
fatty acids 105
  absorption 147, 149
  and amino acids, aerobic metabolism 59–60
feedback systems 5–7
  hormone control 438
female reproductive system 532–539
  development 581
  disorders 556–558
  see also menstrual cycle
femur 467
  bone marrow 169
  curvature 482
fenestra ovalis (oval window) 418
fenestra rotunda (round window) 418
fenestrated capillaries 217
fermentation, colon 150
ferritin 178
fertility awareness methods, contraception 551
fertilization 531, 535, 539, 562–564
fetus 567
  antibodies 280

circulation 570, 576, 577
  drugs, viruses on 589
  haemoglobin 307, 309, 577
  hormones from 570
fever 7, 518, 521
fibre (diet) 106–109, 160
fibres, connective tissue 71
fibrillation 213
fibrinogen 79, 169, 170, 171, 184
  imbalances 196
fibrinolysin, semen 530–531
fibrinolysis 185
fibrinolytic enzymes 195
fibrin stabilizing factor 184
fibroblasts 181
  cartilage 73
fibro-cartilage 74
fibrocytes 79, 82
fibrosis, lungs 317
fibrous pericardium 203
fibrous tissue 71–72
fibula 468
fight and flight 647
filaments, cytoskeleton 25–26
filiform papillae 420
filling time (ventricles) 229
filtration 17
  cell membranes 20
  kidneys 325, 331–332
filtration pressure, kidneys 328
fingerprints 510
fissuring, tongue 156
5-hydroxytryptamine (serotonin) 267, 367, 391
fixator muscles 486
fixed cells, connective tissue 71
fixed joints 468, 469
fixed macrophages 268
flagella 26–28
flat bones 457
flat foot 484
flatulence 150
floating ribs 464
flower-spray endings, muscle spindles 490
fluid balance 96–97
fluid-mosaic model 15
fluids, *see* body fluids
fluoride 109
  dietary 110
  infants, requirements 115
folic acid 108
  deficiency, on fetus 589
  erythropoiesis 177
follicles, ovarian 532
follicle-stimulating hormone 446, 546
  hyposecretion 558
  male 526, 543
fontanelles 577
foot, bones 482–484
foramen magnum 457
foramen ovale 205, 576, 577
foramina, bones 457

forced expiration 299
  FEV$_1$ 302
forced vital capacity 302
Fordham, M., on pain 613
forebrain 356, 369–372
foreskin 531
fossa ovalis 205
fourth ventricle 358
fovea 410
fractures 498
fragile X syndrome 607
fragmentation, chromosomal 607
free radicals 585
freeze-dried factor VIII 188
freezing point, osmolarity 689
frequency, sound, discrimination
  418
fresh frozen plasma 188
friction rub 205
frontal lobes 370
frozen red cell preparations 190
fructose
  absorption 147
  semen 530
frusemide 246
functional capacity, adulthood 582
functional residual capacity (lungs)
  302
fundic region, stomach 135, 137
fundus, uterus 535
fungiform papillae 420
furring, tongue 156
fusiform muscles 473

galactose, absorption 147
gall bladder 140, 152
gallstones 161–162
gametes 29
gametogenesis 539–545
  see also spermatogenesis;
    oogenesis
gamma aminobutyric acid 367
  deficiency 395, 502, 603
gamma-efferent neurons 493
gammaglobulins 170, 272
  imbalances 196
  therapy 162
  see also haemolytic disease of the
    newborn
ganglia
  dorsal roots 353, 383
  neural 353
  sympathetic 389
ganglion cells, retina 413
gases
  blood carriage 306–311
  colon 150
  solubility 303
gas exchange
  blood and tissues 311
  pulmonary 297, 303–304
gastric juice 137, 266
  ionic composition 91
gastric phase, gastric function 138

gastric ulcers 157
gastrin 138, 446
gastritis 156–157
gastrocolonic reflex 151
gastroenteritis 158
gastrointestinal tract 121–163
  ageing 582
  autonomic innervation 390
  defence mechanisms 123, 266
  excretion 323
  hormones 446
  regulation 135
  shift work 671
  stretch receptor theory 122
  water secreted and absorbed
    148–149
gastroscopy 155
gastrulation 565
gate control theory, pain 613,
  615–617
gating mechanisms, neuron cell
  membranes 362
gender differences
  cardiac function 228
  core temperature 518
  pain assessment 626
  see also sex determination
general adaptation syndrome 228,
  238, 647–652
generator potentials, retinal
  receptors 413
genes 2
  for ageing 584–585
  control of 35–38
  expression 37–38
    disorders 588–590
  protein synthesis 29–33
  repression 37–38
gene therapies 609–610
genetic code 30–31
genetic complement 587–588
genetic disorders
  inheritance 601–607
  metabolism 61
genetic engineering 609–610
genetic fingerprinting 610
genetics
  ABO system 187
  see also inheritance; population
    genetics
gene transcription, hormone-
  mediated 436
geniculate nuclei 373
genital herpes 555
genome 595
genotypes 595
  stress response 641
germinal centre, lymph node 260
germinal epithelium 532
germinative matrix, nails 510
germ layers 38
gestation period 525, 572
giant cells, phagocytic 268
gigantism 590

gingivitis 155
glands 430
  subcutaneous 510–511
  see also accessory sex glands
glandular epithelia 68–70
  gastrointestinal tract 124–125
glaucoma 425
glia, see neuroglia
gliding joints 470
Glisson's capsule 151
globin 141, 178, 306–307
globulins, plasma 170, 171
glomerular filtration rate 328, 329,
  334–335
  pregnancy 573
glomeruli 325, 328–329, 331
glomerulonephritis 345
glossitis 156
glossopharyngeal nerve 351, 378,
  406, 421
glottis 295
glucagon 61, 139, 140, 433, 435, 447,
  448
glucocorticoids 433, 444–445
  on mast cells 281
glucose 18, 58, 59
  absorption 147
  anaerobic metabolism 60
  deficiency 61
  homeostasis, role of liver
    153–154
  hormone-mediated release 435
  kidney fluids 325
  membrane transport 18
  plasma levels 172, 690
    control 5–6
  urine 693
glucose-6-phosphate 59
glucostat theory 122
glucuronic acid, bilirubin
  conjugation 178
glycation 586
glyceryl trinitrate 146
glycine, codons for 30
glycocholate (sodium) 141
glycogen 28, 53, 103
glycogenesis 154
glycopeptides, hormonal 431
glycoproteins, glycolipids, cell
  membrane 15
goblet cells 66, 265
goitre 451
Golgi body 14, 22, 23
Golgi cisternae membranes 23
Golgi tendon organs 404, 488–490
gonadotropin-releasing hormones
  543, 546
  hyposecretion 558
gonadotropins 432
  see also follicle-stimulating
    hormone; luteinizing
    hormone
gonads 430, 524, 525
  endocrine function 446

hormones 433
see also ovaries; testes
gonorrhoea, gonococcus 535, 536, 554–555
goose, fats 106
gout 344–345
Graafian follicle 532
gracile fasciculi 375
granular endoplasmic reticulum 23
granular layer, epidermis 507
granulation 81, 84
granulocytes 172, 174, 179–180
    population imbalances 192
granulopoiesis 181
Grave's disease 450
gravity
    and oedema 99
    V/Q ratio 305
great vessels 203
grey matter, spinal cord 355, 384–385
growth
    childhood 577–579
    and nutrition 116
    puberty 581
growth factors 449
    see also epidermal growth factor
growth hormone 61, 432, 438, 440–441, 579
    circadian rhythms 662
    disorders 590
growth plates 74
gubernaculum 527
Guillain-Barré syndrome 395
gums, disorders 155
gustation, *see* taste
Guthrie test 602
gyri 355

haem 178, 306, 307
haematocrit 174–175, 189, 690
    pregnancy 572
haematocytoblasts, *see* stem cells, blood production
haematology 188
haematuria 345
haemoglobin 28, 88, 174, 306–309
    blood levels 175, 691
    breakdown 141, 153, 178
    fetus 307, 309, 577
haemolysis 20
    from drugs 288
haemolytic disease of the newborn 198–199
haemophilia 195–196, 604, 607
haemopoiesis 168–169, 175–176
    see also erythropoiesis; leucopoiesis
haemorrhage, vasoconstriction 220
haemorrhoids 160–161
haemosiderin 178
haemostasis 166, 168, 182–185
Hageman factor 184
hair 265, 509–510

hair follicles 509
    sensory receptors 403
hamstrings 486
handedness 370
haploid number 34, 539
haptens 271–272
Hashimoto's thyroiditis 290, 451
Haversian systems 75, 455
hay fever 289
Hayflick number 584
head movements, and eye position 496
healing, wounds 78–82
health 668
health care, shift work 669, 673, 674–675
health education, circadian rhythms 681
hearing 405, 415–420
heart 202–213, 220–221, 224–230
    autonomic innervation 390
    blood flow path 208
    extrinsic innervation 213
    malfunctions 245–247
    septal defects 590
heart attacks, *see* myocardial infarction
heart block (AV block) 212
heart failure 246–247
heart rate
    abnormal 246
    circadian rhythms 660
    regulation 227–228
heart sounds 207–208
heat
    liver 155
    transfer
        by blood 166
        physics 512–513
    see also hot climates
heat exchange, skin 515, 516
heavy chains 272
helper T-cells 276
hemispheres, brain 370
Henry's law 303
heparin 154, 267
hepatic circulation 152, 221
hepatic duct 140–141
hepatic portal vein 149, 151
hepatic triad 152
hepatic veins 152
hepatitis, viral 162
    on fetus 589
hepatoportal circulation 221
hepatosplenic stage, blood production 168
Hering-Breuer reflex 312
hernia, inguinal 556
heroin, on fetus 589
herpes simplex virus 521
    on fetus 589
herpes simplex virus (type 2) 555
Hertz (unit) 416
heterografts 290

heterozygous genotypes 599
hexachlorethane 421–422
hexoses 52
hiatus hernia 156
hiccoughing 314
hilum, lymph node 260
hindbrain 356, 375–377
hinge joints 470
hippocampus 372, 382
    emotions 383
histamine 180, 267
    cytotoxic reactions 288
histocompatibility antigens 290
histology 64
    gastrointestinal tract 124–126
HIV 269, 286–287
Hodgkin's lymphomas 285
'hole in the heart' 577
holism, phenomenological 639, 664
holistic care 627
holocrine glands 69
home and work conflicts 644–645
home diaries, pain 631
homeostasis 1, 2–7
homografts 290
homologous alleles 597
homozygous genotypes 598, 599
horizontal cells, retina 413
hormones 428–453
    abnormal function 450–452
    definition 430–431
    fate 322
    female reproductive cycle 545–550
    from fetus 570
    gastrointestinal 138
    and metabolism 61
    neuroendocrine 400–401, 439
    spermatogenesis regulation 543–545
    of stress 444
    see also endocrine glands, system
hospital admission
    circadian rhythms 677–682
    and pain 619
hot climates 515–517
    sweat 518–519
human albumin, for infusion 188
human chorionic gonadotropin 546, 549, 568, 570
human development 561–582
human immunodeficiency virus (HIV) 269, 286–287
human immunoglobulin, for infusion 188
human lymphocytic antigens (HLAs) 290
human milk 112–116
human specific globulin, for infusion 188
humerus 465
humoral immunity 270, 278–279
    development 280
hunger 117

hunger centre 121–122
Huntington's chorea 395, 502, 603
hyaline cartilage 74
hyaluronic acid 469
hyaluronidase 72
hybridoma cells 282
hydrocele 556
hydrochloric acid 87
    gastric juice 137–138
hydrocorticosteroids, adrenal
    cortex, circadian rhythms
    662–663
hydrogen carbonate, *see*
    bicarbonate
hydrogen ions 87–89
    excretion 331
    regulation 98, 343
hydrolases 23
hydrolysis 53, 127
hydronephrosis 345
hydrophilia, hydrophobia 13
hydrostatic pressure
    capillaries, oedema 99
    renal capillaries 328
hydroxybutyrate dehydrogenase,
    plasma levels 172
5-hydroxytryptamine (serotonin)
    267, 367, 391
hymen 536
hyoid 464
hypercalcaemia, constipation 161
hypercapnia 316
hypercholesterolaemia 118–119, 656
    shift work 672
hypergammaglobulinaemia 196
hyperglycaemia 61
hyperkalaemia, on myocardium
    228
hyperlipidaemia, familial 602–603
hypermetropia 423
hypernatraemia, on myocardium
    228
hyperpolarization 362, 363
hypersecretion, hormones 450–451
hypersensitivity reactions 287–291
hypertension 236, 248–249
    renal failure 344
    and stress 650
hyperthermia 521
hyperthyroidism 450–451
hypertonic solutions 19
hyperventilation 316–317
hypocapnia 316
hypodermic injections 72
hypogammaglobulinaemia 196
hypogastric arteries 577
hypoglossal nerve 378
hypokalaemia 159
    constipation 161
    on myocardium 228
hypophysis, *see* pituitary gland
hypoproteinaemia 170, 196
    oedema 99, 196
hyposecretion, hormones 451

hyposplenism 285
hypotension 236, 249
hypothalamic-pituitary axis
    438–441
hypothalamus 373, 438–440
    aggressive and sexual behaviours
    383
    circadian rhythms 666
    and food intake 121–122
    hormones 432
    neurosecretory cells 429
    portal system 221
    temperature 7
    thirst 117
hypothermia 521
    on action potentials 395
hypothyroidism, hypotension 249
hypotonic solutions 20
hypoventilation 316, 317
hypovolaemic shock 249
    burns 520
hypoxaemia 304
hypoxia 58, 316
    anaemia 118
    central nervous system 242–243,
    501
    intracellular 34
    see also altitude hypoxia
hypoxic hypoxia 316

ibuprofen 621
IgE antibodies 180
ileocaecal valve 124
ileostomy 160
ileum 139
    absorption 145–146, 147–149
    histology 126
ilium 467
illness, on circadian rhythms
    676–677
illness behaviour 655
imagery, treating pain 624
images, edges 413
immune deficiency diseases 286
    see also AIDS
immune system 257–258
    ageing 582
immunity, *see* non-specific
    immunity; specific immunity
immunization 258, 279, 284
immunogens 271
immunoglobulins 170, 272
    see also haemolytic disease of the
    newborn
immunological competence 280–281
immunological escape 282
immunological surveillance 281
immunosuppressant therapy
    290–291
immunotherapy 40
implantation, zygote 565
impotency 558
imprint theory, circadian rhythms
    667

inborn errors of metabolism 61
inbreeding 607
incisors 131, 580
inclusions, cytoplasmic 12, 28
income, and stress 643
incompetence, heart valves 208
incomplete dominance 598, 603
incontinence, faecal 161
incus 416
independent assortment, Mendelian
    inheritance 600
indirect clinical measures of pain
    631
individualism, stress response
    641–642, 644, 650
indomethacin 621
industrial accidents, shift work 672
inert elements 47
infant formulas 115–116
infant respiratory distress
    syndrome 318, 576, 590
infants
    development 577–581
    nutritional requirements 112–116
infarction 195
infection
    active natural immunity 282–283
    conjunctivitis 425
    Fallopian tubes 534–535, 555
    leucocytosis 192–193
    lymphatic system 284–286
    nervous system 392
    otitis media 425
    sinusitis 425
    skin as barrier 512
    urinary tract 346
    see also sexually transmitted
    diseases and specific
    infections
infectious hepatitis 162
inferior olivary nuclei 377
inferior vena cava 208
infertility, male 531, 555–556, 558
inflammation 79, 267, 649
influenza 284
infra-red photocoagulation,
    haemorrhoids 160
infundibulum, Fallopian tube 534
ingestion 122
inguinal hernia 556
inheritance 594–612
    ABO system 187
    genetic disorders 601–607
    see also genetics
inherited clock theory 666
inhibin 446, 527, 544, 553
inhibiting hormones 439–440
inhibitory neurotransmitters 367
    imbalances with excitatory
    neurotransmitters 395–396
inhibitory post-synaptic potentials
    (IPSP) 367
inhibitory synapses, integration
    367–368

initiation, protein synthesis 33
injections, hypodermic 72
injuries, pain 614
inner cell mass 565, 568
innominate bones 465–467
inositol 104
insensible water loss 97
insertions, muscles 473
insomnia 664
inspiration 298
inspiratory reserve volume 301
insulin 61, 139, 140, 433, 447–448
   Arthus reactions 289
   on cells 18
   on fetus 589
intensive care, pain assessment
      624
intercalated discs, cardiac muscle
      77, 210
intercellular fluid 3
intercostal muscles 298, 299
intercostal nerves 312
interferon 270, 276
interleukins
   glucocorticoids on 281
   I-1 275, 281
   I-2 276
interlobular arterioles, liver 152
intermediate filaments 26
internal carotid arteries 358
internal jugular veins 360
internal synchronization 664
International System of Units 687
interneurons, spinal cord 354, 385
interstitial cell-stimulation hormone
      526, 543, 545
interstitial fluid, see tissue fluid
interstitial growth, cartilage 73
interstitial nephritis 345
intervertebral discs 463
intervertebral foramina 460
interviewing patients 682
intestinal phase, gastric function
      138
intracellular calcium 92, 95
intracellular compartment 12
   interchanges with extracellular
      compartment 94
intracellular digestion 24
intracellular fluid 89, 90, 91–92
intracellular messengers 57–58
intrafusal muscle spindles 490
intralobular veins, liver 152
intrauterine devices 552
intrinsic factor of Castle 138
intrinsic pathway, blood
      coagulation 185
intrinsic sugars 104
inulin 335
involuntary muscle, see smooth
      muscle
iodine 45, 109
   deficiency 451
   dietary 110

estimated average requirements
      114
   thyroid uptake 441
ions 45–47, 57, 87
   on myocardium 228
   neurons 361
   receptor excitation 400
iris 408, 414–415
iron 57, 109
   assimilation 154
   deficiency 118, 190
   dietary 110
   erythropoiesis 177
   estimated average requirements
      114
   haemoglobin 307
   intestinal absorption 149
   metabolism 178
   milk feeding 116
   plasma levels 691
      circadian rhythms 662
irregular bones 457
ischaemic heart disease 252–253
   and stress 655–656
ischaemic response, central nervous
      system 216, 231
ischium 467
islets of Langerhans 139–140
isoantigens, blood groups 185
isografts 290
isolation studies, circadian rhythms
      663–664, 665
isometric contractions 478
isotonic contractions 478
isotonic solutions 19
isotopes 45
isovolumetric ventricular
      contraction phase 225
isovolumetric ventricular relaxation
      phase 226
isthmus, Fallopian tube 534

Jacob-Monod operon theory 35–37,
      40
jaundice
   haemolytic disease of the
      newborn 198
   'physiological' 577, 667
jejunum 139
   histology 126
Jenner, Edward 284
jet lag, jet syndrome 676
joints 468–470, 482
   disorders 499–500
   receptors 404
joule (unit) 106
juxtaglomerular apparatus 445
juxtamedullary nephrons 330

kaolin mixtures 159
Kaposi's sarcoma 287
karyotypes 595

keratin 67, 507
keratinized stratified squamous
      epithelia 67
keratohyalin 507
ketones 60
kidneys 321–347
   ageing 582
   blood flow 328
   blood pressure regulation 239
   infection 345
   proximal tubules 66
killer T-cells 275–276
kilocalories 106
kinins 267
Klinefelter's syndrome 606
kneecap 467
knee-jerk 492
knee joint 482
   movements 486
Korotkoff sound 207, 233
Krauss end-bulbs 517
Krebs' cycle 59
Kupffer cells 152, 181
kwashiorkor 119

labia majora, minora 536
labile tissues 78
laboratory slips, haematology 188
labour 572–573
   time of night 677
labyrinthine disease 425
lachrymal ducts 408
lachrymal glands 68, 408
   secretions 266, 408
lactase 144
lactate dehydrogenase, serum
      levels 691
lactation 575–576
   vitamin requirements 113
lactic acid 60
   lysozymes 269
lactiferous ducts, sinuses 538–539
lactogen, placental 570, 575
lacunae, bone 74–75, 455
ladder, see staircase, analgesic
      therapy
lamellae, bone 75
lamina flow 231
lamina propria
   epithelial cell 147
   gastrointestinal tract 125
Langerhans cells 278
language 382
large intestine 123, 149–151
   absorption 147
   disorders 159–161
   histology 126
   regulation 135
   see also colon
laryngeal pharynx 132
larynx 295
lateral corticospinal tract 498
lateral fissure, cerebrum 370
lateral geniculate nuclei 373

lateral spinothalamic tracts 407
lateral umbilical ligament 577
lateral ventricles 358
laxatives, self-medication 680
Lazarus, R.S., on stress 651,
    653–654
lead salts 420
learning 381–382
lecithin 141
left anterior descending branch,
    coronary artery 209
left cerebral hemisphere 370
left coronary artery 209
left-to-right blood shunts 246
left ventricular failure 246
lemnisci 375
lens 410
let-down of milk 575
lethal alleles 599
leucocytes 21, 167, 172, 174,
    178–181
    counts 692
    population imbalances 191–193
    urine 693
leucocytosis 191–192
leucopenia 191–192
leucopoiesis 181
leukaemias 39, 192, 193
levers, musculoskeletal 485
levodopa 395, 396
life, characteristics 1–2
life change units 642
life events 642–644
lifting objects, muscle action 493
ligaments 71, 469
    injuries 500
    yellow elastic tissue 72
ligamentum venosum 577
ligation
    Fallopian tubes 551
    haemorrhoids 160
light, intensity control 414–415
light chains 272
light refraction 410–411
limbic system 372
    conditional learning 381
    emotions 383
    olfaction 422
limb withdrawal reflex 386
lining epithelia 65–67
linoleic acid, linolenic acid 105
lipases 23, 132, 144
    alimentary 142, 143
    gastric 137
lipids 53–55
    cell membranes 13
    chyme 141
    dietary 105–106, 116
    emulsification 141
    and hunger 122
    inclusions 28
    metabolism 294–295
    serum levels 691
lipid-soluble molecules 15

lipofucin 585
lipogenesis 154
lipoproteases 147
lipoproteins 584
    serum levels 691
liposuction 73
liver 149, 151–155
    disorders 161, 162, *see* also
        hepatitis, viral
lobules, liver 151
lock and key theory
    antibodies 273
    enzymes 50
London Hospital pain observation
    chart 629
long bones 456
long-chain fatty acids, absorption
    147, 149
long-loop feedback systems,
    hormone control 438
longsightedness 423
loop diuretics 330
loop of Henle 330, 331, 336–337
loose areolar connective tissue
    72
LSD, on fetus 589
lubrication, synovial fluid 469
lumbar curve 482
lungs 294, 295
    at birth 576–577
    excretion 323
    fibrosis 317
    function 297
    stretch receptors 312
    surface area 297
    see also pulmonary...
luteal phase 549–550
luteinizing hormone 7, 446, 546
    hyposecretion 558
    male 526, 543, 545
lymph 75
    flow rate 258
    formation 263
lymphatic pumps 258
lymphatic system 94, 256–257,
    258–263
    imbalances 284–286
    obstruction 99, 258, 286
lymphatic vessels 258, 263
lymph nodes 258–259
    cortex 260
    enlargement 285
lymphoblasts 175
lymphocytes 71, 79, 174, 180
    counts 192, 692
    production 181, 270–271
    response 257, 274–275
    spleen 263
    steroids on 281
lymphoedema 258, 286
lymphoidal system 258–263
lymphokines 275, 276
lymphomas 285–286
lymphotoxins 275

lysergide, lysergic acid
    diethylamide, on fetus 589
lysis 20
    immune response 274
lysosomes 14, 22, 23–24
    secondary 269
lysozymes 24, 266, 269
lysyltaurine 420

macrophage-activating factor 276
macrophage-chemotaxic factor 276
macrophages 71, 181, 267, 268
    antigen-presenting cells 274–275
    monokines 278
macrophenotypes 645
macula, vestibular apparatus 405
magnesium 57
    dietary 110
    estimated average requirements
        114
    intestinal absorption 149
malabsorption, vitamin K 194
male reproductive system 526–532
    development 581
    disorders 555–556
malignant tumours 38–40
malleus 416
malnutrition 118, 170
Malpighian corpuscles 325
maltase 144
mammary glands, *see* breasts
mandible 460
Mantoux test 289
manubrium 463–464
marginal artery 209
mast cells 71, 267, 276
    cytotoxic reactions 288
    glucocorticoids on 281
master gland, *see* anterior pituitary
    gland
mastication 131
maternal antibodies 257–258, 280,
    282, 577
matrix, cartilage 70
maturation, *see* human
    development
maximal oxygen consumption rate
    315
McCaffery, M., on pain 614, 628
McGill-Melzack pain questionnaire
    629–631
mealtimes 664–665
mean arterial pressure 234
mean corpuscular volume 691
measurement, units of 687–689
mechanical digestion 127
mechanical methods, birth control
    552
mechanoreceptors 402, 403
medial geniculate body 420
medial geniculate nuclei 373
median lemniscus 377, 495
mediastinum 202

medulla 134
  kidney 330
medulla oblongata 375–377
  cardiac centres 213
  dorsal column nuclei 495
  respiratory centres 312
  vasomotor centre 220
  vomiting centre 157–158
megakaryocytes 175, 182
megaloblasts of Ehrlich 168
meiosis 34, 539, 540, 597, 599
Meissner's capsules, corpuscles 403,
    510
Meissner's plexus 125
melanin 28, 508
  inheritance 598
melanocytes 507–508
melanocyte-stimulating hormone
    432, 440–441, 508
melanoma 521
melatonin 448–449, 666–667
membrane potentials, resting 95
membranes, epithelial 77–78
membrane threshold, neurons 362
membranous urethra 529
memory 381–382
memory B-cells 279
memory T-cells 277
menarche 581
Mendelian inheritance 599–600
Ménière's syndrome 425
meninges 379–380
meningitis 392
menisci 469
menopause 550, 583–584, 591
menstrual cycle 7, 545–549
  disorders 556–557
  vagina, mucus 551
Merkel's discs 403, 507
merocrine glands 69
mesencephalon 356, 373–375
mesenteries 126, 138–139
mesoblastic stage, blood production
    168
mesoderm 565, 567
messenger RNA 29, 31
messengers
  intracellular 57–58
  see also second messengers
metabolic acidosis 158, 159
metabolic alkalosis 158
metabolism 48–51
  and nutrition 101
  rates 505
    circadian rhythms 660
    increasing 515
  wastes 293–294
    excretion 321–347
    transport 166
metachromal rhythm 27
metastases 38–39
metatarsals 468
metencephalon 356
methane, molecule 48

methyldopa, cytotoxic reactions
    288
micelles 147
microcirculation 216–218
microfilaments 26
microglia 355
microphages 180, 268
microtubules 26
microvilli, small intestine 139
micturition 333, 351
midbrain 356, 373–375
  nuclei 497
middle cerebral artery 359
  CVA 394
middle ear 416–417
mifepristone (RU-486) 553
migration, cells 79
migration inhibitory factor 276
milieu intérieur 2–3
milk, human 112–116
Milkhail, A., definition of stress 639
milk teeth 131, 580, 581
mineralocorticoids 433, 445
minerals 57
  dietary 109–110
  estimated average requirements
    114
mini-pill 552
miraculin 420
mitochondria 14, 24–25
  cardiac muscle 210
  size 12
  spermatozoa 541
mitogenic factor, cellular immunity
    276
mitosis 33–34, 539, 596–597
mitral valve 206, 224, 226
  disease 208
mixed glands 70, 140, 430
mobility, lack 454
modality, sensory stimuli 399–400
molar solutions 688
molar teeth 131, 580
mole (unit) 688
molecules 47–48
monitors, see sensory receptors
monoblasts 175
monoclonal antibodies 282
monocytes 174, 181, 278
  counts 192, 692
monoglycerides 105
monosaccharides 52, 102, 104
  absorption 147
monosomy 606
mons pubis 536
morphine 621
  on fetus 589
morula 38, 564
mosaicism 606–607
motilin 144–145
motor cortex 370, 497
motor disorders 393
motor end plates (neuromuscular
    junctions) 477

motor neurons 351
  spinal cord 385
motor output, central 496–498
motor units 485–486
mountaineers 191
mouth
  disorders 155
  innervation 135
  physiology 128–132
  see also oral absorption
movements 1
  cilia 27
  control 486–498
  muscle spindles 493–494
mucous membranes 78
  defence mechanisms 264,
    265–266
  gastrointestinal tract 124–125
  ileum 145
  small intestine 139
mucus 28, 265–266
  gastritis 157
  goblet cells 66
  large intestine 150
  small intestine 139
mucus cells, gastric glands 137
Müllerian ducts 567
Müllerian-inhibition substance 567
multiple sclerosis 394, 395, 501
mumps 156
  fetus 589
murmurs, heart 208
muscarinic receptors 391
muscle fibre defect 500
muscle spindles 404, 490–494
muscle thick fibres 26
muscle tissue 76–77
  see also cardiac muscle; skeletal
    muscles; smooth muscle
muscular arteries 216
muscularis externa 125–126
muscularis mucosa 125
musculoskeletal pumps 219, 243
musculoskeletal systems 454–504
music, for pain 623–624
mutagens 39, 588
mutations 561, 597–598
  ageing 585
  inheritance of 601–605
  in populations 608
myasthenia gravis 290, 395, 501
myelencephalon 356
myelin 349
  on conduction velocity 364
  loss 394, 395
myeloblasts 175
myelocytes 175
myeloid stage, blood production
    168–169
myeloid stem cells 175
myelomeningocoele 589
myenteric plexus, oesophagus 134
myocardial infarction 247, 252, 253,
    656

myocardial infarction *cont.*
  circadian rhythms 677
  shift work 672
myocardium (cardiac muscle) 77,
    205, 210, 470
  oxygen requirements 293
myofibrils 77, 474
myofilaments 474–475
myometrium 535
myopia 423
myosin 26, 77, 475, 476

nails 265, 510
napping 682
  shift work 675
nasal cavity 295
  olfactory epithelium 421
nasolachrymal ducts 457–460
nasopharynx 132
natriuretic factor, *see* atrial
    natriuretic factor
natural immunity 282–283
natural killer lymphocytes 277–278
natural methods, contraception 551
natural selection 608
nausea 157
nearsightedness 423
neck cells, *see* mucus cells, gastric
    glands
necrosis 195
negative feedback 5–6
Neisseria gonorrhoeae, *see*
    gonorrhoea
neonates 576–577
  circadian rhythms 667
  immunological competence 280,
    577
  nutritional requirements 112–116
  see also haemolytic disease of the
    newborn
neoplasms 38–40
nephrons 325, 328–329
nerve deafness 425
nerve fibres, types 365
nerve growth factors 393
nerve roots 383
nerves 349
  connection to muscle 485–486
  nomenclature 353–354
nervous system 348–398
  ageing 582
  disorders 392–396
  embryonic development 566
  function 360–369
    development 579–580
  vs hormonal system 429
  see also central nervous system
nervous tissue 75–76
neural tube 566
neuroendocrine hormones 400–401,
    439
neurogenic shock 250
neuroglia 76
  cells 354, 364

neurohypophysis, *see* posterior
    pituitary
neurolemmocytes (Schwann cells)
    349, 354, 364
neuromodulators 229, 617
neuromuscular disorders 501
neuromuscular junctions 477
neurons 76, 348
  function 360
  loss 393
  mitochondria 25
  pain-transmitting 615
  selective permeability 18
  structure 351–353
neuropeptides 367
neurosecretory cells 429
neurosurgery, for pain 622
neurotransmitters 360, 365–367, 429
  autonomic system 391
  excitatory 229, 366–367
  imbalances 395–396
  inhibitory, pain control 617
neutralization, bacterial toxins 273
neutrons 44–45
neutrophils 174, 179–180, 267
  counts 192, 692
  cytotoxic reactions 288
  leucocytosis 180
newborn, *see* neonates
niacin (nicotinamide) 59, 108
nicotinamide adenine dinucleotide
    59
nicotine
  birth weights 590
  on fetus 589
nicotinic receptors 391
night admission wards, community
    care 681–682
nipple 538
nitrogen
  blood urea, serum levels 690
  dietary 104, 105
  partial pressures in respiratory
    gases 305
nociceptors 402, 403, 615
nocturia 662, 678
nodes of Ranvier 364
noise 416, 668
non-A, non-B hepatitis 162
non-disjunction 605–606
non-Hodgkin's lymphomas 285–286
non-pigmented granular
    dendrocytes 509
non-specific immunity 257, 264–269
non-specific urethritis 555
non-steroidal anti-inflammatory
    drugs 621
non-striped muscle, *see* smooth
    muscle
non-volatile sources, hydrogen ions
    88
noradrenaline 227, 238, 367, 391,
    446
  addiction 653

deficiency, depressive illness 396
  hypertension 650
  neurotransmitter for melatonin
    release 666
normal saline 20
Norplant 552
nose, *see* nasal cavity
nucleases 23
  alimentary 142, 143–144, 144
nuclei (atomic) 44
nuclei (brain) 356
  cerebral 371–372
  medulla oblongata 495
  midbrain 497
  see also named nuclei
nuclei (cells) 11–12, 28–29
  cell homeostasis 34
nucleic acids 56
  dietary 111
  see also DNA; RNA
nucleolus 28
nucleoplasm 28
nucleosidases, nucleotidases,
    alimentary 142, 144
nucleotides 29–30
nucleus of tractus solitarius 421
null cells (killer T-cells) 275–276
numerical scales, pain 629
nursing staff
  and pain 619, 626–627
  see also health care, shift work
nutrients, excess 322–323
nutrition 1, 2, 11, 101–120
  embryonic development 588–590
  placental function 570
  standards 111

obesity 118
  children 579
  puberty 581
obligatory excretion 322
oblique muscle layer, stomach 137
obstructive airway disease 317
occipital lobes 371
oculomotor nerve 351, 378, 408
Oddi, sphincter of 139
odontoid process 463
odour 421
oedema 99
  hypoproteinaemia 99, 196
  peripheral 247
  see also lymphoedema
oesophageal stage, deglutition 134
oesophagus 132–133
  disorders 155
  histology 126
oestrogens 7, 433, 434, 539, 546
  adrenal 445
  breasts in pregnancy 575
  exogenous, on fetus 589
  labour 572–573
  ovarian 446, 548–549
  role in development 581
offensive behaviours 383

oil-soluble molecules 15
olecranon process 465
olfaction, *see* smell, sense of
olfactory bulb, glomeruli 422
olfactory nerve 378, 422
oligodendrocytes 355, 364
oligospermia 556
olivary bodies 377
olive oil 106
oncotic pressure 93, 328
  and oedema 99
oogenesis 542
oogonia 542
open-loop feedback systems,
    hormone control 438
operator genes 36
operon theory (Jacob and Monod)
    35–37, 40
opioids
  endogenous 617
  on fetus 589
  therapy 620–622
opsin 412
opsonization 274
optic disc 408
optic nerve 378, 405
optics, eye 410–411, 423–424
optimization of immune adherence
    269
oral absorption 146
oral contraceptives 552
orange juice example 16
organelles 11, 12, 22–28
  turnover 37
organic compounds 48
organic disease, and stress 655–656
organizations, distressors 644
organ systems 2
orgasm 537
  ejaculation 531
origins, muscles 473
oropharynx 132
osmolality
  blood 691
  ions on 94–95
  urine 693
osmolarity 689
  urine and plasma 337
osmoreceptors 98, 338–339, 399, 441
osmosis 17, 18–20
osmotic pressure 89
  units 689
  urine 330
  see also oncotic pressure
ossein 74
osseous connective tissue, *see* bone
ossicles 416–417
ossification 74
osteoarthritis 499
osteoblasts, osteoclasts 74, 455
osteocytes 74, 82, 455
osteogenic cells 455
osteomalacia 109, 499
osteomyelitis 499

osteons 455
osteopetrosis 499
osteoporosis 498–499
otitis media 425
otoliths 405, 488
oval window 418
ovarian cycle 545
ovaries 524, 532–533
  cysts 557
  endocrine function 446
  hormones 433
  malignant tumours 557
  oogenesis 542
overhydration 99, 336, 338
ovulation 535, 549, 562
  temperature 551
ovum 11
  nucleus 563–564
  size 12
oxygen
  blood carriage 307–309
  debt 60
  molecule 47
  movement 16
  partial pressures
    air 303
    blood 691
    chemoreceptors 423
    respiratory gases 305
    tissues 311
  requirements 293
    exercise 294, 315
    heart 208, 209–210
    kidneys 331
    lungs 297
    pregnancy 573
  transport 169
oxygen-haemoglobin dissociation
    curve 308–309, 313
oxyntic cells, gastric glands
    137–138
oxytocin 432, 441, 546
  labour 573
  lactation 575

'pacemaker' tissue, *see* conductive
    tissue
Pacinian corpuscles 403
packed cell volume, *see* haematocrit
packed red cells 190
pain 400, 613–636
  acute 614
  assessment 624–627
  chronic 614–615
  clinical measurement 628–632
  via spinal cord 385
painmeter (pain thermometer) 629
pain-producing substances 615
pain threshold 614
palliative coping methods 655
palm oil 106
pancreas 70, 139–140, 430
  disorders 158

  endocrine function 447–448
  hormones 433
pancreatic juice 143–144
  ionic composition 91
pancreozymin, *see* cholecystokinin-
    pancreozymin
pantothenic acid 108
papillae
  dermal 510
  tongue 420
papillary muscles 206
papilloma virus, and cancer 39
papovavirus 521
paracetamol 621
paracrine secretions 430
paranasal sinuses 460
paraphimosis 556
parasympathetic nervous system
    387, 390–391
  coronary blood flow 210
  deglutition 134
  heart 213, 227, 229
  small intestine 144
parathyroid glands 443–444
  hormones 342, 432, 443–444
paraurethral glands 536
paraventricular nuclei 338
parenteral feeding 158
parietal cells (stomach) 137–138
parietal lobes 370
parietal peritoneum 126
Parkinson's disease 395, 396, 502
parotid glands 129, 156
pars distalis 440
partial antigens (haptens) 271–272
partial pressures 303
  tissues 311
  values 305
  see also named gases
parturition, *see* birth
passive immunity 280
  artificial 284
  natural 282
passive transport, cell membranes
    16–20
patella 467
pathogens 257
patient-controlled analgesia 625
pavement epithelia, *see* squamous
    epithelia
Pavlovian conditioning 129–130
pectoral girdle 465
pedigree analysis 609
pelvic girdle 465–467, 482
pelvic inflammatory diseases 555
penicillin
  antigenicity 272
  capillary fragility 194
  haemophilia 196
  syphilis 554
penile urethra 529
penis 531
  disorders 556
pennate muscles 473

pentasomy XXXXX 606
pentoses 52
pepsin 137, 142
pepsinogen 137, 142
peptic ulcers 157
  shift work 671
peptidases, alimentary 142, 144
peptides 55
  hormonal 431
perception
  adaptation to shift work 673
  environmental stressors 651,
    652–653
perceptual learning 381
perfusion 92
pericarditis 205
pericardium 203–205
perilymph 418
perimysium 471–473
perineum 536–537
perineurium 349
Periodic Table 44
periosteum 74
peripheral arterial disease,
    circadian rhythms 677
peripheral nervous system 350–354
peripheral resistance 231–323
  on blood flow 230
  regulation 235
peristalsis
  oesophagus 134
  small intestine 140
  stomach 137
peritoneum 78, 126
peritonitis 150, 160
  from salpingitis 535
permanent teeth 131, 580–581
permanent tissues 78
permeability, selective 15, 18
permease, E. coli 36, 37
pernicious anaemia 138
  tongue 156
personality types 653
  pain assessment 625
petechiae 194
pethidine 621
pH 88–89, 166
  acid-base regulation 342
  blood 91, 691
  enzymes 95
  fluid compartments 90
  large intestine 150
  small intestine 139, 141
  urine 693
  vagina 536
phagocytes 79
  steroids on 281
phagocytosis 17, 21, 179, 267–269
  in spleen 262
phagosomes 21, 24, 269
phalanges 465, 468
pharynx 132, 295
  disorders 155
phase shifts, circadian rhythms 668

phasic receptors 401–402
phenindione 195
phenomenological holism 639, 664
phenotypes 38, 595
  polygenic 598
  stress response 641
phenylalanine hydroxylase 601–602
phenylbutazone 194
phenylketonuria 61, 601–602
phenylthiocarbamide 420
pheromones 430, 511
phosphates 95
  excretion 342
  fluid compartments 90
  intestinal absorption 149
  intracellular 92
  plasma levels 172
phospholipids 105
  cell membranes 13
phosphorus 57, 109
  dietary 110
  estimated average requirements
    114
phosphorylases 435
photocoagulation, infra-red,
    haemorrhoids 160
photoreceptors 402
phrenic nerve 312, 350
physical activity levels 106, 116
physical stressors 644
physiological dead space 300–301
'physiological' jaundice 577, 667
physiological stress 638
physiology, definition 1
pia mater 380
pigments
  skin 508
  visual 405, 412
piles (haemorrhoids) 160–161
pill, the (oral contraceptives) 552
piloerection 514
pineal gland 448–449, 666–667
pinna 416
pinocytosis 17, 21
pinosomes 21, 24
pitch 416
pituitary-adrenocortical axis, stress
    650
pituitary gland 440
  hormones 432
  hypothalamic-pituitary axis
    438–441
  portal system 221
pivot joints 470
placebos 620
placenta 568–570
  separation 573–575
placental lactogen 570, 575
plantar calcaneonavicular ligament
    484
plants, proteins 105
plaque (teeth) 155
plaques, atheromatous 194,
    250–251

plasma 3, 89, 90, 167, 169–172
  interchanges with interstitium
    92–94
  values 690–692
plasma cells 180, 278–279
plasma components, for infusion
    188, 196
plasmalemma, plasma membrane,
    see cell membranes
plasma protein fraction, for
    infusion 188
plasma proteins 75, 94, 154,
    169–172
  calcium binding 341
  homeostatic failures 196
plasma thromboplastin antecedent
    184
plasma volume 691
plasmin, seminal 530
platelet actomyosin 182
platelet coagulation factors 184, 185
platelet phase, haemostasis 182–183
platelets 168, 174, 182
  blood coagulation 7
  clumping 185
  counts 691
  population imbalances 193–194
pleura 295, 298
plexuses 352
ploidy 34, 539, 605–606
pneumonia 318
  on fetus 589
  Pneumocystis carinii 287
pneumotaxic centre 312
polar bodies 543, 563–564
polarization
  neuron membranes 361
  water molecule 57
poliomyelitis 501
  on fetus 589
polycyclic sleep 682
  see also napping
polycythaemia 189, 190–191
polygenic inheritance 604–605
polygenic phenotypes 598
polymodal receptors 400
polymorphonucleocytes 179
polyneuritis 501
polypeptidases, pancreatic 143
polypeptides 55
polyribosomes 29
polysaccharides 53, 102–104
polyunsaturated fats 54–55, 105
pons varolii 375
  nuclei, REM sleep 381
popliteal pulse 233
population drift 608
population genetics 607–608
pores, see channels
porphyrins, haem 307
portal blood vessels, hypothalamic-
    pituitary 439
portal veins 221
  see also hepatic portal vein

positive feedback 7
 labour 573
posterior cerebral artery 359
 CVA 394
posterior interventricular artery 209
posterior pituitary 440, 441
 hormones 432
posterior spinocerebellar tract 407
posterior spinothalamic tracts 495
post-lunch dip 660, 661–662
post-ovulation phase, menstrual
 cycle 549–550
post-synaptic inhibition 369
 pain control 617
post-synaptic neurons 365
post-translational changes, ageing
 586
postural reflexes 493
posture 454, 479–480
 control 486–498
 sense 404–405
potassium 95
 action potentials 394
 dietary 110
 estimated average requirements
  114
 excretion 327
 fluid compartments 90
 intestinal absorption 149
 kidney fluids 325
 on myocardium 228
 neurons 18, 361, 362, 367
 plasma levels 172, 691
  adaptation to shift work
   673–674
 reabsorption 331
 regulation 98, 340–341, 445
 urine 693
  circadian rhythms 662
poultry, fats 106
PQ interval (PR interval), ECG 213
precapillary sphincters 216,
 217–218, 243
precipitation 274
prefixes 694–695
pregnancy 524–525, 549–550
 abortion 553
 breast changes 538
 haemorrhoids 160
 leucocytosis 192
 maternal physiology 572
 nutrition 116–117
 vitamin requirements 113
premature babies, surfactant 300
premenstrual syndrome 557
prenatal diagnosis 608–609
preoptic nuclei 338
pre-ovulation phase 548–549
prepuce 531
presbyopia 423
pressure
 air, middle ear 416
 units 689
pressure sores 520

presynaptic inhibition 367
 pain control 617
primary hypertension 249
primary immune responses
 279–280
primary oocytes 542
primary somatosensory cortex 370,
 495–496
primary structure, proteins 56
primary visual cortex 371
PR interval, ECG 213
proaccelerin (coagulation factor)
 184
problem-focused coping 654
procarboxypolypeptidase 143
processes, bones 457
progeria 584
progesterone 539, 546, 549–550
 breasts in pregnancy 575
 labour 572–573
 role in development 581
progesterone-only pill 552
progestins 433
programme theory of ageing
 584–585
prolactin 432, 440–441, 546
 lactation 575
prolymphocytes 175
promonocytes 175
promoter genes (operator genes) 36
proprioception 404–405, 487–490
prorennin 137
prosencephalon 356, 369–372
prostacyclin 195
prostaglandins 434, 449
 dysmenorrhoea 557
 female 546
 inflammation 267
 labour 573
 pain 615
 semen 530
prostate gland 530, 531
 disorders 556
proteases 23, 49, 132
 pancreatic 143
protein binding, calcium 170, 341
protein kinases 435
proteins 55–56
 cell membranes 13–15
 deficiency 119
 dietary 104–105
 erythropoiesis 177
 estimated average requirements
  112
 fluid compartments 90
 kidney fluids 325
 plasma levels 691–692
 size 12
 synthesis, genes 29–33
 see also plasma proteins
proteinuria 345
prothrombin 169, 170, 184
 deficiency 196
protons 44

proximal convoluted tubules 66,
 329, 331
pruritus, renal failure 519
pseudo-epithelia 67
pseudohermaphroditism 558
pseudo-organic disease 655
pseudopodia 21, 269
pseudo-stratified epithelia 67–68
psoriasis 521
psychic factors, breathing 314
psychogeriatric patients, urine
 output 678
psychological stress 638, 651
psychological stressors 644
psychological subjectivity, pain
 618–619
psychophysiological homeostasis 4
psychophysiological imbalances,
 shift work 670–671
psychophysiological subjectivity,
 stress 641–642
psychosomatic pain,
 electrocardiogram 626
ptyalin (salivary amylase) 131, 142
puberty 581–582, 645
 disorders 590
pubis 467
pulmonary capillaries 303–304
pulmonary circulation 221
 blood gases 303
 neonate 576
pulmonary infarction 195
pulmonary oedema 99, 246
pulmonary trunk vessel 208
pulmonary valve 206
pulmonary veins 208
pulmonary ventilation (respiratory
 minute volume) 301
pulse 233–234
 shock 249
pulse pressure 233–234
pump failure, see cardiogenic
 shock; heart failure
pumps (membrane transport) 20,
 92
pumps (skeletomuscular) 219, 243
pupil 414–415
Purkinje fibres 211
purpura 194
pus 83
P-wave, ECG 212
pyelonephritis 345
pyloric region, stomach 136
pyloric sphincter 134–135, 136, 137
pyramidal pathways 497–498
pyramids 375, 498
pyrexia 7, 518, 521
pyridoxine 108
 role in erythropoiesis 177
pyrogens 180
pyruvic acid 59

QRS complex, ECG 212
QT interval, ECG 213

quadriceps femoris 486

radiation (heat) 512–513
radioisotopes 45
    carbon 45
    iodine, thyroid uptake 441
radioulnar joints 469
radius 465
rapid eye movement sleep 380, 381
    shift work 671
reabsorption 329–330, 330–331
    electrolytes 337
    kidneys 327
reactivity, non-self materials 271
receptor fields 401
receptor-mediated endocytosis 17, 21
receptors 57–58
    interpretation of activity
        406–407
    sensory 6, 399–405
recessive alleles 598
recessive inheritance
    autosomal 601–603
    sex-linked 603–604
recombinant DNA technology 609
recombination 600
recommended daily amounts,
    nutrition 111
rectum 150
    histology 126
    pain 626
red blood cells, see erythrocytes
red cell mass, pregnancy 572
red muscle 484
red nucleus 374
red pulp, spleen 262
reduction division (meiosis) 34,
    539, 540, 597, 599
reflexes
    atrial 227
    conditioned 129–130
    gastrocolonic 151
    Hering-Breuer 312
    postural 490–493
    spinal 386
refraction, light 410–411
refractory state, neurons 363
regulator genes 36
reinforcement, neural development
    580
Reissner's membrane 418
relational learning 382
relaxation techniques 351, 652
    hypertension 248
    pain 623
relaxin 467, 546, 550, 570, 573
releasing hormones 439–440
remodelling, bone 480
REM sleep, see rapid eye
    movement sleep
renal artery and vein 324
renal clearance 334–335
renal failure
    acute 345–346

chronic 344, 345
    sweat 519
renal nerves, efferent 324
renin 239, 247, 445
    hypertension 248
renin-angiotensin-aldosterone axis
    445
rennin 137, 580
repression, genes 37–38
repressor genes 36
reproduction 524–560
    development 581–582
request forms, haematology 188
residual volume 302
    pregnancy 573
resistance, see peripheral resistance
resistance stage, general adaptation
    syndrome 647–649
respiration 1
    aerobic 9, 24
    anaerobic, erythrocytes 176
    cellular 58–60
    transport of gases 166
    see also breathing
respiratory centres 312, 377
respiratory distress syndrome
    adult 318
    infant 318, 576, 590
respiratory epithelia 265
respiratory gases
    partial pressures 305
    units 689
respiratory minute volume
        (pulmonary ventilation) 301
respiratory quotient 294–295
respiratory system 9, 293–320
    autonomic innervation 390
    neural control 311–314
response-based definition, stress
    638–639
resting membrane potentials 95,
    361
restrictive lung disorders 317
rest rooms, hospital wards 678
rete testis 529
reticular formation 374–375, 381
reticulin fibres 71, 72
reticulocytes 175
    counts 189, 692
reticuloendothelial system
    erythrocyte destruction 177
    liver 152, 153
    monocytes 181
retina 408
    receptor activation 411–413
retinal artery thrombosis 195
retinene 412
retirement 643
Rhesus blood groups 187, 198–199
rheumatic fever 208
rheumatoid disease 290, 500
rhodopsin 412
rhombencephalon 356, 375–377
Rhone Valley survey, shift work 673

rhythm methods, contraception 551
riboflavin 108
    erythropoiesis 177
ribonucleases, alimentary 143–144
ribosomes 22, 29, 33
ribs 464
rickets 499
right cerebral hemisphere 370
right coronary artery 209
right heart failure 247
right lymphatic duct 258, 263
right-to-left shunts 246, 576, 577
Rivinus's ducts 129
RNA 31
road traffic accidents, shift work
    673
rods 410, 411–413
root hair plexuses 403
roots (verbal) 696–698
rotational shift work patterns 669,
    674–675
rough endoplasmic reticulum 23
round window 418
rubella, on fetus 589
rubrospinal tract 498
Ruffini organs 517
RU-486 (mifepristone) 553
running 484
rupture of spleen 285

saccades 415
saccule 404–405, 488
sacral nerves 387
sacrum 460
St Vitus' dance (Huntington's
    chorea) 395, 502, 603
saline, normal 20
saliva 128–130, 266
    amylase 131, 142
    ionic composition 91
salivary glands 128–129
    autonomic innervation 390
    disorders 156
Salmonella endotoxins, haemolysis
    288
salpingitis 534–535, 555
salt, appetite for 117, 420
saltatory conduction 364
salts 87
    see also minerals
samples, circadian rhythms 680–681
sarcolemma 77, 474
sarcoma 39
sarcomeres 475
sarcoplasm 77, 474
satiety 117
satiety centre 122
saturated fats 54, 105, 116
    as stressors 655–656
scala media 418
scala tympani 418
scala vestibuli 418
scapula 465
scarlet fever, on fetus 589

scars 83
scavenger macrophages 181
Schwann cells 349, 354, 364
SCID (severe combined immunodeficiency) 287
sclera, eye 408
scoliosis 500
scrotum, swellings 556
seasonal affective disorder 660–661
sebaceous glands 509
sebum 265, 509
secondary follicles, lymph node 260
secondary immune responses 277, 279–280
secondary oocyte 543, 562
secondary sexual characteristics 545, 581–582
secondary structure, proteins 56
secondary tumours 39
second messengers 435–436
second-order neurons, spinal cord 384
secretin 138, 144, 433, 446
secretion 21, 322
    kidneys 327
    liver 154
secretory cells, endoplasmic reticulum 23
secretory epithelia 64
secretory phase, menstrual cycle 549–550
segmentation, small intestine 140
segregation of alleles 599
selection, in populations 608
selective permeability 15, 18
self-medication, adverse drug reactions 680
self vs non-self 271, 289
Selye, Hans
    definition of stress 638–639
    see also general adaptation syndrome
semen 524, 530–531
semicircular canals 404, 488
semilunar valves 206–207, 224
    see also aortic valve; pulmonary valve
seminal vesicles 530–531
seminiferous tubules 527, 539
senescence, see ageing
senses 399–427
    ageing 582
sensitivity 1–2
sensorimotor development 579–580
sensory association area 370
sensory function
    control of movements 495–496
    homeostasis 422–423
sensory neurons 351
    from muscle spindles 490
sensory receptors 6, 399–405
septa, cardiac 203, 205
    defects 590
    see also foramen ovale

septicaemia, shock 250
serotonin 267, 367, 391
serous membranes, serosa 78, 126
serous pericardium 203
serous secretions 68
Sertoli cells 527–529, 543–544
serum 172
    values 690–692
    see also anti-sera
serum hepatitis 162
sesamoid bones 457
set-points, variation 7
severe combined immunodeficiency 287
sex chromosomes, disorders 606
sex determination 566–567
    see also gender differences
sex hormones
    adrenal 445
    gonads 433, 446
sex-linked recessive inheritance 603–604
sex organs, male, autonomic innervation 390
sexual act
    female 537
    male 531–532
sexual behaviour 383, 415
sexually transmitted diseases 553–555
sexual reproduction
    inheritance mechanism 599
    see also reproduction
sexual stimulation, autonomic effects 391
shift maladaptation syndrome 673
shift work 669–675
shingles, on fetus 589
shivering 515
shock 249–250, 650
    anaphylaxis 288
    burns 520
short bones 456
short-chain fatty acids, absorption 147
shortsightedness 423
short-term memory 381–382
shoulder blade (scapula) 465
'show' (birth) 573
shunts
    cardiac 246
    left-to-right 246
    right-to-left 576–577
    ventilation/perfusion ratio 317
    see also arterial-venous anastomoses
sickle-cell anaemia 603
sick syndrome (Selye) 647
simple diffusion 16–18
simple epithelia 65–67
sinoatrial node 210–212, 224
sinuses
    lymph node 260

venous 220
    see also dural sinuses
sinusitis 425
sinusoids, liver 151–152
SI units 687
skeletal connective tissue 73–75
skeletal muscles 76–77, 470–479
    blood flow 241, 244–245
    contraction 475–478
    disorders 500–501
    fatigue resistance 484–485
    histology 474–475
    nomenclature 471
    oxygen requirements 293
    relationship to bone 485
skeletomuscular pumps 219, 243
skeletomuscular systems 454–504
skeleton 457–470
    ageing 582
    disorders 498–500
    functional development 579
Skene's glands (paraurethral glands) 536
skin 506–512
    ageing 582
    AV anastomoses 218, 516
    blood flow, exercise 244
    defence mechanisms 264, 265, 512
    disorders 519–521
    excretion 323, 512
    oxygen requirements 293
    pigmentation, inheritance 598
    repair 79–81
    subcutaneous connective tissue 72
    T-cells, interactions with 278
    temperature 661
    see also cutaneous receptors
skull 457–460
    see also cranium
sleep 380–381
    shift work 671–672
sleep-wake cycle 663–664
sliding filament theory, muscle contraction 476–477
slow muscle fibres 484, 615, 616
slow-wave sleep 380, 381
small intestine 123, 138–139, 147–149
    defence mechanisms 266
    digestive secretions 144
    disorders 158–159
    histology 126
    physical digestion 140
    regulation 135, 144–145
smallpox
    on fetus 589
    vaccination 284
smell, sense of 406, 421–422
    loss 425
smoking
    birth weights 590
    on fetus 589

smooth endoplasmic reticulum 23
smooth muscle 77, 470
  arteries 214
sneezing 265, 314
Snellen tests 410
social class, pain assessment
  625–626
socializing
  hospital wards 678
  and shift work 670
social readjustment rating scale 642
social stressors 642–644
sociopsychological subjectivity of
  pain 618–619
sociopsychophysiological
  subjectivity of stress 641–642
sodium 45, 46–47, 94–95
  balance 96
  depletion 117
  dietary 110
  estimated average requirements
    114
  excretion 327
    effect of GFR 329
  fluid compartments 90
  kidney fluids 325
  on myocardium 228
  neurons 18, 361, 362
  plasma levels 172, 692
  reabsorption 330
  regulation 98, 339–340, 445
  urine 693
    circadian rhythms 662
sodium bicarbonate 57
sodium chloride 57
sodium glycocholate 141
sodium/potassium/ATPase pump
  20, 92
sodium taurocholate 141
solar plexus 389
soluble fibre 107–108
soma 353
somatic mutation theory, ageing
  585
somatic nerves 350
  vs autonomic nerves 392
somatosensory cortex, primary 370,
  495–496
somatostatin 140, 433, 448
somatotrophin, see growth
  hormone
sorbitol 104
sound 415–416
  bone conduction 419
  frequency discrimination 418
spasms, pain 623
specialization, cells 63–64
special senses 400, 405–406,
  408–422
specific heat 514
specific immunity 257–258, 269–275
speech 382
  frontal lobes 370
spermatogenesis 526, 539–541

hormones, regulation 543–545
spermatogonia 539–540
spermatozoa 25, 541
  counts 531, 556
  fertilization 563
spermicidal agents 552
spermiogenesis 540–541
sphincters 123, 473
  anal 150, 151
  of Oddi 139
  pyloric 134, 135, 136, 137
  urethral 332, 333
sphygmomanometers 232–233
spina bifida 588–590
spinal canal 385
spinal cord 354–355
  ascending pathways 407
  blood supply 360
  functional anatomy 383–386
spinal muscular atrophies 501
spinal nerves 351
spine, see vertebral column,
  vertebrae
spines, bones 457
spinocerebellar tracts 495, 496
  posterior 407
spinothalamic tracts 407, 495
spiritual centre 449
spirometry 301–303
spleen 261–263
  erythrocyte destruction 177–178
  rupture 285
splenectomy 285
splenomegaly 178, 285
spondylitis 500
spongy bone 74, 455
squamous epithelia 65
  stratified 67
stable factor, coagulation 184
stable tissues 78
stagnant hypoxia 316
staircase, analgesic therapy 620
stapedius 418
stapes 416, 418
staphylococcal infections, skin
  damage 265
starch 53, 103
  digestion 131–132
Starling's law of the heart 229, 247
starvation 119
stem cells
  blood production 175
  lymphocytic 261, 270
stenosis, heart valves 208
Stenson's ducts 129
stercobilin 141, 178
stercobilinogen 178
sterility, male 531, 555–556, 558
sterilization 551
sternum 463–464
steroids 16, 433, 434
  adrenal 444–445
  immunosuppressant therapy 290
  mechanism of action 436

stress 281
  as synotoxic hormones 649
stimuli
  hormone release 436–437
  stress as 637
stomach 123
  absorption 146
  disorders 156–158, 257
  histology 126
  physiology 134–138
  regulation 135
  see also gastric juice
stomatitis 156
stones, see calculi, renal; gallstones
storage, liver 154
straight tubules, testis 529
strap muscles 473
stratified epithelia 67–68
stratum lucidum 507
stratum spinosum 507
streptokinase 195
streptomycin, on fetus 589
stress 637–658
  hormones of 444
  and immunity 281
  personality types 653
stress appraisal model (Lazarus)
  653–654
stressor scales 642–643
stress syndrome (general
  adaptation syndrome) 228,
  238, 647–652
stress threshold 651
stretch receptors 404
  lungs 312
stretch receptor theory,
  gastrointestinal 122
stretch reflexes 492–493
striated, striped muscle, see skeletal
  muscles
strokes, see cerebrovascular
  accidents
stroke volume 228–229
strong acids 87
strong opioids 621
structural genes 36
Stuart factor 184
St Vitus' dance (Huntington's
  chorea) 395, 502, 603
subarachnoid space 379–380
subclinical infection, active natural
  immunity 283
subcutaneous connective tissue 72,
  510–511
subdural space 379
subjectivity
  activity-rest cycles 665
  pain 618–622
  stress 641–646
sublingual administration 146
sublingual glands 129
submandibular glands 129
submucosa, gastrointestinal tract 125
substance P 367, 616, 617

substantia gelatinosa 385, 615
substantia nigra 374
succus entericus 144
suckling (breast feeding) 112–116, 441, 575–576, 580
sucrase 49, 144
sucrose 52
suction lipectomy 73
sudoriferous glands, *see* sweat glands
suffixes 695–696
sugar alcohols 104
sugars 52–53
suicide bags, *see* lysosomes
suicide rates, circannual 660–661
sulci (cerebral cortex) 355
sulphonamides 194
sulphur 57
superior sagittal sinus 360
superior vena cava 208
suppressor T-cells 277
suprachiasmatic nucleus 413–414, 666
suprarenal glands, *see* adrenal glands
surface area 18, 512
    burns 520
    vs volume 33
surface phagocytosis 269
surfactant 300, 576
surgery
    birth control 551
    circadian rhythms 681
    for pain 622
sustentacular cells (Sertoli cells) 527–529, 543–544
sutures, cranium 460, 469, 577
swallowing, *see* deglutition
sweat 265
    excretory function 512
    hot climates 518–519
    ionic composition 91
    production 516–517
    volumes 97
sweat glands 68, 510–511
    autonomic innervation 390
symbols 699
sympathetic nervous system 387–391, 647
    adrenal medulla 446
    coronary blood flow 210
    exercise 244, 389–390
    heart 213, 227, 229
    heart failure 247
    heat conservation 514
    pain 623
    pupil dilation 414–415
    salivary glands 129
synapses 353, 365
    integration 367–369
    transmission disorders 395–396
synaptic conduction 365–367
synchronization 664
    internal 664

syncope 249
    see also fainting; vasovagal attacks
syncytium
    functional, cardiac muscle 210
    skeletal muscle fibres 474
synergistic muscles 486
synotoxic reactions 649
synovial joints 468, 469–470
synovial membranes 77, 469
syphilis 554
    on fetus 589
Système Internationale 687
systemic arterial pressure, *see* blood pressure
systemic circulation 221
systole 224
    atria 226
    ventricles (cardiac) 225–226, 226
systolic pressure 231

T3 (tri-iodothyronine) 441–442
T4 (tetra-iodothyronine) 441–442
tachycardia 246
talus 482
target tissues, lack of response, hormones 451–452
tarsals 468
taste 406, 420–421
    loss 425
taurocholate (sodium) 141
teaching, circadian rhythms 681
tears 266, 408
tectorial membrane 418
tectospinal tract 498
tectum 373
teeth 131
    development 580–581
    disorders 155
tegmentum 373–375
telencephalon 356
temperature 61, 505–506, 517–518
    on action potentials 395
    adaptation to shift work 673
    cardiac function 228
    cell membrane transport 15
    circadian rhythms 660–662
        illness 677
    conduction velocity, axons 364
    and hunger 122
    ovulation 551
    receptors 517
    regulation 512–518
    set-points 7
    testes 527
temporal lobes 371
tendons 71, 77, 471
    Golgi organs 404, 488–490
tensor tympani 418
teratogens 588
terminal cisternae 477
tertiary structure, proteins 56
testes 524, 526–529
    descent 567, *see also* cryptorchidism

disorders 556
endocrine function 446
hormones 433
    see also spermatogenesis
testicular feminization syndrome 558
testosterone 433, 543, 545, 546
    role in development 581
tetanus 265
    anti-serum 170
tetany 478, 501
tetra-iodothyronine 441–442
tetralogy of Fallot 246
thalamus 372–373, 407, 413, 420
thalidomide, on fetus 589
thermodilution 230
thermogenesis 515
thermoreceptors 402, 403
thermoregulation 218
    role of blood 166
thiamin 108
third ventricle 358
thirst 117, 129, 239
thoracic duct 147, 258, 263
thready pulse, shock 249
threshold levels, sensory receptors 401
threshold membrane potentials 95
thrombin 185
thrombocytes, *see* platelets
thrombocytopenia 193–194
thrombocytosis 193
thrombokinase 184
thromboplastin 184
    tissue thromboplastin 185
thrombosis 194–195
    atherosclerosis 251–252
    dissolution therapy 195
thrombosthenin (platelet actomyosin) 182
thymosin 261, 270
thymus 261, 270
    absence 286
    hormones 448
    hypertrophy 285
thyroglobulin 441
thyroid gland 441–443
thyroid hormones 432, 434, 441–443
    cold climate 515
    deficiency 590
    growth 579, 580
    mechanism of action 435–436
    see also thyroxine
thyroiditis, Hashimoto's 290, 451
thyroid-stimulating hormone (thyrotropin) 432, 442
thyrotoxicosis 109
    thymus hypertrophy 285
thyroxine 61, 432
    heart rate 228
    hypersecretion 450–451
tibia 468
tibiofibular joints 469, 482
tidal volume 301

time-dependence of control
mechanisms 5
time zones, travel across 676
tinnitus 425
tissue autoregulation, blood flow
242–243
tissue differentiation 594
diseases 587–590
tissue factor, blood coagulation
184–185
tissue fluid 3, 89–90
interchanges with plasma 92–94
vs plasma 169
tissue pressure, lymph flow rate 258
tissues 63–85
tissue typing 290
T-lymphocytes 180, 260, 261,
269–270, 275–278
type IV hypersensitivity 289
tolerance, immune 280–281
tongue 130–131
disorders 155–156
papillae 420
tonic receptors 401–402
tonsillitis 156
total lung capacity 302
touch, treating pain 624
toxins 257
bacteria, neutralization 273
toxoids 283–284
toxoplasmosis, on fetus 589
trabeculae, thymus 261
trace elements 44, 87
dietary 110
trachea 295
cartilage 133
tractus solitarius, nucleus of 421
training (exercise) 245
transactional model of stress 646
transaminases, serum levels 692
transamination 37, 153
transcellular fluids 89, 91, 100
transcendental meditation 652
transcription, genes 31, 32
errors 585
hormone-mediated 436
transcutaneous electrical nerve
stimulation 617, 622–623
transducers 400
transfer factors, cellular immunity
276
transferrin 170
transfer RNA 29, 31, 33
transfusions
ABO system 186–187
for anaemia 190
incompatible 288
supplies for 196–198
transgenics 609
transient ischaemic episodes 394
transitional epithelia 67
translation 31, 32–33
errors 585
translocation 607

transplantation
cytotoxic reactions 288–289
rejection 290
transport
by blood 166
cell membranes 15–21
transverse sinuses 360
transverse tubules, skeletal muscle
fibres 474
trauma, central nervous system
movement disorder 501
neuron loss 393
travel across time zones 676
treppe 478
tricarboxylic acid cycle 59
trichromatic theory 412
tricuspid valve 205
tricyclic antidepressants 396
trigeminal nerve 378
triglycerides 53–54, 105, 143
trigone 332
tri-iodothyronine 441–442
tripeptides 55
absorption 147
triplets (codons) 30, 32
triple X syndrome 606
trisaccharides 102–103
trisomies 605–606
trochlear nerve 378, 408
trophectoderm 565, 568
trophoblasts 565
tropic hormones 431, 439
tropomyosin 476
troponins 476
true connective tissues 71–72
true ribs 464
trypsin 142, 143
trypsinogen 142
T-tubules, skeletal muscle fibres 474
tubercles, bones 457
tuberculosis
bacilli 269
on fetus 589
Mantoux test 289
tubular glands 69
tubules (nephrons) 325, 328–329
tubulin 26
tumour necrotic factor 278
tumours 38–40
endocrine glands 451
lymphatic system 284–286
tunica albuginea
ovary 532
testes 527
tunica externa, interna 214
tunica media 182
veins 219
turbulent flow 231
Turner's syndrome 606
T-wave, ECG 212
twitch 478
2,3-diphosphoglycerate 309, 315
tympanic membrane 416
typhoid fever, on fetus 589

tyrosine, synthesis disorder 601

ulcerative colitis 160
ulcers
skin 520
see also peptic ulcers
ulna 465
ulnar nerve 465
ultraviolet light, neonatal jaundice
198
umbilical cord 570–571
umbilical vessels 577
unconscious patients, care 682
underground cave studies, sleep-
wake cycle 663–664, 665
'unit' membranes 13
units of measurement 687–689
see also decibel; joule
universal donors, recipients 187
unsaturated fats 54–55
unstriated muscle, *see* smooth
muscle
upright posture 480–481
uraemia, *see* renal failure, chronic
urate, *see* uric acid
urea 154, 322
clearance 693
diffusion 16–17
kidney fluids 325
plasma levels 172, 690
urine 337–338, 693
ureters 324, 331
urethra 332
male 529
uric acid
excess 344–345
plasma levels 172
urinary bladder 332–333
control, children 667
epithelia 67
infections 346
urinary system, autonomic
innervation 390
urination 333, 351
urine 324–327
circadian rhythms 662
components 693
osmotic pressure 330
output, psychogeriatric patients
678
regulation 336–338
urobilinogen 141, 178
urokinase 195
uterus 535
utricle 404–405, 488

vaccines, vaccination 258, 279,
283–284
vacuoles 22
vagina 536
mucus, menstrual cycle 551
vagus nerve 351, 354, 378, 387, 421
dorsal nucleus 379
to heart 227

valence, antigens 272
vallate papillae 420
valves
    heart 205–207, 208, 224, 226
    veins 219
variable regions, antibodies 273
varicose ulcers 219
varicose veins 219
vasa recta 337
vascular collapse, *see* shock
vascular phase, haemostasis 182
vascular shock 250
vascular system 202, 214–223
    skin healing 81
vas deferens 529
vasectomy 551
vasoconstriction 214, 220, 232
    hypovolaemic shock 249
    pulmonary 306
vasodilation 214, 232
    inflammation 267
vasomotor centre, medulla
    oblongata 220
vasopressin, *see* antidiuretic
    hormone
vasovagal attacks 250
    see also fainting; syncope
vegetable fats 106
veins 218–220
    layout (fig.) 223
velocity, blood flow 241
venous blood, haemoglobin 308
venous pressure 234–235
venous return 229
venous sinuses 220
    see also dural sinuses
venous thrombosis 195
ventilation/perfusion ratio 304–306
    shunts 317
ventral geniculate nuclei 373
ventral nerve roots 383
ventricles (brain) 358
ventricles (cardiac) 205, 208
    hypertrophy, ECG 213
    systole 225–226, 226
ventricular end diastolic volume 224
venules 219
verbal rating scales, pain 628
vertebral arteries 358, 359
vertebral column, vertebrae
    460–463
    posture 481–482
vertebral foramina 383, 460
vestibular apparatus 404–405, 488,
    496
vestibular glands 536
vestibulocochlear nerve 378, 419
vestibulospinal tract 498
Victoria, Queen, haemophilia A 607
villi, small intestine 139, 145
viruses
    and cancer 39
    on fetus 589

hepatitis 162
size 12
skin diseases 521
visceral peritoneum 126
viscosity, blood 692
vision 405, 408–415
    disorders 423–425
visual acuity 410
visual adaptation 412
visual analogue scale, pain
    628–629
visual cortex, primary 371
visual fields 410
visual pigments 405, 412
visual purples 412
visual signals, interpretation 413–414
vital capacity 302
Vitallograph 302
vitamin A, toxicity 109
vitamin B6, *see* pyridoxine
vitamin B12 109
    absorption 138
    erythropoiesis 177
vitamin C (ascorbic acid) 108
    erythropoiesis 177
    semen 531
vitamin D 155, 342
    deficiency 499
    toxicity 109
vitamin E, erythropoiesis 177
vitamin K
    antagonists 195
    coagulation of blood 194
vitamins 57, 109
    assimilation 154
    estimated average requirements
        113
    synthesis in colon 150
    see also fat-soluble vitamins;
        water-soluble vitamins
vitreous humour 408–410
volatile sources, hydrogen ions 88
voltage, neuron membranes 361
volume, *vs* surface area 33
voluntary muscle, *see* skeletal
    muscles
VO₂max (maximal oxygen
    consumption rate) 315
vomiting 157–158
    shock 249
vulva 532, 536
walking 482–484
    knee joint 487
wandering cells 71, 181
wandering macrophages 268
warfarin 195
warts 521
washed red cells, for infusion 190
wasting, hypotension 249
water 57, 87, 94
    absorption 147
    alimentary secretion and
        absorption 148–149

balance 96–97
    in food 111
    movement between
        compartments 92–94
    obligatory excretion 322
    pH 88
    plasma 171
    reabsorption 331
    regulation 97–98, 336–339
        disorder 451
    total body, pregnancy 573
waters, *see* amniotic fluid
water-soluble vitamins 108
    absorption 147
    assimilation 154
water vapour, partial pressures in
    respiratory gases 305
wax 425
weak acids 87
weak opioids 621
weaning 116
Wernicke's area 382
wet suits 514
Wharton's ducts 129
white blood cells, *see* leucocytes
white fibro-cartilage 74
white fibrous tissue 71–72
white matter, spinal cord 354,
    383–384
white muscle 485
white pulp, spleen 262
wind chill 513
wisdom teeth 131, 580–581
Wolffian ducts 567
work
    distressors 644
    see also shift work
work performance, shift work 672
wound healing 78–82
wrist 465

xenografts 290
xenophobic responses 280
xiphisternum 463

yearly rhythms 660–661
yellow elastic tissue 72
yellow elasto-cartilage 74
yellow spot (fovea) 410
Yerkes-Dodson, on stress 646
yolk sac 571
    blood islands 168
zeitgebers 664–666
    hospital wards 678
zinc
    dietary 110
    estimated average requirements
        114
Z-lines 476
zygomatic bones 460
zygote 11, 524, 535, 539
    formation 562–564
zymogen cells 137